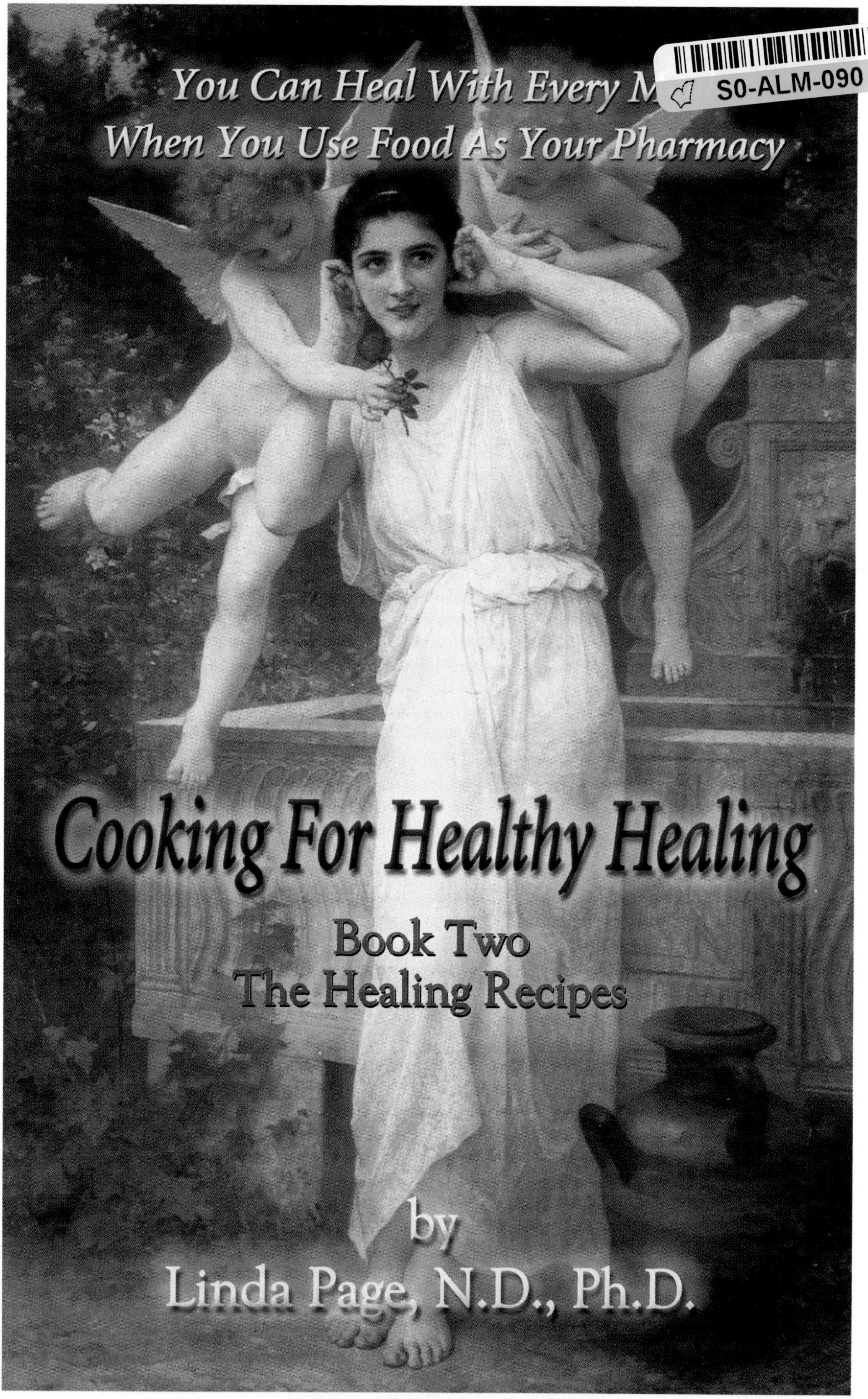

You Can Heal With Every M
When You Use Food As Your Pharmacy

Cooking For Healthy Healing

Book Two
The Healing Recipes

by
Linda Page, N.D., Ph.D.

Linda Page N.D. Ph.D.

Long before natural foods and herbal formulas became a "chic," widely accepted method for healing, Dr. Linda Page was sharing her extensive knowledge with those who dared to listen.

Through what some would call an accident of fate but she calls a blessing, she was compelled to research alternative avenues of healing. Sequestered in a hospital with a life-threatening illness, watching her 5-foot frame wither to 69 pounds, her hair drop out, and her skin peel off, doctors told her they had no cure. With only a cursory knowledge of herbs, she began a frantic research process of testing herbal formulas and healing food combinations on herself. She read voraciously about herbal healing. Good friends shopped for herbs and she began to formulate the many compounds which would eventually save her life, revitalize her health and restore beautiful new hair and skin. It was that incident that led her to seek her degrees in Naturopathy and Nutrition.

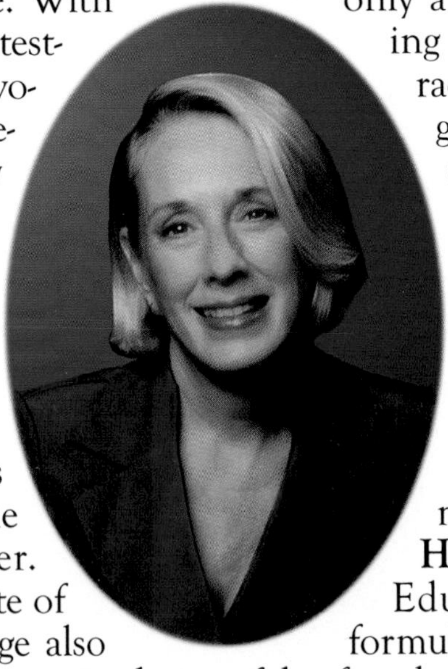

A prolific author and educator, Dr. Page has sold over a million books including **Healthy Healing, Cooking For Healthy Healing, How To Be Your Own Herbal Pharmacist, Party Lights, Detoxification** and a popular series of books which address specific healing therapies for topics like menopause, male and female energy, colds and flu and cancer. **Healthy Healing** is a textbook for course work at UCLA, The Institute of Educational Therapy, and Clayton College of Natural Health. Dr. Page also formulated over 250 herbal formulas for Crystal Star Herbal Nutrition. She received one of the first herbal patents in the United States for her formulas that help balance hormones to ease menopausal symptoms.

Dr. Page is an Adjunct Professor at Clayton College of Natural Health. She has appeared weekly on a CBS television station with a report on natural healing; she has been featured on national CBS television; she is a principle speaker at national health symposiums and conventions; she is featured regularly in national magazines; she appears on hundreds of radio and television programs, and websites like WebMD. Dr. Page also leads educational healing tours around the world.

Today, Dr. Page delights in having come full circle. "I feel I am living my dream. I am so grateful that knowledge of healing through herbal formulas and good foods is becoming so widespread. I see it as an opportunity for people to seize the power to heal themselves. Knowledge is power. Whether one chooses conventional medicine, alternative healing avenues, or combines them both in a complementary process, the real prescription for healing is knowledge."

Dr. Page is a member of The American Naturopathic Medical Association, The California Naturopathic Association, The American Herbalists Guild, The American Botanical Council and The Herb Research Foundation.

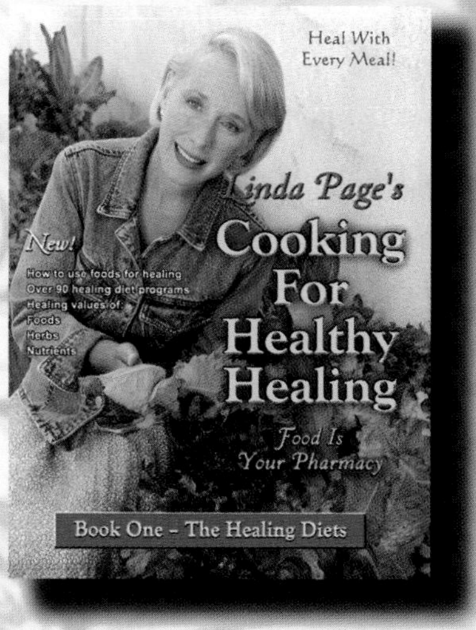

Be sure to add the companion book to your set:

Cooking For Healthy Healing
Book One
The Healing Diets

Discover the healing secrets of foods, herbs, spices, green foods and more. There are 80 healing programs, all cross referenced to Book Two - The Healing Recipes.

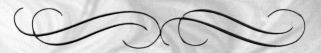

Other Books By
Linda Page, N.D., Ph.D.

Healthy Healing
A Guide To Self-Healing For Everyone

How To Be Your Own Herbal Pharmacist

Detoxification

Stress & Energy

Party Lights

The Healthy Healing Library Series

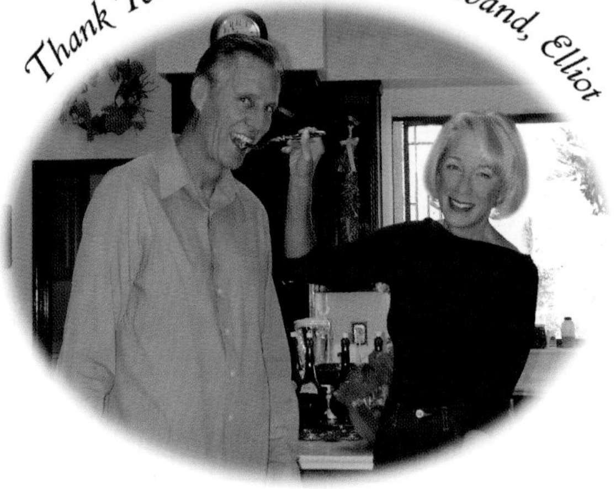
Thank You To My Dear Husband, Elliot

For being the loving life partner that he is.
For all the lively comments, and all the hours of proofreading and analysis.
For taste-testing his way through the recipes,
and never getting to have the same thing twice....even when he liked it!

Thanks also to:
Barbara Howard - Marketing Director, Cover Design, Graphic Design, Editor
Sarah Abernathy - Editor, Research, Prepress Director, Graphics
Kim Tunella - Research, Drafting
Jim Rector - In-house Sales Processing, Customer Service

Publisher's Cataloging-in-Publication
(Provided by Quality Books, Inc.)

Rector-Page, Linda G.
Linda Page's cooking for healthy healing. Book two, The healing recipes : food is your pharmacy.
p. cm.
Includes bibliographical references and index.
ISBN: 1884334822

1. Diet therapy--Popular works. 2. Cookery for the sick. 3. Cookery (Natural foods) 4. Nutrition--Popular works. I. Title. II. Title: Cooking for healthy healing III. Title: Healing recipes

RM219.R43 2002 641.5′631
QB101-201461

Traditional Inc. Wisdom

Published by Traditional Wisdom, Inc.
Printed in the United States of America

Testimonials

Read what other people say about Linda Page!

Dear Linda,

I have worked with Cooking For Healthy Healing, with good results. It is a wonderfully helpful book! I have found your book extraordinarily helpful and the menus and recipes are delicious! Thank you!

Sincerely,
Ms. Anne L.
Sarasota, FL

Dear Linda,

I believe everyone can benefit from periodic detoxification, but it must be done with care. In your book, Detoxification, you bring together comprehensive individualized detox programs that are safe and effective.

Sincerely,
Randy Ruben Baker, M.D.
Soquel, CA

Dear Linda,

Your video, "Unleashing The Healing Power of Herbs," is a joy to watch. It is visually beautiful, well organized and very informative! Thank you for your important work and for keeping us all educated about natural healing!

Sincerely, Mrs. M. Engles, Charleston, SC

Dear Linda,

Almost three years ago Healthy Healing became my "bible" and most frequently given gift. There is no need for trips to the drugstore in this household!

Sincerely,
C.M.
San Francisco, CA

Dear Linda,

Your book, How To Be Your Own Herbal Pharmacist is an excellent resource on how herbal nutrition can enhance your health. Thank you for this book that can empower people and help them to live healthier lives.

Sincerely,
Bernie Seigel, M.D.
Author - Love, Medicine & Miracles

A personal letter to my readers.....

Before our "modern age," food was pretty wholesome. People were close to their gardens and farms, and animals and natural resources. Today, we live in a man-made jungle of food substances instead of foods - many of them highly processed, devoid of nutrients, full of hidden fat, chemical-laced, and sugar-drenched.

It doesn't stop there. The hottest topic in the food industry today is functional foods. Manufacturers are creating new "pharmafoods" (often low-nutrient foods like margarine or pastries) by packing them with a slew of vitamins, minerals, herbs and isolated plant essences. In the first half of 1999 alone, functional foods were a $62 billion industry!

It's all in the name of health. The claims are exuberant.... the new foods can fight heart disease, stress, weight gain, even cancer. But, is this stuff really good for you? Make no mistake about it. These aren't Nature-made foods. They're man-made foods.

By stuffing these foods with substances - even natural ones - that aren't a normal part of the food, are we making our foods into drugs? The food is being sold as, say, a muffin. But is it a real muffin, or a medicated muffin?

What's the difference? An essential nutrient is something your body needs but cannot make for itself. Nutrition, like foods and herbs, provides your body with essential nutrients, elements it needs and can use to heal. There is no such thing as an essential drug. A drug can't combine with your body to restore and revitalize.

Nature's whole, ready-to-use medicines are often the only "prescription" your body needs to get better. Nature is, after all, the perfect pharmacy. Many foods and herbs are such highly complex medicines that they are almost micro-pharmacies in themselves.

Still, the world has changed! The explosion of enthusiasm and interest in plant medicine means everybody wants to get on the bandwagon. The sales of herbal products alone increased by more than 100% since 1994. Yet just a few short years ago, practically every medical expert was calling food and herbal healing worthless, demonizing herbalists, calling all naturopaths quacks.

The American public has changed this view from the grass roots up. The rise of individual, personal health care has begun. Clearly, Americans want to take more responsibility for their health and that of their families. But that means lots of answers to thousands of questions are going to be needed.

We don't completely understand exactly how foods and herbs work. They are foods. They are medicines. We may never fathom their intricacies.

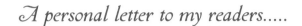

We feel uncomfortable when something isn't logical. But Nature isn't logical. The way natural healing works isn't logical either. It just doesn't "fit" into the way western Science sees and understands things. Science breaks things down and takes them apart in order to measure and understand them. There's nothing wrong with that, as long as we realize it isn't the only way... especially when we're dealing with an incredible, whole human person who is so much more than a lab test or a blood panel.

The truth is, people aren't logical either.... healers need to pay much more attention to the whole person for healing to be long-lasting.

If we can't understand it, can it work to heal us? Our scientific culture relies totally on things like lab tests and substances that are man-made because they fit into our ability to understand. "Scientific" medicine attacks anything that can't be specifically isolated, broken down, peeled apart or synthesized. It discounts the value of something it can't understand, believing that something can't possibly work if we can't understand it.

It doesn't even matter if the natural, whole substance works. A "silver bullet" must be identified so that it can be synthesized and manufactured. Even advanced medical techniques, like genetic science, work this way.

I believe only the whole food can give the whole benefit. Many plants can only work in their whole form. While single plant elements can be tested and measured, a lab can only give a partial answer about a highly complex living thing. When we take one out of the literally hundreds of elements in a plant and say, "That's it, that's what this plant is good for," we lose. It's never the whole story. Healing foods and herbs are never just one plant for one problem.

If we make our foods and herbs into drugs, will we get unwanted side effects, adverse reactions, drug interactions, even addictions that are the downside of drugs?

I had to learn the hard way, but it made me a firm believer in the old way, in the traditional way of herbal healing. Isolating constituents or boosting certain plant elements changes the balance of the plant and the protective factors it has built in.

But foods and herbs are so much more than a test or a scientific measurement. Plants are the only medicines I know of that treat the whole person, not just their symptoms... I believe God shows his face to us in natural healers.

I say, let foods and herbs do what they do so well.... heal and balance from the inside out, naturally and safely. Use them in their whole form as medicinal foods.

Health for each of us is personal. To approach it impersonally, only through big business, science and government means that your health is bound to lose.

Linda

About this Book....

Food is potent medicine. Your diet can literally transform your body.

Wholesome food not only fuels your body, eating wholesome foods can also help solve your health problems. Your diet can keep your energy levels up and stress levels down, your skin, hair, and nails healthy, your complexion glowing, your eyes bright, and your bones and muscles strong. It can fine-tune mental awareness and prevent disease from taking hold. A poor diet and junk foods produce lethargy, illness, and indifference.

Good food is good medicine. It is the prime factor for changing your body chemically and psychologically. A good diet is even a key to higher consciousness. A well-nourished system opens body receivers and transmitters for higher energies. By creating new balance in a body where there was imbalance, a clean healthy body allows the beauty of the spirit to shine through.

The food you eat changes your weight, your mood, the texture and look of your body, your outlook on life, indeed the entire universe for you.... and therefore your future. Eating right is the first step to the health and balance of your universe. This book is about getting back to the basics... because basics are basics, like classics are classics, for a reason.

The book you hold in your hands took me seventeen years to write. It's the result of an enormous amount of work in using foods as medicine. All the recipes and diet plans were tested again and again, first through the Rainbow Kitchen restaurant and juice bar I owned in the early eighties, to the diet programs I developed for Country Store Natural Foods and Crystal Star Herbal Nutrition, to the highly focused healing diets of today using foods as Nature's Pharmacy.

Through all this time, the results were clear and undeniable..... Foods and herbs (we have to remind ourselves that herbs are foods) can indeed heal – even serious diseases – sometimes dramatically. Foods and herbs can prevent some health problems from happening at all and many illnesses from developing further. The secret is using foods and herbs to change body chemistry. Drugs can't do it. Only foods and herbs can do it. This two book set tells you how.

The history of the world would be entirely different if the human diet had been different. Our children are literally formed from, and become, the nutrients (or poisons) within us. Not only are we what we eat, our children are as well, before and after birth. The pattern for the immune system and inherited health of your children and grandchildren is laid down by you.

Healthy parents = healthy children.
Healthy grandparents = healthy grandchildren.
and thus the world.
That's how important diet is!

How to Use this Book....

Good food can be great medicine!

All the advances made by modern medicine still don't address chronic diseases very well; they don't address disease prevention at all.

Sometimes food can be your best medicine... even for serious diseases. We tend to think that the healing powers of foods are subtle or mild, without the overwhelming potency of drugs. Yet healing doesn't always need to deal a hammer blow.... even for serious problems.

As new research advances the science of nutrition, there's an enormous thirst for information about how to use it. Most people are actively trying to eat better. Organic foods are mainstream today. But most people don't know HOW to use foods as medicine. This two book set can help you navigate the healing path easily and effectively. It's all a matter of the way you direct what you eat.

You'll have everything you need to do it yourself, day by day, and succeed.

–Detailed **STEP-BY-STEP DIETS** for a wide range of illnesses and health problems.

–A large **FOOD and NUTRIENT DIGEST,** with the important elements and healing properties of hundreds of foods and herbs so you can build your own target diet.

–RECIPES and MENU PLANS for every health problem in the book.

–Over **1000 RECIPES** to choose from to keep your diet interesting and focused on healing.

In the 1930's, at the height of the scientific love affair with orthodox medicine, the Nobel prize winning doctor, Albert Schweitzer said, *"the doctor of the future will be oneself."* He already saw the limitations of drugs and surgery-based healing. He knew that immune strength was the only real way to prevent disease.

In fact, the immune system of each one of us is so entirely unique to us, that it may be impossible for a laboratory to ever develop a drug to activate immunity. Only foods or herbs, that combine with each person individually, and work with each person's distinctive enzymes at the deepest levels of each person's body, can do the job for immune response.

Medicines from foods and herbs work just the opposite from drugs. They nourish the body and enhance the immune system. Drugs function outside the system, usually operating to overwhelm a harmful organism. Today's orthodox medicine is "heroic medicine," largely developed in wartime for emergency wartime requirements. It's a patching up system. It isn't supportive or nourishing; it's often risky over the long term; and it doesn't stimulate immune response.

Yet, I feel we need both types of medicine. Drugs can stop an emergency and stabilize your body to give your immune system a chance to take over.

Clearly, orthodox medicine has saved many lives. Just as clearly, alternative medicine has prevented much illness. Use the delicious recipes in this book to put yourself on the path to the best health you've ever had!

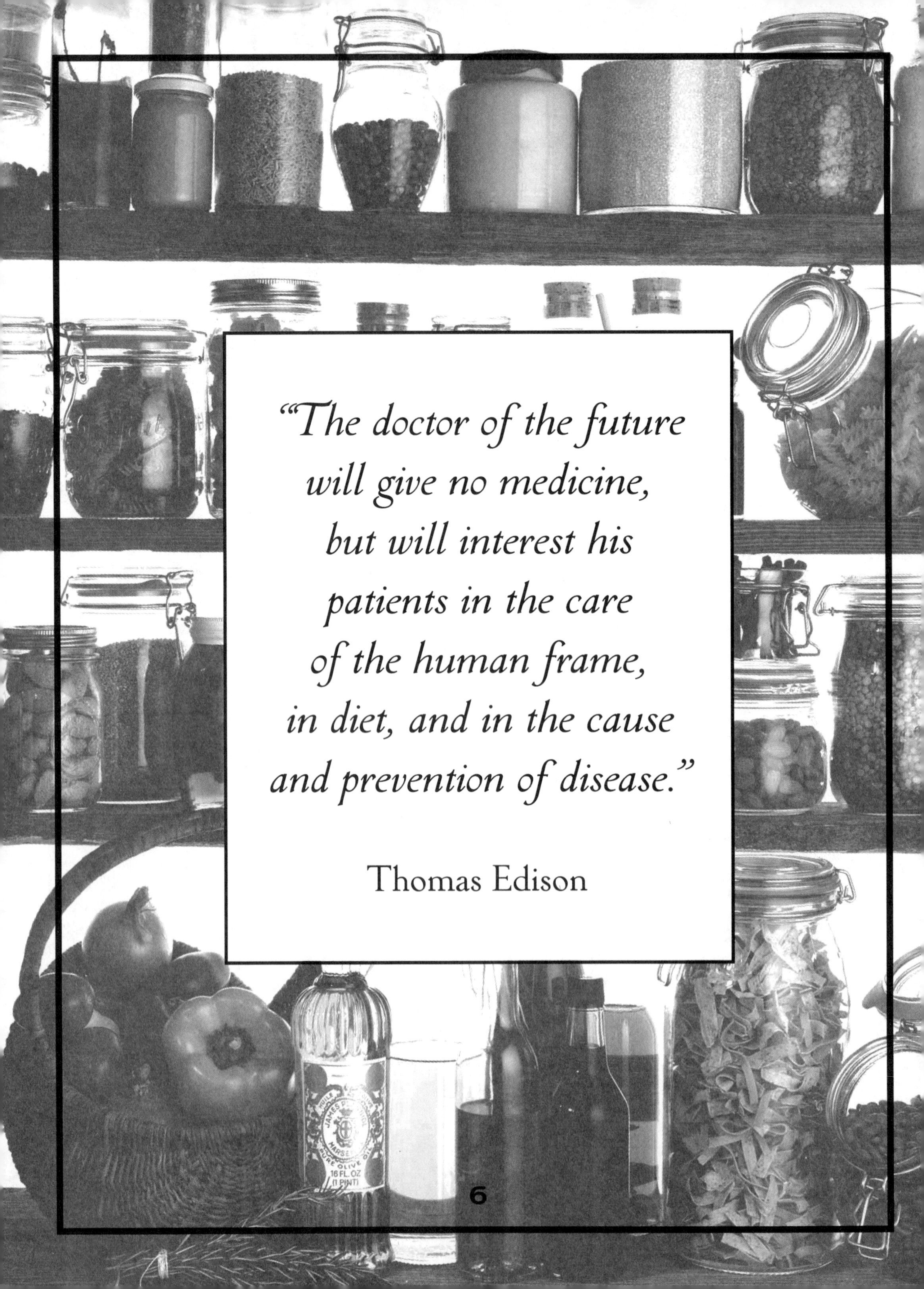

"The doctor of the future
will give no medicine,
but will interest his
patients in the care
of the human frame,
in diet, and in the cause
and prevention of disease."

Thomas Edison

Table of Contents

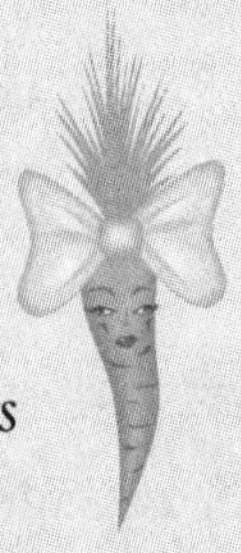

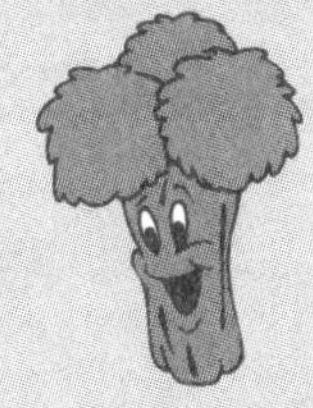

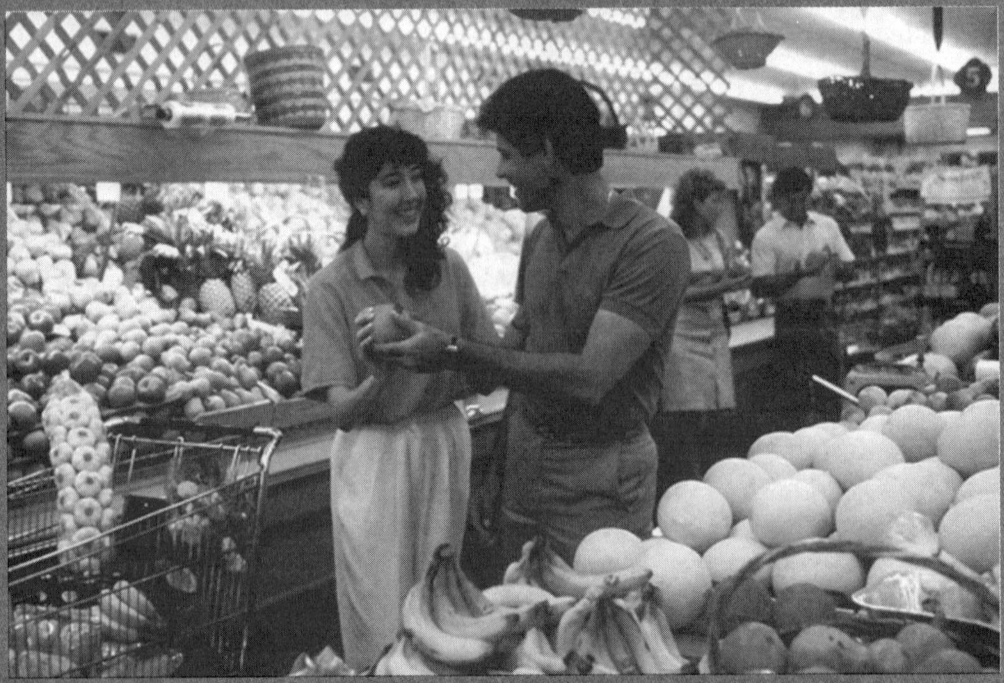

About the Healing Recipes

The healing recipes in this book are simply prepared, to preserve as much food value as possible. They're loaded with taste, balance and high nutrition. Most include a nutritional analysis that identifies specific nutrients you can use to enhance your healing program.

The recipes are easily adaptable - I know that the best dishes for you are ultimately your own creations. But knowing the basics, the seeds of cooking for health so to speak, makes it easier. As you see your health improve, try adapting the recipes to accelerate your program.

This is a healing cookbook, so the recipe sections are loosely framed to reflect the stages of a healing program. For example, the first four or five sections have body cleansing, liquid, fresh, morning and macrobiotic foods. The middle recipe sections generally help your body rebuild and maintain health. The last two sections offer recipes for healthy feasting and entertaining.

As you progress through the recipe sections, you may find your tastes tending toward the dishes in the back of the book. Consider it a sign that your body is probably getting better.

Care is an important ingredient - flavor your food with an abundant portion. Care for your diet and that of your family adds a quality that can't be equalled. A loving feeling creates an atmosphere of warmth in the kitchen, for the person who prepares it, and for those who eat it. Preparing food for a healing diet allows you to work with the most central elements of health, and gives you a chance to express caring within yourself and for others.

I've developed these delicious recipes over more than two decades of working with healing foods. They really produce results. Make them a part of your menu even after your health problems are solved.

Using the Healing Recipes

Every recipe in this book has several healing benefits.

Decide what you want your diet to do for your health today. Then choose a recipe with the health benefits you need and the type of meal you want to eat. It couldn't be simpler.

Here's an example:

You've decided to boost your brain power and enhance your memory ability. Follow these easy steps:

1: Look up the BRAIN POWER BOOSTER DIET on page 281 of the "Cooking For Healthy Healing Diet Book".
2: Follow the step-by-step diet for at least one month.
3: Browse through one or more of the recommended RECIPE SECTIONS listed with the diet.
4: Zero in on the SPECIFIC RECIPES that list brain power as one of the benefits.
5: Choose one or more that appeal to your taste buds.
6: Make the recipe; eat it; feel better.

That's all there is to it! You'll never be bored during your healing diet. There are over 1000 recipes in this book. Check out other recipes to vary your diet and your meal plans and still get the memory enhancing results you want.

Get ready for a treat from these recipes - lots of treats. Even though you may be on a "healing diet," there is a lot of variety. Whole foods combine easily and naturally. It's really hard to make a bad meal when you are eating naturally. While you are on a healing diet, cook from scratch whenever possible, so that you control the quality of your diet all the way.

Most people notice that they don't have to overstuff their bodies with "empty" calorie foods to feel satisfied. Their appetites become keen for lean, whole foods. You, too will find yourself eating things that you like and that agree with you, eating only when you are hungry, and eating a little less than possible.

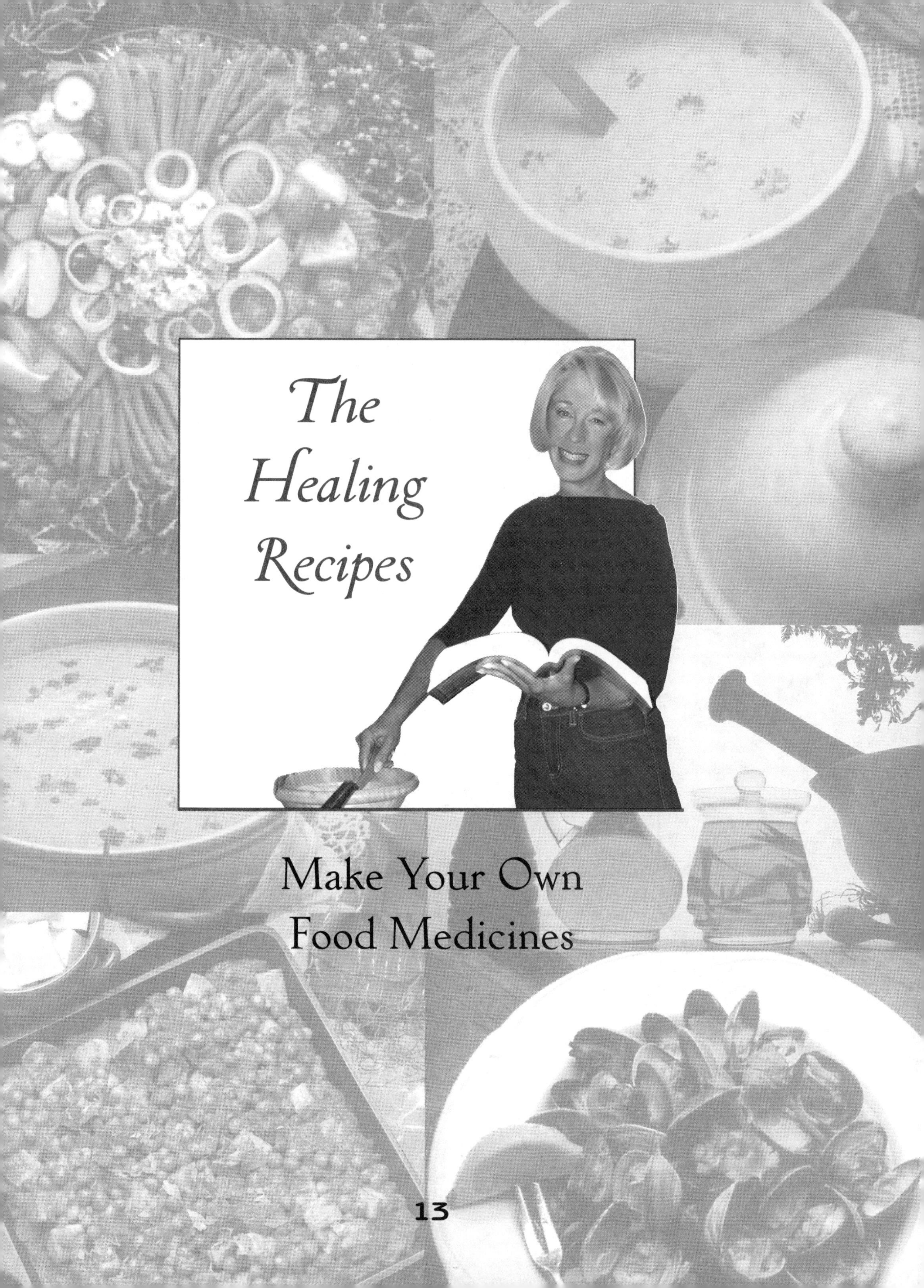

The Healing Recipes

Make Your Own Food Medicines

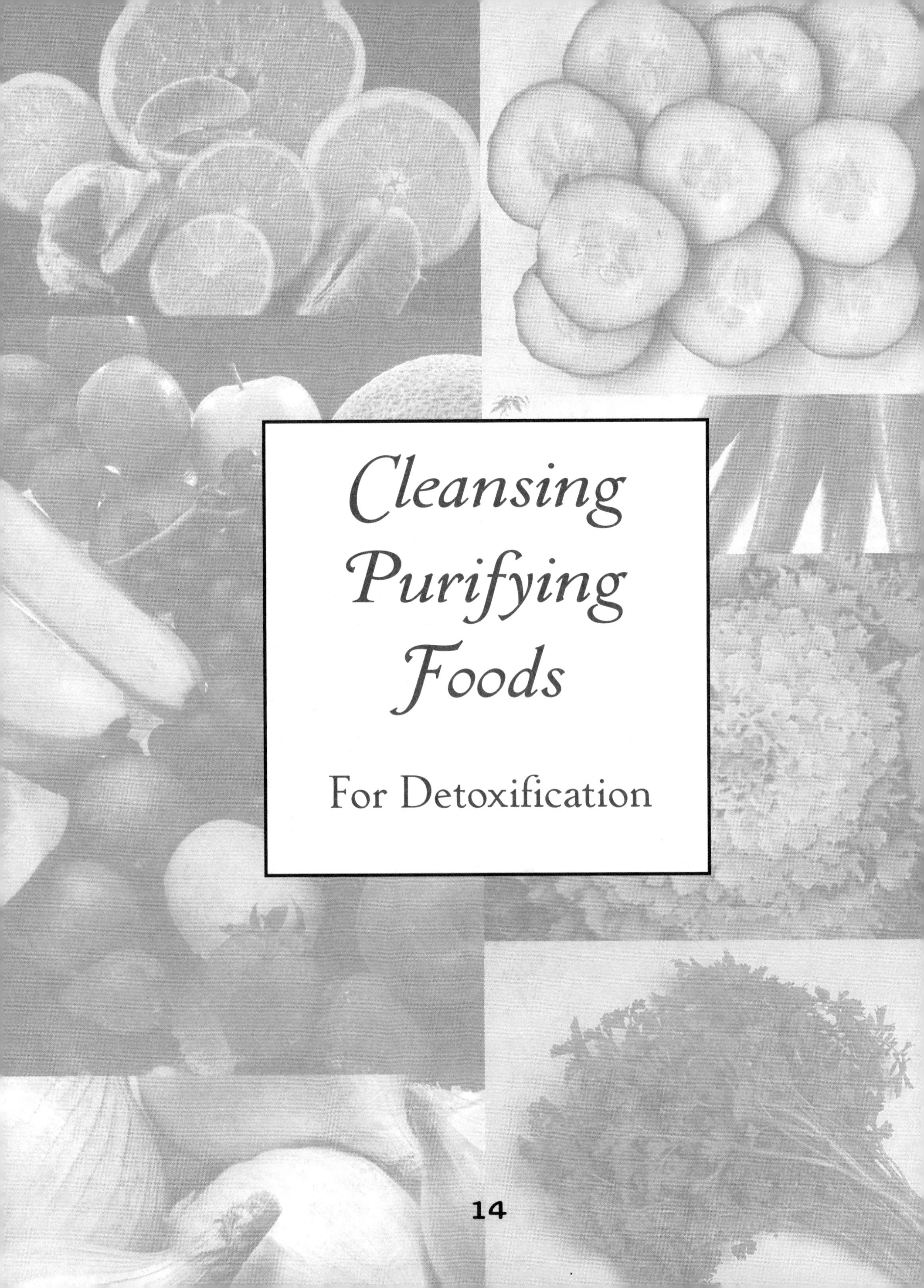

Cleansing Purifying Foods

For Detoxification

Cleansing & Purifying Foods

The recipes in this section are carefully targeted for detoxification, cleansing and purifying. Each detox recipe is targeted with food ingredients that help the body normalize from the daily assault from pesticides, chemical pollutants and heavy metals, and toxins from drugs, caffeine and nicotine.

For best results, cleansing foods should be organically grown and eaten fresh. Only fresh foods and juices retain the full complement of nutrients and plant enzymes that Mother Nature offers.

- **Fruit juices** eliminate wastes quickly and reduce cravings.
- **Fresh vegetable juices** carry off excess body acids, and are rich in nutrients that satisfy your body's needs with less food.
- **Chlorophyll-rich foods** have a molecular structure close to human plasma; taking in chlorophyll-rich foods is like giving yourself a mini transfusion.
- **Herb teas and mineral drinks** provide energy and cleansing at the same time, without having to take in solid food for fuel.
- **Sea greens** act as the ocean's purifiers and they perform much the same for your body, also largely made up of salt water.

How do you use cleansing foods?

Our bodies are designed to be self-healing organisms. Healing is allowed to occur through cleansing. Cleansing foods and juices are crucial to the success of your detox plan.

—Cleansing foods keep your body chemistry balanced and body processes stable while you detox. Mother Nature cleans house dramatically during a detox. You may eliminate accumulated poisons and wastes rapidly, causing headaches, slight nausea and weakness as your body purges; reactions are usually temporary and disappear along with the waste and toxins.

—Cleansing foods regulate the speed of your detox so your body doesn't cleanse too fast or dump too many toxins into your bloodstream all at once. Cleansing foods keep you from re-poisoning yourself during the detox process.

—Cleansing foods support your nutrition and energy levels while you detox, so you don't become too hungry or too tired. New healthy tissue starts building right away when these foods are taken in.

Remember these easy cleansing watchwords:

1: The day before you begin your detox, eat green salads and fresh fruits, and drink plenty of healthy liquids, so that the upcoming body chemistry changes will not be uncomfortable. A gentle herbal laxative taken the night before is beneficial.

2: Avoid all dairy products and cooked foods during a cleanse.

3: Drink 6 to 8 eight oz. glasses of water daily to keep your body flushing out the toxins your tissues are releasing.

4: Conserve outward activity. Focus your mind on internal cleansing - allow your energy to concentrate on inner vitality.

5: Bathe twice daily while cleansing, to remove toxins coming out on the skin. Dry brush your skin with a natural bristle brush for five minutes before a bath or shower, until skin is pink and glowing. Use a body scrub or natural "salt glow" for best results. Take an enema during the cleanse, to remove old, encrusted waste from the colon and to allow the juices and raw foods to do their best work. (See page 571, *How To Take An Enema* in the Cooking For Healthy Healing Diet Book for directions.)

6: Take daily fresh air walks with deep breathing to enhance aerobic activity. Sunbathe early in the morning every day possible for increased purification and fortifying vitamin D.

Cleansing and Purifying Recipe Sections

Cleansing Fruit Drinks

Fruit juices are like a quick car wash for your body. Their high water and sugar content speed up metabolism to release wastes quickly. Their alkalizing effects help reduce cravings for sweets. However, their rapid absorption means the pesticides and chemicals sprayed on fruits can enter your body rapidly. Eat organically grown fruits whenever possible. Wash fruit well if commercially grown. Fruits and fruit juices have their best nutritional effects when taken alone. Eat them before noon for best energy conversion and cleansing benefits.

Make all drinks in a blender. Add everything to the blender, blend, and drink.

STOMACH CLEANSER and BREATH REFRESHER

This recipe works for: Digestive Disorders, Weight Control, Waste Management
For 2 drinks:

Juice 1 bunch Grapes, I basket Strawberries, 3 Apples cored, and 4 sprigs Fresh Mint. Add $^1/_2$ teasp. Acidophilus Powder if desired.

Nutrition per serving: 190 calories; 4gm protein; 44gm carbohydrate; 7gm fiber; trace fat; 0 choles.; 186mg calcium; 19mg iron; 19mg magnesium; 425mg potass.; 35mg sodium; Vit. C 58mg; Vit. E 1 IU.

HEMORRHOID and VARICOSE VEIN TONIC

This recipe works for: Waste Management; Arthritis Diseases; Cardio-Pulmonary
For 1 drink:

Juice 1 cup pitted Cherries, 1 bunch Grapes, $^1/_4$ Pineapple, $^1/_2$ cored Apple, and $^1/_4$-inch slice Ginger Root.

Nutrition per serving: 224 calories; 2gm protein; 55gm carbohydrate; 5gm fiber; trace fat; 0 choles.; 36mg calcium; 1mg iron; 36mg magnesium; 591mg potass.; 4mg sodium; Vit. C 38mg; Vit. E 1 IU.

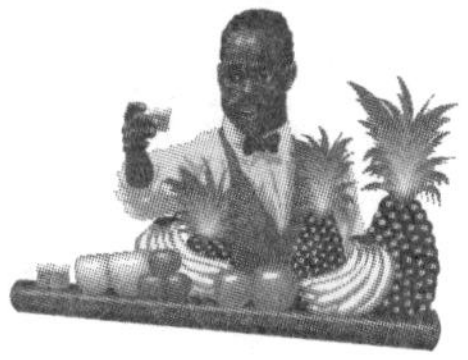

GINGER AID for PROSTATE HEALTH

This recipe works for: Men's Diets; Digestive Disorders; Cardio-Pulmonary
For 1 drinks:

Juice 1 Lemon, 1-inch slice Fresh Ginger Root, and 1 large bunch Green Grapes. —Fill glass with Sparkling Water.

Nutrition per serving: 184 calories; 2gm protein; 46gm carbohydrate; 4gm fiber; 0 fat; 0 choles.; 32mg calcium; 2mg iron; 2mg magnesium; 550mg potass.; 6mg sodium; Vit. C 46mg; Vit. E 6 IU.

GINGER - LEMON CLEANSE for ALLERGIES

This recipe works for: Allergies - Asthma, Weight Control, Respiratory Infections
For 2 drinks (a day's supply):

Juice 1-inch slice Fresh Ginger Root, 1 Lemon, 6 Carrots with tops, 1 Apple, cored.

Nutrition per serving: 165 calories; 3gm protein; 40gm carbohydrate; 9gm fiber; trace fat; 0 choles.; 73mg calcium; 2mg iron; 41mg magnesium; 867mg potass.; 4mg sodium; Vit. C 41mg; Vit. E 3 IU.

DIURETIC MELON MIX

This recipe works for: Kidney Problems, Weight Control, High Blood Pressure
A morning drink for diuretic activity; on an empty stomach 3 times daily.
For 1 quart:

Juice 3 cups Watermelon Cubes, 2 cups Persian Melon Cubes, 2 cups Honeydew Cubes.

APPLE CLEANSE for MUCOUS CONGESTION

This recipe works for: Kidney Problems, Weight Control, High Blood Pressure
For 1 drink:

Juice 2 large Apples, seeded, and $^1/_2$ teasp. grated Horseradish, 2 TB Lemon Juice.

BLADDER INFECTION CLEANSER

This recipe works for: Kidney Problems, Immune Power, Fatigue Syndromes
For 2 drinks:

Juice 4 Apples, $^1/_2$ cup Cranberries, $^1/_2$ teasp. Vitamin C powder.

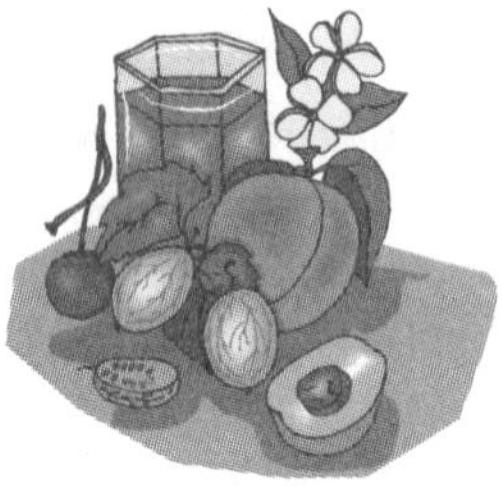

BLOOD CLEANSER - BUILDER

This recipe works for: Immune Compromised Disease, Overcoming Addictions, Liver - Organ Healing, Cancer
For 4 large drinks:

Juice 2 bunches Grapes or 2 cups Grape Juice, 6 Oranges or 2 cups Orange Juice, and 8 Lemons peeled or 1 cup Lemon Juice.
—Stir in: 2 cups Water and $^1/_4$ cup Honey.

Nutrition per serving: 174 calories; 2gm protein; 45gm carbohydrate; 1gm fiber; trace fat; 0 choles.; 25mg calcium; 1mg iron; 25mg magnesium; 418mg potass.; 4mg sodium; Vit. C 91mg; Vit. E 1 IU.

ARTHRITIS - BURSITIS RELIEF

This recipe works for: Arthritis Problems, Controlling Cancer, Sports Nutrition
For 2 drinks:

Juice 3 Oranges, peeled, $^{1}/_{4}$ Pineapple or Mango, and $^{1}/_{2}$ Apple, cored.

Nutrition per serving: 146 calories; 2gm protein; 37gm carbohy.; 5gm fiber; 1gm fats; Vit. E .5mg; 0mg cholesterol; 91mg calcium; 31mg magnesium; 480mg potass.; 3mg sodium; trace zinc.

CONSTIPATION CLEANSER

This recipe works for: Colon Problems, Digestive Disorders, Skin Problems
For 1 drink:

Juice 1 firm Papaya, $^{1}/_{4}$- inch slice Ginger Root, 2 Prunes and 1 Pear.

Nutrition per serving; 267 calories; 3gm protein; 67gm carbo.; 11g fiber; 1g good fats; 0 cholesterol; 107mg calcium; 1mg iron; 54mg magnesium; 1173mg potassium; 11mg sodium; Vit. C 197mg; Vit. E 7 IU.

ACNE DETOX

This recipe works for: Skin Problems, Kidney Problems, Digestive Disorders
For 1 drink:

Juice 2 slices Pineapple, $^{1}/_{2}$ Cucumber, $^{1}/_{2}$ Kiwi, and $^{1}/_{4}$-inch slice Ginger Root.

PURIFYING VITAMIN C-FLUSH

This recipe works for: Respiratory Infections, Immune Power, Childhood Diseases
For 2 drinks:

Juice 1 cup sliced Strawberries, 1 cup Orange Juice, 1 Kiwi peeled, $^{1}/_{2}$ cup Mango or Pineapple Chunks, $^{1}/_{4}$-inch slice peeled Ginger Root, and $^{1}/_{4}$ tsp. Vitamin C Crystals.

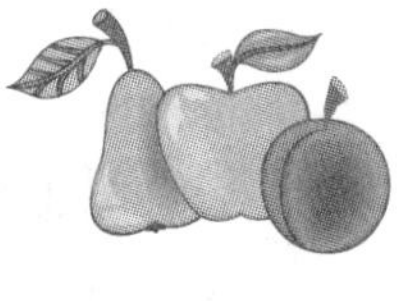

Nutrition per serving: 91 calories; 2gm protein; 20gm carbohy.; 3gm fiber; 2gm fats; vit. E 1.3 IU; 0mg cholesterol; 32mg calcium; 22mg magnesium; 404mg potass.; 32mg sodium; 1mg zinc.

Effective, healing single fruit juices:

1: **Black Cherry juice** for gout and rheumatism; 2: **Cranberry juice** for bladder and kidney infections; 3: **Grape and Citrus juices** for high blood pressure; 4: **Pineapple-Coconut juice** for fatigue and nerves; 5: **Canteloupe** for allergies; 6: **Apple juice** for fatigue.

Body Balancing Vegetable Juices

Vegetable juices are wonderful nutrient sources. They contain large amounts of vitamins; they are high in minerals. They are excellent for mucous cleansing and rebalancing the body quickly. They are full of enzymes for assimilation. Some have over 1000 of the known enzymes necessary for human cell response. Vegetable juices are potent fuel in maintaining good health, yet don't come burdened by the fats that accompany animal products. Those included here have been used with therapeutic success for many years.

Should you get a juicer? Juicers are expensive appliances, but they can really boost the nutrient and cleansing power of your drinks. A juicer juices all of a fruit or vegetable (even rinds, stems, peels, seeds) to give you up to 95% of the plant's nutritive value. Juicer juices accelerate your cleanse and noticeably enhance your energy level. A good juicer essentially pre-digests fresh fruits and vegetables for almost immediate assimilation by your body.

Champion, JuiceMan and Acme are all good juicers for a detox program.

POTASSIUM JUICE

This recipe works for: almost every health problem where cleansing is needed.

The single most effective juice for cleansing, neutralizing acids and rebuilding the body. It is a blood and body tonic that provides rapid energy and system balance.

For one 12-oz. glass:

Juice in the juicer 3 Carrots, 3 Stalks Celery, 1/2 Bunch Spinach, and 1/2 Bunch Parsley.
—Add 1 to 2 teasp. Bragg's Liquid Aminos if desired.

Nutrition per serving: 136 calories; 6gm protein; Vit. C 73mg; Vit. E 4mg; 30gm carbo.; 3gm fiber; trace fats; 0 cholest.; 211mg calcium; 2mg iron; 122mg magnesium; 1602mg potassium; 244mg sodium; 1mg zinc.

POTASSIUM ESSENCE BROTH

This recipe works for: almost every health problem where cleansing is needed.

Make this broth in a soup pot. It is an ideal source of minerals and electrolytes.

For a 2 day supply: Cover with water in a soup pot- 4 Carrots, 3 Ribs Celery, 2 Potatoes with skins, 1/2 Bunch Parsley, 1/2 Head Cabbage, 1 Onion, and 1/2 Bunch Broccoli.

—Simmer covered 30 minutes. Strain and discard solids.

—Add 2 tsp. Bragg's Liquid Aminos or 1 tsp. Miso. and 2" piece Sea Greens (any kind). Store in the fridge.

Nutrition per serving: 66 calories; 4gm protein; Vit. C 39mg; Vit E 1mg; 15gm carbo.; 6gm fiber; trace fats; 0 cholest.; 84mg calcium; 1mg iron; 53mg magnesium; 713mg potassium; 32mg sodium; 1mg zinc.

PERSONAL BEST V-8

This recipe works for: Immune Power, Fatigue / Candida Syndromes, Anti-Aging.
A high vitamin/mineral drink for normalizing body balance.
For 6 glasses:

Juice 6 to 8 Tomatoes (or 4 cups Tomato Juice), 3 to 4 Green Onions with tops, $^1/_2$ Green Pepper, 2 Carrots, 2 Ribs Celery with leaves, $^1/_2$ Bunch Spinach, washed, $^1/_2$ Bunch Parsley, 2 Lemons, peeled, (or 4 TBS. Lemon Juice).
—Add 2 teasp. Bragg's Liquid Aminos and $^1/_2$ teasp. ground Celery Seed.

Nutrition per serving; 59 calories; 3 gm protein; Vit. C 145mg; Vit. E 4mg; 13gm carbo.; 4gm fiber; trace fats; 137mg calcium; 67mg magnesium; 4mg iron; 1214mg. potassium; 195mg. sodium; 2mg. zinc.

IMMUNE ENHANCER

This recipe works for: Immune Power, Immune Compromised Disease, Cancer
For 2 drinks:

Juice $^1/_2$ Bunch Parsley, 1 Garlic Clove, 6 Carrots, 3 Stalks Celery with leaves, 2 Tomatoes, 1 Bell Pepper, a dash of Hot Pepper Sauce (or Cayenne Pepper), 4 Romaine Leaves, 1 Stalk Broccoli. —Add 1 teasp. Miso Paste mixed with a little water.

Nutrition per serving; 126 calories; 6gm. protein; Vit. C 62mg; 27gm. carbohydrate; 9gm. fiber; trace fats; 0 cholesterol; 70mg. calcium; 42mg. magnesium; 2mg. iron; 984mg. potassium; 128mg. sodium; 1mg. zinc.

GENTLE DIVERTICULITIS-COLITIS DETOX

This recipe works for: Waste Management, Fatigue Syndromes, Colon Cancer
For 2 large drinks (a day's supply):

Juice 4 handfuls greens: 1 Spinach, 1 Parsley, 1 Kale, and 1 Parsley, 2 large Tomatoes, $^1/_4$ head Green Cabbage, 4 Carrots w/ tops, 1 Garlic Clove and 2 stalks Celery with leaves.

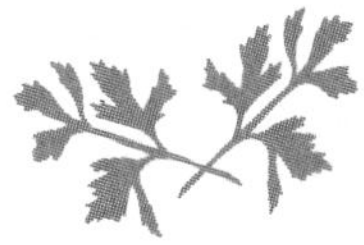

KIDNEY FLUSH

This recipe works for: Bladder-Kidney Problems, Immune Compromised Disease
For four 8-oz. glasses:

Juice 4 Carrots with tops, 1 Cucumber with skin, 4 Beets with tops, 1 handful Spinach Leaves, and 4 Celery Stalks with leaves. —Add 2 teasp. Bragg's Liquid Aminos.

Nutrition per serving: 88 calories; 4gm protein; 19gm carbohydrates; 6gm fiber; trace fats; 0 cholesterol; 77mg calcium; 2mg iron; 55mg magnesium; 1310mg potassium; 260mg sodium; Vit. C 22mg; Vit E 1 IU.

RESTORATIVE BLOOD TONIC

This recipe works for: Recovery from Surgery, Female Balance, Healthy Pregnancy
An amazingly simple, but effective Chinese medicine restorative for women.
For 8 drinks:

Simmer 35 Black Dates and 5 slices peeled Fresh Ginger in 8 cups Water. —Stir in 1 teasp. Royal Jelly (or 1 TBS. royal jelly mixed with honey) and 1 TB Sesame Tahini. —Sip throughout the day for several weeks.

DAILY CARROT JUICE CLEANSE

This recipe works for: Stress and Exhaustion, Fatigue Syndromes, Anti-Aging
For 2 large drinks:

Juice 4 Carrots, 1/2 Cucumber, 2 Ribs Celery w/ leaves and 1 TB chopped Dry Dulse.

Nutrition per serving: 79 calories; 3gm protein; 18gm carbohydrate; 6gm fiber; trace fats; 0 cholesterol; 67mg calcium; 1mg iron; 34mg magnesium; 698mg potassium; 88mg sodium; 1mg zinc.

PROSTATE SEDIMENT CLEANSER

This recipe works for: Men's Problems, Liver and Organ Healing, Anti-Aging
For 2 large drinks (a day's supply):

Juice 2 large handfuls mixed dark green leaves, especially Spinach, Kale, Collards and Dandelion Leaves, and 3 Tomatoes, 2 dropperful squirts of Echinacea Extract.

Nutrition per serving: 79 calories; 4gm protein; 16gm carbohydrate; 6gm fiber; trace fats; 0 cholesterol; 91mg calcium; 3mg iron; 60mg magnesium; 846mg potassium; 63mg sodium; Vit. C 81mg; Vit. E 5 IU.

HEALTHY MARY TONIC

This recipe works for: CardioPulmonary Health, Brain Boosting, Immune Power
A virgin mary is really a healthy veggie drink when you make it fresh.
For 4 drinks:

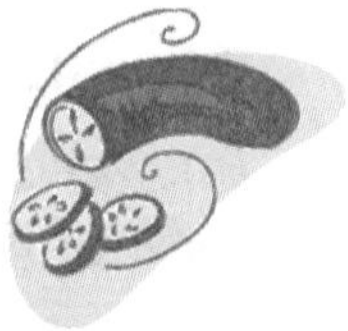

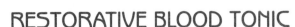

Juice 3 cups Water, 1/2 Green Bell Pepper, 2 Large Tomatoes, 2 Celery Stalks with leaves, 1 Green Onion with top, and 1 handful Fresh Parsley.
—Add 1 TBS. crumbled, dry Sea Greens, (any kind), or 1 teasp. Kelp Powder.

Nutrition per serving: 70 calories; 3gm protein; 14gm carbohydrate; 4gm fiber; trace fats; 0 cholesterol; 70mg calcium; 2mg iron; 41mg magnesium; 984mg potassium; 129mg sodium; Vit. C 61mg; Vit. E 1IU.

ARTHRITIS RELIEF DETOX

This recipe works for: Arthritic Diseases, Liver - Organ, Bone Building, Anti-Aging
For 1 large drink:

Juice a large handful Spinach, a large handful Parsley, a large handful Watercress, 5 Carrots with tops, 3 Radishes. —Add 1 TBS Bragg's Liquid Aminos.

Nutrition per serving: 207 calories; 10gm protein; 44gm carbohydrate; 14gm fiber; trace fat; 0 choles.; 279mg calcium; 7mg iron; 137mg magnesium; 4937mg potass.; 879mg sodium; Vit. C 147mg; Vit. E 7iu.

EXCESS WATER RETENTION CLEANSER

This recipe works for: Kidney Disease, High Blood Pressure, Weight Control
For 1 large drink:

Juice 1 Cucumber, 1 Beet, 1/2 Apple, seeded, and 4 Carrots with tops.
—Add a 2-inch piece fresh Daikon Radish or soak slivers of dried Daikon and add.

HIGH BLOOD PRESSURE REDUCER

This recipe works for: Circulatory Diseases, Sugar Imbalances, Skin and Hair
For 1 large calcium/magnesium drink:

Juice 2 Garlic Cloves, 1 handful Parsley, 4 Carrots w/ tops, 1 Cucumber, 2 Stalks Celery and 2 squirts Siberian Ginseng Extract.

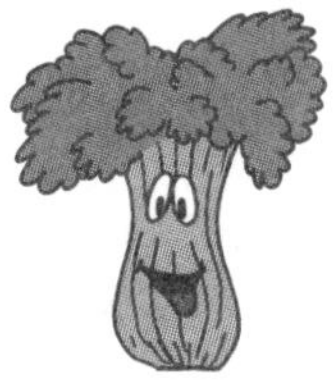

REDUCE HIGH CHOLESTEROL

This recipe works for: Weight Control, Sugar Imbalances, Circulatory Diseases
For 2 drinks:

1 large handful Parsley, 5 Carrots with tops, 2 Apples, and 1/2 tub Alfalfa Sprouts.

SWEEP THE COBWEBS BRAIN BOOSTER

This recipe works for: Stress and Exhaustion, Brain Boosting, Anti-Aging
For 1 large drink:

Juice 1 bunch Parsley, 4 Carrots, a 1-inch piece fresh or preserved Burdock or Ginseng Root, and 2 Stalks Celery. —Add 2 squirts Ginkgo Biloba Extract if desired.

BLADDER INFECTION DETOX

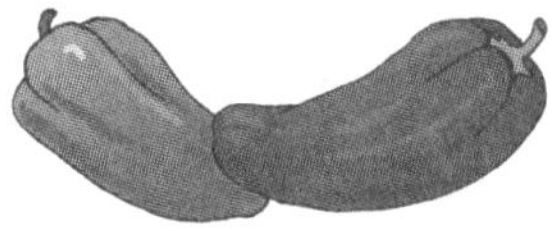

This recipe works for: Bladder Infection, Prostate, PMS-Menopause Symptoms
For 2 drinks (a day's supply):

Juice 3 Broccoli Flowerets, 1 Garlic Clove, 2 Large Tomatoes, 2 Ribs Celery with leaves, and 1 Green Bell Pepper. —Add 2 squirts Echinacea-Goldenseal Extract if desired.

Nutrition per serving: 107 calories; 3gm protein; 22gm carbohydrate; 4gm fiber; trace fat; 0 choles.; 34mg calcium; 7mg iron; 48mg magnesium; 337mg potass.; 142mg sodium; Vit. C 17mg; Vit. E 1 IU.

CONSTIPATION CONGESTION CLEANSE

This recipe works for: Waste Management, Digestive Disorders, Arthritis Diseases
For 2 large drinks (a day's supply):

Juice 1/4 head Green Cabbage, 3 Ribs Celery with leaves, and 5 Carrots with tops.

ECZEMA-PSORIASIS CLEANSER

This recipe works for: Skin Disease, Liver-Organ Imbalance, Prostate Problems
For 1 large drink:

Juice 1 Tomato, 1 Cucumber, 2 Stalks Celery, 1 handful each: Parsley and Watercress.

MAGNESIUM MIGRAINE CLEANSE

This recipe works for: Circulatory Diseases, Fatigue Syndromes, Arthritis Diseases
For 1 large drink:

Juice 1 Garlic Clove, 1 handful Parsley, 5 Carrots, 2 Ribs Celery, with tops.

HIGH PROTEIN SPROUT COCKTAIL

This recipe works for: Surgery Recovery, Sugar Imbalances, Weight Control
This usable protein juice is especially good for ending a cleanse.
For 2 drinks:

Juice 3 cored Apples with skin, 1 tub (4-oz.) Alfalfa Sprouts and 6 Sprigs Fresh Mint.

Nutrition per serving: 185 calories; 6gm protein; 41gm carbohydrate; 10gm fiber; trace fat; 0 choles.; 268mg calcium; 28mg iron; 27mg magnesium; 283mg potass.; 52mg sodium; Vit. C 16mg; Vit. E 1 IU.

Energizing Green Drinks

I believe green drinks are critical to the success of every cleansing program. Green drinks are potent fuel in maintaining human energy and good health. They are an amazing source of life giving nutrients, rich in chlorophyll, vitamins, minerals, proteins and enzymes.

Some green drinks have almost twice as much protein as wheat germ, with five times the amount of minerals. Green drinks also have anti-infective properties, carry off acid wastes, neutralize body pH, and are excellent for mucous cleansing. They can help clear the skin, cleanse the kidneys, and purify and build the blood.

Chlorophyll is the key to green therapy.

The most therapeutic ingredient of all fresh green plants and green superfoods (like chlorella and spirulina), is chlorophyll. Chlorophyll is the pigment that plants use to enable photosynthesis — absorbing the sun's light energy, then converting it into earth and plant energy. This energy is transferred into our cells and blood when we eat chlorophyll-rich greens.

Chlorophyll might be called the "blood" of plants. The chlorophyll molecule is remarkably similar to human plasma, except that it carries magnesium in its center instead of iron. Thus, green foods help human bodies build red blood cells. In essence, eating any of the chlorophyll-rich foods is almost like giving yourself a "mini-transfusion" to help treat illness, enhance immunity and sustain well-being.

Chlorophyll is a primary aid for organ detoxification, helping to neutralize and remove drug deposits, normalize blood composition and release system toxins. Anti-bacterial qualities make chlorophyll valuable for treating colds, inner-ear infections and inflammation. Chlorophyll-rich foods help maintain your body's acid/alkaline balance — to help clear skin, cleanse the kidneys and restore healthy glands. Gland secretions stimulate the immune system to set up a disease defense environment.

Chlorophyll may be one of our best health protectors against some chemical warfare weapons, especially heavy metal build-up, because it can bind with several heavy metals to help eliminate them. A new U.S. Army study reveals that a chlorophyll-rich diet can double the lifespan of animals exposed to lethal radiation.

CANDIDA YEAST CLEANSER

This recipe works for: Colon - Digestive Disorders, Candida and Fatigue Syndromes
For 2 drinks:

Juice 1 Bunch Parsley, 2 Cloves Garlic, 6 Carrots, 2 Stalks Celery, and 3 Kale Leaves.
—Add 1 tsp. Miso Paste mixed with 2 TBS Water, and $^1/_2$ tsp. Barley Green powder.

Nutrition per serving: 135 calories; 5gm protein; 29gm carbohydrate; 10gm fiber; trace fat; 0 choles.; 161mg calcium; 4mg iron; 63mg magnesium; 1125mg potass.; 246mg sodium; Vit. C 97mg; Vit. E 3 IU.

OVERWEIGHT DETOX and APPETITE SUPPRESSANT

This recipe works for: Skin and Hair Problems, Stress Exhaustion, Weight Control
For 1 drink:

Juice 1 large handful dark greens like Spinach, Kale or Parsley, 1 Stalk Celery with leaves, 1 Carrot, 1 Bell Pepper, 1 Tomato, and 1 Broccoli Floweret.
—Add 1 TB dry Sea Greens (any type) and 1/2 teasp. Spirulina Powder.

Nutrition per serving: 161 calories; 10gm protein; 33gm carbohydrate; 12gm fiber; trace fat; 0 choles.; 243mg calcium; 5mg iron; 145mg magnesium; 1712mg potass.; 296mg sodium; Vit. C 243mg; Vit. E 5 IU.

INTENSE PARSLEY CLEANSE

This recipe works for: Colon - Digestive Disorders, Overcoming Addictions, Cancer
A rapid blood cleanser.
For 2 large drinks (a day's supply):

Juice 1 bunch Parsley, 6 Carrots, 1/2 Apple and 2 squirts Siberian Ginseng Extract.

SKIN CLEANSING TONIC

This recipe works for: Digestive Disorders, Skin Problems, Surgery Recovery
Deep greens to cleanse, nourish and tone skin tissue from the inside.
For 1 drink:

Juice 1 Cucumber with skin, 1/2 bunch Fresh Parsley, 4-oz. tub Alfalfa Sprouts, and 3 Sprigs Fresh Mint. —Add 1/2 teasp. Chlorella or Spirulina Granules.

Nutrition per serving: 91 calories; 22gm protein; 19gm carbohydrate; 3gm fiber; trace fat; 0 choles.; 276mg calcium; 13mg iron; 156mg magnesium; 615mg potass.; 78mg sodium; Vit. C 23mg; Vit. E 3 IU.

DIABETES BLOOD BALANCER

This recipe works for: Sugar Imbalances, Candida - Fatigue Syndromes, Cancer
For 1 large drink:

Juice 3 Romaine Lettuce Leaves, 5 Carrots with tops, 2 handfuls Fresh Green Beans, and 2 Brussels Sprouts.
—Add 1 tsp. Miso Paste dissolved in water and stir.
—Add 1/2 tsp. Spirulina Pwdr. and 1 tsp. Siberian Ginseng Extract.

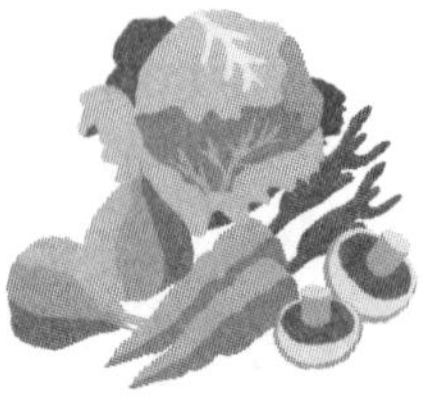

Nutrition per serving: 130 calories; 6gm protein; 29gm carbohydrate; 7gm fiber; trace fat; 0 choles.; 108mg calcium; 3mg iron; 63mg magnesium; 1324mg potass.; 253mg sodium; Vit. C 111mg; Vit. E 3 IU.

STRESS CLEANSE

This recipe works for: Mental Energy, Liver - Organ Problems, Stress Exhaustion
For 1 drink:

Juice 1 small handful each Parsley and Watercress, 2 Stalks Celery, 1 Carrot, $^1/_2$ Bell Pepper, 1 Tomato and 1 Broccoli Floweret. —Add $^1/_2$ teasp. Barley Green powder.

Nutrition per serving: 111 calories; 6gm protein; 24gm carbohydrate; 8gm fiber; trace fat; 0 choles.; 141mg calcium; 56mg iron; 67mg magnesium; 1208mg potass.; 145mg sodium; Vit. C 195mg; Vit. E 5 IU.

HEMORRHOIDS and VARICOSE VEINS TONER

This recipe works for: Bowel Problems, Liver-Organ Problems, Digestive Disorders

Vitamin C, calcium and bioflavonoids boost collagen production which helps new more elastic tissue to form.

For 2 large drinks (a day's supply):

Juice 3 handfuls dark greens- Kale Leaves, Parsley, Spinach, or Watercress, 5 Carrots with tops, 1 Green Bell Pepper and 2 Tomatoes. —Add $^1/_2$ tsp. Chlorella Granules.

GLAND and ORGAN CLEANSER

This recipe works for: Liver - Organ Problems, Skin Problems, Arthritis Diseases
For 2 drinks:

Juice 4 Apples, 2 Stalks Celery, 1 Beet, 1 bunch Watercress, 1 Lemon, 1 Scallion with top, $^1/_2$ teasp. Spirulina Granules.

Nutrition per serving: 134 calories; 13gm protein; 9gm carbohydrate; 2gm fiber; trace fat; 0 choles.; 108mg calcium; 7mg iron; 69mg magnesium; 237mg potass.; 55mg sodium; Vit. C 61mg; Vit. E 1 IU.

SUPER SPROUT PROTEIN DRINK

This recipe works for: Sports Nutrition, Sugar Imbalances
For 2 drinks:

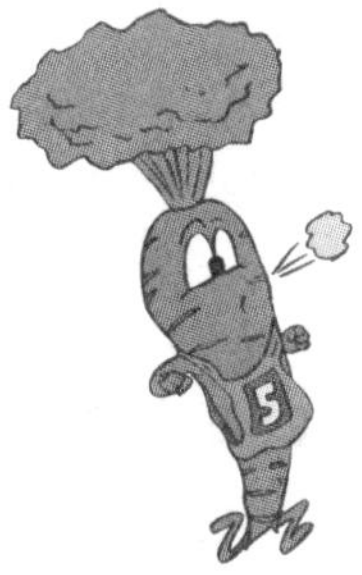

Juice 1 cup each Buckwheat Sprouts, Sunflower Sprouts, Alfalfa Sprouts, Mung Bean Sprouts (or 4 cups Mixed Sprouts), 1 Carrot, 1 Stalk Celery, $^1/_2$ Cucumber, 1 Scallion with top, 2 TBS. Sauerkraut, and 1 teasp. Siberian Ginseng Extract.

Nutrition per serving: 135 calories; 6gm protein; 41gm carbohydrate; 9gm fiber; trace fat; 0 choles.; 268mg calcium; 28mg iron; 26mg magnesium; 284mg potass.; 529mg sodium; Vit. C 16mg; Vit. E 3 IU.

Enzyme Therapy Drinks

Detoxification drinks have a powerful effect on the body's recuperative powers because of their rich, easily absorbed nutrients. Fresh juices contain proteins, carbohydrates, chlorophyll, mineral electrolytes and healing aromatic oils. But most important, fresh juice therapy makes available large amounts of plant enzymes to every cell in our bodies, an integral part of the healing restorative process.

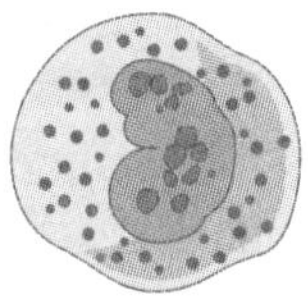

Nothing gets done in our bodies without enzymes. They are the activity components of life. They cause every chemical reaction in our bodies. They play a vital part in breaking down foreign matter (like toxins) as well as food. Enzymes and mineral electrolytes (which restore peristaltic bowel activity) are major contributors in moving toxins out of our systems instead of allowing them to build up and poison us. When your diet is full of cooked foods without enzymes, or microwaved foods which destroy enzymes, or low residue, processed foods (which have a higher tendency to stagnate and putrefy), the process of internal decay develops far more rapidly.

GOLDEN ENZYME THERAPY DRINK

This recipe works for: Skin Problems, Circulatory Problems, Digestive Disorders
For 2 drinks:

Juice 3 cups Pineapple Cubes, 4 Carrots, 1 TB. Honey, 1 half-inch peeled Ginger Root.

PINEAPPLE CARROT COCKTAIL

This recipe works for: Surgery Healing, Sports Nutrition, Digestive Disorders
Natural sources of bromelain, beta carotene and vitamin A.
For 2 drinks:

Juice 1 Pineapple skinned and cored, 4 Carrots, 1 handful fresh snipped Parsley.

Nutrition per serving: 277 calories; 4gm protein; 67gm carbohydrate; 6gm fiber; trace fat; 0 choles.; 136mg calcium; 28mg iron; 82mg magnesium; 1179mg potass.; 81mg sodium; Vit. C 86mg; Vit. E 3 IU.

VEG and VINEGAR STOMACH-DIGESTIVE CLEANSER

This recipe works for: Bowel Problems, Liver-Organ Problems, Digestive Disorders
For one 8-oz. glass:

Juice $^1/_2$ Cucumber with skin, 2 TBS Apple Cider Vinegar, a pinch Ground Ginger and a pinch Cardamom Powder. —Add enough cool Water to make 8-oz.

ENZYME COOLER

This recipe works for: Liver Problems, Digestive Disorders, Healthy Pregnancy
An intestinal balancer to help lower cholesterol, clean the intestinal tract.
For 2 drinks:

Juice 1 Apple cored, 1 Pineapple skinned and cored; 2 Lemons peeled, 1 half-inch piece peeled Ginger Root, and $^1/_2$ tsp. Acidophilus Powder.

Nutrition per serving: 76 calories; 2gm protein; 46gm carbohydrate; 6gm fiber; trace fat; 0 choles.; 38mg calcium; 1mg iron; 44mg magnesium; 455mg potass.; 4mg sodium; Vit. C 71mg; Vit. E 1 IU.

GREEN ENZYMES to LOWER CHOLESTEROL

This recipe works for: Liver Problems, Circulatory Problems, Sugar Imbalances
For 4 drinks:

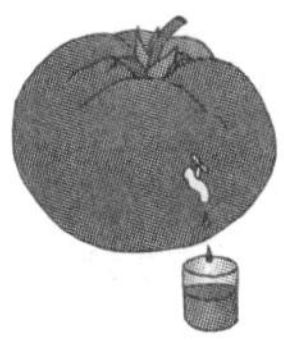

Juice 4 ripe Tomatoes, 4 Celery Stalks, $^1/_2$ Daikon Radish, 1 bunch Parsley, 1 small bunch Spinach, $^1/_4$ tsp. Cayenne Pepper 1-inch Slice Fresh Ginger.

Nutrition per serving: 141 calories; 8gm protein; 31gm carbohydrate; 6gm fiber; trace fat; 0 choles.; 93mg calcium; 3mg iron; 80mg magnesium; 769mg potass.; 154mg sodium; Vit. C 25mg; Vit. E 1 IU.

ENZYME ENERGY TONIC

This recipe works for: Sress Exhaustion, Women's Problems, Sugar Imbalances
A good afternoon pick-me-up juice during a 3 to 7 day cleanse.
For 2 drinks:

Juice 1 cups each: Alfalfa, Broccoli, Sunflower and Radish Sprouts, 1 large Carrot, 1 Stalk Celery with leaves, and 3 TBS Raw Sauerkraut.

EVER GREEN DRINK

This recipe works for: Allergies and Asthma, Respiratory Infections, Arthritis
A personal favorite for taste, mucous release and enzymatic action.
For 1 drink:

Juice 1 Apple with skin, 1 tub (4-oz.) Alfalfa Sprouts, $^1/_2$ Fresh Pineapple skinned/cored, 1 teasp. Spirulina or Chlorella Granules, 4 sprigs Fresh Mint.

Nutrition per serving: 351 calories; 13gm protein; 74gm carbohydrate; 14gm fiber; 1mg fat; 0 choles.; 560mg calcium; 1mg iron; 272mg magnesium; 596mg potass.; 118mg sodium; Vit. C 44mg; Vit. E 1 IU.

Body Normalizing Hot Broths and Tonics

Broths are satisfying, body alkalizing, pH balancing nutrition during a cleanse. They are simple, easy, can be taken hot or cold, and provide a means of "eating" and being with others at mealtime without going off your liquid diet. This is more important than it might appear, since solid food, taken after your body has released all its solid waste, but before the cleanse is over, may drastically reduce your success.

Hot tonics are neither broths nor teas, but unique combinations of purifying, energizing vegetables, fruits and spices. Tonic ingredients provide noticeable synergistic activity when taken together — with more medicinal benefits than any one ingredient alone. Take them morning and evening for best results.

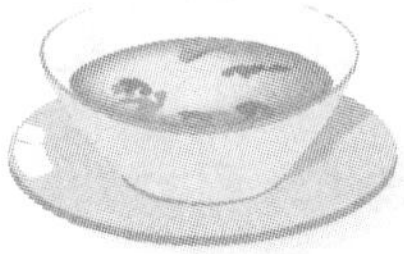

REVITALIZING TONIC

This recipe works for: Liver Problems, Overcoming Addictions, Brain Boosting
A good tonic for any kind of hangover. Effective hot or cold. Works every time.
Enough for 8 drinks:

Whirl in the blender: 1 1/2 cups Water, 1 cup chopped Onions, 2 Ribs Celery chopped, 1 Bunch Parsley chopped, 2 TBS snipped fresh or dried Basil, 2 teasp. Hot Pepper Sauce, 1 teasp. Rosemary, 1/2 teasp. Fennel Seeds, and 2 teasp. Bragg's Liquid Aminos.

—Pour into a large pot with 48-oz. Knudsen's Spicy Veggie Juice. Bring to a boil and simmer for 30 minutes. Use hot or cool.

Nutrition per serving: 33 calories; 3gm protein; 8gm carbohydrate; 4gm fiber; 2mg fat; 0 choles.; 60mg calcium; 1mg iron; 27mg magnesium; 916mg potass.; 113mg sodium; Vit. C 24mg; Vit. E 1 IU.

MACROBIOTIC PURIFYING SOUP

This recipe works for: Asthma and Allergies, Compromised Immunity, Cancer
May be used for the start of almost any healing diet.
For 6 cups:

Toast in a large pan until aromatic (about 5 minutes): 2/3 cup Lentils, 2/3 cup Split Peas, 2/3 cup Brown Rice and 2 Cloves Garlic minced.

—Add 1 chopped Onion, 1 chopped Carrot, 1 Rib Celery, chopped, 3 cups Onion or Veggie Broth, 3 cups Water, 1 teasp. Turmeric Powder, 1/2 teasp. Lemon-Pepper and 1/2 teasp. Ginger Powder. Simmer gently 1 hour stirring occasionally.

Nutrition per serving: 341 calories; 13gm protein; 74gm carbohydrate; 14gm fiber; 1mg fat; 0 choles.; 24mg calcium; 1mg iron; 71mg magnesium; 446mg potass.; 88mg sodium; Vit. C 24mg; Vit. E 1 IU.

PURIFYING MINERAL BROTH

This recipe works for: Illness Recovery, Fatigue Syndromes, Arthritis Diseases
For 6 cups:

Sauté briefly in 2 TBS Canola Oil: $\frac{1}{4}$ cup chopped Celery, $\frac{1}{4}$ cup snipped Daikon Radish, $\frac{1}{4}$ cup chopped Leeks, $\frac{1}{2}$ cup Broccoli chopped and $\frac{1}{2}$ cup grated Carrots.

—Add 6 cups Mineral Rich Enzyme Broth (pg. 33), 2 TBS snipped Lemon Peel, 2 teasp. Bragg's Liquid Aminos, $\frac{1}{4}$ cup snipped Parsley. —Heat for 1 minute, and serve hot.

Nutrition per serving: 33 calories; 8gm protein; 3gm carbohydrate; 1gm fiber; 2g fat; 0 choles.; 18mg calcium; trace iron; 7mg magnesium; 433mg potass.; 86mg sodium; Vit. C 15mg; Vit. E 1iu.

VIRUS FIGHTER BROTH

This recipe works for: Illness Recovery, Respiratory Infections, Immune Diseases
For 2 bowls:

Cover with water in a pot: $\frac{1}{4}$ Daikon Radish, chopped with leaves, $\frac{1}{4}$ Burdock Root, chopped, 1 Carrot, chopped. Soak and sliver 3 dry Shiitake Mushrooms. Save soaking water and add to soup pot.

—Simmer one hour. —Add 2 squirts Echinacea or Usnea Extract.

ONION - MISO ANTIBIOTIC BROTH

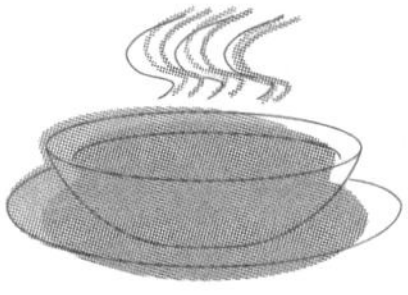

This recipe works for: Allergies - Asthma, Respiratory Infections
For 6 small bowls of broth:

Sauté 1 chopped Onion in $\frac{1}{2}$ tsp. Sesame Oil for 5 minutes. Add 1 Stalk Celery with leaves; sauté 2 minutes. Add 1-qt. Vegetable Broth. Simmer covered 10 minutes.

—Add 4 TBS Miso and 2 chopped Green Onions. Remove from heat; whirl in blender.

Nutrition per serving: 49 calories; 3gm protein; 7gm carbohydrate; 1gm fiber; trace fat; 0 choles.; 20mg calcium; 1mg iron; 9mg magnesium; 84mg potass.; 239mg sodium; Vit. C 3mg; Vit. E trace.

GARLIC TONIC BROTH

This recipe works for: Cold and Flu Recovery, Immune Diseases, Immune Power
Enough for 6 servings:

Bring to a boil, lower heat and simmer for 20 minutes: 6 cups Water, 2 small Heads Garlic, separated, 1 Large Onion, quartered, 2 Stalks Celery, diagonal cut, $\frac{1}{2}$ teasp. Curry Powder, pinch Saffron Threads, $\frac{1}{2}$ cup chopped Fresh Parsley, $\frac{1}{2}$ teasp. dry Sage, and snipped dry or granulated Sea Greens to taste.

—Let cool slightly and puree in blender.

IMMUNE PROTECTION BROTH

This recipe works for: Cancer Recovery, Fatigue Syndromes, Immune Diseases
For 6 large servings (a week's supply):

Soak in water to cover: 1-oz. dry Maitake Mushrooms, 1-oz. dry Shiitake Mushrooms, 4 TBS dry snipped Sea Greens (any kind), 1-oz. Astragalus Bark and 1-inch piece Ginger Root. Sliver mushrooms; discard astragalus and ginger. Save soaking water.

—Simmer 8 cups Water, add soaking water, 4 TBS Pearled Barley, 4 TBS Organic Brown Rice and 2 cups chopped Organic Leafy Greens (any kind). Simmer 30 minutes. Drink hot. Store in fridge and reheat.

Nutrition per serving: 103 calories; 3gm protein; 22gm carbohydrate; 3gm fiber; 2g fat; 0 choles.; 34mg calcium; 1mg iron; 49mg magnesium; 334mg potass.; 19mg sodium; Vit. C 35mg; Vit. E trace.

MISO, GREEN TEA and MUSHROOM HEALING BROTH

This recipe works for: Illness Recovery, Compromised Immune Diseases
For 2 large servings:

Steep 2 TBS Green Tea Leaves, a 2-inch piece Lemongrass, 2 TBS snipped Sea Greens in 1 cup Water. Add 3 cups Dry Shiitake Mushrooms, soaked and slivered (save mushroom soaking water)

—Sizzle 1 Garlic Clove, minced, and 1/2 Small Onion, diced in 1 tsp. Olive Oil, and 1 tsp. Sesame Oil. Add 3 cups Vegetable Stock, bring to a boil and add 1/4 cup shredded Carrots. Add 1 TB Miso Paste, Mushroom Soaking Water and 1/4 tsp Cayenne Pepper.

—Cook five minutes. Add green tea mix, simmer gently 5 minutes.

Nutrition per serving: 141 calories; 9gm protein; 31gm carbohydrate; 6gm fiber; 1g fat; 0 choles.; 98mg calcium; 3mg iron; 79mg magnesium; 760mg potass.; 154mg sodium; Vit. C 25mg; Vit. E 1 IU.

HERB and VEGETABLE IMMUNE BOOSTER BROTH

This recipe works for: Illness Recovery, Fatigue Syndromes, Arthritis Diseases
For 4 cups of broth:

Heat 3 cups Mineral Rich Enzyme Broth (page 33) in a pot. Add and heat gently: 2 TBS Miso dissolved in 1 cup Water, 1 TB Nutritional Yeast, 2 TBS chopped Green Onions, 1/2 cup Tomato Juice and 1/2 teasp. <u>each:</u> dry Basil, Thyme, Savory and Marjoram.

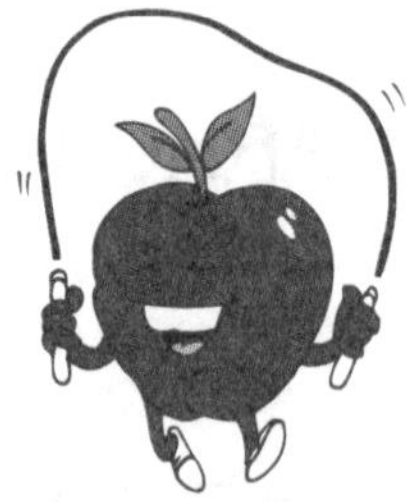

Nutrition per serving: 33 calories; 2gm protein; 3gm carbohydrate; 3gm fiber; 2g fat; 0 choles.; 6mg calcium; 1mg iron; 28mg magnesium; 322mg potassium; 139mg sodium; Vit. C 6mg; Vit. E 1 IU.

CIRCULATION STIMULANT TONIC

This recipe works for: Cardio-Pulmonary Disease, Immune Compromised Diseases
For 4 drinks:

Heat 15 minutes: 1 cup Cranberry Juice, 1 cup Orange Juice, 2 TBS Honey, 6 Cloves, 6 Cardamom Pods, 1 Cinnamon Stick, 4 TBS Raisins, 4 TBS Almonds, chopped, and 1 teasp. Vanilla. —Remove cloves, cardamom and cinnamon stick. Serve hot.

BODY BALANCING APPLE BROTH

This recipe works for: Cold / Flu Recovery, Chronic Respiratory Infections, Arthritis
This broth also alkalizes body pH and helps lower serum cholesterol.
For 4 drinks:

Sauté $^1/_2$ chopped Red Onion and 2 minced Cloves Garlic in 1 tsp. Canola Oil for 5 minutes. —While sautéing, blend in the blender, 1 small Red Bell Pepper, 2 Tart Apples, cored, 1 Lemon partially peeled, 2 TBS Parsley and 2 cups Knudsen's Low Sodium Very Veggie-Spicy Juice. Add onion mix to blender and puree. Heat gently. Take hot.

Nutrition per serving: 93 calories; 2gm protein; 20gm carbohydrate; 3gm fiber; 1g fat; 0 choles.; 36mg calcium; 1mg iron; 28mg magnesium; 404mg potassium; 32mg sodium; Vit. C 86mg; Vit. E 3 IU.

SPRING CLEANSE CARROT SOUP

This recipe works for: Cold and Flu Recovery, Immune Power
For 6 bowls:

In a soup pot, sauté 1 minced Onion in 2 TBS Olive Oil until translucent. —Add 8 cups Water, 1 cup fresh Watercress Leaves, $^1/_4$ cup fresh Basil Leaves, $^1/_2$ cup fresh Dandelion or Nettles Leaves, 4 diced Carrots and 3 TBS White Miso. Cook 30 minutes.

MINERAL RICH ENZYME BROTH

This recipe works for: Bone Building, Allergies and Asthma, Sugar Imbalances
For 6 cups of broth:

Put in a large soup pot: 3 sliced Carrots, 2 Potatoes diced, 1 cup chopped fresh Parsley, 2 Stalks Celery with tops, 1 large chopped Onion.

—Add 6 cups Water, and bring to a boil. Reduce heat and simmer for 30 minutes. Strain and add 1 teasp. Horsetail Extract and 1 TB Bragg's Liquid Aminos.

Nutrition per serving; 60 calories; 2gm protein; 17gm carbohydrate; 3mg fiber; trace fats; 0 cholesterol; 41mg calcium; 1mg. iron; 25mg magnesium; 915mg potassium; 143mg sodium; Vit. C 86mg; Vit. E 3 IU.

MINERAL-RICH AMINOS DRINK

This recipe works for: Bone Building, Sports Nutrition, Cancer-Immune Diseases

A complete, balanced vitamin/mineral electrolyte drink — rich in greens, amino acids and enzymes. Whirl dry ingredients in the blender, then mix about 2 TBS powder into 2 cups of hot water for 1 drink. Let flavors bloom for 5 minutes before drinking. Sip over a half hour period for best assimilation.

Enough powder for 8 drinks:

Add 4 to 6 packets Miso Soup Powder, 1 TB crumbled Dry Sea Greens (any type), 1 TB Red Star Nutritional Yeast, $^1/_2$ cup Soy Protein Powder, 1 packet Instant Ginseng Tea, 2 TBS Bee Pollen Granules, 1 teasp. Spirulina Granules, 1 teasp. Acidophilus Powder, 2 TBS Fresh Parsley Leaf. —Add 1 teasp. Bragg's Liquid Aminos to each drink if desired.

Nutrition per serving; 60 calories; 6gm protein; 17gm carbohydrate; 3mg fiber; trace fats; 0 cholesterol; 41mg calcium; 1mg. iron; 25mg magnesium; 915mg potassium; 143mg sodium; Vit. C 86mg; Vit. E 3 IU.

COLD DEFENSE CLEANSER

This recipe works for: Colds, Flu - Immune Recovery, Immune Power, Allergies

Make this broth the minute you feel a cold coming on. It may prevent it.

Heat for 2 drinks:

Simmer gently 5 minutes: 1$^1/_2$ cups Water, 1 TB Honey, 1 tsp. Garlic Powder, $^1/_2$ tsp. Cayenne, 1 tsp. Ground Ginger, 3 TBS Brandy, 1 TB Lemon Juice.

—Add 1 dropperful Echinacea Extract just before taking. Best in small sips.

Nutrition per serving; 91 calories; 1gm protein; 11gm carbohydrate; trace fiber; trace fats; 0 cholesterol; 4mg calcium; trace iron; 5mg magnesium; 52mg potassium; 1mg sodium; Vit. C 6mg; Vit. E trace.

COLDS and FLU TONIC to CLEAR HEAD CONGESTION

This recipe works for: Colds, Flu - Immune Recovery, Headaches

For 2 drinks:

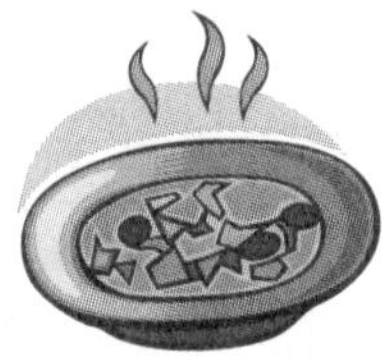

Toast in a dry pan until aromatic: 4 minced Cloves Garlic or 2 teasp. Garlic-Lemon-Sesame Seasoning (page 487), $^1/_4$ tsp. Cumin, $^1/_4$ teasp. Black Pepper, $^1/_2$ tsp. Hot Mustard Powder.

—Add 1 TB Olive Oil and stir in. Toast a little to blend.

—Add 1 cup Water, 1 teasp. Turmeric, $^1/_2$ teasp. Sesame Salt, $^1/_2$ teasp. Ground Coriander or 1 TB fresh Cilantro, 1 cup cooked Split Peas or 1 cup frozen Peas.

—Simmer gently for 5 minutes, and whirl in blender. Very potent.

Nutrition per serving; 170 calories; 9gm protein; 23gm carbohydrate; 4mg fiber; 4 fats; 0 cholesterol; 34mg calcium; 2mg. iron; 38mg magnesium; 379mg potassium; 540mg sodium; Vit. C 3mg; Vit. E 1 IU.

GREEN BROTH with ECHINACEA and ASTRAGALUS

This recipe works for: Fatigue Syndromes, Cancer Recovery, Respiratory Infection
Makes 8 cups

Heat 2 TBS Olive Oil in a soup pot. Add and sizzle: 6 minced Cloves Garlic, 1 diced Leek (white and light green parts only), 5 sliced Scallions, 1 diced Fennel Bulb.

— Add 6 cups Vegetable or Organic Chicken Stock, 1 cup chopped Green Cabbage, 1 cup sliced Broccoli. Simmer 10 minutes. — Add 2 cups frozen Peas, 4 cups sliced Spinach Leaves (for EFA's), 1 handful chopped Fresh Parsley, 1 tsp. Astragalus Extract and 1 tsp. Echinacea Extract, 1 teasp. Lemon-Pepper. Serve immediately.

Nutrition per serving; 144 calories; 8gm protein; 24gm carbohydrate; 6g fiber; 3 fats; 0 cholesterol; 93mg calcium; 3mg iron; 80mg magnesium; 772mg potassium; 154mg sodium; Vit. C 55mg; Vit. E 3 IU.

MUCOUS CLEANSING CHICKEN SOUP

This recipe works for: Asthma, Flu - Immune Recovery, Respiratory Infections

Your grandmother was right. Hot chicken broth has immune stimulants and really does clear out chest congestion faster. This is an Oriental version I like.

For 2 large bowls of broth:

Simmer 3 cups strained homemade Chicken Broth and $^1/_2$ cup Bean Sprouts.

—Add and simmer 10 minutes: 1 cup shredded Chicken, 2 thin slices Ginger, 2 TBS Tamari, $^1/_2$ cup sliced Carrots. —Add $^1/_2$ cup fresh Pea Pods and $^1/_2$ cup shredded Chinese Cabbage. Heat 3 minutes. —Serve with dashes Tamari or Bragg's Liquid Aminos.

Nutrition per serving; 119 calories; 29gm protein; 6gm carbohydrate; 2mg fiber; 0 fats; 0 cholesterol; 44mg calcium; 2mg iron; 41mg magnesium; 399mg potassium; 622mg sodium; Vit. C 26mg; Vit. E 1 IU.

Two-Day Single Food Cleansers

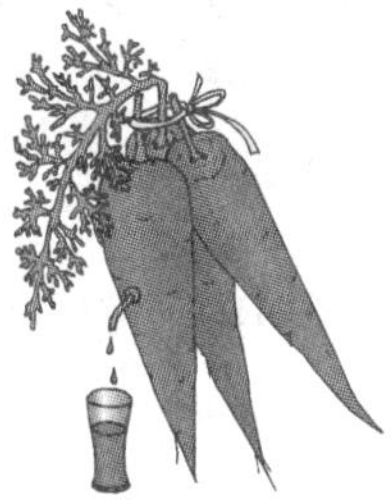

Short mono diets are sometimes highly effective in balancing body chemistry for special problems. Use them for 1 or 2 days, at the end of a liquid diet, and before you take other solid foods.

• **Carrots/Carrot Juice**: for stomach and digestive balance; very beneficial in a diet for arthritis and colon inflammation.

• **Grapefruit/Citrus Fruit**: to stimulate an exhausted liver for better metabolism, and for heavy mucous elimination from the lungs.

• **Apples/Apple Juice**: for digestive and colon problems, lowering blood pressure and cholesterol, and balancing body pH.

• **Grapes/Grape Juice**: use as a blood cleanser, heart tonic and energy source.

Purifying Sea Greens

Sea greens boost every cleansing program. Sea plant chemical composition is very close to human plasma. It can balance your body at the cellular level, purify your blood from the effects of an unhealthy lifestyle, and strengthen your body against environmental toxins. Sea greens reduce excess fluids and fats, and work to transform toxic metals into harmless salts that your body can eliminate. The natural iodine in sea plants reduces radioactive iodine-131 in the thyroid by almost 80%. Sea greens outpace the healing powers of their land-based cousins, broccoli and cabbage.

Sea plants like kelp, dulse, wakame, kombu, nori and sea palm, and marine superfoods like spirulina and chlorella are a veritable medicine chest of healing nutrients. Ounce for ounce, sea greens are higher in essential nutrients than any other food group. They are vigorous sources of proteins, enzymes, antioxidants and amino acids with whole cell availability. Sea plants offer your body basic building blocks for strength and balance, regulate body fluid osmosis, fortify nerve synapses, improve digestion and circulation, help reduce cholesterol and regulate blood sugar levels.

Sea plants are especially rich in minerals like iodine and potassium, have all forty-four trace minerals, substantial amounts of the carotenes and B vitamins (the only vegetarian source of measureable B-12), and are full of chlorophyll, essential fatty acids, octacosonal for tissue oxygenation, and soluble fiber.

Two tablespoons of dry, minced sea greens daily is a therapeutic dose.

MINERAL RICH ENERGY GREEN

This recipe works for: Strong Bones-Teeth, Hair, Skin and Nails, Weight Control
For 4 drinks:

Mix up in the blender: 1/2 cup Amazake Rice Drink, 1/2 cup Oats, 2 TBS Bee Pollen Granules, 1 packet Instant Ginseng Tea Granules, 2 packets Barley Grass or Chlorella Granules, 2 TBS Gotu Kola Leaf, 2 TBS Alfalfa Leaf, 1 TB Dandelion Leaf, 1 TB crumbled, dry Dulse (or any sea green), and 1 teasp. Vitamin C Crystals with Bioflavonoids.

—Mix 2 TBS into 2 cups of Hot Water per drink. Let flavors bloom for 5 minutes before drinking. —Add 1 tsp. Lemon Juice or 1 tsp. Bragg's Liquid Aminos if desired.

SEA GREENS SUPREME

Sprinkle this delicious sea greens blend on your salad, soup, pizza or rice. Just barely whirl the dry ingredients in the blender so there are still sizeable chunks. They expand in any recipe with liquid, and when heated turn a beautiful ocean green color.

1 cup snipped dry Dulse, 1/2 cup snipped dry Nori or Sea Palm, 1/4 cup snipped dry Kombu, 1/2 cup toasted Sesame Seeds, 1/4 cup snipped dry Wakame, 1/4 cup toasted Walnut Pieces.

HIGH VITAMIN C GAZPACHO

This recipe works for: Asthma, Flu - Immune Recovery, Respiratory Infections
A classic gourmet favorite with healing activity. Whirl all in the blender and chill.
For 6 servings:

Simmer 2 Cloves Garlic in 1 cup Water til aromatic. —Add 5 medium Tomatoes, 4 Green Onions, 1/2 Green Pepper diced, 1/2 Cucumber diced, 2 TBS crumbled dry Sea Greens (any kind), 4 Sprigs Parsley, 2 TBS Lemon Juice and 1 tsp. Bragg's Liquid Aminos.

Nutritional analysis: per serving; 46 calories; 2gm protein; 10gm carbohydrate; 3gm fiber; trace fats; 0 cholesterol; 39mg calcium; 1mg iron; 28mg magnesium; 443mg potassium; 48mg sodium; trace zinc.

WATERCRESS and SEA GREENS BROTH

This recipe works for: Liver and Organ Recovery, Respiratory Infections
For 2 bowls:

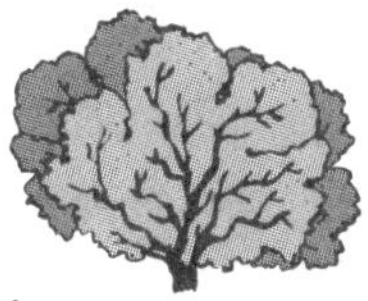

—Blender blend ingredients til smooth: 1/2 cup Water, 1 handful fresh Watercress, 1 cup chopped Mixed Greens, 4 TBS Green Onion minced, 1/2 cup Sunflower Sprouts, 1/4 tsp. Cayenne Pepper. Heat gently.

SEA GREENS and MISO SPECIAL BROTH

This recipe works for: Immune Power, Weight Control, Female-Male Balance
For about 4 bowls:

Bring 4 cups Water to a simmer. Add 4 TBS White Miso, 2 chopped Green Onions, 8-oz. diced firm Tofu, and 6 TBS dry snipped Wakame. Simmer for 2 minutes. — Remove from heat and add 1/2 cup Soy Mozzarella Cheese in small cubes. Sprinkle on 3 teasp. Nutritional Yeast Flakes. Let flavors bloom 30 seconds and serve.

Nutrition per serving; 133 calories; 13gm protein; 9gm carbohydrate; 2mg fiber; 0 fats; 0 cholesterol; 164mg calcium; 7mg iron; 69mg magnesium; 237mg potassium; 655mg sodium; Vit. C 2mg; Vit. E 1 IU.

MINERAL-RICH ALKALIZING ENZYME SOUP

This recipe works for: Strong Bones, Digestive Disorders, Immune Diseases
For 4 soups:

Put in a pot with 1 1/2 quarts of cold water: 2 Potatoes chunked, 1 Onion chunked, 2 Carrots sliced, 1 Stalk Celery with leaves sliced, 1 handful Spinach, and 4 TBS chopped dry Dulse. Add 1 teasp. Bragg's Liquid Aminos. Simmer 30 minutes. Strain.
—Add 2 TBS soaked Flax Seed or Oat Bran if there is chronic constipation.

Cleansing Salads and Dressings

A simple salad is the best way to begin and end a liquid detox diet. A small salad the night before prepares your body and starts the cleansing process. A salad on the last night of your cleanse begins the enzymatic activity of digestion again. Cleansing salads may be used any time you want to put less strain on your digestive system.

Fruits are wonderful for a quick system wash. Their high natural water and sugar content speeds up metabolism to release wastes rapidly. Fresh fruit has an alkalizing effect in the body, and is high in vitamins and nutrients. The way you eat fruits is as important as which fruits you eat. Eat fruits alone or with other fruits for their best healing and nutrition effects. With a few exceptions, eat fruits before noon to take advantage of your body's best energy conversion and cleansing benefits.

MORNING FRESH FRUITS and YOGURT

This recipe works for: Circulatory Problems, Digestive Disorders, Immune Power
For 4 salads:

Chop fruit in a bowl: 1 Banana, 1 Peach or Pear, 1 Apple, 1/4 Fresh Pineapple, 1 Orange.
—Mix in 2 TBS Raisins, 2 TBS toasted Sunflower Seeds and 1/2 cup Lemon/Lime Yogurt.
—Top with 2 TBS Ginger Granola and extra snips of Crystallized Ginger if desired.

MID-MORNING FRUIT TREAT

This recipe works for: Cancer, Digestive Disorders, Stress Effects
For 6 salads:

Chop together in a bowl: 4 Bananas, 2 Pears, 3 cups Grapes, 2 Peaches, 4 Nectarines. —Blend fruit pieces with 1 cup Raisins, 4 TBS Coconut Shreds, and 4 TBS chopped Crystallized Ginger. Pour on top.

Nutrition per serving; 310 calories; 4gm protein; 74gm carbohydrate; 7g fiber; 4 fats; 0 cholesterol; 39mg calcium; 2mg iron; 55mg magnesium; 966mg potassium; 9mg sodium; Vit. C 26mg; Vit. E 3 IU.

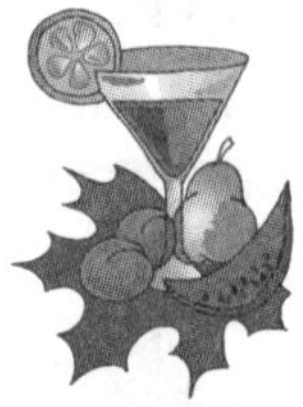

MORNING MELON SALAD

This recipe works for: Bladder Disorders, Digestive Disorders
For 4 salads:

Remove rinds and cube melons in a bowl: 1/2 Honeydew, 1/2 Casaba, 1/2 Cantaloupe, and 1/2 Persian Melon. —Make a sauce by blending some melon mix and pour over.

PINEAPPLE ENZYME SUNDAE

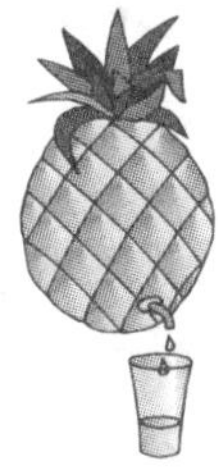

This recipe works for: Male Balance, Digestive Disorders, Cancers
For 6 salads:

Toss in a bowl: 3 cups chopped Fresh Pineapple, 3 cups chopped Fresh Apricots, 12 Fresh Strawberries, and 6 TBS chopped Toasted Almonds.

SPRING CLEANSE SALAD

This recipe works for: Liver - Organ Detox, Arthritis Disorders, Immune Power
For 2 salads:

Chop together in a bowl: 1 Peach, 1 Nectarine, 1 Apricot, and 12 Cherries pitted.

BASIC FRUIT CREAM DRESSINGS

Keep sauces and dressings simple for cleansing fruit salads. Make them in the blender and pour them over the fruit just before you're ready to eat.

Blend 1 or 2 small pieces of the same fruit you used in salad. Add 1 TB Honey. For a thin sauce, add $^1/_2$ cup Water. For thicker sauce, add 1 Banana or $^1/_2$ Avocado.

<u>Fresh vegetable salads are Mother Nature's superfoods</u>:

Massive research validates what natural healers have known for decades. The more fruits and vegetables you eat, the less your risk of disease. People who eat plenty of vegetables have half the risk for cancer as people who eat few vegetables. Most studies show that even moderate amounts of vegetables make a big difference. Eating certain vegetables twice a day, instead of twice a week, can cut the risk of lung cancer by 75%, even for smokers. The evidence is so overwhelming that some researchers are starting to view fruits and vegetables as powerful preventive "drugs" that could substantially wipe out cancer. The healing power of vegetables works both raw and cooked. It is not always true that raw vegetables are better. Even though some fragile anticancer agents, like indoles and vitamin C, are destroyed by heat, a little heat makes beta carotene more easily absorbed. I frequently recommend lightly cooked vegetables because their action is gentler, especially if your body is very ill or your digestion is impaired.

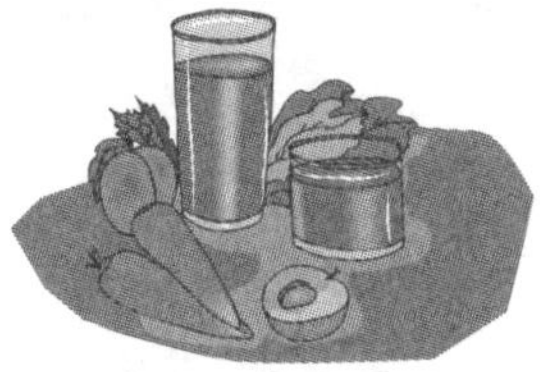

—**<u>What is a serving of fresh vegetables</u>?** One serving is $^1/_2$ cup of cooked or chopped vegetables, 1 cup of leafy greens, or 6-oz. of vegetable juice. Only 10% of Americans eat that much every day.

SHREDDED SALAD SUPREME

This recipe works for: Skin, Hair and Eyes, Digestive Disorders, Liver Power

More of the "essence" of veggies is released during the grating process.

For 1 large salad:

1 cup each: grated Carrots, Cabbage and Zucchini, 2 snipped Scallions, 1 handful Fresh Parsley, 3 TBS Toasted Sesame Seeds. —Use with Mustard Garlic Dressing (page 40).

Nutrition per serving; 267 calories; 12gm protein; 25gm carbohydrate; 10g fiber; 15g fats; 0 cholesterol; 279mg calcium; 6mg iron; 173mg magnesium; 1200mg potassium; 87mg sodium; Vit. C 89mg; Vit. E 5 IU.

EVERGREEN SALAD

This recipe works for: Skin, Hair and Eyes, Digestive Disorders, Liver Power

For 2 salads:

Mix 2 cups chopped mixed Greens (romaine, endive, chicory, spinach), 1 handful each Watercress Leaves, Parsley and Chives minced, and 2 cups Green Onions, minced.

—Mix together juice of 1/2 Lemon, 1 TB Dijon Mustard, 1 TB Sesame Seeds, and 1 TB Toasted Sesame Oil. Pour over salad.

Nutrition per serving; 154 calories; 6gm protein; 13gm carbohydrate; 5g fiber; 10g fats; 0 cholesterol; 174mg calcium; 4mg iron; 76mg magnesium; 711mg potassium; 244mg sodium; Vit. C 7mg; Vit. E 3 IU.

CUCUMBER BODY FLUSH SALAD

This recipe works for: Skin, Hair and Eyes, Bladder-Kidney Disorders, Weight Loss

For 6 large salads:

Slice and divide on salad plates 2 large Cucumbers and 3 large Tomatoes, 1/2 cup Celery sliced, and 1 Red Pepper, finely chopped. —Blend for a dressing: 1 Clove Garlic, 2 TBS snipped Chives, 1/2 Lemon, and 2 teasp. minced dry Sea Greens (any type).

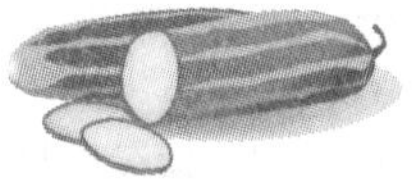

FRESH GOULASH SALAD

This recipe works for: Chronic Infections, Surgery Recovery, Arthritis Diseases

For 4 salads:

Toss 1 cup diced Tomatoes, 1 cup grated Zucchini, 1 cup Corn Kernels, 4 TBS chopped Bell Pepper, 4 TBS snipped Green Onion, pinches Thyme, Basil, Oregano and Marjoram.

—Make a fresh goulash sauce: blend 1 Tomato, pinch Cayenne Pepper, 4 TBS Sunflower Seeds, and juice of 1/2 Lemon. Pour over the salad.

WILD SPRING HERB and FLOWER SALAD

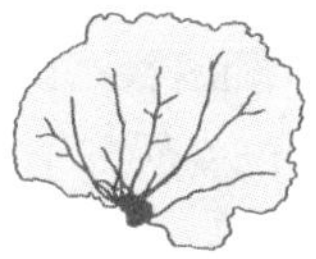

This recipe works for: Chronic Infections, Immune Power
For 6 salads:

Toss together: 1/2 head each Romaine, Frisé Greens, Red Leaf Lettuce, 1/3 cup young Nasturtium Leaves, 1/2 cup Arugula Leaves, 1/4 cup Sweet Violets, 1/3 cup Sweet Violet Leaves, 1/4 cup Fresh Dandelion Leaves, 1/4 cup Orange Mint Leaves, 1/4 cup Lemon Balm Leaves, 2 tsp. snipped Dill Weed and 2 TBS toasted Sea Greens.

—Drizzle with 2 TBS Olive Oil and 2 TBS Balsamic Vinegar.

SPINACH and SPROUT SALAD

This recipe works for: Hair, Skin and Eyes, Weight Control, Brain Booster
For 2 salads:

Wash and toss together 1 small bunch Spinach Leaves, 8-oz. fresh Mung Bean Sprouts, and 2 Cakes Tofu diced or 4-oz. fresh sliced Mushrooms.

—Toss with 2 TBS Toasted Sesame Oil, 2 TBS Brown Rice Vinegar, 2 teasp. Tamari, 2 teasp. minced Crystallized Ginger, and 1 teasp. Sesame Salt. Chill.

Nutrition per serving; 339 calories; 22gm protein; 16gm carbo.; 6g fiber; 23g fats; 0 cholesterol; 277mg calcium; 14mg iron; 158mg magnesium; 626mg potassium; 848mg sodium; Vit. C 23mg; Vit. E 1 IU.

CARROT and CABBAGE SLAW

This recipe works for: Digestive Disorders, Cancer, Waste Management
For 2 salads:

Whirl 1/2 head Chinese Cabbage and 1 Carrot in a food processor. Cover and chill.

—Mix the dressing: 2 tsp. Honey, 3 TBS Tarragon Vinegar, 1 tsp. Crystallized Ginger minced, 1 Green Onion minced, 1/4 tsp. Sesame Salt. Toss and chill to marinate.

FOUR MUSHROOM IMMUNE BOOSTER

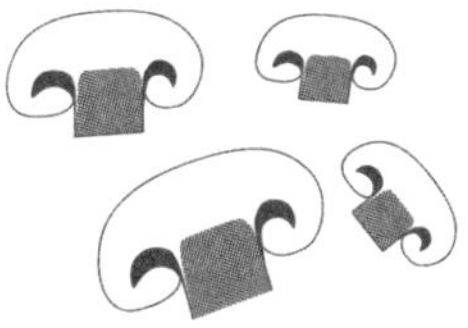

This recipe works for: Infections, Cancer, Immune Power
For 6 salads:

Sizzle for 3 minutes: 1 TB Sesame Oil with 2 Garlic Cloves minced and 2 tsp. minced Pickled Ginger. —Add 3-oz. Oyster Mushrooms, 3-oz. Shiitake Mushrooms, 3-oz. Maitake Mushrooms and 3-oz. Portobellas, and 2 TBS Balsamic Vinegar. Sizzle 4 minutes.

—Add 1/4 cup Tamari, 1/4 cup Seasoned Stock and simmer 2 minutes. —Finely slice 3 heads Belgian Endive, 1/2 head Red Leaf Lettuce, and 1 head Raddichio. —Divide between salad plates; pile on mushroom mix. Sprinkle with Dulse Flakes.

SESAME-MUSHROOM MEDLEY

This recipe works for: Liver - Organ Healing, Gland Imbalances, Sugar Imbalances
For 6 salads:

Toss everything in a bowl: 1 lb. Mixed Mushrooms sliced, 1 Red Bell Pepper diced, 1 bunch Scallions sliced, 1 teasp. Coriander, 2 TBS Toasted Sesame Oil, pinch Cayenne Pepper, and 3 TBS each toasted Black and White Sesame Seeds.

—Drizzle on 1 TB Tamari, 2 TB Lime Juice and 1 TB Sake Wine.

Nutrition per serving; 98 calories; 4gm protein; 6gm carbo.; 2g fiber; 8g fats; 0 cholesterol; 21mg calcium; 2mg iron; 39mg magnesium; 363mg potassium; 142mg sodium; Vit. C 29mg; Vit. E 1 IU.

MUSHROOMS and GREENS

This recipe works for: Liver-Organ Healing, Cancer, Reduced Immune Diseases
For 2 to 4 salads:

Toss together with 4 TBS Balsamic Vinegar: 2 cups Spinach Leaves, 4 TBS minced Green Onions, 2 Beets with tops in matchsticks, and 2 cups thin-sliced Mushrooms.

Nutrition per serving; 35 calories; 1gm protein; 2gm carbo.; 1g fiber; 2g fats; 0 cholesterol; 17mg calcium; 1mg iron; 15mg magnesium; 435mg potassium; 86mg sodium; Vit. C 15mg; Vit. E 1 IU.

MAKE a RAINBOW SALAD

This recipe works for: Liver - Organ Healing, Digestive Disorders, Hair and Skin
Serve salad on a round platter with each veggie as a "rainbow color arc."
For 6 salads:

Prepare each vegetable separately. Thin-slice 2 cups Purple Cabbage and 2 cups Broccoflower. Grate 3 small Zucchini, 2 Beets, 4 Carrots, 3 Crookneck Squash.

—Toss 3 TBS toasted Sesame Seeds, 3 TBS Toasted Sesame Oil, 2 TBS Tamari and 1 teasp. Garlic Powder and 1 teasp. New Chapter GINGER WONDER Syrup.

SWEET and SOUR CUCUMBERS

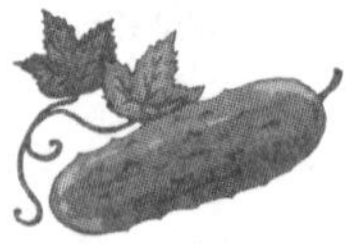

This recipe works for: Digestive Disorders, Hair and Skin
For one salad:

Slice 1 Cucumber and 1/4 Red Onion.
—Mix the dressing: 2 teasp. Olive Oil, 2 teasp. Honey, 3 teasp. Raspberry Vinegar.
—Top with 1 tablespoon of Lemon Yogurt.

SPROUTS PLUS

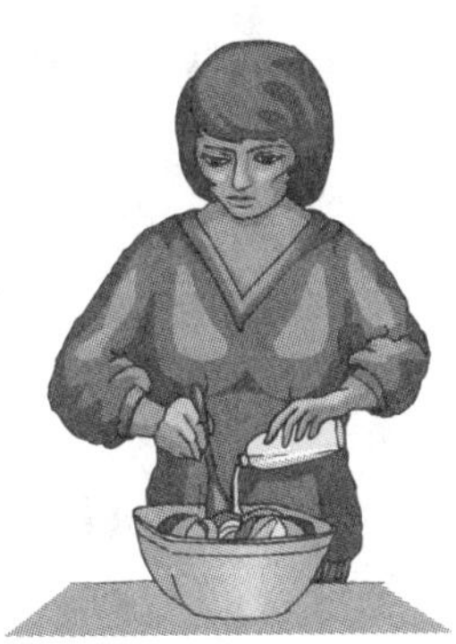

This recipe works for: Arthritis, Healthy Pregnancy
For 2 salads:

Toss together 1 tub Alfalfa Sprouts, 2 cups Grated Carrots, 1 cup minced Celery, 3 pinches Lemon Zest.

SWEET and SOUR MIXED SALAD

This recipe works for: Digestive Disorders, Hair and Skin, Bladder-Kidney Infection
For two large delicious salads:

Slice 1 Cucumber and 1/2 Green or Red Bell Pepper very thin. —Heat together until aromatic: 3 thin slices Red Onion, 1 teasp. Honey, 1/4 cup Seasoned Vinegar, and 1 teasp. Fresh Daikon Radish. Toss with veggies. —Mix the dressing: 6 TBS Olive Oil, 4 TBS Lime Juice, 1/4 cup Tomato Juice, and 1 teasp. Sesame Salt. Toss with veggies.

Nutrition per serving; 242 calories; 2gm protein; 17gm carbo.; 2g fiber; 11g good fats; 0 cholesterol; 38mg calcium; 1mg iron; 37mg magnesium; 438mg potassium; 542mg sodium; Vit. C 41mg; Vit. E 5 IU.

CARROT and LEMON SALAD

This recipe works for: Digestive Disorders, Hair and Skin, Sugar Imbalances
For 2 salads:

Grate 2 cups Carrots. Toss with 2 TBS Raisins, and 2 teasp. fresh minced Mint. —Mix together 2 TBS Lemon Juice, 1 TB Canola Oil, 1/4 teasp. 5 Spice Powder, 1 TB fresh minced Parsley, pinch Lemon Zest and a pinch of Stevia Leaf. Spoon over carrots.

Nutrition per serving; 140 calories; 4gm protein; 20gm carbo.; 4gm fiber; 7g good fats; 0 cholesterol; 41mg calcium; 1mg iron; 22mg magnesium; 458mg potassium; 41mg sodium; Vit. C 21mg; Vit. E 5 IU.

Make fresh, simple dressings for your cleansing veggie salads.

VEGETABLE SPICE CREAM

Blend almost any vegetable or veggie mix with seasonings to make a low fat, cleansing dressing for salads. Make in the blender; add a little water to help blend. Option: Use avocado to bind after liquefying other ingredients.

Blend any Vegetable chopped, 1 TB Dulse Flakes, 1 TB Tamari, 1 TB Olive Oil. —Add 1/2 teasp. <u>each</u>: powdered Garlic, Ginger and Mustard.

NO OIL TAMARI LEMON

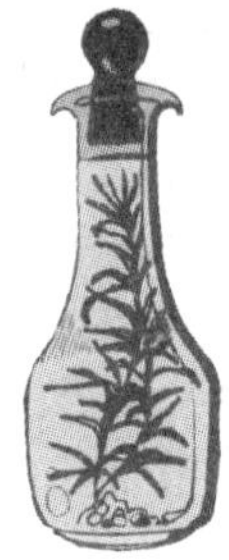

Whisk 2 TBS Lemon Juice, 1 TB Tamari, 1 TB Honey, 1 teasp. Sesame Seeds, and 1 teasp. minced Crystallized Ginger.

LOW FAT ITALIAN

Whisk together 1 TB chopped Parsley, 2 teasp. Wine Vinegar, pinch Garlic-Lemon Seasoning, 2 teasp. Lemon Juice, 2 teasp. Olive Oil, and 1 TB White Wine.

MUSTARD GARLIC DRESSING

Blender blend $^1/_2$ cup toasted Walnuts, 2 TBS Tahini, 1 TB Dijon Mustard, 1 Lemon, peeled, 1 teasp. Garlic minced, 1 teasp. Tamari, and a little Water to thin slightly.

ARIZONA GUACAMOLE DRESSING

Blend 2 Avocados, 6 to 8 Dried Tomatoes, cut into pieces, 2 Green Onions, 1 Lemon peeled, 1 clove fresh Garlic, 1 TB Tamari, and Water to blend.

BALSAMIC HONEY FRENCH

Whisk together 1 cup Balsamic Vinegar, 2 TBS Honey, 1 pinch Dry Mustard, 2 pinches Lemon-Pepper, and 4 TBS Canola Oil.

SUNFLOWER SEED CREAM

Blender blend 1 cup Sunflower Seeds, $^1/_2$ Lemon peeled, $^1/_2$ tsp. Tamari, $^1/_2$ tsp. Dulse Flakes, 1 sprig <u>each</u> fresh Basil and Sage, and 3 TBS Water.

HONEY - MUSTARD DRESSING

Blender blend 2 TBS Olive Oil, 1 tsp. Dijon Mustard, 1 TB Raspberry Vinegar, 1 tsp. Dried Dill, 1 tsp. Honey, and $^1/_4$ tsp. Lemon-Pepper. Chill.

Herb Teas For Detoxification

Herbal teas are the most time-honored of all natural healing mediums. I view herb teas as high mineral drinks during a cleanse that provide energy without having to take in solid proteins or carbohydrates for fuel. Essentially body balancers, teas have mild detoxification properties that are easily used by your body. The important volatile oils in herbs are released by the hot brewing water, and when taken in small sips throughout a cleanse, they flood the tissues with concentrated nutritional support to accelerate regeneration and release of toxic waste. In general, herbs are more effective when taken together, in combination, than when used singly.

How to take herbal teas for best results in your detox program:

1) Use a glass, ceramic or earthenware pot. Stainless steel is okay, but aluminum lessens herbal effects, and the metal may wash into the tea and your body.

2) Pack a small tea ball with loose herbs.

3) Bring 3 cups of cold water to a boil. Remove from heat. Add herbs, and steep covered (10 to 15 minutes for a leaf - flower tea, 25 minutes for a root - bark tea).

4) Keep lid tightly closed during steeping and storage. Volatile herbal oils are the most valuable part of the drink, and will escape if left uncovered.

5) Drink teas in small sips over a long period of time rather than all at once, to allow the tissues to absorb as much of the medicinal value as possible.

6) Take 2 to 3 cups of tea daily for best medicinal effects.

GINGER ALE for CLEANSING and DIGESTION

This original 1920's home remedy tea works amazingly well to eliminate infection during a cold, flu or fever. I like it better than today's ginger ale as part of a detox.

For 1 quart:

Simmer 3 cups Water for 5 minutes. Add 2 teasp. fresh grated Ginger Root, 1 teasp. dry Red Raspberry Leaf, 1 teasp. dry Sassafras Root, and 1 teasp. dry Sarsaparilla Root, broken. —Let steep 15 minutes. Strain and add 1 cup Sparkling Mineral Water just before serving. Add 3 fresh Lemon Slices if desired.

Nutrition per serving; 79 calories; 2gm protein; 18gm carbo.; 4g fiber; 2g fats; 0 cholesterol; 67mg calcium; 1mg iron; 35mg magnesium; 698mg potassium; 87mg sodium; Vit. C 25mg; Vit. E 1 IU.

APPLE and ALOE STOMACH CLEANSER

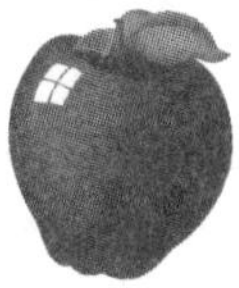

This recipe works for: Digestive Disorders, Immune Boosting

For one 8-oz. glass:

Whirl in the blender: 1 Apple, 2 TBS Aloe Vera Juice Concentrate and $^1/_4$ teasp. each: Ground Ginger, Ground Coriander, Ground Cinnamon. —Add enough Water to make 8-oz.

ROOT BEER REVITALIZER

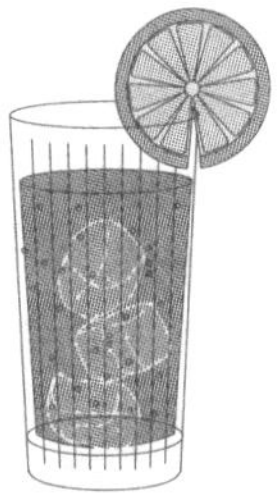

This recipe works for: Colon-Digestive Disorders, Liver-Organ Healing
Old-fashioned, decidedly delicious medicine for cleansing.
For 4 glasses:

Make up the dry blend: 3-oz. dry SASSAFRAS BARK pieces, 2 teasp. fresh grated GINGER ROOT, 2-oz. dry SARSAPARILLA ROOT, 1 TB ground CINNAMON, 1-oz. DANDELION ROOT, 2 teasp. ORANGE PEEL, 1-oz. BURDOCK Root.
—Add 4 TBS. dry mixture to 1-qt. water. Simmer for 15 to 20 minutes. Strain.

My favorite herb tea for a good detox is **GREEN TEA,** an unfermented tea rich in flavonoids with antioxidant and anti-allergen activity. Green tea has a long history in the Orient as a beneficial body cleanser. Its anti-oxidant polyphenols do not interfere with iron or protein absorption, and as with other plant antioxidants like beta carotene and vitamin C, green tea polyphenols work at the molecular level, combatting free radical damage to protect against degenerative disease.

Other herbal choices for specific problems:

A tea combination for blood cleansing: *red clover, pau d' arco, nettles, sage, alfalfa, milk thistle seed, echinacea, horsetail, gotu kola and lemongrass.*

A tea combination for mucous cleansing: *mullein, comfrey, ephedra, marshmallow, pleurisy root, rose hips, calendula, boneset, ginger, and fennel seed.*

A tea combination for the bowel and digestive system: *senna leaf, papaya leaf, fennel seed, peppermint, lemon balm, parsley, calendula, hibiscus and ginger.*

A tea combination for gentle bladder and kidney flushing: *uva ursi, juniper berries, ginger and parsley.*

A tea combination for stress headache: *rosemary, mint, catnip, chamomile.*

A tea combination for removing congestion from chest and sinuses: *marshmallow root, mullein, rose hips and fenugreek seed.*

A tea combination for releasing body energy: *gotu kola, peppermint, red clover and cloves.*

A tea combination for warming against aches and chills: *wild cherry bark, licorice root, rose hips and cinnamon.*

A tea combination for restoring bowel and colon regularity: *fennel seed, flax seed, fenugreek seed, licorice root, burdock root and spearmint.*

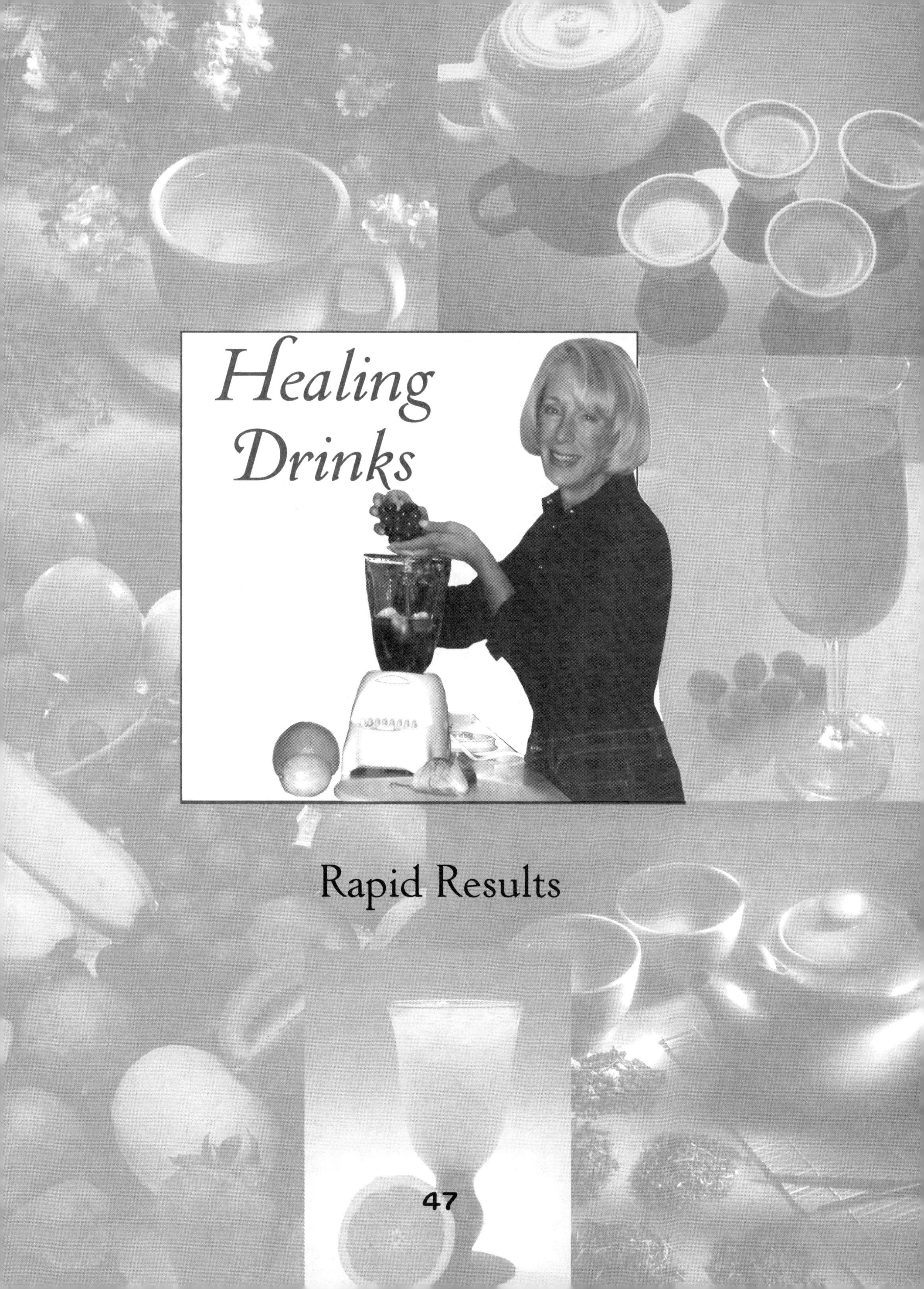

Healing Drinks

Rapid Results

Healing Drinks

Liquids are a fast, easy way to take usable nutrients into your body. They are the least concentrated form of nutrition, but have the great advantage of easy assimilation; they break down and flush out toxins quickly. They lubricate and flood your tissues with therapeutic nutrients in a gentle, often delicious way. In fact, since many natural liquids are rich in minerals, proteins and chlorophyll (nutrients often deficient in our bodies), the drinks in this section, even though rich in medicinal qualities sometimes taste better than anything else. Your body often craves what it needs most.

About Milk: Almost no milk is used in healing recipes, because of its clogging, mucous-forming properties. Pasteurized milk is a pretty dead food for rebuilding body nutrition. Even raw milk is often difficult to assimilate for someone with allergies, asthma, or respiratory problems. But there are delicious, healthy substitutes that can be used in cooking: soy milk, almond milk, rice milk, plain yogurt mixed with water or white wine, kefir, tahini, and more. These foods are more flavorful than milk in almost every case. They have richness without fat, digestibility without clogging, and taste without excess mucous formation. See *"Food Exchanges - Milk Substitutes,"* page 136 in the COOKING FOR HEALTHY HEALING DIET BOOK and *"Dairy Free Cooking"* page 259 in this book.

About Water: I can't say enough good things about drinking plenty of water every day. Water lubricates the body, flushes out waste and toxins, hydrates the skin, regulates body temperature, acts as a shock absorber for joints, bones and muscles, supplies natural earth minerals, and dissolves organic minerals, vitamins, proteins and sugars for body assimilation. Water cleanses the body inside and out. Concern about the lack of purity in our water supply is leading many people to buy bottled water. See *"About Water,"* page 58, in the COOKING FOR HEALTHY HEALING DIET BOOK for more about water.

About Black Teas: Black teas contain caffeine and tannins, but differ from coffee in the amount and kind of caffeine they have. Black teas, do not raise blood cholesterol, or lower vitamin C levels, and can be useful in counteracting depression. In addition, cold wet black tea bags placed over the eyelids are proven eye brighteners, and help clear red, tired eyes.

About Green Tea: green tea leaves are dried without fermentation, do not interfere with iron or calcium absorption, and have some of the same spirit lifting qualities as black teas. Japanese green tea is an especially good blood cleansing tea. Refrigeration is advised for long-term storage of green teas. See *"About Black and Green Tea,"* page 68 in the COOKING FOR HEALTHY HEALING DIET BOOK for more.

About Coffee Substitutes: These are grain or chicory based drinks, roasted and ground, often with a little molasses or herbs added for flavor. They are caffeine-free, and some of the newest ones, ROMA - Celestial Seasonings, RAJA's CUP - Maharishi Ayurveda, and DANDY BLEND - Goosefoot Acres are delicious.

About Herb Teas: The herb teas in this section may enjoyed any time as pleasureable drinks as well as for their healing qualities. If you need to restrict your caffeine, but still want a little uplifting energy, these teas are caffeine-free and fill the bill. My favorite single herb teas are peppermint, spearmint, licorice, rose hips, hibiscus, and lemon grass. Spices like cinnamon, nutmeg, cloves, lemon peel and star anise are wonderful brewed as teas, and may be taken alone or mixed with other spices and herbs for exotic tastes. Blend herb and spice teas with fruit juices for tang. They are at their best as sun-brewed, iced drinks.

How to make Sun Tea: For 1 gallon. Use 10 to 12 tea bags or 8 to 10 TBS loose tea to a gallon jar. Place in the sun or a sunny window, and let steep 5 or 6 hours until tea is twice as dark and strong as you usually like it. Fill with ice cubes, let chill a minute and serve.

Healing Drink Recipe Sections

Energy Drinks

Need quick, reliable energy? The drinks in this section are unique combinations of vegetables, fruits and spices with significant energizing qualities. I've carefully combined the ingredients so they'll provide noticeable synergistic action together - with more medicinal benefits than the specific foods alone. I've even targeted some of the drinks to specific body areas that commonly suffer from fatigue. Try them - I know you'll feel the difference in your energy levels - especially in your long term stamina. Morning and evening are the best times to take these drinks.

AMINOS ENERGY

This recipe works for: Anti-Aging, Cancer Diets, Immune Breakdown Diseases
Enough for 8 drinks:

Whirl ingredients in the blender, then mix about 2 TBS of the powder into 2 cups of hot water for 1 drink. Let flavors bloom for 5 minutes before drinking. Sip over a half hour period for best assimilation.

4 to 6 packets Miso Soup Powder (Edwards & Son Co. makes a good one), 1 TB crumbled Dry Sea Greens (any type), $^1/_2$ cup Soy Protein Powder, 1 packet Instant Panax Ginseng Tea, 1 packet Instant Siberian Ginseng Tea, 1 packet Effervescent Vitamin C, 2 TBS Bee Pollen Granules, 1 teasp. Spirulina Granules, 1 TB Nutritional Yeast Flakes.
—Add 1 teasp. Bragg's Liquid Aminos to each drink if desired.

Nutrition per serving: 65 calories; 7gm protein; 6gm carbohydrate; 1gm fiber; trace fat; 0 choles.; 53mg calcium; 5mg iron; 13mg magnesium; 90mg potass.; 594mg sodium; Vit. C 125mg; Vit. E 3 IU.

CHICKEN-CHILI RESPIRATORY SYSTEM TONIC

A Latin-Asian healing broth. Serve hot in small bowls. Potent congestion clearing.
This recipe works for: Foods for Men, Circulatory Healing, Respiratory Infections
For 4 drinks:

Combine in a pot: 4 cups organic Chicken Broth, 1 to 2 small Jalapeño Chilies, stemmed, seeded, thin-sliced, 1 small handful fresh Cilantro Leaves, 4 shredded fresh Lemon or Lime Peels, 4 slices fresh, peeled Ginger Root. Simmer for 15 minutes. Strain into a bowl. —Add 2 TBS Lemon or Lime Juice, a few more Cilantro Leaves, 2 sliced Scallions.

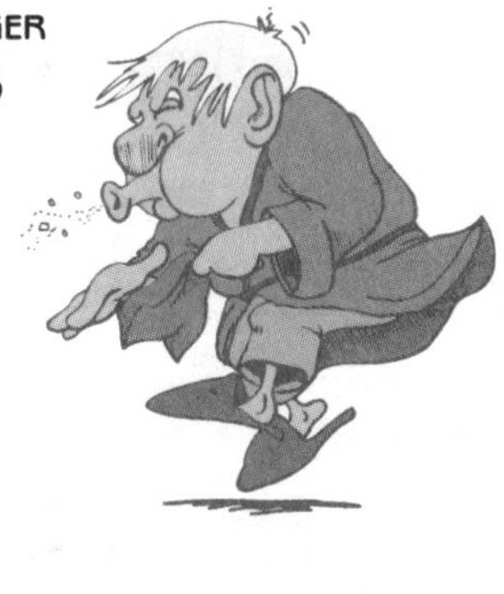

Nutrition per serving: 83 calories; 4gm protein; 13gm carbohydrate; 7gm fiber; 2gm fat; 0 choles.; 54mg calcium; 1mg iron; 12mg magnesium; 133mg potass.; 304mg sodium; Vit. C 42mg; Vit. E trace.

DEEP ENERGY MUSHROOM TONIC

This recipe works for: Immune Response, Cancer Diets, Liver and Organ Healing
For 4 drinks:

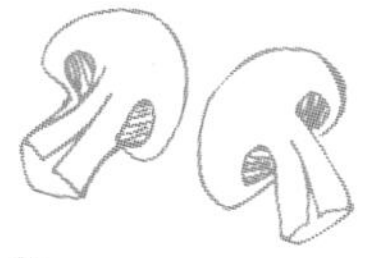

Combine 4 cups Water, 4 sticks Astragalus Bark, 1 cup soaked, slivered Shiitake Mushrooms, $^1/_2$ cup soaked Chinese Tree Mushrooms (Asian food stores) and $^1/_3$ cup Black Beans in a soup pot. Bring to boil and simmer 20 min. —Add $^1/_2$ cup Brown Rice and simmer 20 minutes more. —Add $^1/_2$ cup chopped Carrots, $^1/_2$ cup Spinach Leaves and simmer.

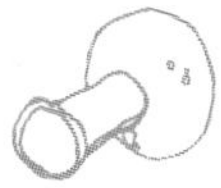

Nutrition per serving: 161 calories; 7gm protein; 32gm carbohydrate; 5gm fiber; 1gm fat; 0 choles.; 29mg calcium; 6mg iron; 65mg magnesium; 258mg potass.; 19mg sodium; Vit. C 3mg; Vit. E 1 IU.

HIGH PROTEIN SOUP

This recipe works for: Immune Response, Fatigue Syndromes, Holistic Recovery
For 2 to 3 large bowls:

Blend smooth 1 cup mixed Nuts and Seeds, 1 cup grated mixed Vegetables (summer squash, zucchini, carrots, celery, peas, etc.), 1 cup Mung or Alfalfa Sprouts, 3 TBS. Onion minced, $^1/_2$ teasp. Garlic Powder, 1 teasp. Tamari, $^1/_4$ teasp. Cayenne Pepper, and 1 to 2 cups Water to thin to desired consistency.

Nutrition per serving: 307 calories; 16gm protein; 17gm carbohydrate; 5gm fiber; 22gm fat; 0 choles.; 70mg calcium; 3mg iron; 135mg magnesium; 518mg potass.; 113mg sodium; Vit. C 9mg; Vit. E 11 IU.

CIRCULATION ENERGY TONIC Energize against aches and chills.

This recipe works for: Heart and Circulation, Bladder Problems, Recovery
For 4 drinks (2 day's supply):

Heat gently for 15 minutes: 1 cup Cranberry Juice, 1 Cinnamon Stick, 1 cup Orange Juice, 4 TBS Raisins, 2 TBS Honey, 4 TBS Almonds chopped, 4 to 6 Whole Cloves, 1 teasp. Vanilla, 4 to 6 Cardamom Pods —Remove spices. Serve hot.

POTENT MENTAL ENERGY TONIC

This recipe works for: Brain Boosting, Anti-Aging, Overcoming Addictions
For 2 drinks:

Heat gently for 15 minutes: 1 teasp. Butter, pinch Dry Mustard, 2 Whole Cloves, 1 teasp. fresh grated Ginger, 1 Cinnamon Stick, 2 Cardamom Pods, pinch Cumin Powder or 1 teasp. Cumin Seeds, 2 cups Orange Juice, pinch Cayenne. —Heat all together for 15 minutes. Remove solid spices and serve in small cups.

RESTORATION TONIC

This recipe works for: Brain Boosting, Allergy-Asthma, Overcoming Addictions

This is right out of the movies...minus the valet and the raw egg. You know, where smoke comes out of your ears after one sip. Revitalizes your brain and body if you have a hangover. Effective hot or cold. Works every time.

For 8 rejuvenating drinks:

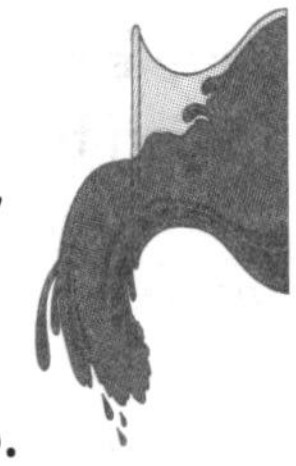

Mix in the blender: One 48-oz. can Tomato Juice or Knudsen's Spicy Very Veggie Juice, 1 cup mixed, chopped Green, Yellow, and Red Onions, 2 Ribs Celery chopped, 1 Bunch Parsley chopped, 2 TBS. chopped fresh Basil (or 2 teasp. dried), 2 teasp. Hot Pepper Sauce, 1 teasp. Rosemary Leaves, $^1/_2$ teasp. Fennel Seeds, $1^1/_2$ cups Water, 1 teasp. Tamari.

—Pour into a large pot. Bring to a boil and simmer for 30 minutes.

Nutrition per serving: 46 calories; 2gm protein; 11gm carbohydrate; 2gm fiber; trace fat; 0 choles.; 39mg calcium; 1mg iron; 25mg magnesium; 422mg potassium; 88mg sodium; Vit. C 54mg; Vit. E 1 IU.

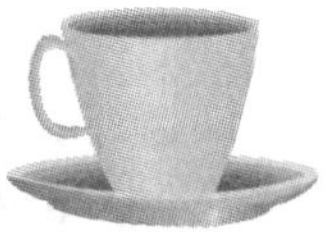

Caffeine Substitutes

<u>**Need to cut down on your caffeine**</u>? Try these unique energizers for your healing program. They have kick without caffeine.

MOCHA MOCHA COFFEE SUBSTITUTE

This recipe works for: Brain Boosting, Stress Relief, Heart-High Blood Pressure

Try 1 to 2 teasp. per cup of this caffeine-free mix. Steep and strain like a tea. You can find the ingredients in your health food store.

For about 24 cups:

Mix: 1 cup Carob Chips, 1 cup Barley Malt Powder, 1 cup Roast Chicory Granules.

—Add $^1/_2$ cup Cinnamon <u>Chips</u>, $^1/_2$ cup Allspice <u>Berries</u>, $^1/_2$ cup Licorice Root <u>Pieces</u>.

—Add $^1/_4$ cup Whole Cloves, $^1/_4$ cup Cardamom Pods and flavoring drops of Vanilla.

CHAI TEA Like a spicy latte without the caffeine. Good hot or iced.

This recipe works for: Candida Syndromes, Allergy-Asthma, Digestive Disorders

For about 2 cups:

Steep 2 rounded teaspoons of Your Favorite Tea for 10 minutes in 2 cups Hot Water. Steam 6-oz. dairy-free Soy Milk or Rice Milk til hot. Add to tea.

—Add small pinches of ground Ginger, ground Cinnamon, ground Cardamom.

—Add 2 to 3 drops Vanilla and a pinch of Fructose. Let sit 5 minutes.

HOMEMADE ROOT BEER Buy herb ingredients at a health food store.

This recipe works for: Food for Men, Liver-Organ Healing, Sugar Imbalances
Wild west boys took swigs of this when they needed some "quick draw" energy.
Use about 4 TBS for one pot:

Steep in 1 quart steaming water for 20 to 30 minutes: 3-oz. SASSAFRAS BARK pieces, 3-oz. SARSAPARILLA ROOT pieces, 3-oz. LICORICE ROOT pieces, 3-oz. FENNEL or ANISE SEED, 1-oz. roasted DANDELION ROOT, 1-oz. BURDOCK ROOT, $^{1}/_{2}$-oz. GINGER ROOT pieces, $^{1}/_{2}$-oz. CHINESE STAR ANISE, $^{1}/_{4}$-oz. LEMON PEEL pieces.

CAFFEINE FREE GINGER TEA Try to have a little ginger every day.

This recipe works for: Brain Boosting, Fatigue Syndromes, Stress Relief
For 1 pot:

Steep in 1-qt. steaming water for 15 minutes: 1 handful PEPPERMINT LEAF, 1 handful ROSE HIPS, 1 TB fresh sliced GINGER ROOT, 1 TB ORANGE PEEL, 2 tsp. ROSEMARY LEAVES.

HOT JULEPS A good afternoon pick-me-up. Good hot or iced.

The recipe works for: Stress Reactions, Digestive Disorders, Colon-Bowel Health
For about 2 drinks:

Steep together in 2 cups HOT WATER for 10 minutes: 3 PEPPERMINT TEA BAGS (or 2 cups strong peppermint tea), juice of 2 ORANGES, 2 tsp. HONEY, 2 pinches STEVIA LEAF.

Herb Teas for Your Healing Program

Blending your own therapy teas can be a rewarding experience for your health. This section has some basic complementary herbs to get you started, and examples of traditional blends valuable for a healing diet. (See CLEANSING & PURIFYING FOODS, page 45 for brewing instructions.)

<u>Mints are tiny miracles for healing</u>. They help digestion; they purify; they fight harmful bacteria; they soothe and relax. See the COOKING FOR HEALTHY HEALING DIET BOOK, THE FOOD PHARMACY DIGEST, page 518 for info on each mint. *Peppermint, Spearmint, Wintergreen* and *Lemon Balm* are delicious by themselves and boost the activity of other herbs.

Lemon-y herbs are purifiers. They normalize body pH; they cleanse and neutralize toxins; they're full of vitamin C; they stimulate the liver. *Lemon Grass, Lemon Peel and Orange Peel* blend well with other herbs.

Berries are balancers and toners. They stimulate circulation; they're full of vitamin C and bioflavonoids; they balance pH. Berries have high amounts of vitamin C. *Hawthorn Berries, Juniper Berries and Rose Hips* add a tangy taste.

Sea greens teas are like hot broths. They provide a wealth of minerals and weight loss benefits. *Dulse, Wakame, Sea Palm amd Kombu* are some of my favorites.

Blossoms are soothing healers. They relax stress; they sooth eruptions and rashes; they neutralize acidity; they gently purify. *Red Clover, Calendula (Marigold), Yarrow and Chamomile* often taste as good as they look.

Roots and barks add substance. They provide foundation nutrients like minerals; they boost immune response; they're good for your glands. *Cinnamon, Licorice Rt., Wild Cherry Bark and Ginger Root add spice to a tea.*

Leafy herbs add lift. They're full of antioxidants; they stimulate and protect; they are tonics. *Green tea, Stevia leaf, Rosemary and Raspberry* add oomph to your blend.

Cooking with tea is exploding in the gourmet world. Teas can add exotic, different flavors to a recipe, and I think it's a wonderful way to incorporate herbal benefits into your meals.

Even though it's a hot new cuisine, you need to be careful when using medicinal tea to target therapy needs. Cooking herbs neutralizes many of their subtle medicinal functions. It certainly kills the plant enzymes. Sometimes it's okay in the case of roots and barks, but it's the reason I'm so careful to pour boiling water over herbs and steep them rather than boil them when I'm making a medicinal tea.

A couple of ways I've successfully used this technique.... Let's add tea to rice as an example. It's a tasty and very effective method of using tea for medicinal benefits. I cook the rice with slightly less water as needed, then add about half a cup of tea to 2 or 3 cups of hot rice and let it steam in.

Adding herbs to your veggie steamer for the final 5 minutes of cooking is a delicious way to get their healing volatile oils into your steamed vegetables.

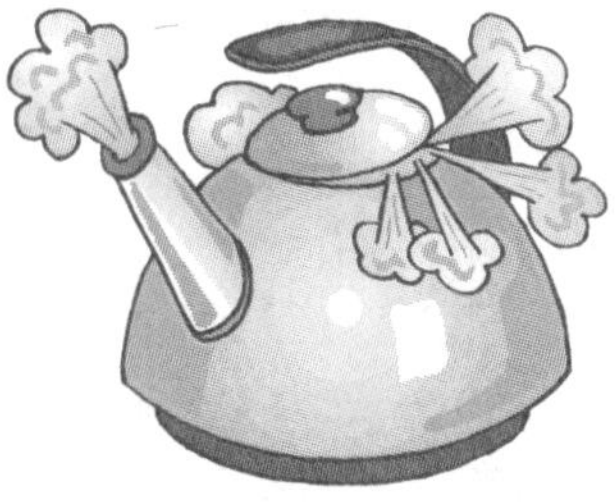

Check out the simple medicinal blends on the next few pages to make for your healing program.
Use one small packed tea ball for 4 cups of tea.

RELAXING TEA for STRESS and HEADACHE

This recipe works for: Stress Reactions, Digestive Disorders, Insomnia
Enough for 4 cups:

1 teasp. Rosemary, 1 teasp. Spearmint, 1/2 teasp. Catnip, 1/2 teasp. Chamomile Flowers.

DIURETIC TEA for GENTLE BLADDER FLUSHING

This recipe works for: Bladder - Kidney Disorders, Prostate Health
Enough for 4 cups:

1 teasp. Uva Ursi, 1 teasp. Juniper Berries, 1/2 teasp. Ginger, 1/2 teasp. Parsley Leaf.

AFTER DINNER MINT TEA for GOOD DIGESTION

This recipe works for: Liver Health, Digestive Disorders, Insomnia
Enough for 4 cups:

1 teasp. Peppermint, 1 teasp. Hibiscus, 1/2 teasp. Papaya Leaf, 1/2 teasp. Rosemary.

ENERGY TEA for FATIGUE

This recipe works for: Stress Reactions, Digestive Disorders, Insomnia
Enough for 4 cups:

1 teasp. Gotu Kola, 1 teasp. Peppermint, 1 teasp. Red Clover, 1/2 teasp. Cloves.

CARDAMOM ICED TEA for LIVER HEALTH

This recipe works for: Digestive, Colon - Bowel Disorders, Liver - Organ Health
Enough for 1 pitcher:

Add 18 Darjeeling Tea Bags and 18 Cardamom Pods to 6 cups Lukewarm Water in a pitcher. Let sit for 12 hours.
—Strain; add 6 TBS Honey, or 3 TBS Fructose, and 6 TBS Lemon Juice.
—Pour into glasses of crushed ice. Top with 6 Sprigs Fresh Mint.

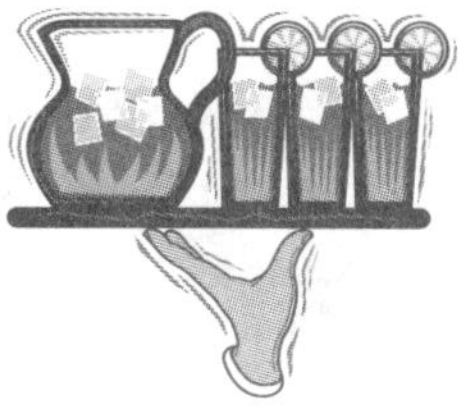

Note: Make herbal iced tea right. Add 2 extra teaspoons of loose tea (or 2 more tea bags) to the pot for iced tea to stand up to the watering effect of the ice. Let the tea steep about 10 minutes longer than for hot tea. Pour over ice in chilled glasses.

Smoothies, Frosts and Slushes

There is nothing like fresh, frosty fruit for rich refreshment. Smoothies have been popular ever since the juice bars of the California sixties. Blender blended, these drinks taste decadently sinful, but are a wonderful way to get your fresh fruit for the day while satisfying sugar cravings. Frosts and slushes are partially frozen drinks that really taste like dessert. The key to perfect taste as well as convenience is keeping cut-up fruits, especially the bananas, **in the freezer** - so you can pop them in the blender any time. (You can add 4 or 5 ice cubes during blending instead of freezing the bananas, but it won't taste quite as rich).

SIX FRUIT SMOOTHIE

This recipe works for: Brain Boosting, Allergy-Asthma
For 6 drinks:

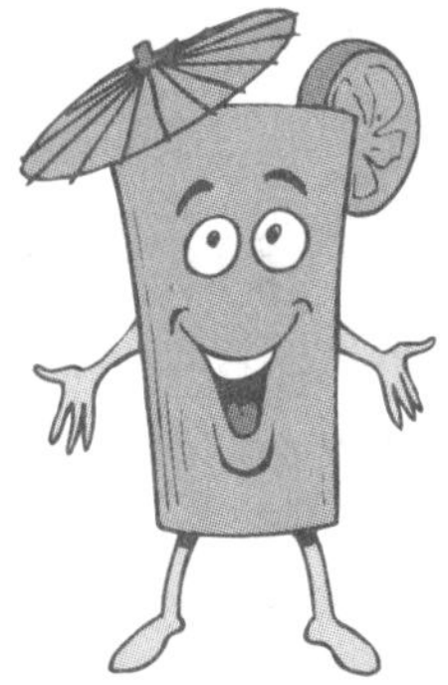

Blend til smooth: 4 Frozen Bananas chunked, 1/2 Fresh Pineapple chunked, 1/2 pint Strawberries, 2 cups Orange Juice, 3 TBS Maple Syrup, 1 TB Cranberry Juice Concentrate, 1 TB Lemon Juice, 10 Ice Cubes and enough cold water to blend smooth.

CRAN-APPLE FROST

This recipe works for: Bladder Disorders, Fatigue Syndromes, Allergies-Asthma
For 3 tall drinks:

Blend til smooth: 2 cups Cranberry Juice, 2 cups Apple Juice, 2 small Frozen Bananas in chunks, 2 TBS Honey, 1/4 cup Rice Dream or Vanilla Soymilk, 1 TB Lemon Juice and 4 Ice Cubes. Top with Nutmeg sprinkles.

Nutrition per serving: 289 calories; 2gm protein; 71gm carbohydrate; 2gm fiber; 1g fat; 0 choles.; 129mg calcium; 2mg iron; 23mg magnesium; 688mg potassium; 40mg sodium; Vit. C 596mg; Vit. E trace.

FRESH BERRY SLUSH

This recipe works for: Circulatory Disorders, Healthy Pregnancy, Female Balance
For 4 tall drinks:

Blend til smooth: 1/2 pint basket Raspberries, 1/2 pint Strawberries (or other favorite berries), 2 cups mixed Berry Juice or Orange Juice, and 4 TBS Honey. Drop in 10 Ice Cubes and blend til frosty. Sprinkle on Cinnamon.

TAHITI SWEETIE

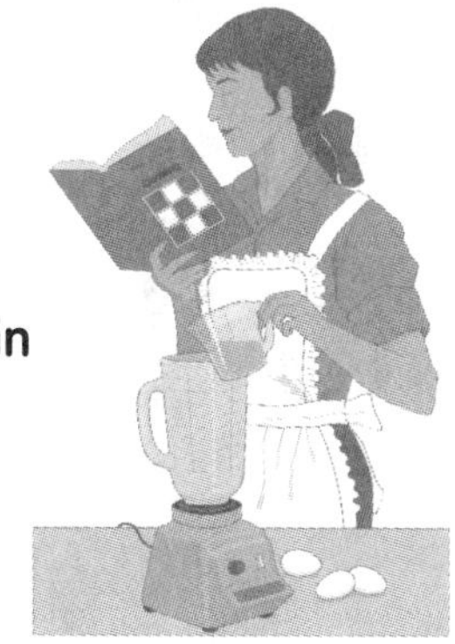

This recipe works for: Illness Recovery, Digestive Disorders
For 2 drinks:

Blend til smooth: 1/2 cup fresh Pineapple Chunks, 1 Frozen Banana in chunks, 1/2 Papaya chunked, 2 cups Vanilla Soymilk or Rice Milk.
—Add a few drops Vanilla or Coconut Extract or Almond Extract.
—Top with 1/4 cup Toasted Coconut Shreds.

Nutrition per serving: 247 calories; 8gm protein; 46gm carbohydrate; 4gm fiber; 4gm fat; 0 cholesterol; 426mg calcium; 4mg iron; 33mg magnesium; 528mg potassium; 3mg sodium; Vit. C 58mg; Vit. E 1 IU.

APRICOT ORANGE CREAM

This recipe works for: Arthritis, Cancer Healing, Digestive Help, Hypoglycemia
For 1 large drink:

Blend smooth: 4 fresh Apricots halved, 1 Orange, peeled and sectioned, 1 Frozen Banana chunked, 1 TB chopped Almonds, 1 TB Shredded Coconut, extra Orange Juice.

GINGER-MANGO FROST

This recipe works for: Circulation Disorders, Digestive Disorders, Weight Loss
For 2 drinks:

Blend smooth: 1 ripe Mango, peeled, chunked, 1 cup crushed Ice, 1/2 cup Low-Fat Vanilla, or Piña Colada Yogurt, 1/2 cup Pineapple Juice, 1 tsp. minced Crystallized Ginger.

Nutrition per serving: 148 calories; 4gm protein; 35gm carbohydrate; 3gm fiber; 1gm fat; 0 cholesterol; 126mg calcium; 1mg iron; 27mg magnesium; 384mg potassium; 43mg sodium; Vit. C 36mg; Vit. E 1 IU.

ELIOTT'S HEALING GREEN SMOOTHIE

This recipe works for: Sports Nutrition, Weight Control, Liver - Organ Health
For 2 drinks:

Blend til smooth: 1 cup Cranberry Juice, 1 cup Apple Juice, 2 TBS Aloe Vera Juice Concentrate, 1 tsp. each Green Kamut Powder, Green Magma Powder, Beta Carrot Powder 1 tsp. Royal Jelly, 1 Banana, 1 Apple, and 1 Orange. Add water if necessary.

Nutrition per serving: 262 calories; 3gm protein; 63gm carbohydrate; 5gm fiber; 1gm fat; 0 cholesterol; 83mg calcium; 2mg iron; 33mg magnesium; 748mg potass.; 30mg sodium; Vit. C 481mg; Vit. E 1 IU.

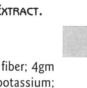

Stress Easing Coolers

Healthy coolers are wonderful on a hot day or after exertion to keep you hydrated and energized. Each of the following recipes makes a BIG PITCHER to keep in the fridge.

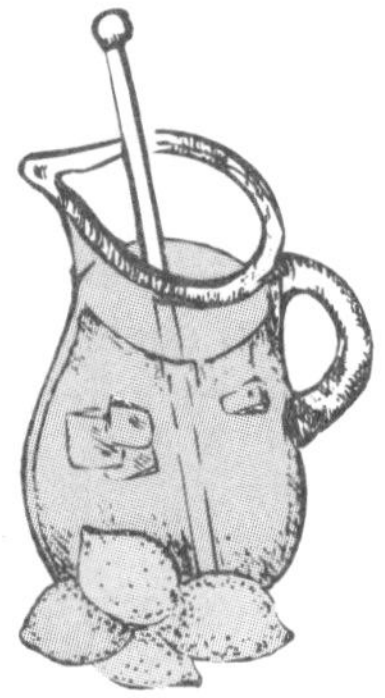

STRAWBERRY APPLE LEMONADE

This recipe works for: Stress Reactions, Weight Control, Hair, Skin

Pour into a large pitcher: $1^1/_2$ quarts organic APPLE JUICE, $1^1/_2$ cups LEMON JUICE, 1 cup sliced STRAWBERRIES. Chill and pour over ice.

EASY HAWAIIAN PUNCH

This recipe works for: Stress Reactions, Weight Control, Hair, Skin and Nails

Pour into a large pitcher: $1^1/_2$ cups PINEAPPLE-COCONUT JUICE, 1 cup PAPAYA JUICE, $^1/_4$ cup ORANGE JUICE, 2 TBS LIME JUICE.

KIWI-LIME SPARKLE

This recipe works for: Digestive Health, Circulation DIsorders, Liver-Organ Health

Pour in a pitcher: 4 cups peeled KIWI chunks, 4 TBS fresh LIME JUICE and the slivered peel of 1 LIME, 3 TBS minced CRYSTALLIZED GINGER. Fill pitcher with SPARKLING WATER.

HIBISCUS ICED TEA

This recipe works for: Respiratory Infections, Weight Control, Anti-Aging

Add 24 bags (1 box) HIBISCUS TEA to 8 cups WATER and let sit for 5-6 hours in a sunny spot until quite dark red. Remove tea bags.
—Add $^1/_2$ cup HONEY, $^1/_4$ cup LIME JUICE and 1 LIME sliced in circles.
—Serve over Ice.

MELONS and MINTS ICED RELAXER

This recipe works for: Bladder Infections, Weight Control, Anti-Aging, Skin, Hair

Blender blend: 1 cup CANTALOUPE chunks, 2 cups HONEYDEW MELON chunks, 2 cups WATERMELON chunks, $^1/_4$ cup LEMON JUICE, $^1/_2$ cup chopped FRESH MINT (reserve sprigs for garnish), 2 cups SPARKLING WATER.

Herbs and wines make beautiful music together! For a different gourmet drink, try your next wine cooler with herbs and spices.

LEMON MINT SANGRIA

This recipe works for: Stress Reactions, Weight Control, Circulatory Health
For 4 servings:

Combine in a pitcher: 1 bottle Dry White Wine, $^{1}/_{2}$ cup White Grape Juice, 1 10-oz. bottle Sparkling Water, 3 TBS Sherry, 4 Sprigs Fresh Mint or 3 Spearmint Tea Bags, peel of 1 Lemon in slivers and 2 TBS Lemon Grass.
—Let steep 4 hours. Top serve, remove lemon peel, lemon grass and tea bags.
—Float Kiwi rounds and Mint Sprigs on top.

Nutrition per serving: 164 calories; 1gm protein; 8gm carbohydrate; 1gm fiber; 0 fat; 0 choles.; 92mg calcium; 8mg iron; 19mg magnesium; 148mg potass.; 23mg sodium; Vit. C 53mg; Vit. E 1 IU.

HIBISCUS WINE COOLER

This recipe works for: Sports Nutrition, Weight Control, Liver - Organ Health
For 1 pitcher:

Place 10 to 12 Hibiscus Tea Bags in a large pitcher. Pour over $1^{1}/_{2}$ cups steaming hot water. Let steep 5 minutes. Remove bags and let cool.
—Add 1 bottle Blush Wine, 2 cups Apple Juice, or Sparkling Grape Juice to fill pitcher.
—Add 12 ice cubes. Float Grape Halves or Lemon Slices on top.

Nutritive Meal Replacement Drinks

Meal replacement drinks are popular with dieters and sports enthusiasts. High quality, nutrient dense protein powders, they have large amounts of added vitamins, minerals and electrolytes. For **weight loss**, meal replacement drinks reduce calorie and food quantity while keeping nutrition balanced and adequate. For **athletes**, especially those on training diets with three or more meals a day, meal replacement drinks boost calorie, protein and amino acid intake without accompanying fats.

Making your own meal replacement drinks addresses your specific diet needs. Check out the foods and food supplements in the *Digest* sections of the COOKING FOR HEALTHY HEALING DIET BOOK. Decide on the foods and nutrients you want. Put them in the blender or a soup pot for a customized, quick, liquid meal. Use the five examples here for inspiration.

NON-DAIRY PROTEIN MEAL REPLACEMENT

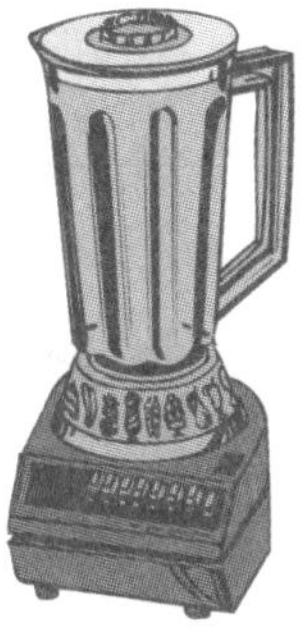

This recipe works for: Illness Recovery, Hypoglycemia
For 2 large drinks:

Blender blend: 1 cup sliced Strawberries, 1 sliced Banana, 1 cup Papaya chunks, 1 cup Pineapple-Coconut Juice, 8-oz. Vanilla Soy Milk or Rice Milk, 2 TBS Sweet Cloud Syrup or Barley Malt, 2 TBS toasted Wheat Germ.

ATHLETE'S HEAVY DUTY PROTEIN DRINK

This recipe works for: Sports Nutrition, Weight Control, Food for Men
For 2 drinks:

Blend in the blender: 1 cup Water, 1 cup Yogurt any flavor, 1 cup Vanilla Rice Dream or Vanilla Soymilk, 1 Banana, sliced, 1 Egg, 2 TBS Nutritional Yeast, 1 TB Toasted Wheat Germ, 2 TBS Peanut Butter, 2 teasp. Bee Pollen Granules, 2 teasp. Spirulina, or Green Superfood Powder of your choice.

Nutrition per serving: 404 calories; 21gm protein; 58gm carbohydrate; 5gm fiber; 12g fat; 0 choles.; 430mg calcium; 5mg iron; 95mg magnesium; 818mg potass.; 208mg sodium; Vit. C 6mg; Vit. E 5 IU.

MORNING and EVENING FIBER DRINK

This recipe works for: Sports Nutrition, Weight Control, Liver - Organ Health

For daily regularity; use as needed with confidence in its efficiency, without concern about dependency. Take 1 tablespoon in 8-oz apple juice, morning and bedtime.

Blend dry in the blender: 4-oz. Oat Bran or Rice Bran, 1-oz. Acidophilus Powder, 2-oz. Flax Seed, $^1/_2$-oz. Fennel Seed, $^1/_2$-oz. Apple Pectin Powder, 1-oz. Psyllium Husk Powder.

Nutrition per serving: 49 calories; 3gm protein; 10gm carbohydrate; 4gm fiber; 2g fat; 0 choles.; 75mg calcium; 2mg iron; 46mg magnesium; 161mg potass.; 13mg sodium; Vit. C .3mg; Vit. E trace.

HIGH PROTEIN and EFA'S COCONUT MILK DRINK

This recipe works for: Sports Nutrition, Childhood Energy, Fatigue Syndromes
For 3 drinks:

Blend in the blender: 2 cups chopped fresh Pineapple, 1 15-oz. can Unsweetened Coconut Milk, 1 Banana, $^1/_2$ cup Orange Juice together and pour over ice.

Nutrition per serving: 381 calories; 4gm protein; 30gm carbohydrate; 4gm fiber; 30g fat; 0 choles.; 40mg calcium; 5mg iron; 95mg magnesium; 661mg potass.; 20mg sodium; Vit. C 43mg; Vit. E 1 IU.

DIETER'S MID-DAY MEAL REPLACEMENT DRINK

This recipe works for: Sports Nutrition, Weight Control, Immune Power

This drink is good-tasting and satisfying. It is full of foods that help raise metabolism, cleanse and flush out wastes, balance body pH, and stimulate enzyme production. Blend a dry batch in the blender. Use 1 tablespoon per glass. Drink slowly.

Makes enough for 10 drinks:

Blender blend: 6 TBS Rice Protein Powder, 4 TBS Oat Bran, 2 TBS Bee Pollen Granules, 2 TBS Flax Seed, 2 teasp. Spirulina Powder or Green Superfood Blend of your choice, 2 teasp. Fructose, 1 teasp. Acidophilus Powder, $^1/_2$ teasp. Lemon Peel Powder, $^1/_2$ teasp. Ginger Powder.

Nutrition per serving: 46 calories; 4gm protein; 6gm carbohydrate; 1gm fiber; 1g fat; 0 choles.; 48mg calcium; 3mg iron; 15mg magnesium; 68mg potass.; 47mg sodium; Vit. C trace; Vit. E trace.

SWEET, LOW-FAT PROTEIN DRINK

Also rich in vitamin C, potassium and antioxidants.

Enough for 2 large drinks:

Blender blend: 1 cup Vanilla Soymilk or Rice Dream, 2 Bananas, 3 ripe Kiwis, 1 cup Pineapple-Coconut Juice, 1 cup Seedless Grapes, 2 TBS Honey.

Nutrition per serving: 471 calories; 8gm protein; 99gm carbohydrate; 6gm fiber; 8g fat; 0 choles.; 267mg calcium; 4mg iron; 96mg magnesium; 1202mg potass.; 27mg sodium; Vit. C 143mg; Vit. E 3 IU.

Tips to make high nutrient drinks count:

—If you want it cold and refreshing, use frozen fruit and frozen fruit juice concentrates instead of ice. Using fruit juice concentrates means you won't need honey or other sweeteners. My favorite is apple juice concentrate.

—Use yogurt instead of milk for tang (and friendly flora).

—For a velvety texture, add your chosen protein or superfood powders last, then blend just until they disappear. Over-blending can make your drink too thick to drink. A vial of liquid ginseng, an ounce of wheatgrass juice or a teaspoon of green food powder really rev up nutrient value and add intriguing flavors.

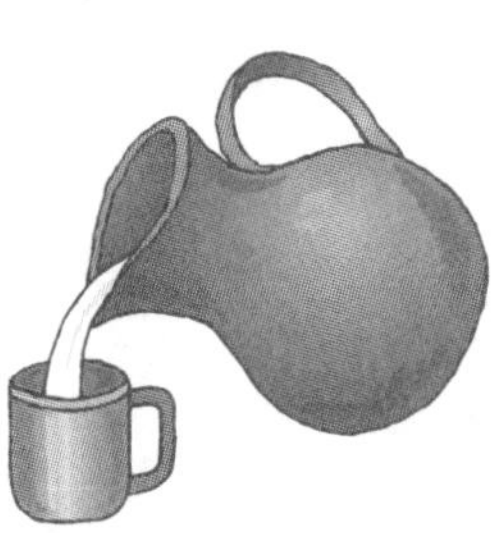

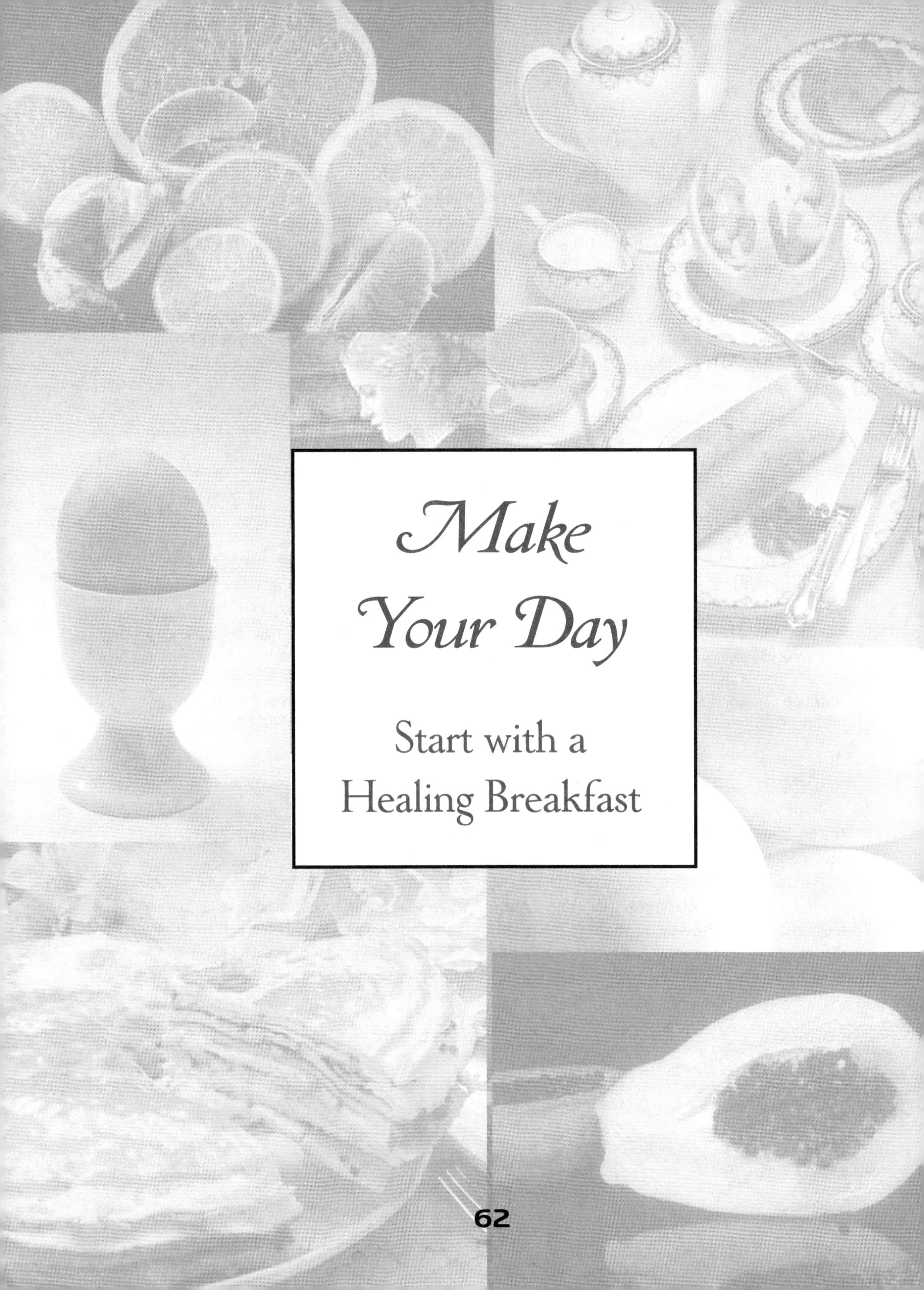

Make Your Day

Start with a Healing Breakfast

Rise and Shine!

Healing Foods For Breakfast and Brunch

Most of us realize that breakfast is important for our day's health. But morning nutrients are more than just early fuel. They are a key factor in a healing diet. Foods taken on rising, at breakfast and mid-morning, lay the foundation for daily body chemistry balance. Ideally, your body needs to get about one third of its daily nutrients in the morning. Healing progress can be noticeably accelerated through conscious attention to the nutrients you eat before noon. Today we can target breakfast for our healing needs.

Breakfast at its best is comforting, energizing food after your body's night of fasting and cleansing. But a good breakfast takes some thought. A heavy, high fat meal leads to a sluggish day; a sugar-filled breakfast leads to jitters, then a mid-morning slump; a caffeine breakfast leads to nervousness and hyperactivity.

If you don't eat breakfast at all, your body won't have the fuel it needs for good mental and physical performance.... and both will suffer. Breakfast may be even more important for kids than it is for adults. New studies show that a solid, low-glycemic meal in the morning can positively affect hyperactivity and bad behavior in children during the day.

Morning foods are linked with our earliest awareness of good nutrition - whole grain granolas, brans, fruits, nut butters, yogurt, protein drinks and breakfast teas. As new research reveals even more about the value of these foods, we're adding other healthy food categories to "breakfast," like whole grain sandwiches, pitas and chapatis, brown rice or cous-cous with spices, vegetables and sea greens, soy foods, sweet tahini and low-fat hummus. Eggs, yogurt and kefir all sustain mental energy throughout the day. Nuts, like almonds and cashews; seeds, like flax and sesame; sprouts, like alfalfa, sunflower and clover for breakfast add anti-cancerous, immune boosting properties. They help convert beta carotene into vitamin A, and compliment vitamin D and calcium.

Here's what a healing breakfast can do for you:

—You'll stimulate and establish your body's chemistry for the next 24 hour period - especially important for immune response.

—You'll fuel your liver function to better metabolize fats and to form healthy red blood cells.

—New tests show that people who eat breakfast have generally lower cholesterol levels than people who don't.

—You'll establish broad spectrum enzyme production through the pancreas for better tolerance of food sensitivities and to increase your assimilation of nutrients.

—A good breakfast goes to your head. Your brain and memory functions make maximum use of food fuel in the morning.

—If you have hypoglycemia, a good solid breakfast is almost a must. The body's glycogen supply can be maximized in the morning hours for better sugar tolerance and energy use.

—Breakfast is your day's best opportunity to get high fiber foods like whole grains and fruits, for regularity and body balance.

—Your metabolism is at its highest in the morning to help you burn calories faster. Low-fat, high energy breakfast foods help keep you away from junk foods and unconscious nibbling all day.

Breakfast and Brunch Recipe Sections

Morning Drinks

You must have protein to heal. The new breed of protein drinks are a great way to get protein without meat or dairy, bulk or excess fat, yet they offer a real energy boost.

NON-DAIRY MORNING PROTEIN DRINK

This recipe works for: Allergies, Food for Men, Recovery, Respiratory Infections
For 2 drinks:

Blender blend until mixed: 1 cup Strawberries or Kiwi chunks, 1 Banana sliced, 1 cup Apple Juice, 1 cup fresh Papaya or Pineapple chunked, 8-oz. Rice Dream or Vanilla Soymilk, or Vanilla Yogurt, 1 TB Bee Pollen Granules, 2 pinches Ginger Powder.

Nutrition per serving; 153 calories; 4gm protein; 32gm carbo.; 3gm fiber; 2gm fats; 0 cholesterol; 27mg calcium; 2mg iron; 46mg magnesium; 515mg potassium; 20mg sodium; Vit. C 44mg; Vit. E 1 IU.

MORNING ORANGE SHAKE

This recipe works for: Immune Power, Cancer Control, Fatigue Syndromes
For 2 drinks:

Blender blend: 2 Oranges peeled and sectioned, 2 TBS Vanilla Yogurt, 1 Frozen Banana chunked, 1 teasp. Vanilla, $^1/_4$ cup Orange Juice, 1 TB Toasted Wheat Germ.

Nutrition per serving; 160 calories; 5gm protein; 36gm carbo.; 4gm fiber; 1gm fats; 0 cholesterol; 88mg calcium; 1mg iron; 47mg magnesium; 593mg potassium; 11mg sodium; Vit. C 91mg; Vit. E 1 IU.

HAWAIIAN MORNING SMOOTHIE

This recipe works for: Digestive Disorders, Female Balance, Heart Health
For 4 drinks:

Blender blend: 1 small can Papaya Nectar, 1 cup Vanilla Rice Milk or Soy Milk, 1 cup Orange Juice, 2 Frozen Bananas, 2 pinches Ginger Powder, 1 tsp. Spirulina Powder.

BETA-CAROTENE SHAKE

This recipe works for: Cancer Control, Immune Breakdown Diseases
For 2 drinks:

Blender blend: 10-12 Fresh Apricots pitted, $^1/_2$ large, peeled, seeded Papaya, 4 Ice Cubes, 10-12 Fresh Mint Leaves, 1 tsp. Spirulina Powder.

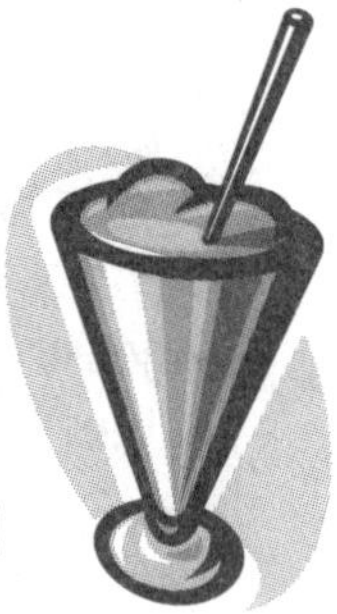

HONEY-ALMOND PROTEIN DRINK

This recipe works for: Food for Men, Anti-Aging, Stress - Exhaustion Syndromes
For 2 drinks:

Blender blend: $^1/_2$ cup Almonds, $^1/_3$ cup Honey, 1 cup Apple Juice, 2 drops Almond Extract, $^1/_4$ teasp. Vanilla Extract, 1 TB Toasted Wheat Germ, 1 tsp. Spirulina Powder.

Nutrition per serving; 442 calories; 9gm protein; 70gm carbo.; 4g fiber; 16gm fats; 0 cholesterol; 106mg calcium; 3mg iron; 117mg magnesium; 482mg potassium; 35mg sodium; Vit. C 3mg; Vit. E 13 IU.

PRE-MORNING WORKOUT SMOOTHIE

This recipe works for: Cancer Control, Immune Disease, Sports Nutrition
For 2 large drinks:

Blender blend: 1 Frozen Banana, 2 cups Apple Cider, 1 cup Fresh Fruit (I like pineapple or berries), $^1/_4$ cup Peanut Butter or $^1/_2$ cup Almonds, 1 TB Bee Pollen Granules, 1 TB toasted Wheat Germ, 1 tsp. Spirulina Powder or a favorite Green Superfood Powder.

Nutrition per serving; 458 calories; 12gm protein; 64gm carbo.; 7g fiber; 20gm fats; 0 cholesterol; 126mg calcium; 4mg iron; 155mg magnesium; 955mg potassium; 48mg sodium; Vit. C 21mg; Vit. E 5 IU.

WINTER MORNING WARM-UP *while you stretch out.*

This recipe works for: Food for Men, Arthritis, Sports Nutrition
For 2 large drinks:

Blender blend: 1 Frozen Banana, 2 cups Apple Cider, 1 cup Fresh Fruit (I like pineapple or berries), $^1/_4$ cup Peanut Butter or $^1/_2$ cup Almonds, 2 pinches Cinnamon, 1 tsp. Spirulina Powder or your favorite Green Superfood Powder.

Healing Teas in the Morning

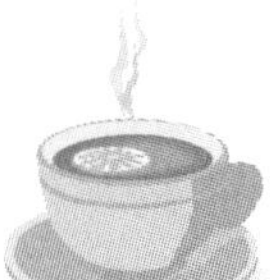

Black, green or herbal teas in the morning can satisfy the need for a little lift at the beginning of the day - with little or no caffeine. My favorite morning black teas are Darjeeling, English Breakfast and Earl Grey (available caffeine-free). Green tea is a proven body cleanser. Taken in the morning, it stimulates better digestion and liver health all day. (See **About Black and Green Teas** in the DIET BOOK page 68.)

Good herbal teas to drink in the morning include red raspberry for body balance, gotu kola for mental energy, and ginseng teas for vitality.

FRESH LEMON MINT TEA a caffeine-free wake-up call.

This recipe works for: Liver and Organ Health, Immune Power, Digestive Disorders
For 4 cups:

Combine: 1 handful chopped fresh Mint Leaves, half a handful of chopped fresh Lemon Mint Leaves or fresh Lemon Grass, and 1/3 cup peeled, chopped Fresh Ginger in a large teapot. Cover with 4 cups Boiling Water.
—Steep 20 minutes. Add 6 TBS Fresh Lemon Juice and 6 TBS Maple Syrup or Honey.

Nutrition per serving: 95 calories; 2gm protein; 24gm carbo.; 1g fiber; 0g fats; 0 cholesterol; 46mg calcium; 1mg iron; 16mg magnesium; 205mg potassium; 12mg sodium; Vit. C 33mg; Vit. E 1 IU.

HOT APPLE and SPICE TEA

This recipe works for: Digestive Disorders, Liver Health
For 4 cups:

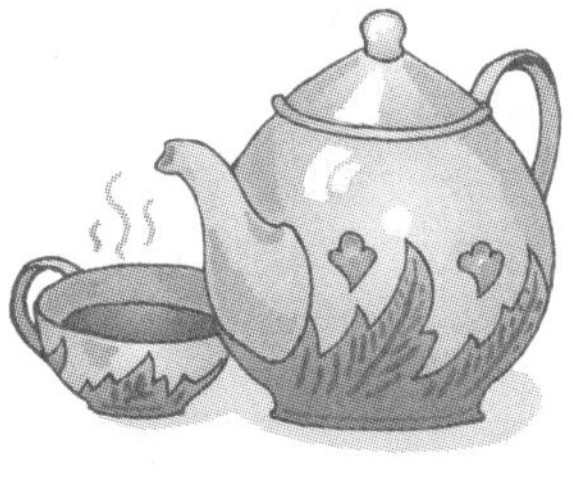

Simmer in a large pan for 10 minutes: 4 cups Apple Cider, 1 Cinnamon Stick, 10 Whole Cloves, 3 slices Crystallized Ginger, and 6 Cardamom Pods. Strain out solids.

GREEN TEA CLEANSER good hot or cold; full of antioxidants, Vitamin C

This recipe works for: Liver and Organ Health, Immune Power, Digestive Disorders
Make cinnamon honey - drop a cinnamon stick in a jar of honey and leave it.
For 4 cups:

Steep together in a large teapot for 15 minutes: 4 cups Water, 1 handful loose Green Tea, or 5 to 6 Green Tea bags, 1 TB Burdock Root Pieces, 3 slices Crystallized Ginger, 1 TB Gotu Kola Herb, 1 TB Hawthorn Berries, and 1 TB Orange Peel. Strain out solids. Add 1 TB cinnamon-steeped Honey if desired.

MORNING IMMUNI-TEA

This recipe works for: Respiratory Infections, Immune Power, Liver - Organ Health
For 4 cups:

Steep in a large teapot for 20 minutes: 4 cups Water, 3 slices peeled fresh Ginger Root, 2 TBS dried Sage Leaves, or half a handful Fresh Sage Leaves. Strain. Pour into cups. Add 15 drops Echinacea Root Extract and 15 drops Milk Thistle Seed Extract.

Nutrition per serving; 10 calories; 0gm protein; 1gm carbo.; 1g fiber; 0gm fats; 0 cholesterol; 46mg calcium; 0mg iron; 13mg magnesium; 35mg potassium; 1mg sodium; Vit. C 2mg; Vit. E trace.

Start Your Day with Fruit

As you plan your day's nutrition, think of fruits as rich in skin vitamins like vitamin-A, vitamin K, vitamin C and bioflavonoids, full of enzymes for digestion and cleansing, and rich antioxidant sources to fight the free radical assault you're going to face today. (In a normal day, our bodies take over 10,000 free-radical hits.) Fruits provide plenty of minerals you'll need, too, like potassium, magnesium and calcium. (See *About Fruits*, in the Cooking for Healthy Healing Diet Book, page 20-21 for more info.)

HIGH PROTEIN FRUIT BREAKFAST MIX

This recipe works for: Respiratory Infections, Immune Power, Liver - Organ Health
Each mix makes enough for two.

For enzymes and skin tone: mix together $^{1}/_{2}$ cup <u>each</u>: Fresh Chopped Papaya and Fresh Chopped Strawberries.
—Add $^{1}/_{4}$ cup <u>each</u>: Toasted Sliced Almonds, Toasted Sesame Seeds, chopped Prunes, and chopped Dried Papaya or Pineapple. Mix in $^{1}/_{4}$ cup Vanilla Yogurt.

OR

For regularity and minerals: mix together $^{1}/_{2}$ cup <u>each</u>: Fresh Sliced Grapes and fresh sliced Pineapple.
—Add $^{1}/_{4}$ cup <u>each</u>: Toasted Chopped Walnuts, Toasted Sunflower Seeds, chopped Dried Prunes and Raisins. Mix in $^{1}/_{4}$ cup Vanilla Yogurt.

Mix the high nutrient topping in a small bowl and pour over either fruit mix.
2 TBS Toasted Wheat Germ, 2 TBS chopped Crystallized Ginger, 2 teasp. Honey, 2 teasp. Lecithin Granules, 2 teasp. Lemon Juice, 2 teasp. Nutritional Yeast Flakes

Nutrition per serving; 466calories; 14gm protein; 63gm carbo.; 9gm fiber; 21gm fats; 1 cholesterol; 178mg calcium; 4mg iron; 156mg magnesium; 744mg potassium; 41mg sodium; Vit. C 52mg; Vit. E 9 IU.

SMOOTH PRUNES

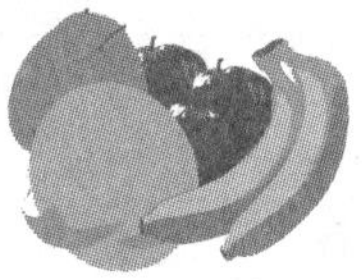

This recipe works for: Colon - Bowel and Digestive Health
For 4 bowls:

Soak 2 cups Pitted Prunes in water in the fridge until soft, or overnight.
—Blender blend with 1 pint Plain or Vanilla Yogurt, 1 TB Honey, and $^{1}/_{2}$ tsp. Vanilla.
—Whirl until smooth, and mound in small open bowls. Sprinkle with Nutmeg.

Nutrition per serving; 208 calories; 8gm protein; 42gm carbo.; 7g fiber; 2gm fats; 7 cholesterol; 249mg calcium; 1mg iron; 43mg magnesium; 643mg potassium; 88mg sodium; Vit. C 4mg; Vit. E 1 IU.

GINGER GRAPEFRUIT with TOASTY MERINGUE TOP

This recipe works for: Arthritis, Weight Loss, Female Balance
Topping for 4 grapefruit halves:

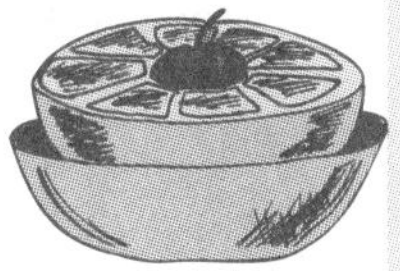

Whip 2 Egg Whites to soft peaks. Add 1/4 cup Thin Honey and 1/4 teasp. Powdered Ginger and whip to meringue consistency.
—Spread meringue on grapefruit halves, and bake at 300° for 15 to 20 minutes.

Nutrition per serving; 109 calories; 2gm protein; 27gm carbo.; 2g fiber; 0g fats; 0 cholesterol; 16mg calcium; 0mg iron; 12mg magnesium; 195mg potassium; 24mg sodium; Vit. C 47mg; Vit. E trace.

MORNING LUNG TONIC PEARS for chest congestion seasons.

This recipe works for: Respiratory Infections, Liver - Organ Health, Digestive Health
For 2 servings:

Core and slice 2 Hard Winter Pears.
—Drizzle each pear with 2 teasp. Honey, and sprinkle with 1/2 teasp. Ground Cardamom. Bake or broil until brown and caramelized.

YOGURT CHEESE TOPPING for FRUIT or GRANOLA

Great on fresh fruits, granola or hot cereal, toast or bagels.

Make fresh yogurt cheese the night before. Simply spoon a pint or more of Plain Yogurt onto a large cheesecloth square. Tie up the ends of the square and loop over your kitchen sink faucet to drain into the sink overnight. Store airtight in the fridge.

Mix together in a small bowl: 1/2 cup Yogurt Cheese, 1 TB Light Honey, 1 TB Lemon Juice, grated Zest of 1 Fresh Lemon.

Nutrition per serving; 187 calories; 7gm protein; 38gm carbo.; 2gm fiber; 2gm fats; 7mg cholesterol; 252mg calcium; 0mg iron; 26mg magnesium; 360mg potassium; 89mg sodium; Vit. C 35mg; Vit. E trace.

BREAKFAST FRUIT SALAD

This recipe works for: Recovery, Weight Loss, Skin, Female Balance, Anti-Aging
Eat as is, or top waffles or French toast with a spoonful instead of syrup or butter.
For 4 servings:

Peel and slice 3 Peaches. Toss with 2 baskets Blueberries and a small basket of Strawberries, sliced. —Drizzle with 4 TBS Honey, and sprinkle with Ground Cardamom.

BREAKFAST BANANA SPLIT with STRAWBERRY SYRUP

This recipe works for: Skin, Hair, Nails, Female Balance, Childhood Health
For 2 servings:

Place on a pieplate: 2 Bananas, sliced lengthwise. Drizzle with Honey. Sprinkle with Lemon Juice. Broil til topping bubbles, about 2 minutes.
—Make the STRAWBERRY SYRUP: blender blend 1 cup fresh sliced Strawberries with 2 teasp. Honey, 1 teasp. Cinnamon and 2 teasp. Arrowroot Powder. Transfer to a saucepan and bring to a rolling boil, stirring constantly. Remove from heat as soon as the syrup begins to thicken. Top bananas just before serving. Sprinkle with Granola.

HONEYDEW with FROSTY BLUEBERRIES

This recipe works for: Circulation Disorders, Respiratory Problems, Arthritis
For 4 servings:

Heat in a saucepan: $^1/_2$ cup Honey and $1^1/_2$ teasp. Vanilla. When honey bubbles, remove from heat, let cool slightly. Then gently stir in to coat 1 cup Blueberries.
—Lift berries from honey with a slotted spoon and place in a tray to freeze for 30 minutes (no more). —Cut a Honeydew in quarters. Place each quarter on a salad plate. Divide berries between melon pieces. Sprinkle with minced Crystallized Ginger.

NEW ENGLAND CRANBERRY- HONEY COMPOTE

This recipe works for: Bladder - Kidney Disorders, Female Balance, Arthritis
For about 6 cups:

Stir til blended in a saucepan: 4 cups Apple Juice and $^1/_2$ cup Honey, 1 pound Dried Mixed Fruit, 1 cup Cranberry-Apple Juice, $^1/_2$ cup Raisins, 2 Cinnamon Sticks, 6 thin Lemon Slices and 6 thin Orange Slices. Simmer til tender, about 25 minutes.
—Add $^1/_2$ cup Cranberries (fresh or frozen). Simmer for 5 more minutes.
—Remove from heat. Cover, chill; top with toasted chopped Walnuts.

GREEN TEA FRUIT BOWL

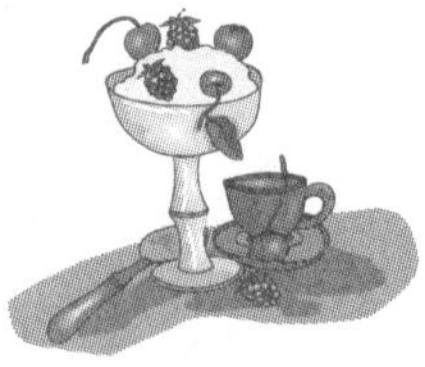

This recipe works for: Organ Health, Female Balance, Sugar Imbalance
For 2 servings:

Build this in layers in a glass bowl: Cover bottom of bowl with Granola. Gently spread on Vanilla Yogurt, and smooth it with the back of a spoon. Cover with toasted Sun Seeds. Top with Apple Slices, then smooth on another thin coat of yogurt.
—Blend a half pint of Raspberries with a half cup Green Tea. Pour over and sprinkle with toasted slivered Almonds.

Breakfast Grains and Cereals

Breakfast is one of the best times to eat your grains. Their solid, satisfying, but low-fat nutrition can power you all day. Whole grains are full of plant protein and complex carbohydrates to add fiber to your diet and to stabilize your blood sugar. Whole grains are one of the best food sources of B-vitamins and vitamin E.

Your health food store has a wide range of gourmet grains you can use. Try amaranth, barley, buckwheat, brown rice, quinoa, oats, millet, triticale, spelt or cous-cous. Make a blend (for better amino acid balance), or use a single grain as you like.

My Personal Favorite: I like brown rice in the morning. It is an efficient source of protein and B vitamins that works well for a brown rice cleanse or for weight loss. I sprinkle my brown rice with 2 tablespoons (usually more) of snipped dry sea vegetables. I top it with fresh shredded carrots and spinach (for EFA's). I stir in some sesame seeds and sprinkle it all with tamari sauce. It's my perfect breakfast.

BASIC BREAKFAST GRAINS

This recipe works for: Sugar Imbalances, Female Balance, Food for Men
For 4 servings:

Heat 1 cup Apple Juice and 1 cup Water. Add 1 cup your choice of Whole Grains. (see above for suggestions). Reduce heat to medium, cover and cook until liquid is absorbed, about 25 minutes.

—Serve hot with a handful of Toasted Sliced Almonds and Toasted Sunflower Seeds, dashes of Cinnamon and a handful of Raisins.

—Serve cold with 1 or 2 teasp. Honey and Fruit Yogurt to taste.

Nutrition per serving; 301 calories; 10gm protein; 46gm carbo.; 6g fiber; 9gm fats; 0 cholesterol; 58mg calcium; 3mg iron; 103mg magnesium; 439mg potassium; 8mg sodium; Vit. C 23mg; Vit. E 2 IU.

ISLAND GRANOLA Make this the night before to let flavors blend.

This recipe works for: Fatigue Disorders, Female Balance, Stress and Exhaustion
For 6 servings:

Prepare a nut and seed mix once a week: Toast <u>1 cup each</u> Shredded Coconut, chopped Almonds, Pumpkin Seeds and Sunflower Seeds in a 250° oven until golden brown. —Store in an airtight container.

—Chop in chunks and put in a bowl with a cover: 1 Mango, $^{1}/_{2}$ Fresh Pineapple, 1 Papaya, 2 Bananas, $^{1}/_{2}$ cup Raisins, 2 cups Pineapple-Orange Juice.

—Add 2 cups Rolled Oats, 1 tsp. Vanilla, generous sprinkles Cinnamon and Nutmeg.

—The next morning, add 1 cup of the nut and seed mix; divide among bowls.

Make Your Own Custom Granola:

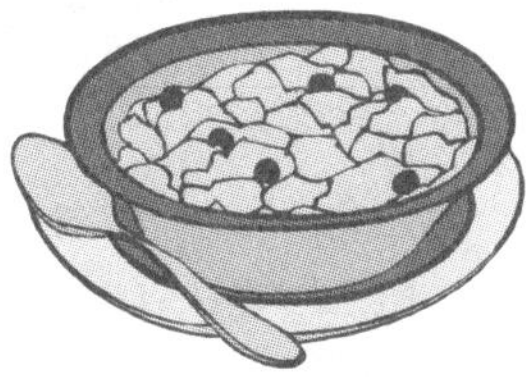

Granola is an oven-roasted hearty blend of whole grains, nuts, seeds and dried fruits, lightly coated with honey, maple syrup or molasses and an unsaturated oil. Real granola is robust, nutritious and delicious. Unfortunately most mass-market granolas have partially hydrogenated oils (trans fats) instead of high quality oils, sugar or corn syrup instead of natural sweeteners, sulfur dried fruits and all kinds of sugary bits added. The recipes on this page take you back to the original, wholesome, high-density energy foods. Store air-tight to maintain crispness. Either recipe makes enough for 10 breakfasts for 2 people.

REAL GRANOLA Tip: buy ingredients in bulk from your health food store.

This recipe works for: Skin and Hair, Female Balance, Healthy Pregnancy
Enough for 20 servings. Preheat oven to 150°.

Mix in a big bowl: 8 cups Rolled Oats, 2 cups Toasted Wheat Germ, 1 cup Shredded Coconut, 1/2 cup Grapenuts Type Cereal, 2 cups Chopped Almonds, 1 cup Sesame Seeds.

—Blender blend next 4 ingredients, and pour over first mixture: 1/2 cup Canola Oil, 1/2 cup Maple Syrup, 1/3 cup Apple or Pear Juice, 2 teasp. Vanilla or Almond Extract.

—Spread on baking sheets. Bake on low in oven for 1 hour until crunchy and golden. Stir every 10 minutes.

—Add 1 cup Chopped Dates, Dried Cherries, Dried Blueberries or Raisins.

Nutrition per serving; 417 calories; 14gm protein; 48gm carbo.; 8g fiber; 3gm fats; 0 cholesterol; 76mg calcium; 5mg iron; 166mg magnesium; 433mg potassium; 36mg sodium; Vit. C 3mg; Vit. E 10 IU.

ORIGINAL OLD-FASHIONED GRANOLA

This recipe works for: Sugar Imbalances, Waste Management, Food for Men
Enough for 20 servings. Preheat oven to 250°.

Mix together in an extra large bowl: 6 cups Rolled Oats, 2 1/2 cups Toasted Sunflower Seeds, 1 cup Toasted Pumpkin Seeds (pepitas), 2 cups Toasted Wheat Germ, 1/4 cup Sesame Seeds, 1/2 cup Shredded Coconut, 1 cup Walnut Pieces, 2 cups Sliced Almonds.

—Warm in a pan: 1/2 cup Canola Oil, 1 1/2 cups Honey. Pour over granola and toss.

—Spread on two 11 x 17 jelly roll pans; bake for 25 minutes. Remove and stir.

—Reduce oven temperature to 150°. Stir every 10 minutes or so.

—Return to the large bowl and add 4 cups Dried Chopped Fruits, like Raisins, Currants, Apricots, Dates and Pitted Prunes.

—Toss to blend and let cool before storing.

Nutrition per serving; 580 calories; 15gm protein; 77gm carbo.; 10gm fiber; 27gm fats; 0 cholesterol; 78mg calcium; 4mg iron; 159mg magnesium; 714mg potassium; 8mg sodium; Vit. C 3mg; Vit. E 1 IU.

IMMUNE SUPPORT BREAKFAST Make up and store airtight.

This recipe works for: Allergies - Asthma, Waste Management, Immune Power
Use about 1/2 cup dry mix per serving:

Mix together in a large bowl: 2 cups each: Rolled Oats, Rolled Barley, Oat Bran, 1 cup Toasted Sunflower Seeds, 1/2 cup Dried Cherries, 1/2 cup Dried Blueberries, 1 cup Chopped Almonds, 1/2 cup Lecithin Granules, 1/2 cup Ground Flaxseeds, and 1/2 cup Raisins.
—Soak amount you need in Vanilla Soymilk, Rice Milk or Apple Juice to moisten.

Nutrition per serving; 292 calories; 10gm protein; 41gm carbo.; 7gm fiber; 14gm fats; 0 cholesterol; 112mg calcium; 3mg iron; 129mg magnesium; 389mg potassium; 7mg sodium; Vit. C 1mg; Vit. E 12 IU.

APPLE COUS-COUS for BREAKFAST Light and satisfying

This recipe works for: Sugar Imbalances, Colon Health, High Blood Pressure
Makes about 4 cups:

Make 3 cups cous-cous according to package directions. Set aside.
—Sizzle 3 TBS chopped Almonds and 1/2 cup chopped Carrots for 3 minutes in 1 TB Canola oil. Season with 2 pinches each Herb Salt and Curry Powder.
—Top with 1/2 cup Chopped Apple and 2 TBS Raisins.

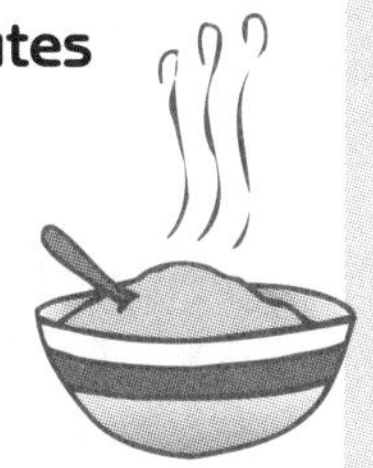

NON-DAIRY APPLE RAISIN OATMEAL

This recipe works for: Allergies - Asthma, Childhood Health, Bone Building
Serves 2:

Bring 2 Cups Water to a boil. Add 1 Cup Oatmeal and stir for 4 or 5 minutes. Remove from heat. Divide in two bowls.
—Top with Banana Slices and Raisins. Drizzle on 1 TB Honey and 1/2 cup Apple Juice.

BREAKFAST RICE with FRESH TOMATOES

This recipe works for: Men's Health, Allergies- Asthma, Weight Control
Makes 4 servings:

Bring to boil in a pot: 6 cups Organic Chicken or Vegetable Stock, 1 cup chopped Fresh Tomatoes, 1/2 teasp. Lemon-Pepper Seasoning. Add 2 cups Jasmine Rice, bring to a boil, cover and simmer until water is absorbed.
—Stir in 3 TBS Tamari or Teriyaki Sauce and 2 TBS Parmesan Cheese. Serve hot.

Nutrition per serving; 373 calories; 10gm protein; 77gm carbo.; 2gm fiber; 2gm fats; 2mg cholesterol; 74mg calcium; 5mg iron; 34mg magnesium; 235mg potassium; 702mg sodium; Vit. C 9mg; Vit. E 2 IU.

Healthy Breakfast Breads

There's a lot more to breakfast breads than bagels, doughnuts and Danish pastries. Whole grain breads are packed with solid low-fat nutrition you can use all day.

TOASTED WHEAT GERM MUFFINS high in fiber

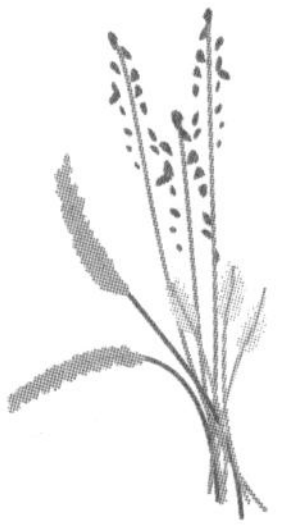

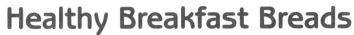

This recipe works for: Men's Health, Colon Health, Heart Health
For 12 muffins: Preheat oven to 375°.

Combine 1 cup Toasted Wheat Germ, 1/2 cup Plain Yogurt and 1/2 cup Water. Let stand 1 hour. Mix in 1 Egg and 2 TBS Canola Oil.

—Mix in 1 cup Whole Wheat Pastry Flour, 4 teasp. Baking Powder, and 1/2 teasp. Sea Salt. Fill lecithin-sprayed or paper-lined muffin tins 2/3 full.

—Bake 20 minutes until a toothpick inserted in the center comes out clean.

RAISINS and OATS MUFFINS

This recipe works for: Heart and High Blood Pressure, Arthritis, Cholesterol
For 6 big deli-style muffins, oil 6 pyrex custard cups, and bake at 375°.

Combine dry ingredients: 1 cup Unbleached Flour, 1/2 cup Whole Wheat Pastry Flour, 1 cup Grapenuts or Raisin Bran Cereal, 1 cup Rolled Oats, 1 1/2 teasp. Baking Soda —Form a well in the center, and pour in 1 cup Plain Yogurt, 1/2 cup Honey, 1 Egg, 1/4 cup Canola Oil, 1/2 cup Raisins.

—Stir until lumpy, and bake 25 minutes until a toothpick comes out clean.

Nutrition per serving; 431 calories; 11gm protein; 75gm carbo.; 6gg fiber; 12gm fats; 30mg cholesterol; 110mg calcium; 4mg iron; 76mg magnesium; 379mg potassium; 420mg sodium; Vit. C 2mg; Vit. E 5 IU.

CRANBERRY APPLE NUT BREAD

This recipe works for: Overcoming Adictions, Fatigue Syndromes, Women's Health
Makes 4 loaves. Preheat oven to 350°F. Lightly oil and flour 4 small loaf pans.

Sift together: 3 cups Whole Wheat Pastry Flour, 1/2 cup Wheat Germ, 1 1/2 tsp. Baking Powder, 1 tsp. Baking Soda, and 1/2 tsp. Salt.

—In another bowl: mix 4 TBS Canola Oil, 3/4 cup Turbinado or Brown Sugar, 2 Eggs, 1 cup Orange Juice.

—Fold in 2 cups Chopped Cranberries, 1 cored, Chopped Apple, 1 tsp. Grated Orange Peel and 2/3 cup Chopped Walnuts.

—Pour the batter into loaf pans and bake for 40 to 45 minutes, or until a toothpick inserted into the center comes out clean. Remove from pans and let cool.

MOLASSES SPICE BREAD

This recipe works for: Heart Health, Liver and Organ Health, Digestive Health
For 16 squares. Preheat oven to 350°F. Lightly oil an 8-inch square baking pan.

Combine 2 cups Whole Wheat Pastry Flour, 1/2 cup Date Sugar, 1 1/2 teasp. Baking Soda, 2 teasp. Ground Ginger, 1 teasp. Cardamom, 3/4 teasp. Cinnamon, 1/2 teasp. Salt.

—Fold in 2 Eggs, 1/2 cup Unsulphured Molasses, 2 TBS Fresh Grated Ginger, 1/2 cup Apple Juice, and 1/4 cup Vegetable Oil.

—Pour batter into pan and bake for 25 to 30 minutes. Let cool completely before removing from pan. Cut into 16 squares before serving.

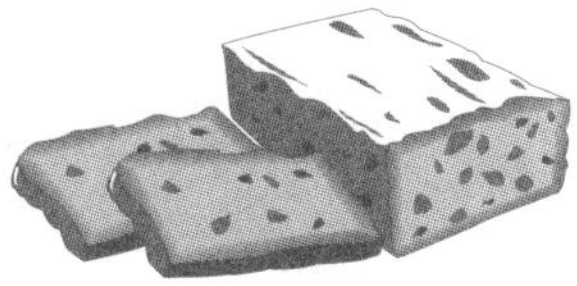

EVERYTHING BANANA BREAD

This recipe works for: Heart Health, Children's Health, Sports Nutrition
For 10 slices. Preheat oven to 350°F. Lightly oil a 9x5-inch loaf pan.

Stir together: 2 cups Unbleached Flour, 1 cup Whole-Wheat Pastry Flour, 2 tsp. Baking Powder, 1 tsp. Baking Soda, 1 tsp. Ground Cinnamon, 1/2 tsp. Salt, 1/4 tsp. Nutmeg, 2 tsp. Chinese Five-Spice Powder and 1 tsp. Ground Ginger.

—Mash 3 very Ripe Bananas and fold in.

—Gently stir in 1/3 cup Canola Oil, 3/4 cup Maple Syrup, 1 TB Lemon Juice, 1 tsp. Grated Lemon Zest, 3/4 tsp. Lemon Extract, 1/4 cup Poppy Seed, 1/3 cup Raisins.

—Scrape batter into prepared loaf pan and gently smooth top with spatula. Bake for 1 hour, or until toothpick inserted in middle comes out clean. Cool in pan 30 minutes, then invert onto wire rack to cool completely.

Nutrition per serving; 321 calories; 5gm protein; 57gm carbo.; 4gm fiber; 9gm fats; 0 cholesterol; 154mg calcium; 3mg iron; 56mg magnesium; 335mg potassium; 310mg sodium; Vit. C 6mg; Vit. E 3 IU.

BERRY-OAT MUFFINS

This recipe works for: Bone Building, Stress - Exhaustion, Immune Power
Makes 12 muffins. Preheat your oven to 350°F. Oil a 12-cup muffin tin.

Combine in a bowl: 1/2 cup Canola Oil, 1/2 cup Turbinado Sugar, 1 Egg, 1/2 cup Plain Non-fat Yogurt, 1 cup Whole Wheat Pastry Flour, 2 cups Rolled Oats, 1 tsp. Baking Powder, 1/2 tsp. Baking Soda, 1/4 tsp. Ground Cinnamon, 1 cup Fresh Berries (any kind).

—Fill buttered muffin cups.

—Bake 25 to 30 minutes. Let cool about 5 minutes.

Nutrition per serving; 207 calories; 5gm protein; 24gm carbo.; 3gm fiber; 10mg fats; 17mg cholesterol; 276mg calcium; 1mg iron; 40mg magnesium; 164mg potassium; 99mg sodium; Vit. C 3mg; Vit. E 5 IU.

EASY HONEY BREAKFAST BREAD Much better than a Danish

This recipe works for: Fatigue Syndromes, Immune Power, Heart Health
For 12 servings: Preheat oven to 375°F.

Mix together just to moisten: $^1/_4$ cup Canola Oil, 2 Eggs, $^1/_2$ teasp. Salt, 1 cup Whole Wheat Pastry Flour, $^1/_2$ cup Barley Flour, 1 $^1/_2$ teasp. Baking Soda, $^3/_4$ cup Honey, 3 TBS Maple Syrup, 1 teasp. Almond Extract.
—Fold in $^1/_2$ cup Plain Low-Fat Yogurt, $^1/_2$ cup Chopped Dates, $^1/_2$ cups Chopped Walnuts. Batter will be very light.
—Pour batter into a lecithin-sprayed round baking pan. Top with $^1/_4$ cup Chopped Walnuts, and bake for 35 minutes until springy when touched. Serve in wedges.

Nutrition per serving; 240 calories; 4gm protein; 38gm carbo.; 3g fiber; 9g fats; 36mg cholesterol; 40mg calcium; 1mg iron; 32mg magnesium; 182mg potassium; 267mg sodium; Vit. C 2mg; Vit. E 3 IU.

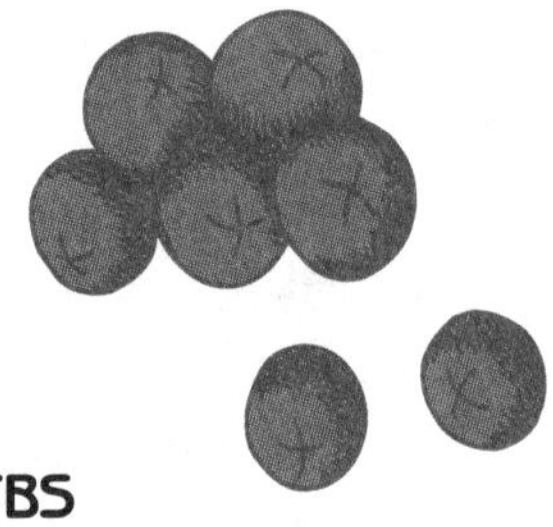

BREAKFAST BLUEBERRY CRISP

This recipe works for: Allergy Reactions, Immune Power
Makes 4 to 6 servings. Preheat oven to 350°F.

Combine: 2 cups Cooked Brown Rice, $^3/_4$ cup Rice Milk, 2 TBS Brown Sugar, 2 TBS Honey, 1 TB Canola Oil, 1 tsp. Cinnamon. Fold in 2 Sliced Bananas and 2 cups Fresh or Frozen Blueberries.
—Put into an 8-inch square baking pan and cover with foil. Bake 30 minutes. Cool slightly before serving.

Nutrition per serving; 202 calories; 3gm protein; 42gm carbo.; 3g fiber; 3gm fats; 0mg cholesterol; 70mg calcium; 1mg iron; 42mg magnesium; 240mg potassium; 11mg sodium; Vit. C 10mg; Vit. E 1 IU.

HOT CORN STICKS healthy portable energy food.

This recipe works for: Food for Men, Sports Nutrition, Immune Power
Makes 14 sticks: Preheat oven to 450°F.

Sift into a bowl: 1 cup Unbleached Flour, $^3/_4$ cup Yellow Cornmeal, 2 tsp. Baking Powder, 4 TBS Brown Sugar, $^1/_2$ tsp. Salt.
—Gently stir in $^3/_4$ cup Rice Milk, 4 TBS Canola Oil, and 1 Egg.
—Generously spray 2 cast iron "ear of corn" pans with lecithin spray.
—Fill pans $^3/_4$-full. Bake about 20 minutes, until golden brown. Serve hot, or remove from pan, cool and wrap tightly in foil for traveling. Reheat before serving.

Nutrition per serving; 112 calories; 2gm protein; 16gm carbo.; 1g fiber; 4gm fats; 15mg cholesterol; 75mg calcium; 1mg iron; 11mg magnesium; 42mg potassium; 137mg sodium; Vit. C 0mg; Vit. E 1 IU.

Soy Protein for Breakfast

Soy foods like soy milk, tofu, tempeh and soy protein powder offer excellent vegetarian sources of protein for morning fuel.

GREEN TEA, FRUIT and SOY SHAKE

This recipe works for: Strong Bones, Female Balance, Cancer Control
For 1 large serving:

Blender blend until smooth: 1/2 cup Vanilla Soy Protein Powder or 3/4 cup Vanilla Low-fat Soy Milk, 1/2 cup Orange Juice or Apple Juice, 1 cup Chopped Strawberries, 1/2 cup Brewed Green Tea, 1 Banana, 1/2 cup Low-fat Vanilla Yogurt, 2 TBS Lemon Juice.

HIGH PROTEIN TOFU PANCAKES

This recipe works for: Strong Bones, Recuperation, Fatigue Syndromes
For 18 easy pancakes: Preheat a griddle or cast iron skillet until a drop of water skitters on the surface.

Blender blend: 1 cup Vanilla Yogurt, 1 teasp. Baking Powder, 1/2 cup Water, 2 pinches Salt, 3 Eggs, 1/2 cup Buckwheat Flour, 1/2 cup Barley Flour, 1 TB Canola Oil, 16-oz. Very Fresh Tofu, mashed, 2 TBS Maple Syrup, 1 1/2 teasp. Vanilla.

—Whirl til smooth, and pour on the hot griddle in 1/3 to 1/2 cup circles. Flip when bubbles appear and stack on a serving platter. Serve with Maple Syrup or Apple Juice.

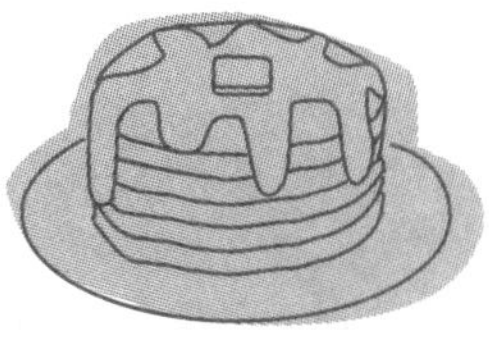

Nutrition per serving; 142 calories; 6gm protein; 21gm carbo.; 6gm fiber; 4gm fats; 36mg cholesterol; 117mg calcium; 3mg iron; 43mg magnesium; 178mg potassium; 76mg sodium; Vit. C 1mg; Vit. E 1 IU.

NO DAIRY BREAKFAST PIZZA unusual, delicious, great for kids

This recipe works for: Female Balance, Allergies, Fatigue Syndromes
For 10 to 12 pieces: Preheat oven to 425°. Heat a round pizza pan in the oven until the batter is ready.

Blender blend batter briefly: 1 3/4 cups Plain or Vanilla Soy Milk, 2 Eggs, 2 TBS Canola Oil, 2 cups Buckwheat Pancake Mix. —Spray the hot pizza pan with lecithin spray, and pour on the batter. —Sprinkle with 1/2 cup <u>each</u>: Granola, Chopped Pecans, Raisins. —Bake 12 to 15 minutes until brown at the edges. Cut in wedges. Serve with Maple Syrup or Apple Juice.

Nutrition per serving; 212 calories; 6gm protein; 24gm carbo.; 1g fiber; 11gm fats; 56mg cholesterol; 155mg calcium; 1mg iron; 38mg magnesium; 269mg potassium; 189mg sodium; Vit. C 1mg; Vit. E 1 IU.

BAKED APPLES with LEMON BALM and TOFU

This recipe works for: Sugar Imbalances, Fatigue Syndromes, Heart Health
Makes 8 servings. Preheat oven to 375°F. Have a glass baking dish ready

Partially core 4 Large Granny Smith Apples, about 1 $^1/_2$ inches in diameter. Remove top $^3/_4$ of the core but leave the bases intact. Stuff each apple hole with a few Raisins, a few Pumpkin Seeds and a few Sunflower Seeds. Fill holes with water. Put apples in the baking dish and pour $^3/_4$ cup boiling water around them.

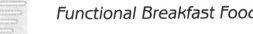

—Bake uncovered for 35 minutes, rotating the dish after 20 minutes. Apples turn yellow when done.

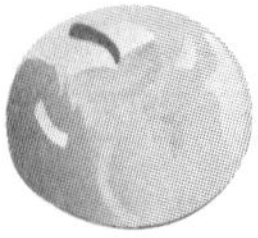

—Whisk an 8-oz. package Soft Silken Tofu with 4 tsp. Maple Syrup, 2 TBS minced Lemon Peel and $^1/_2$ tsp. Nutmeg. When the apples are baked, cut each in half vertically and top each half with the tofu mixture. Garnish with Raisins and Sunflower Seeds.

TAHINI TOFU BREAKFAST STICKS

This recipe works for: Men's Health, Colon Health, Heart Health
For 8 slices: Preheat oven to 400°F. Oil a baking tray.

Slice 1 lb. Tofu in 8 slabs. Cut slabs in half lengthwise. Place slabs on oiled tray.

—Combine in a bowl: $^1/_4$ cup Sesame Tahini or Almond Butter, $^1/_4$ cup Chickpea Miso and 1 TB Soy Bacon Bits. Spread half the sauce on each slab. Sprinkle with Toasted Wheat Germ, and bake until crusty, or under a broiler for 1 minute. Turn slabs and spread on rest of sauce. Sprinkle with more Wheat Germ. Bake or broil until crusty.

Nutrition per serving; 159 calories; 13gm protein; 8gm carbo.; 2g fiber; 9gm fats; 0mg cholesterol; 139mg calcium; 7mg iron; 97mg magnesium; 244mg potassium; 323mg sodium; Vit. C 2mg; Vit. E 1 IU.

TOFU SCRAMBLE

This recipe works for: Heart-Cholesterol Health, Weight Loss, Liver - Organ Health
Freeze and thaw tofu first for tastiest results.
For 4 servings:

Crumble in a bowl 1-lb. frozen, thawed Low-fat Tofu. Drain well.

—Heat 1 TB Olive Oil and sauté for 5 minutes: 1 Small Onion, sliced, $^1/_4$ cup Shiitake Mushrooms, soaked and sliced, and $^1/_2$ cup diced Yellow Pepper until aromatic.

—Add Tofu, 1 tsp. Tamari, 1 tsp. Sesame Salt and sauté 5 minutes longer, until peppers are just tender and tofu is golden. Serve hot as is or on whole grain toast.

Nutrition per serving; 225 calories; 19gm protein; 12gm carbo.; 2g fiber; 13g fats; 0mg cholesterol; 238mg calcium; 12mg iron; 119mg magnesium; 432mg potassium; 618mg sodium; Vit. C 25mg; Vit. E 1 IU.

Healthy Breakfast Eggs - It's An Art

Eggs are finally getting the "break" they deserve as researchers learn how to consider the whole food and not just its parts in their findings. Recent studies show what the health food world has long known; that an egg's cholesterol content is balanced by its lecithin and phosphatides. Eggs are still one of nature's premier foods.

BOUILLION POACHED EGGS Easy gourmet eggs like the pros do it.

This recipe works for: Heart-Cholesterol Health, Weight Loss, Fatigue Syndromes
For 2 breakfast servings:

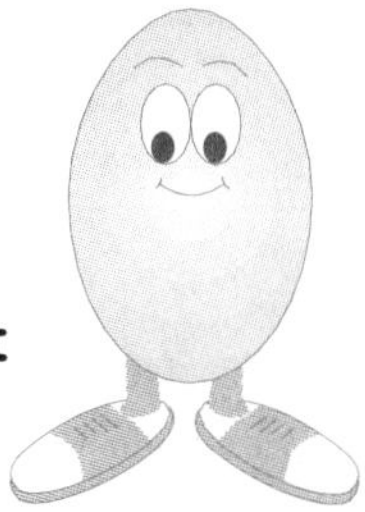

Heat 1 quart water and 1 TB White Vinegar in a heavy skillet to boiling. Add 2 Vegetable or Chicken Bouillon Cubes.

—Crack an Egg into a teacup, lower the cup into the broth - let the egg slide out. Repeat three times. Cook to medium firm, for 3 minutes. Lift eggs out gently with a slotted spoon. Serve immediately... on Toast or Fresh Watercress.

SCRAMBLED EGGS SPECIAL

This recipe works for: Weight Control, Anti-Aging, Brain Booster
For 4 servings: Heat a griddle or skillet til a drop of water skitters on the surface.

Braise $^1/_4$ cup Minced Onion in 2 TBS Vegetable Broth and 2 TBS White Wine until brown and aromatic.

—Meanwhile, whirl in the blender 6 Eggs, 6 Parsley Sprigs (or 2 teasp. Parsley Flakes), $^1/_2$ teasp. Sesame Salt, $^1/_3$ cup Low Fat Cottage Cheese, $^1/_4$ teasp. Lemon-Pepper and 1 teasp. Dijon Mustard. —Pour onto hot onion sauté and cook slowly, stirring frequently but gently until eggs are set.

Nutrition per serving; 139 calories; 14gm protein; 2gm carbo.; 1g fiber; 8gm fats; 320mg cholesterol; 56mg calcium; 1mg iron; 11mg magnesium; 144mg potassium; 397mg sodium; Vit. C 3mg; Vit. E 1 IU.

HUEVOS RANCHEROS FRITTATA Rich tasting, but low-fat

This recipe works for: Men's Health, Sports Nutrition, Brain Booster
For 6 small portions: Preheat oven to 350°F.

Arrange a 7-oz. can Whole Green Chilies face open in a single layer in a 3-qt. baking dish. Sprinkle with 1 cup Low Fat Cheddar, 1 cup Low Fat Jack, and 1 TB Chopped Green Olives. Repeat layers of cheeses and olives.

—Beat 3 Eggs, 1 cup Plain Yogurt and 1 Diced Tomato together in a bowl. Pour over cheeses, and bake for 30 minutes until edges begin to brown. Sprinkle on more Chopped Tomato and drizzle on Mild Salsa.

EASY VEGETABLE HERB FRITTATA

This recipe works for: Men's Health, Immune Breakdown, Brain Booster
For 8 wedge portions: Preheat oven to 350°F.

Sauté 1/4 cup Minced Red Onion in 1 TB Canola Oil and 1 TB Balsamic Vinegar.
—Add 1 cup Chopped Fresh Tomatoes and turn off heat.
—In the blender, whirl 8 Eggs, 1/4 cup Plain Low-Fat Yogurt and 1 teasp. Italian Herbs. Pour over tomatoes in the skillet. Sprinkle with 1/2 cup Chopped Bell Pepper, 1/4 cup Minced Black Olives, and 1 cup Grated Low-Fat Mozzarrella Cheese.
—Bake for 15 minutes until eggs set. Top with Snipped Parsley and cut in wedges.

Nutrition per serving; 147 calories; 10gm protein; 4gm carbo.; 1g fiber; 10gm fats; 222mg cholesterol; 142mg calcium; 1mg iron; 15mg magnesium; 174mg potassium; 169mg sodium; Vit. C 19mg; Vit. E 3 IU.

SCRAMBLED EGGS with BABY SHRIMP extra protein to heal

This recipe works for: Men's Health, Weight Loss, Brain Boosting, Recovery
For 4 servings:

Mix briefly in a bowl: 6 Eggs, 2 Green Onions, minced, 1/2 teasp. Salt. Heat 1 TB Canola Oil, 1 TB Raspberry Vinegar and 2 TBS White Wine and sizzle egg mixture til hot.
—When hot, add Onion-Egg mix and 2 pinches White Pepper. Stir until half cooked.
—Add 5 to 6-oz. cooked Small Shrimp. Stir and lift gently until set. Serve hot.

Nutrition per serving; 191 calories; 18gm protein; 3gm carbo.; 1g fiber; 11gm fats; 389mg cholesterol; 63mg calcium; 2mg iron; 26mg magnesium; 222mg potassium; 470mg sodium; Vit. C 3mg; Vit. E 3 IU.

ZUCCHINI OPEN-FACE OMELET nice and spicy

This recipe works for: Fatigue Syndromes, Men's Health, Recovery
For 4 to 5 wedges: Preheat oven to 350°F. Use a cast iron or oven-ready skillet.

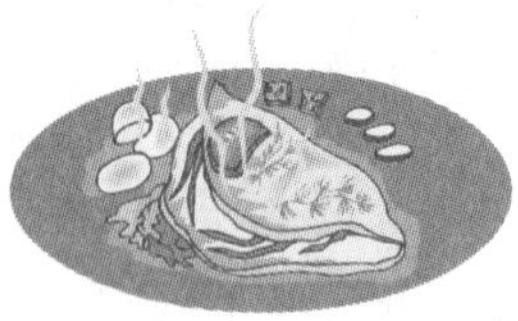

Sauté half a Bell Pepper chopped, 2 Medium Zucchinis chopped, 1 teasp. Sesame Seeds over medium high heat in 1 TB Canola Oil and 2 TBS Vegetable Broth for 5 minutes.
—Whirl in the blender: 6 Eggs, 2 TBS Plain Yogurt, 1 1/2 teasp. Herb Salt.
—Add to skillet and cook for 2 minutes, until eggs just set on the bottom.
—Put skillet in the oven and bake for 4 minutes until eggs set on the top.
—Cut in wedges. Top with ARIZONA GAUCAMOLE (pg. 44).

Nutrition per serving; 200 calories; 19gm protein; 2gm carbo.; 2g fiber; 12gm fats; 380mg cholesterol; 66mg calcium; 4mg iron; 26mg magnesium; 325mg potassium; 466mg sodium; Vit. C 23mg; Vit. E 2 IU.

Make Your Own Breakfast Bars

Bars are everywhere today - but most of them I've seen are still full of fat and sugar (even in health food stores). Bars are great fast breakfast food. They can be almost a complete, nutritious meal. If you're on a healing diet, you might want to make your own so you can control the ingredients. Just make a batch when you have time and you'll have a week or more of hurry-up breakfasts.

TRIPLE FIBER BARS

This recipe works for: Sports Nutrition, Men's Health, Recovery
For 36 bars: Preheat oven to 375°. Lightly coat a 9 x 13 pan with canola spray.

Mix the dry ingredients in a bowl: 1 cup Oat Bran, $\frac{1}{2}$ cup Whole Wheat Flour, 4 TBS Brown Sugar, $\frac{1}{2}$ teasp. Baking Soda, 3 cups Rolled Oats, and 2 TBS Bee Pollen Granules.

—Mix the wet ingredients until fluffy in another bowl: 4 TBS Butter, $\frac{1}{2}$ cup Canola Oil, $\frac{1}{2}$ cup Honey, 2 TBS Maple Syrup, 1 Egg, 1 teasp. Vanilla.

—Combine all ingredients together until just blended. Add 1 cup Pitted Prunes, chopped, $\frac{1}{2}$ cup Chopped Walnuts. Spoon into baking dish and smooth top. Bake for 25 minutes until golden. Cool on racks. Cut in bars.

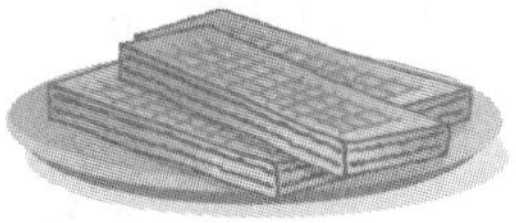

FAT-FREE APPLESAUCE BARS

This recipe works for: Childhood Nutrition, Sugar Imbalances, Heart Health
For 18 bars: Preheat oven to 350°. Lightly coat a square pan with canola spray.

Mix the dry ingredients together: $\frac{1}{2}$ cup Unbleached White Flour or Wholewheat Pastry Flour, $\frac{1}{2}$ cup Date Sugar, 6 TBS Fructose, 6 TBS Unsweetened Cocoa, $\frac{1}{2}$ teasp. Salt and 2 handfuls Raisins.

—Whisk together in a separate bowl: 3 Egg Whites, $1\frac{1}{2}$ teasp. Vanilla, $\frac{1}{4}$ teasp. Cinnamon, $\frac{1}{4}$ teasp. Nutmeg and $\frac{1}{2}$ cup Applesauce.

—Combine the two sets of ingredients. Spread in prepared pan. Bake for 30 minutes, until springy in the center when pressed. Cool 10 minutes. Cut into bars.

BREAKFAST FRUIT NACHOS

This recipe works for: Childhood Nutrition, Men's Health, Weight Control
For 18 wedges: Preheat oven to 375°F.

Split 3 Pita Breads horizontally and cut each in 6 wedges. Toast on baking sheets briefly to crisp. Spread half with Raspberry Preserves and the other half with Orange Marmalade. Top with Granola sprinkles and a Pineapple Wedge. Sprinkle on Grated Cheddar. Broil 2 to 3 minutes until cheddar melts.

THICK and CHEWY ORANGE GRANOLA BARS

This recipe works for: Childhood Nutrition, Cancer Control, Heart Health
For 36 bars: Preheat oven to 350°F. Lightly coat a 9 x 13 pan with canola spray.

Combine crust ingredients, and press into bottom of baking pan: 1 cup Whole Wheat Pastry Flour, (or 1/2 cup Unbleached Flour, 1/4 cup Oat Flour and 1/4 cup Barley Flour), 1/4 cup Fructose and 1/4 cup Date Sugar (or 1/2 cup Brown Sugar), 6 TBS Butter.

—Bake for 10 minutes until pale gold in color. Remove and set aside for filling.

—Combine filling ingredients, and spread on top of crust: 1/2 cup Honey, 2 cups Orange Granola, 1 cup chopped Dates, 2 Eggs, 1/2 cup Butter, 1/2 cup Canola Oil, 1/2 teasp. Salt, 1 cup Shredded Coconut, 1 teasp. Baking Soda, 1 teasp. Nutmeg, 1 1/2 teasp. Vanilla, 1/2 cup Chopped Almonds.

—Bake for 35 minutes.... done, but still chewy. Cut in bars.

PINEAPPLE DATE C-BARS fruit juice sweetened, high vitamin C bars

This recipe works for: Allergy-Asthma, Sugar Imbalances, Digestive Problems
For 24 bars: Preheat oven to 350 °F. Lightly coat a square pan with canola spray.

Simmer filling ingredients until liquid is absorbed: 1 cup packed chopped Dates, 3/4 cup Pineapple Juice and 1/2 cup Crushed Pineapple drained. Set aside.

—Mix the bar layer ingredients: 1 1/2 cups Oats, 1 1/2 cups Oat Flour, 2 teasp. Baking Powder, 2 teasp Apple Pie Spice, 1 1/2 teasp. Vanilla, 1 Egg, 1 TB Honey or Apple Juice, and 4 TBS Butter.

—Pat half of the bar layer mix into the prepared pan. Top with all the filling mix. Sprinkle on rest of the bar layer mix. Pat down to smooth. Bake for 30 minutes. Let stand for 1 hour after removing from the oven for a moister, sweeter bar.

Nutrition per serving; 87 calories; 2gm protein; 16gm carbo.; 2g fiber; 2gm fats; 5mg cholesterol; 40mg calcium; 1mg iron; 27mg magnesium; 119mg potassium; 32mg sodium; Vit. C 1mg; Vit. E trace.

FRUIT and NUT BARS

This recipe works for: Sports Nutrition, Sugar Imbalances, Children's Health
For 36 bars: Preheat oven to 350 °F. Lightly coat a 9 x 13 pan with canola spray.

Mix together: 1 cup Oat Flour (blender enough rolled oats to make a cup), 3 cups Rolled Oats, 1 very Ripe Banana, mashed, 1 cup Apple Juice, 1 cup Unsweetened Shredded Coconut, 1/4 cup Date Sugar, 1/2 cup Chopped Almonds, 1/4 cup Sesame Seeds. Spread half on bottom of baking pan.

Pour a 20-oz. can Unsweetened Crushed Pineapple with juice and 1 1/2 cups Chopped Dates in a saucepan and cook until thickened. Spread over the bottom crust. Top with remaining oat mixture and bake for 30-40 minutes.

The Best Brunches

Our high stress, fast paced lifestyles relegate brunch to holidays, vacations and special occasions. That's too bad because brunch (late-morning) foods are elegant, light, healthy and energy boosting. Most of us need more nutrients before noon for better energy conversion. If you find yourself constantly getting mid-morning food cravings, it may be your body's way of telling you it needs fuel for mental and physical energy, blood sugar balance and a higher metabolic rate.

Brunch is a good place to add more fiber from fruits and whole grain breads to clear colon congestion, lower cholesterol and unclog arteries. It's a good place to add more protein from soy, legumes or eggs for faster healing. Healthy brunch foods can keep you from overeating or binging on fats and sugars later, important for weight control. Include a cup of green tea or herb tea with any brunch to maximize healing benefits. The recipes in this section are healthy with a cultured, polished flair.

TROPICAL FRUIT PLATTER with STRAWBERRY SAUCE

This recipe works for: Women's Health, Respiratory Infections, Weight Control
Makes 12 servings:

Whirl in a blender: 2 cups Strawberries, hulled, 1 TB Honey and 2 TBS Orange Juice.

—On a large platter, overlap slices of each fruit, peeled, cored, quartered lengthwise, and cut crosswise into $^{1}/_{4}$-inch slices: 1 Large Pineapple, 1 large Ripe Papaya, 6 Medium Kiwi.

—Drizzle strawberry sauce attractively over fruit. Garnish with 6 Whole Strawberries. Cut each berry into 4 or 5 slices from tip to, but not through, and flare slightly.

Nutrition per serving; 72 calories; 1gm protein; 18gm carbo.; 2g fiber; 0 fats; 0mg cholesterol; 25mg calcium; 1mg iron; 26mg magnesium; 319mg potassium; 4mg sodium; Vit. C 85mg; Vit. E 1 IU.

SCRAMBLED EGGS with SMOKED SALMON

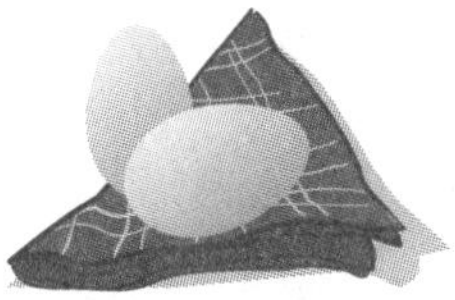

This recipe works for: Women's Health, Stress, Brain Boosting,
Makes 6 brunch servings: Use a non-stick skillet.

Whisk in a bowl: 12 Eggs, $^{1}/_{2}$ tsp. Salt, $^{1}/_{2}$ tsp. Lemon-Pepper.

Heat 3 TBS Canola Oil over medium-high heat. Add eggs. Using a wooden spoon, stir until eggs are almost set, about 5 minutes.

—Gently fold in 6-oz. Thinly Sliced Smoked Salmon, cut into $^{1}/_{2}$-inch wide strips. Stir just until eggs are set, about 1 minute. Transfer eggs to platter.

—Dot hot eggs with 8-oz. well-chilled Low Fat Cream Cheese, cut in small cubes. Sprinkle with Snipped Fresh Chives.

Nutrition per serving; 310 calories; 22gm protein; 4gm carbo.; 1g fiber; 22gm fats; 450mg cholesterol; 96mg calcium; 2mg iron; 19mg magnesium; 239mg potassium; 630mg sodium; Vit. C 1mg; Vit. E 5 IU

BROCCOLI FRITTATA

This recipe works for: Women's Health, Fatigue Syndromes, Heart Health
Makes 8 servings. Preheat oven to 325°F. Oil a quiche pan or round cake pan.

Steam 2 cups Broccoli Florets until crisp-tender; remove from heat and set aside.
—Heat 1 TB Olive Oil and 1 TB Balsamic Vinegar over medium-high heat. Sauté $^1/_2$ cup fine-chopped Sweet Onion and $^1/_2$ cup chopped Red Bell Pepper for 5 minutes, stirring often, until soft. Remove from heat.
—Mince broccoli; stir into onion and pepper. Mix in $^1/_4$ cup Parmesan, 1 cup Crumbled Feta Cheese, $^1/_4$ cup Toasted Wheat Germ, $^1/_4$ teasp. Nutmeg and $^1/_4$ tsp. Paprika.
—In a bowl, beat 6 Eggs and stir into vegetables, then pour into prepared dish.
—Bake 30 minutes until eggs set. Remove and serve warm, cut into wedges.

Nutrition per serving; 151 calories; 10gm protein; 5gm carbo.; 1g fiber; 10gm fats; 175mg cholesterol; 152mg calcium; 1mg iron; 24mg magnesium; 182mg potassium; 211mg sodium; Vit. C 33mg; Vit. E 3 IU.

FANCY FRESH HERB SCONES

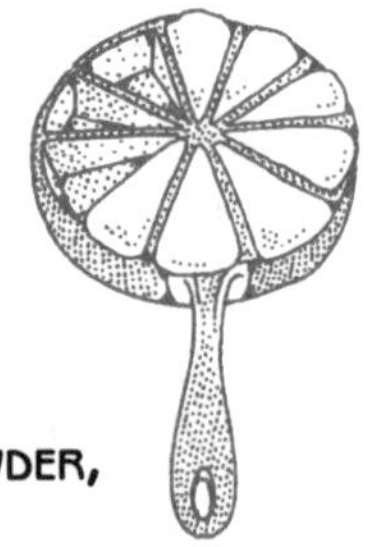

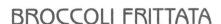

This recipe works for: Skin and Hair, Women's Health, Weight Loss
Makes 16 scones: Preheat oven to 375°F.

In a large bowl, stir together 2 cups Unbleached Flour, 1 TB Baking Powder, $^1/_4$ cup Parmesan Cheese, 1 teasp. Lemon-Pepper.
—In another bowl, combine $^1/_4$ cup Plain Yogurt, $^1/_4$ cup Water, $^1/_3$ cup Olive Oil, 1 Egg, 2 tsp. Lemon Juice, 1 Clove Garlic minced, 2 TBS snipped Fresh Chives and 2 TBS snipped Fresh Basil. Add the liquid to the dry mixture, stirring to make a soft dough. Knead a few times on a lightly floured surface.
—Cut the dough in half and pat each half into an 9 inch round on an oiled cookie sheet. Cut each circle into eight wedges but do not separate. Brush tops with a Plain Yogurt and Water glaze. Sprinkle with 1 TB Fennel Seed and 1 TB Cumin Seed.
—Bake for 20 minutes until lightly browned. Cool on a wire rack for 5 minutes, then wrap loosely in a dish towel for 20 minutes to allow flavors to develop.

BRUNCH POLENTA

This recipe works for: Skin, Hair, Nails, Bone Building, Blood Sugar Balance
For 4 servings: Preheat oven to 350°F. Use a heavy pot.

Bring 1 cup Chicken Broth to a boil. Add $^1/_2$ cup Polenta and stir til it masses together and pulls away from sides of the pan, 10 minutes. Stir in $^1/_4$ cup Grated Parmesan, 1 TB Olive Oil, and 2 pinches <u>each</u> Pepper and Salt. Spoon half the mixture into four individual ramekins or custard cups. Make an indentation in the middle and crack 1 Egg into each. Cover with rest of polenta. Cover with more Parmesan. Place ramekins on baking sheets; bake until cheese browns, 10 minutes. Serve hot.

BRUNCH FRUIT CUPS

This recipe works for: Anti-Aging, Brain Boosting, Fatigue Syndromes
Makes 30 appetizer servings:

Cut 2 cups Seedless Grapes in half. Peel 1 Pear and 1 Kiwi and cut into matchsticks.
—In a bowl, gently mix fruits, $^1/_2$ cup Seasoned Rice Vinegar, $^1/_4$ cup snipped Fresh Basil, and $^1/_2$ lb. shelled Cooked Tiny Shrimp, well-drained.
—Spoon into 30 rinsed, chilled Butter Lettuce Leaves and arrange on a platter.

Nutrition per serving; 27 calories; 2gm protein; 3gm carbo.; 1gm fiber; 1gm fats; 14mg cholesterol; 8mg calcium; 1mg iron; 6mg magnesium; 70mg potassium; 18mg sodium; Vit. C 4mg; Vit. E 1 IU.

GREEK ISLANDS EGGPLANT OMELET

This recipe works for: Fatigue Syndromes, Bone Building, Food For Men
Makes 8 servings: Preheat broiler.

Place 3 one-lb. Eggplants in a baking pan. Pierce them all over with a fork. Broil until their skins blacken and flesh feels very soft to touch, turning occasionally, about 25 minutes. Cool, stem and peel. Transfer to a bowl and mash.
—Heat 2 TBS Olive Oil and 1 TB Red Wine in a heavy skillet over medium heat.
—Add 4 Garlic Cloves, minced and 2 Large Onions, sliced. Sauté until golden, about 20 minutes. Set aside.
—Whisk 6 Eggs in large bowl to blend. Stir in $^3/_4$ cup snipped Fresh Parsley, 1 teasp. Lemon-Pepper, 1 tsp. crushed Caraway Seeds, $^1/_2$ tsp. Ground Coriander and the mashed eggplant.

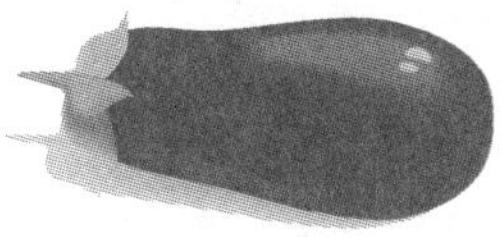

—Heat 2 TBS Olive Oil in large broiler-proof nonstick skillet over very low heat. Add egg mixture, cover and cook until omelet is almost set -15 minutes. Uncover skillet and place under broiler 5 minutes until top is pale gold. Using rubber spatula, loosen omelet with rubber spatula and slide onto plate. Garnish with Lemon Wedges.

GREEN TEA and MINT GRANITA

This recipe works for: Stress, Better Digestion, Weight Control
Makes 4 servings:

Pour 3 cups boiling water over 6 teasp. Green Tea Leaves in a teapot, add $^1/_4$ cup Sugar (or 3 TBS Fructose) and 12 Peppermint Leaves. Allow to steep about 5 minutes. Strain, set over ice water until cool. Freeze in ice cube trays for 3 hours.
—Powder 2 teasp. Green Tea Leaves in a coffee grinder.
—Process a few tea cubes at a time on high in a food processor, until broken into granules; stir in powdered green tea. Serve immediately in chilled glasses, garnished with a Mint Sprig.

PIÑA COLADA FREEZE

This recipe works for: Sugar Imbalance, Good Digestion, Men's - Women's Health
Makes 2 servings: Freeze 1 cup pineapple chunks and 1 banana.

Whirl all ingredients together in a blender until smooth: 1 cup Frozen Pineapple Pieces, 1 peeled, Frozen Banana, 3/4 cup Vanilla Almond Milk, 1/2 cup Frozen Vanilla Yogurt, 1/2 cup Orange Juice. Sprinkle with 3 TBS Toasted Coconut. Serve immediately.

FANCY HASH BROWNS

This recipe works for: Fatigue Syndromes, Men's Health, Immune Power
Enough for 8 servings:

Boil 5 Red Rose Potatoes in water over high heat for 5 minutes. Drain and cool.
—Toast 2 TBS Soy Bacon Bits in a large skillet until aromatic, about 5 minutes.
—Add 2 TBS Olive Oil and 2 Large Sliced Onions, and sauté for 25 minutes, covered until soft and brown. Remove onions and set aside.
—Grate potatoes in a food processor. Add 1/2 teasp. Salt, 1/2 teasp. Lemon-Pepper.
—Put 2 TBS Olive Oil and potatoes in the skillet. Press against bottom and sides to form a crust. Cook 15 minutes on medium heat until brown on the bottom.
—Drizzle on 1 TB Olive Oil, 1/2 teasp. Garlic-Lemon Seasoning and 1 teasp. Rosemary.
—Mix in onions. Run under broiler for 1 minute to brown and crisp. Serve hot.

Nutrition per serving; 134 calories; 3gm protein; 16gm carbo.; 2g fiber; 7gm fats; 0mg cholesterol; 27mg calcium; 1mg iron; 28mg magnesium; 327mg potassium; 138mg sodium; Vit. C 7mg; Vit. E 1 IU

CORN MUFFIN SURPRISE

This recipe works for: Fatigue Syndromes, Recovery, Food For Men
Makes 10 servings: Preheat oven to 350°F. Oil 10 standard muffin-pan cups.

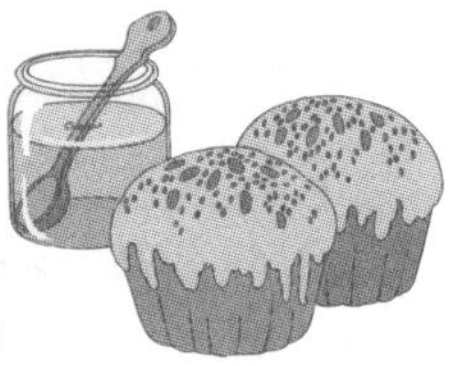

In a bowl, mix together: 1 cup Cornmeal, 1/2 cup Unbleached Flour, 1/2 cup Toasted Wheat Germ, 1 TB Baking Powder, 1/4 cup packed Brown Sugar or 3 TBS Orange Honey.
—In another bowl, mix 2 Eggs, 1 cup Low-Fat Rice Milk, 2 TBS Canola Oil and 1 teasp. Orange Peel Powder. Add wet ingredients to dry and mix just until blended.
—Fill prepared cups half full with batter. Put 1 teasp. Orange Marmalade in each cup and top with remaining batter.
—Bake until tops of muffins are lightly brown, about 20 minutes. Top with a Fresh Orange Peel Curl. Turn muffins out onto wire rack to cool.

Nutrition per serving; 185 calories; 5gm protein; 31gm carbo.; 2g fiber; 5gm fats; 42mg cholesterol; 163mg calcium; 2mg iron; 40mg magnesium; 142mg potassium; 135mg sodium; Vit. C 4mg; Vit. E 3 IU.

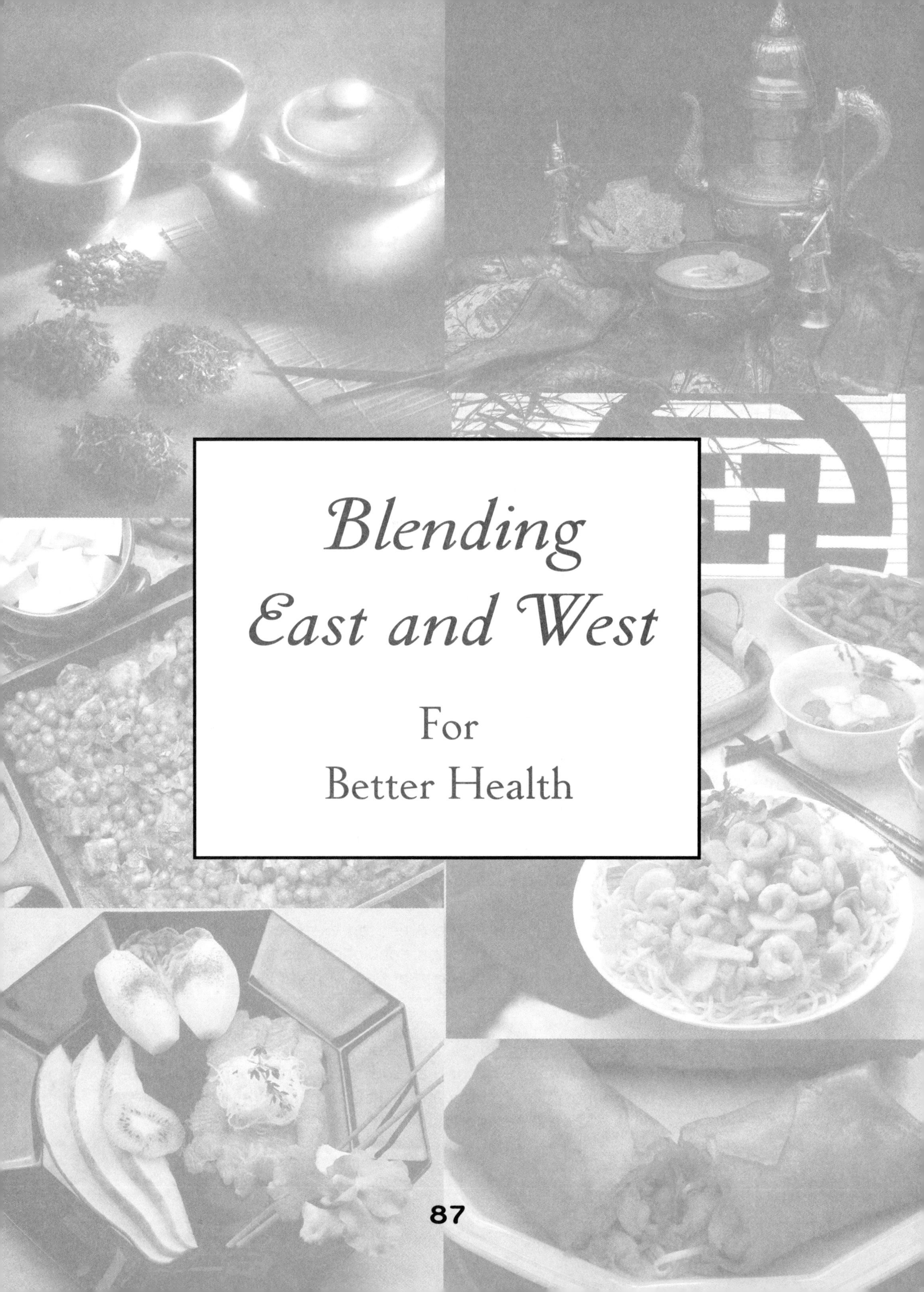

Blending East and West

For Better Health

The Best of East and West

Some call it Pacific Rim style. Some call it California or West Coast-Asian cuisine. Whatever the name, the benefits at the heart of these cuisines are undeniable. Blending Asian and American West Coast cuisines offers more healing advantages than either style alone.

Based on seafood and fish, rice, gourmet noodles, vegetables and fruits, Asian cuisine is nutritiously low in fat, but rich in essential fatty acids, and full of high energy foods. Soy foods like tofu and miso provide animal-free protein and hormone balancing phyotestrogens. Healing mushrooms are plentiful for immune boosting; sea greens naturally detoxify and balance the body.

Asian cuisine offers important support for living in a high stress, polluted environment. Blending it with the best of America's health-conscious West Coast cuisine makes it even healthier.

Asian-West Coast food tantalizes your taste buds and revitalizes your body. Light and flavorful, these are the perfect recipes for anti-aging, cancer protection, immunity, heart health, weight management, glandular balance, mental focus and beauty.

Here are the keys to the East-West blended cuisine:

<u>Less Red Meat:</u> In the American West, turkey, fish and seafood, free of hormones and antibiotics, are the first choices for healthy meat protein instead of beef or pork, which is still popular in most Asian cuisines.

<u>Lower Sodium</u>: West Coast cooking relies more on herbs and spices to enhance flavor than sodium or chemical flavor boosters like monosodium glutamate, linked to headaches, allergic reactions and brain deterioration.

More Enzymes: In the West, foods are cooked very lightly and with less oil. West coasters eat many vegetables raw, keeping beneficial food enzymes intact for smoother digestion.

More Organic, Mineral-Rich Foods: In the West, where the organic foods movement was born, there is more access to pesticide-free fruits and vegetables for healing needs. There is a growing body of evidence today that pesticides lead to cancer, hormone imbalance disorders and learning problems in children. Organic foods retain more healing nutrients (especially minerals) and are easier for our bodies to process than heavily sprayed crops.

—**What's a Stir-Fry?** It's a steam sauté technique used throughout Asia, which is far more healthful than traditional American frying. Stir-frying does wonderful things to food, especially vegetables. It quickly seals in nutrients with short, intense heat, while preserving fresh vitamins and minerals and softening hard-to-digest vegetable cellulose. Stir-frys adapt beautifully to Western tastes and ingredients.

Note: A wide choice of rices make Asian-American cooking sing. Most are interchangeable in your recipes. Try white or brown basmati from India, Texas or California. Red and black rice give recipes a distinct, exotic taste. Jasmine rice is delicious just by itself. Arborio rice is soft for easier digestion. Use sweet rice for desserts or with poultry. Use sushi rice for shapes and molds. Choose brown rice instead of white rice for more B vitamins, minerals and fiber. Or make a blend of rices for your own individual taste. I do.

Blending East and West Recipe Sections

Healing Soups from the Pacific Rim

Asian soups are a good expression of the essence of the East. Light, clear, uncluttered, with depth and unfailing good taste - like many other Oriental arts. They are high in nutrition, and may be taken as any part of a meal - as a first course, main dish, or as a light broth to clear the palate after a strong dish.

I use so many of these in connection with healing diets that it's hard to present just a few, but these will give you a good start. All are dairy free, low in fat, and emphasize body balance. Most may be used as part of a liquid cleansing detox. Feel free to personalize them for your diet.

SHIITAKE MISO SOUP with GINSENG and ASTRAGALUS

This recipe works for: Immune Strength, Men's Health, Respiratory Infections
Makes 8 cups. Use a heavy bottom 4-quart pot.

Sizzle 2 TBS Minced Garlic and 2 TBS Minced Ginger Root in 1 TB Toasted Sesame Oil and 2 TBS Sake (rice wine) until fragrant. Add 1 Minced Leek (white - light green parts only), and sizzle 5 minutes more. Add $^1/_2$ cup Sake or Sherry and bubble 2 minutes.

—Add 7 cups Water, 5 large Astragalus pieces and 8-oz. Fresh Shiitake Mushrooms (stems discarded, caps sliced). Let bubble and simmer uncovered, 10 minutes.

—Whisk in 6 TBS Miso Paste, 1 TB Tamari and 2 TBS Siberian Ginseng Fluid Extract.

—Snip in 2 Scallions and 2 TBS Fresh Watercress or Fresh Cilantro Leaves. Remove Astragalus pieces. Ladle soup into bowls and serve immediately.

Nutrition per serving; 108 calories; 3gm protein; 14gm carbo.; 3gm fiber; 1 gm fats; 0mg cholesterol; 41mg calcium; 1mg iron; 22mg magnesium; 237mg potassium; 594mg sodium; Vit. C 7mg; Vit. E trace.

GREEN TEA - MUSHROOM BROTH with LEMON GRASS

This recipe works for: Fatigue Syndromes, Women's Health, Illness Recovery
Makes 2 servings. Use a 1-quart heavy saucepan.

Brew 2 Green Tea Bags in 3 cups boiling water for 4 minutes. Remove bags.

—Heat 1 tsp. Olive Oil and $^1/_2$ tsp. Toasted Sesame Oil in the saucepan. Add $^1/_4$ cup finely diced Onion and 1 minced Clove Garlic and sizzle 4 minutes. Add 3 cups thinly sliced Brown Mushrooms (like crimini, shiitake, porcini), $^1/_4$ cup shredded Carrot, 2 TBS Light Miso, and a 2-inch piece Lemongrass. Simmer 5 minutes.

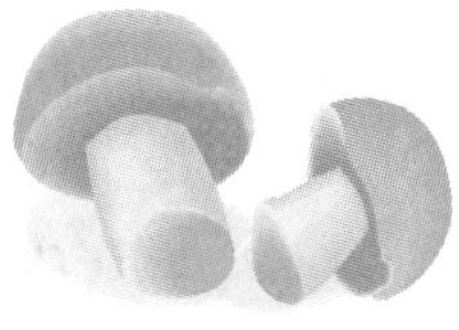

—Remove from heat and add green tea. Let sit for 5 minutes to let flavors bloom.

Nutrition per serving; 203 calories; 6gm protein; 40gm carbo.; 6g fiber; 5 gm fats; 0mg cholesterol; 29mg calcium; 2mg iron; 56mg magnesium; 459mg potassium; 649mg sodium; Vit. C 4mg; Vit. E 1 IU.

BABY ASIAN GREENS SOUP simple, delicious, detoxifying

This recipe works for: Skin, Hair and Nails, Women's Health, Respiratory Recovery
Makes 2 servings. Use a 1-quart heavy saucepan.

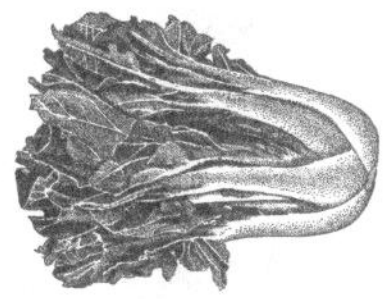

Gently heat 3 cups Organic Chicken Broth. Soak 6 dry Shiitake Mushrooms in $^1/_2$ cup water til soft; then sliver and discard stems. Add mushrooms and soaking water to broth and simmer 15 minutes.

—Add 1 sliced head Baby Bok Choy, and one 4-oz. cake Tofu, diced. Simmer until the bok choy is bright green and tender.

—Remove from heat. Add 6 drops Toasted Sesame Oil, and 1 snipped Scallion.

Nutrition per serving; 144 calories; 13gm protein; 12gm carbo.; 3gm fiber; 5 gm fats; 0 mg cholesterol; 28mg calcium; 4mg iron; 86mg magnesium; 655mg potassium; 103mg sodium; Vit. C 26mg; Vit. E 1 IU.

CHINESE HOT and SOUR SOUP

This recipe works for: Immune Building, Weight Control, High Blood Pressure
Makes 4 servings. Use a 4-quart soup pot.

Heat 4 cups Organic Chicken Broth. Sliver and add 2 Chicken Breast Halves, with skin removed. —Add 1 Onion, sliced and a 1-inch piece Ginger Root, peeled and sliced.

—Soak 6 dry Shiitake Mushrooms in $^1/_2$ cup water til soft; then sliver and discard stems. Add mushrooms and soaking water to broth and simmer 15 minutes.

—Add 1 TB Tamari Sauce, 3 TBS Seasoned Rice Vinegar and 2 TBS Sake or Dry Sherry.

—Add 1 TB Hoisin Sauce and $^1/_8$ teasp. Sambal Hot Chili Paste. Simmer 10 minutes.

—Add $^1/_2$ cup canned Bamboo Shoots, slivered and 2 4-oz. cakes Tofu, diced.

—Beat 3 Eggs in a bowl. Slowly add the eggs in a thin stream to the simmering soup. Gently swirl egg stream. Thinly slice and add $^1/_2$ cup Scallions. Serve hot.

Nutrition per serving; 257 calories; 24gm protein; 14gm carbo.; 3g fiber; 11 gm fats; 180 mg cholesterol; 113mg calcium; 5mg iron; 90mg magnesium; 705mg potassium; 1018mg sodium; Vit. C 6mg; Vit. E 1 IU.

FLUID FLUSHING SOUP Get ingredients from your health food store

This recipe works for: Bladder-Kidney Illness, Weight Loss, High Blood Pressure
Makes 2 servings. Use a 1-quart pot.

For this nutrient-rich broth, wash $^1/_4$ Daikon (Japanese white radish) with leaves, 1 small Carrot, and $^1/_2$ small Burdock Root and 1 large piece dry Astragalus Root. Cut in large pieces. Leave skin on. Place in pot. Add water to cover all vegetables.

—Soak 2 dry Shiitake Mushrooms in $^1/_2$ cup water til soft; then sliver and discard stems. Add mushrooms and soaking water to soup.

—Bring to boil, then cover and simmer for one hour. Strain; add 1 teasp. Bragg's Liquid Aminos if desired and serve hot.

CANCER FIGHTING SOUP Especially good after chemotherapy

This recipe works for: Immune Breakdown Diseases, Cancerous Tumors
Makes 12 servings. Use a gallon pot. Store in the fridge for easy re-use.

Fill the soup pot with 4 qts. Water, 10 Astragalus Sticks and $^1/_4$ cup Pearl Barley.

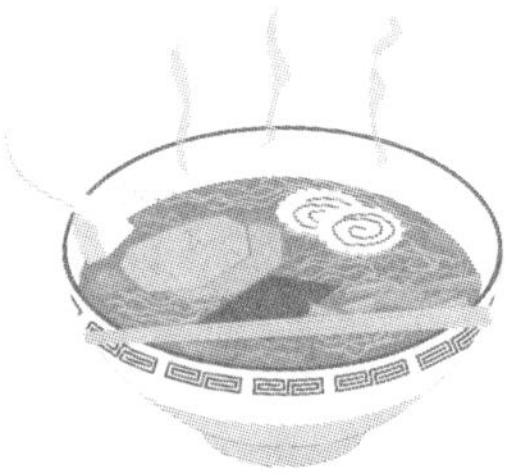

—Soak 10 dry Shiitake Mushrooms in $^1/_2$ cup water til soft; then sliver and discard stems. Add mushrooms and soaking water to soup. Simmer 15 minutes.

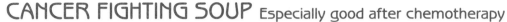

—Add 1 cup each: diced Carrots, diced Beets, diced Yams, diced Broccoli Stems. Simmer for 30 minutes. Remove from heat. Discard Astragalus pieces.

—Stir in 1 dropperful each: Reishi Mushroom extract, Siberian Ginseng extract. Add 1 TB Barley Grass Powder. Eat hot.

MUSHROOM HEAVEN SOUP

This recipe works for: Recuperation and Recovery, Cancers, Infections
For 4 to 6 servings: Use a heavy bottom 4 quart pot.

Dice 1 bunch Scallions and set aside. Remove lower woody stems from 1 bunch or bag of fresh or canned Enoki Mushroom and set aside.

—Soak 8 dry Shiitake Mushrooms in 1 cup water til soft; then sliver and discard stems. Stir 1 TB. Kuzu or Arrowroot into reserved mushroom soaking water. Add to mushrooms, stir to coat and set aside.

Sizzle 1 TB fresh grated Ginger and 1 TB fine minced Garlic in 2 TBS Peanut Oil until fragrant. Add 8-oz.sliced Button Mushrooms and sauté for 5 minutes.

—Add 6 cups Miso Broth and heat gently. Add 2 TBS Tamari, $^1/_4$ cup Sherry or Sake, 3 TB Brown Rice Vinegar, 2 teasp. Honey, and $^1/_2$ teasp. Black Pepper.

—Add one small can sliced Water Chestnuts, the Enoki Mushrooms and the Shiitake mushrooms and soaking water to soup. Simmer 10 minutes.

—Ladle into serving bowls. Top with scallions and small cubes of Soy Cheese.

Nutrition per serving; 163 calories; 6gm protein; 21gm carbo.; 3g fiber; 6 gm fats; 0 mg cholesterol; 44mg calcium; 2mg iron; 33mg magnesium; 470mg potassium; 908mg sodium; Vit. C 9mg; Vit. E 1 IU.

TOFU DUMPLINGS

A tasty addition to any soup, they add protein and make the soup a full meal.
For 4 to 6 dumplings:

Mash everything together and form into balls: 1 LB Fresh Tofu, 1 TB Light Miso, 1 TB Soy Flour, $^1/_2$ teasp. Toasted Sesame Oil, 1 teasp. Arrowroot or Kuzu dissolved in 1 teasp. Water. —Drop balls into a simmering soup, and let bubble for 15 minutes.

FAMOUS SOUP Achieved its fame through many years of requests.

This recipe works for: Arthritis, Anti-Aging, Stress and Exhaustion, Heart Health
For 6 cups:

Toast $^1/_2$ cup sliced Almonds and 1 TB Sesame Seeds in a 350° oven until golden.
—Bring 4 cups organic Chicken Broth or Light Miso Soup to a boil.
—Soak 6 dry Shiitake Mushrooms in $^1/_2$ cup water til soft; then sliver and discard stems. Add mushrooms and soaking water to broth and simmer 15 minutes.

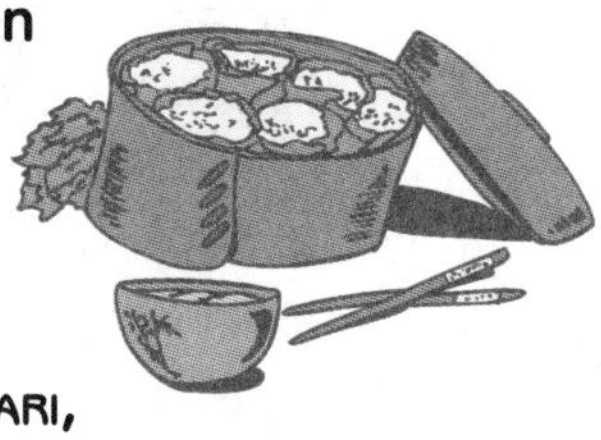

—Add $^1/_4$ cup <u>each</u>: diced Red Onion, diced Celery, diced Carrot and diced Jicama. Simmer gently for 5 minutes til tender crisp.
—Add 2 TBS Sake or Sherry, 1 TB Brown Rice Vinegar, 1 TB Tamari, one 3-oz. pkg. Ramen Noodles, 4-oz. diced Shrimp and 1 pinch Stevia Leaves.
—Bubble for 2 minutes. Remove from heat. Top immediately with 1 cup shaved Iceberg Lettuce or shredded Belgian Endive, and toasted almonds and sesame seeds.

Nutrition per serving; 144 calories; 11gm protein; 11gm carbo.; 3g fiber; 6 gm fats; 41mg cholesterol; 48mg calcium; 2mg iron; 49mg magnesium; 373mg potassium; 528mg sodium; Vit. C 4mg; Vit. E 5 IU.

Healing Salads from the Pacific Rim

Fresh vegetables and greens are a meal mainstay of the cultures all around the Pacific Rim. As salads, they offer unique combinations. But the main delight of these dishes are the distinctive spicy dressings that appeal to western tastes.

SUSHI SALAD Easy to make, with the same great taste of sushi rolls.

This recipe works for: Weight Control, Skin, Hair and Nails, Anti-Aging
For 4 salads:

Toast 1 cup Brown Rice until aromatic in a dry pan, or in a little Peanut Oil until grains are coated. Add 2 cups Water or Non-Fat Chicken Broth. Bring to a boil, cover and simmer about 30 minutes until all liquid is absorbed. Remove from heat.
—Mix and toss with the cooled rice: 2 TBS Seasoned Rice Vinegar, 1 toasted Sushi Nori Sheet, snipped in small pieces, 1 pinch Wasabi Powder or 1 teasp. Wasabi Paste.
—Pile into salad bowls and divide over top: 1 thin sliced Avocado, 3 minced Scallions, 1 cup King Crab pieces.
—Serve with a dab of HOT MUSTARD DRESSING: mix 4 teasp. Chinese Hot-Sweet Mustard, 2 teasp. Tamari, pinch Wasabi Powder or 1 teasp. Wasabi Paste, pinch Lemon-Pepper, 4 TBS Lemon Juice and 6 TBS Olive Oil.

Nutrition per serving; 342 calories; 27gm protein; 44gm carbo.; 11g fiber; 7gm total fats; 141mg cholest.; 305mg calcium; 9mg iron; 234mg magnesium; 3104mg potassium; 319mg sodium; Vit. C 72mg; Vit. E 3 IU.

EASY GINGER SHRIMP SALAD

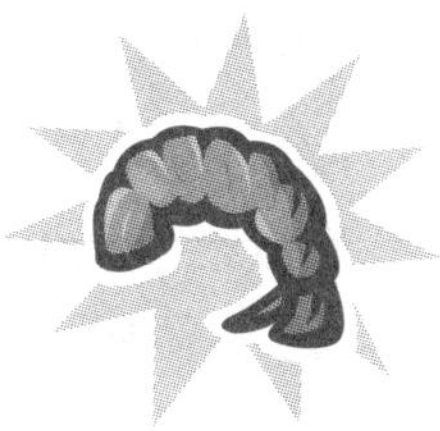

This recipe works for: Heart Health, Circulation, Weight Control
For 6 salads:

Toss together: $1\frac{1}{2}$ LB. cooked Shrimp, drained, 3 TBS Seasoned Rice Vinegar, 2 TBS Pickled Red Ginger, slivered, 1 TB Teriyaki Sauce, $\frac{1}{2}$ teasp. Toasted Sesame Oil. Pile onto rinsed, crisped Asian-style Greens on salad plates.

—Pinch a small cone of Wasabi Paste onto each plate. Dip shrimp in cones.

Nutrition per serving; 123 calories; 24gm protein; 1gm carbo.; 1g fiber; 2 gm total fats; 221mg cholesterol; 51mg calcium; 4mg iron; 44mg magnesium; 267mg potassium; 252mg sodium; Vit. C 4mg; Vit. E 3 IU.

HOT and SOUR SEAFOOD SALAD The perfect opening to a meal.

This recipe works for: Male Health, Waste Management, Digestive Disorders
For 4 to 6 servings:

Sauté in 2 TBS Canola Oil: $\frac{1}{2}$ cup sliced Almonds, 4-oz. Crispy Chinese Noodles and 2 TBS Sesame Seeds until golden brown. Remove and drain on paper towels.

—Add 2 TBS Dry Sherry to pan and sauté 2 cups shelled, split Shrimp, Prawns or Crab Meat briefly, until just opaque and firm, about 2 minutes.

—Shred into a large salad bowl: 2 cups thin sliced Green Cabbage and 2 cups Chinese Cabbage (Nappa). Toss in 4 chopped Scallions with tops and rest of ingredients.

—Toss with an Asian-style dressing: 5 TBS Canola Oil, 6 TBS Brown Rice Vinegar, 4 teasp. Honey, $\frac{1}{2}$ teasp. Lemon Pepper. Serve immediately.

Nutrition per serving; 326 calories; 11gm protein; 20gm carbo.; 3g fiber; 23 gm total fats; 57mg cholesterol; 70mg calcium; 3mg iron; 64mg magnesium; 296mg potassium; 16mg sodium; Vit. C 18mg; Vit. E 9 IU.

QUICK SALMON SALAD I love to use left-over barbecued salmon here.

This recipe works for: Women's Health, Hair, Skin and Nails, Weight Loss
Makes 4 salads: Use a large, lemon-rubbed salad bowl.

Toss about 1 pound cooked, cubed Salmon Filet (skinless) with $\frac{1}{2}$ cup White Wine, and 2 TBS Fresh Lemon Juice.

—Mix together 3 TBS fresh, minced Lemon Mint or Lemon Balm Herb, 1 cup Jicama, peeled and diced, 1 TB Lemon Juice, 1 tsp. Olive Oil, Pepper and Dulse Granules to taste.

—Mix gently with the Salmon and serve on plates covered with a bed of torn Spinach and Endive.

—Top each salad with Red Bell Pepper Rings.

Nutrition per serving; 231 calories; 25gm protein; 6gm carbo.; 3g fiber; 9 gm total fats; 49mg cholesterol; 34mg calcium; 3mg iron; 76mg magnesium; 778mg potassium; 192mg sodium; Vit. C 45mg; Vit. E 7 IU.

QUICK NAPPA - NOODLE SALAD

This recipe works for: *Sugar Imbalances, Bladder Problems, Digestive Disorders*
For 8 salads:

Pour boiling water to cover over one 3-oz. package Ramen Noodles. Let steep for 1 minute only. Drain and toss with 4 cups thin sliced Chinese Cabbage (Nappa) and 1 thin sliced European-style Cucumber. Set aside in a salad bowl.

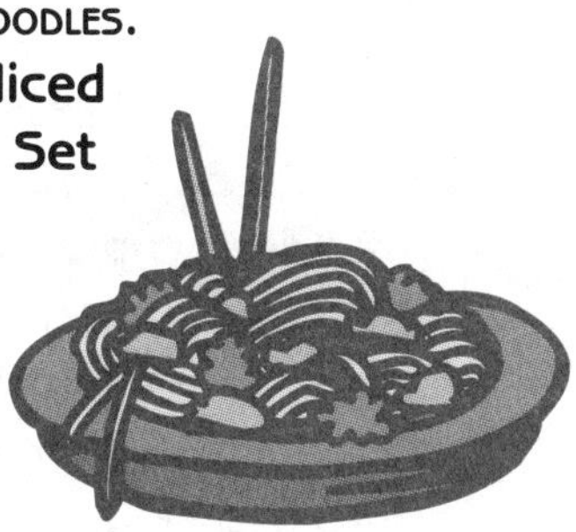

—Sauté 2 TBS Sesame Seeds and 4 minced Green Onions in 2 teasp. Canola Oil and 1 teasp. Sherry for 3 minutes. Remove from heat and set aside.

—Blend the salad sauce in a bowl and pour over cabbage mix: Seasoning Packet from the Ramen Noodles, 3 TBS Brown Rice Vinegar, 2 TBS Canola Oil, 1 TB Honey, 1/4 teasp. Sesame Salt (Gomashio) and 1 teasp. Toasted Sesame Oil.

—Top with green onions and sesame seeds and serve chilled.

Nutrition per serving; 91 calories; 2gm protein; 9gm carbo.; 3mg fiber; 5 gm totl fats; 4mg cholesterol; 31mg calcium; 1mg iron; 28mg magnesium; 198mg potassium; 193mg sodium; Vit. C 15mg; Vit. E 3 IU.

SPICY THAI SALAD with PEANUT SAUCE

This recipe works for: *Male Health, Stress and Energy, Illness Recovery*
For 6 salads: Use a wok.

Sauté 6-oz. peeled Shrimp in 1 TB Peanut Oil and 1 TB White Wine til opaque and firm, about 2 minutes. Remove and set aside.

—Pan roast 1/2 cup Walnut Pieces in the hot dry wok. Turn onto paper towels and set aside.

—Add equal parts water and wine to cover bottom of the hot wok, and add 2 cup shredded Green Cabbage and 12 cups thin sliced Chinese Cabbage (Nappa). Add 1 package (10-oz.) frozen Peas. Toss briefly til shiny and green.

—Remove from heat, mix with shrimp.

Dress with the following PEANUT SAUCE:

Mix together 3 TBS Peanut Butter, 1 TB Brown Rice Vinegar, 2 TBS Peanut Oil, 1/2 teasp. Toasted Sesame Oil, 2 TBS Tamari, 1/4 teasp. Black Pepper, 1 TB Honey.

—Toss the dressing with the salad to coat. Snip 2 Green Onions over top and sprinkle with the Walnuts.

Nutrition per serving; 292 calories; 15gm protein; 23gm carbo.; 9mg fiber; 17 gm total fats; 55mg cholesterol; 98mg calcium; 3mg iron; 98mg magnesium; 612mg potassium; 127mg sodium; Vit. C 61g; Vit. E 7 IU.

CHICKEN TERIYAKI SALAD a perfect Asian-American balance.

This recipe works for: Women's Health, Healthy Pregnancy, Sugar Imbalances
For 6 salads: Use a wok for this salad.

Poach in $^1/_2$ inch Organic Chicken Broth: 3 boneless, Organic Chicken Breasts, skinned and cut in narrow strips, until white and firm. Remove and place in a bowl.

—Julienne 1 Red Bell Pepper and 4 Green Onions and add to bowl with chicken.

—Add 50 to 60 Snow Peas, strung and blanched to bright green in hot water.

—Add 1 cup chopped Cashews, toasted to golden in the oven.

—Blender blend the SPICY-SWEET DRESSING: 2 TBS snipped Parsley, 2 Cloves Garlic, 3 TBS Brown Rice Vinegar, $^1/_2$ cup Tamari, 2 TBS Sake, 4 TBS Sesame Tahini, 1 TB Honey, 4 TBS Canola Oil, 2 tsp. Chinese 5-Spice Powder, 1 tsp. Hoisin Sauce, and 2 tsp. Toasted Sesame Oil. Toss with salad ingredients. Top with toasted Sesame Seeds. Chill.

Nutrition per serving; 229 calories; 20gm protein; 13gm carbo.; 4mg fiber; 10 gm total fats; 44mg cholester.; 97mg calcium; 2mg iron; 47mg magnesium; 654mg potassium; 337mg sodium; Vit. C 33mg; Vit. E 6 IU.

ASIAN TURKEY SALAD with GINGER DRESSING

This recipe works for: Women's Health, High Blood Pressure, Sugar Imbalances
Makes 6 servings:

Make the GINGER DRESSING first: Whisk in a bowl: $^1/_3$ cup Canola Oil, $^1/_4$ cup Brown Rice Vinegar, 1 TB Honey, 1 TB Tamari, $^1/_2$ tsp. Lemon Pepper, $^1/_2$ tsp. ground Ginger Root and 1 teasp. New Chapter''s GINGER WONDER Syrup. Chill for 2 hours.

—Place 4-oz Mung Bean Threads (vermicelli) in hot water for 2 minutes until soft. Drain and set aside.

—Into a large bowl: shred $^1/_2$ Head Lettuce (about 4 cups). Mix in 3 cups cubed cooked Turkey, 2 Stalks Celery and 4 sliced Green Onions.

—Pour Ginger Dressing over lettuce mix. Toss with half the noodles. Place remaining noodles on a large platter. Spoon salad over noodles. Sprinkle with 2 TBS toasted Almonds.

ASIAN CRAB-CUCUMBER SALAD

This recipe works for: Hair, Skin, Nails, Gland Health, Bladder-Kidney Problems
Makes 4 servings:

Toss together 1 diced Red Pepper, 1 large European style Cucumber, diced, a 7-oz. can rinsed, drained Crabmeat and 4 TBS plain, Low-fat Yogurt. Serve on a bed of Baby Asian Greens. Drizzle with Annie's Raspberry Vinaigrette (from your health food store) and sprinkle with 2 teasp. Sesame Seeds. Chill in the fridge.

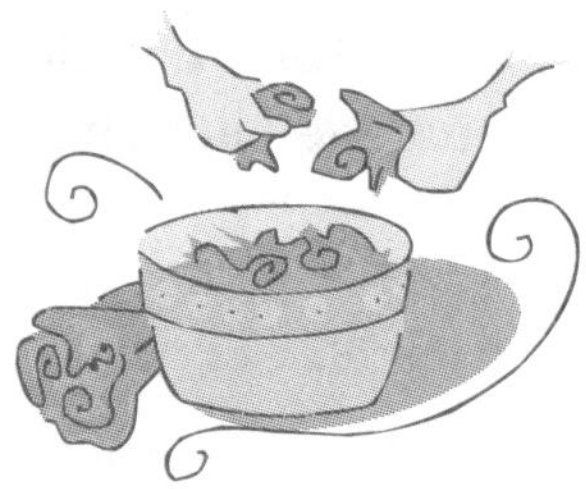

TOASTED ALMOND - GREEN RICE SALAD Loaded with EFA's.

This recipe works for: Women's Health, Bone Building, Brain Boosting, Kid's Health
Makes 6 large servings:

Oven toast $^1/_3$ cup sliced ALMONDS in a 300° oven. Set aside.
—Pan roast 1 cup BROWN RICE until fragrant. Add 2 cups WATER. Bring to a rapid boil. Cover, reduce heat and simmer until water is absorbed, about 30 minutes. Fluff with a fork and chill.
—Wash and mince 6 cups BABY SPINACH and 6 GREEN ONIONS. Mix greens and onion with rice. Mix in 2 TBS SOY BACON BITS. Season with LEMON PEPPER and DULSE GRANULES.
—Mix the ALMOND DRESSING in a bowl and pour over: 5 TBS CANOLA OIL, 4 TBS BALSAMIC VINEGAR, 1 TB HONEY or 2 pinches STEVIA LEAF, and 1 TB DIJON MUSTARD.

Nutrition per serving; 295 calories; 8gm protein; 34gm carbo.; 5mg fiber; 15 gm total fats; 0mg cholester.; 102mg calcium; 3mg iron; 121mg magnesium; 547mg potassium; 1115mg sodium; Vit. C 17mg; Vit. E 7 IU.

THAI SPICY RICE BUFFET SALAD

This recipe works for: Women's Health, Bone Building, Bladder Problems
Makes 6 servings: Preheat oven to 375°F.

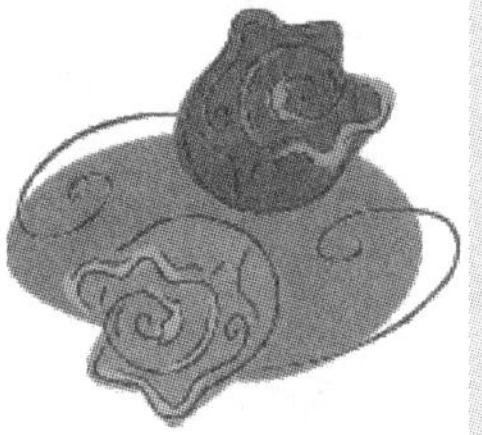

Place 2 cakes FIRM TOFU in a steamer basket over boiling water and steam 15 minutes. Cut into $^1/_2$-inch cubes. Set aside.
—Add 1 cup frozen CORN KERNELS to steamer. Turn off heat and steam 2 minutes. Drain, rinse under cold water and set aside.
—In a large bowl, mix 4 TBS TAMARI, 2 pinches GINGER POWDER, and 2 TBS TOASTED SESAME OIL. Add hot TOFU and toss to coat. Set aside to marinate.
—In a saucepan, bring 2 cups water to a boil. Add 1 cup BROWN BASMATI RICE and $^1/_2$ teasp. salt and return to boil. Cover, reduce heat to low and simmer until water is absorbed, about 35 minutes. Remove from heat and let stand 10 minutes. Transfer rice to a large bowl. Add 3 TBS BROWN RICE VINEGAR, 1 TB SHERRY and fluff with fork.
—Drain tofu; spread on baking sheet. Bake, stirring occasionally, until lightly browned on all sides, about 25 minutes.
—When rice reaches room temperature, add steamed CORN, $^3/_4$ cup thinly sliced CREMINI MUSHROOMS, 2 thinly sliced LEMON CUCUMBERS and baked TOFU. Toss to blend.
—Wash 3 bunches watercress, dry thoroughly in salad spinner or with paper towels. Place in a large bowl and toss with THAI DRESSING: Blender blend til smooth: 4 TBS CREAMY PEANUT BUTTER, 1 TB LIGHT MISO, 1 tsp. minced FRESH GINGER and $^1/_8$ tsp. SAMBAL CHILI PASTE.
—Julienne cut 3 CARROTS. Toss with 1 cup MUNG BEAN SPROUTS. Pile in the center of a large platter. Then place rice salad and watercress on either side of the pile.

Nutrition per serving; 201 calories; 9gm protein; 17gm carbo.; 4mg fiber; 12 gm total fats; 0mg cholester.; 71mg calcium; 4mg iron; 84mg magnesium; 438mg potassium; 754mg sodium; Vit. C 10mg; Vit. E 1 IU.

Stars of the Pacific Rim Seas

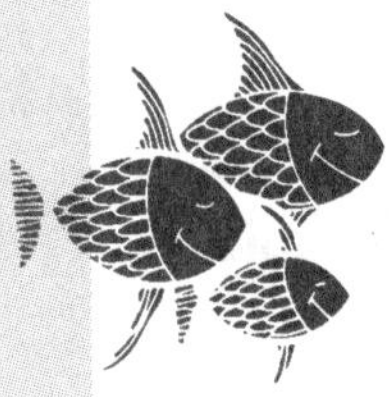

I call foods from the sea "foods for your heart and mind." They're loaded with Omega-3's that reduce unhealthy fats. They're full of potassium and iodine to boost your brain activity. The light, low-fat Pacific Rim way of cooking sea foods optimizes these benefits... and adds others, like essential fatty acids for hair, skin and nails, zinc for men's health and sexuality, and protection against hormone imbalances, important for both men and women. (See also pages 36-37 on Sea Greens Recipes.)

STEAMED ASIAN SALMON with SEA GREENS

This recipe works for: Heart and High Blood Pressure, Boosting Sexuality
Makes 6 servings: Use a wok steamer for best results.

Combine: 2 TBS Golden Miso Paste, 2 teasp. Chinese Hot Mustard, $^1/_2$ teasp. Lemon-Pepper and $^1/_2$ teasp. Dulse Granules. Spread over 6 Salmon Fillets (about 5-oz. each).

—Thinly slice 2 bunches Bok Choy. Pile onto wok steamer tray. Place tray in wok filled with 2 cups boiling water and a 1" piece of fresh Ginger. Cover bok choy with salmon fillets. Thinly slice 1 bunch Scallions. Sprinkle on top of salmon fillets. Cover and steam 10 minutes or until fish flakes easily with fork.

Nutrition per serving; 230 calories; 51gm protein; 5gm carbo.; 1mg fiber; 10 gm total fats; 78mg cholester.; 89mg calcium; 2mg iron; 59mg magnesium; 895mg potassium; 315mg sodium; Vit. C 28mg; Vit. E 1 IU.

WHITE SEA BASS with BRAISED SPINACH Loaded with EFA'S

This recipe works for: Heart and High Blood Pressure, Brain Boosting, Hair, Skin
Makes 4 servings: Use a wok steamer for best results.

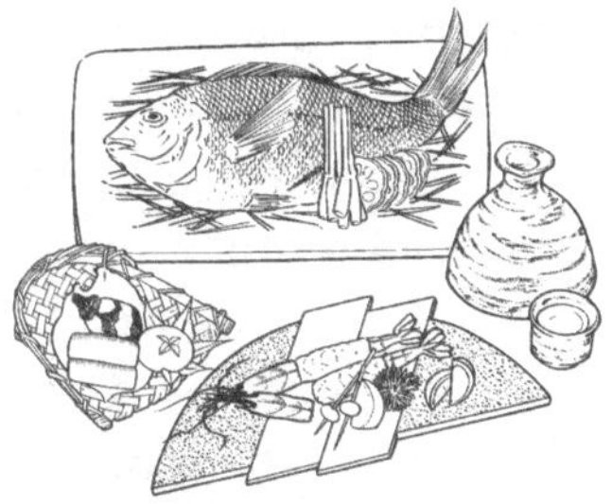

Mix the MISO MARINADE: $^1/_2$ cup Miso Broth, 1 TB fresh, grated Ginger Root, $^1/_2$ cup Sherry, 1 tsp. Chinese Five Spice Powder, 2 TBS Sesame Seed, 6 TBS Tamari, 2 TBS Honey. Pour over 4 boned, skinned White Sea Bass Fillets; cover and let marinate overnight.

—Thinly slice 1 large package Baby Spinach. Pile onto wok steamer tray. Place tray in wok filled with 2 cups boiling water and a 1" piece of fresh Ginger. Cover spinach with marinated fish. Thinly slice 1 bunch Scallions and sprinkle on fish.

—Cover and steam 10 minutes or until fish flakes easily with fork.

Nutrition per serving; 212 calories; 21gm protein; 16gm carbo.; 3mg fiber; 6 gm total fats; 53mg cholester.; 163mg calcium; 5mg iron; 114mg magnesium; 834mg potassium; 617mg sodium; Vit. C 24mg; Vit. E 3 IU.

SWEET GINGER SHRIMP

This recipe works for: Illness Recovery, Brain Boosting, Hair, Skin and Nails
Makes 4 servings: Barbecue on skewers for best results.

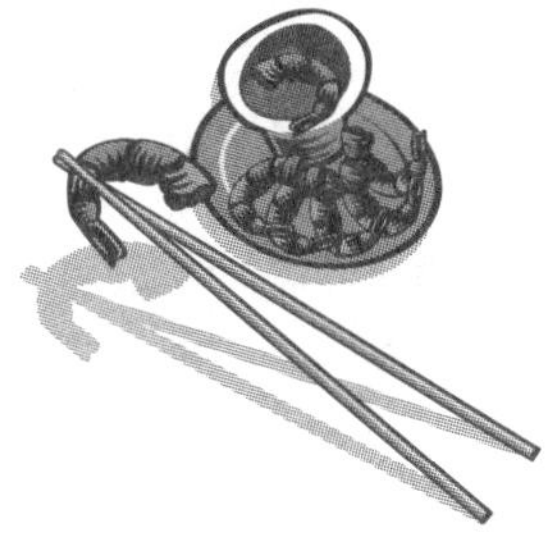

Make a quick marinade: combine 2 TBS Sherry, 2 TBS Tamari, 2 TBS Olive Oil, 1 crushed Clove Garlic, 1 teasp. Chinese 5-Spice Powder and 2 TBS fine-minced Candied Ginger. Coat 16 shrimp with a basting brush, and let marinate for at least 20 minutes. Butterfly and flatten shrimp.

—Parboil 16 Pearl Onions for 5 minutes. Drain.

—Thread shrimp on and onions skewers. Brush with marinade and barbecue for 5 minutes, basting several times, until shrimp turn pink.

RICE PAPER SHRIMP A favorite of American soldiers in Vietnam.

This recipe works for: Illness Recovery, Brain Boosting, Hair, Skin and Nails
For 8 rolls: Made of rice and water only, buy the rice papers in Asian markets.

Make rolls an hour ahead of serving time so rice paper won't crack or fall apart.

—Mix the filling: 1 LB tiny, cooked Salad Shrimp, 1 teasp. Honey or New Chapter's Ginger Wonder Syrup, $^1/_2$ cup Brown Rice Vinegar, 1 TB Lime Juice, $^1/_2$ cup chopped Green Onion, 3 TBS chopped fresh Mint, $^1/_2$ teasp. Sambal Chili Sauce, 3 TBS fresh chopped Cilantro. Chill til you're ready to make the rolls.

—Lay dry Rice Paper Wrappers on a flat surface or cutting board. Brush with water. Let sit 2 minutes to soften. Only work with one or two at a time. Put 1/8 of the filling on the bottom half of each wrapper. Fold bottom up and over. Fold in sides, and roll up into a tight cylinder. Put on a baking sheet, cover well with plastic wrap, and chill.

—Make the DIPPING SAUCE: In a saucepan, mix 1 small minced Carrot, 6 TBS Honey, 1 teasp. crushed Red Pepper or $^1/_4$ teasp. Sambal Chili Sauce, 1 TB Miso Paste, 1 TB Balsamic Vinegar, $^1/_2$ teasp. Garlic Powder, and $1^1/_2$ cups Water. Heat and boil down to 2 cups. Cool and serve on the side for dipping rolls.

Nutrition per serving; 76 calories; 12gm protein; 5gm carbo.; 1mg fiber; 1 gm total fats; 111mg cholester.; 32mg calcium; 2mg iron; 24mg magnesium; 159mg potassium; 140mg sodium; Vit. C 9mg; Vit. E 1 IU.

GRILLED SALMON STEAKS ASIAN STYLE

This recipe works for: Heart Health, Brain Boosting, Hair, Skin and Nails
Makes 4 servings:

Make a quick fresh marinade: $^1/_4$ cup Olive Oil, 3 TBS Tamari Sauce, 2 chopped Scallions, 1 TB snipped, dried Sea Greens (any kind), and 1 TB fresh Ginger, peeled and finely chopped. Rub into 4 fresh Salmon Steaks and marinate for 1 hour in the fridge.

—Grill steaks about 4 minutes per side, basting often with marinade.

GRILLED PRAWNS with VEGGIES and SESAME SAUCE

This recipe works for: Immune Response, Arthritis Syndromes, Anti-Aging
For 4 servings:

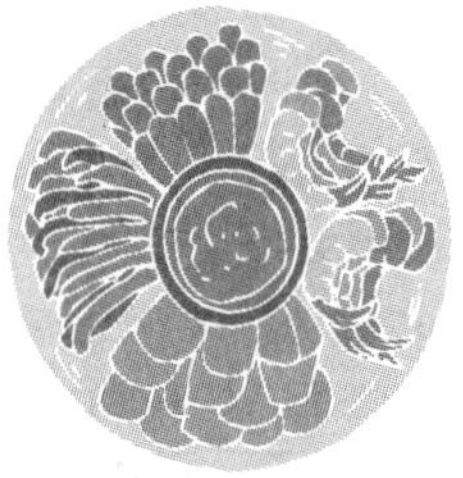

Dry roast $^{1}/_{2}$ cup Sesame Seeds in a pan until golden. Set aside.
—Make a marinade: $^{1}/_{2}$ cup Sake or Sherry, 2 TBS Tamari and 1 TB Toasted Sesame Oil. Use half to marinate 1 LB shelled, butterflied Prawns, and the other half to marinate the 8 sliced Green Onions, 4 small, sliced Zucchini, 8 fresh Shiitake Mushrooms.
—Grill prawns on a griddle until just opaque and tender. Then grill vegetables until seared and tender. Baste twice. Remove from heat immediately. Put prawns and veggies on a platter and keep warm.
—Make the SESAME SAUCE: Whirl in a blender until smooth: toasted sesame seeds, 3 TBS Olive Oil, 4 TBS White Wine, 1 TB Honey, Juice of 1 Lemon, 2 TBS fresh, minced Ginger, pinch Paprika, pinch Garlic Powder. Drizzle over prawns and veggies.

PUMPKIN CRUSTED SALMON with GINGER GREENS

This recipe works for: Men's Health, Health and High Blood Pressure, Anti-Aging
Makes 4 servings:

Make marinade: Mix 2 TBS Tamari, 1 tsp. Toasted Sesame Oil, 3 TBS Peanut Oil. In a skillet, sauté $^{1}/_{2}$ cup Pumpkin Seeds for 2 minutes til golden. Coat 4 8-oz. skinless Salmon Fillets. Pour on marinade. Grill or bake salmon about 8 minutes and set aside.
—Heat 2 TBS. Peanut Oil in a large skillet. Add 1 TB minced Garlic, and 1 TB minced Fresh Ginger and sizzle for a few minutes until fragrant. Add 1 TB Sherry and 3 sliced Baby Bok Choy, and cook 3-4 minutes. Season with Chinese 5-Spice Powder and the Juice of 1 Lime. Divide on 4 warm plates and top with 1 salmon fillet.

SUSHI SHRIMP SALAD

This recipe works for: Brain Boosting, Recovery from Illness, Heart Health
For 6 servings:

Make the SUSHI DRESSING: Combine $^{1}/_{2}$ cup Seasoned Rice Vinegar and 2 TBS minced Fresh Ginger, $^{1}/_{2}$ teasp. prepared Wasabi, and 2 TBS Toasted Sesame Oil.
—In a large bowl, combine 4 cups cooked Brown Rice, 2 cups diced Cucumber, 1 cup thawed frozen Peas, $^{1}/_{2}$ cup thin-sliced Daikon Radish, $^{1}/_{4}$ cup sliced Green Onions and dressing. Gently mix in 1 lb. cooked, peeled Shrimp. Arrange 6 cups rinsed, Fresh Spinach Leaves on a platter and spoon sushi salad into the center. Garnish with Pickled Ginger slices.

Nutrition per serving; 342 calories; 27 gm protein; 44gm carbo.; 12mg fiber; 7 gm total fats; 147mg cholester.; 305mg calcium; 8mg iron; 234mg magnesium; 1094mg potassium; 319mg sodium; Vit. C 72mg; Vit. E 3 IU.

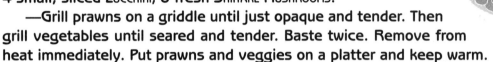

YOSENABE, JAPAN'S CIOPPINO Good with Japanese soba noodles

This recipe works for: Hormone Health, Recovery from Illness, Heart Health
For 8 servings:

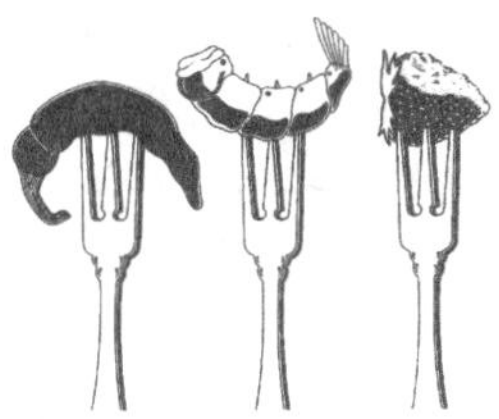

Sizzle in a hot wok 3 TBS PEANUT OIL, 3 CLOVES GARLIC, minced, 2 TBS FRESH GINGER, minced and 1 teasp. TOASTED SESAME OIL and 2 snipped SPRIGS LEMON GRASS til fragrant.

Add and bring to a boil 1 cup bottled CLAM JUICE, 2 LOBSTER TAILS, split and chunked, (or 2 KING CRAB LEGS in big chunks), 1 LB frozen CALAMARI RINGS, 1 dozen fresh CLAMS or OYSTERS, 1 dozen large, shelled PRAWNS, 8-oz. thick SEA BASS in bite size chunks.

—Let bubble a minute while you make the sauce. Mix 1 cup CLAM JUICE, 2 TBS SAKE, 2 TBS OYSTER SAUCE, 1 TB KUZU CHUNKS or ARROWROOT, 1 TB grated LEMON PEEL, 1 teasp. HONEY. Add to YOSENABE and stir in until thickened and glossy.

Nutrition per serving; 246 calories; 30 gm protein; 6gm carbo.; 2mg fiber; 10 gm total fats; 223mg cholester.; 68mg calcium; 5mg iron; 56mg magnesium; 522mg potassium; 633mg sodium; Vit. C 9mg; Vit. E 6 IU.

Health Benefits from Asian Pastas

I never cook with commercial pastas anymore. Asian noodles like soba noodles, bean thread noodles and udon noodles are a delight to cook with, and they are far superior to refined pastas for a healing diet. Low in gluten, low in fat, easily assimilated and less likely to cause food sensitivities - they offer important support during the hard work of healing! Chinese bean thread noodles (also called cellophane noodles), made from mung beans, are ideal for people looking for pasta's heartiness without weight gain. Japanese soba noodles, made with nutrient-rich buckwheat, are lower in fat than traditional ramen. People with wheat-gluten sensitivity do especially well with rice noodles like Japanese udon noodles. You'll love the flavor of the Asian pastas in the following recipes, and your body will love their health benefits.

QUICK STIR-FRY SHRIMP on RAMEN NOODLES

This recipe works for: Fatigue Syndromes, Recovery from Illness, Heart Health
Makes 4 servings: Use a hot wok for best health benefits.

Quickly stir-fry for 3 minutes: 2 sliced ONIONS, 1 thin-sliced RED BELL PEPPER, and 1 cup diagonally sliced CELERY in 2 TBS CANOLA OIL. —Add 1 LB shelled SHRIMP, 1 cup sliced WATER CHESTNUTS, 1 $^1/_2$ cups ORGANIC CHICKEN BROTH, 3 TBS TAMARI, 1 teasp. GINGER POWDER mixed with 2 teasp. HONEY, $^1/_2$ tsp. SALT and simmer 5 minutes. Mix 1 TB ARROWROOT POWDER mixed in 2 TBS WATER. Cook 2 more minutes until hot.

EGG NOODLES with ASIAN VEGETABLES

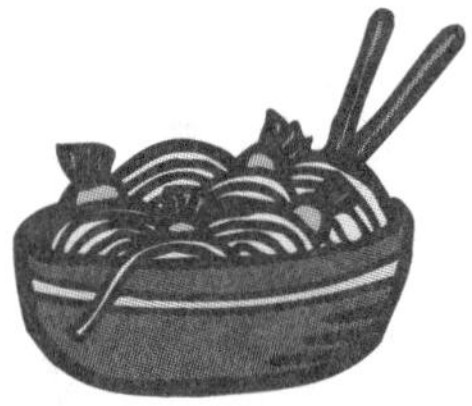

This recipe works for: Circulatory Health, Heart Health
Makes 4 servings: Use a large wok.

Cook 4 oz. Japanese Egg Noodles according to package directions, only 2 to 4 minutes. Don't let them get mushy. Drain and toss with a little Toasted Sesame Oil.
—Mix 4 TBS Water, 2 TBS Tamari, 2 teasp Balsamic Vinegar, 1 teasp Honey, $^1/_2$ tsp. Ginger Powder and 1 teasp Arrowroot Powder in a small bowl. Set aside.
—Heat 1 TB Canola Oil in a wok. Add 2 Scallions, thin sliced, 1 Clove Garlic, minced and 1 teasp minced Crystallized Ginger. Stir until fragrant, about 20 seconds.
—Add 1 cup trimmed Snow Peas, and toss just until they begin to change color, about 10 seconds. Add and toss noodles. Stir in tamari mixture until the sauce is thickened and evenly distributed. Transfer to a serving dish. Serve hot.

Nutrition per serving; 162 calories; 6 gm protein; 26gm carbo.;4mg fiber; 4 gm total fats; 23mg cholester.; 56mg calcium; 2mg iron; 14mg magnesium; 74mg potassium; 251mg sodium; Vit. C 7mg; Vit. E 1 IU.

BEAN THREAD SALAD with CUCUMBERS and CHILIES

This recipe works for: Bladder-Kidney Health, Good Body Chemistry, Hair and Skin
Makes 6 servings:

Bring a large pot of water to a boil. Put in 6-oz. Bean Thread Noodles, and cook 3 minutes. Drain immediately and cool with cold running water. Drain again and cut threads with scissors into 5-inch pieces.
—Put bean threads in a large bowl and toss with 1 large European-style Cucumber, cubed and 2 Carrots cut in matchsticks. Add 1 TB fine minced Ginger, 2 TBS Seasoned Rice Vinegar, 1 teasp. Salt, $^1/_2$ teasp. Pepper and 1 teasp Honey. Toss to mix well.
—In a small skillet, heat 1 TB Canola Oil over high heat. Sauté 4 Whole Cloves Garlic, and 2 dried Red Chilis until fragrant, about 2 minutes. Discard chilis and garlic. Pour hot oil over cucumber blend. Add $^1/_2$ teasp. Toasted Sesame Oil and toss.

FOUR-CABBAGE PASTA SALAD

This recipe works for: Digestive Disorders, Recovery from Illness, Liver Health
Makes 6 servings:

Mix dressing first: Whisk together $^1/_3$ cup Canola Oil, 3 TBS Tamari, 3 TBS Balsamic Vinegar, 1 TB Toasted Sesame Oil, 1 TB grated Fresh Ginger and 1 TB Garlic Granules.
—Cook 8-oz. Japanese Udon Noodles according to package directions. Drain and set aside. —In a large bowl, shred 6 cups mixed cabbages: Salad Savoy, Nappa Cabbage, Green Cabbage and Red Cabbage. Add 3 TBS sliced green onions, and $^1/_3$ cup fresh chopped Cilantro or Watercress Leaves. Add 4 organic shredded Chicken Breast Halves, and the noodles. Toss with dressing; sprinkle with $^1/_4$ cup toasted Sesame Seeds.

FRESH NOODLES and SEA SCALLOPS

This recipe works for: Bone Building, Recovery from Illness, Brain Boosting
Makes 6 servings: Buy fresh noodles in your produce section or Asian food stores.

In a skillet, sauté 1 TB Toasted Sesame Oil, 1 small sliced Onion, and $^{1}/_{2}$ teasp. Garlic Granules in a skillet over medium-high heat until fragrant. Add $^{1}/_{2}$ LB large Sea Scallops, cut in half, and sauté for 2 to 3 minutes until golden on all sides. Remove from pan to stop cooking and set aside.

—In a large pot, bring 4 cups Water and 2 TBS Miso Paste to a boil. Add 1 TB grated Fresh Ginger Root, 1 pinch Paprika, 3 TBS bottled Teriyaki Sauce, and an 8-oz. package fresh Linguine (Lo Mein). Simmer 2 minutes. Stir in a 1 LB bag frozen, Oriental-style vegetables, unthawed, return to a boil and simmer 2 minutes more. Stir in browned Scallops and 2 thinly sliced Scallions just before serving. Serve hot.

BUDDHA'S PASTA and VEGETABLES

This recipe works for: Cancer Healing, Illness Recovery, Liver Health
Makes 6 servings: Use a large wok. Serve as is or over rice.

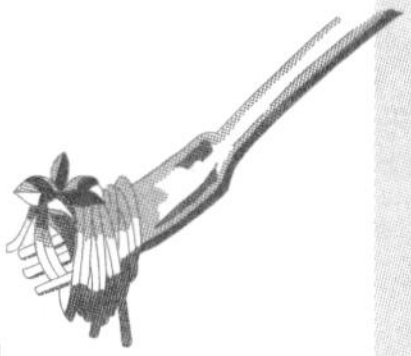

—In a bowl, soak 8 dry Shiitake Mushrooms in $^{2}/_{3}$ cup water til soft; sliver and discard stems. Add sauce ingredients to bowl of mushrooms and soaking liquid: 2 TBS Tamari, 2 tsp. Toasted Sesame Oil, 2 tsp. Honey, $^{1}/_{2}$ tsp. Salt, $^{1}/_{4}$ tsp. Lemon-Pepper. Add to soak 2-oz. dried Bean Thread Noodles, broken into 4-inch pieces. Set aside.

—Heat 2 TBS Canola Oil in wok over high heat. Add 1 tsp. minced Garlic, 1 tsp. minced Ginger; stir-fry 1 minute. Add 3 thin sliced Scallions, 1 thin-sliced Carrot, $^{1}/_{4}$ cup julienned Bamboo Shoots, 1 7-oz. can sliced Water Chestnuts, a 15-oz. can Baby Corn Ears drained, 8-oz. Snow Peas trimmed, 8-oz. Bok Choy, sliced in 2-inch pieces.

—Add 8-oz. Firm Tofu, cut in 1-inch cubes. Stir fry about 2 minutes. Add noodles and mushroom sauce, cover and cook 15 minutes until most of sauce is absorbed.

Nutrition per serving; 265 calories; 9gm protein; 42gm carbo.; 6mg fiber; 9 gm total fats; 0mg cholester.; 129mg calcium; 4mg iron; 68mg magnesium; 461mg potassium; 226mg sodium; Vit. C 27mg; Vit. E 3 IU.

VEGETABLES in NOODLE NESTS

This recipe works for: Men's Health, Recovery from Illness, Women's Health
Makes 6 servings: Buy rice sticks or noodles in Asian food or health food stores.

Soak 1 lb. Rice Noodles or Rice Sticks in cold water to cover 20 minutes.

—Combine 1 tsp. Tamari, 2 TBS Sherry, $^{1}/_{2}$ tsp. Toasted Sesame Oil; drizzle over 2 cakes Firm Tofu, cubed and let marinate while preparing remaining ingredients.

—Heat water to boiling in a large pasta pot. Drain noodles; add to boiling water and cook about 2 minutes. Drain again. Toss with 1 TB Tamari and drops Toasted

Sesame Oil. Arrange a nest of noodles on each of 4 plates.

—In a small bowl, mix 1 TB. Sherry, 1 teasp. Cornstarch and $^1/_4$ tsp. Black Pepper.

—In a wok, sizzle 1 TB Miso Paste and $^1/_2$ cup Water over high heat. Add 1 small jar Roasted Red Bell Pepper Strips, drained, and 1 cup fresh Broccoli Florets. Stir fry until broccoli is tender, about 3 minutes. Add tofu and marinade, 1 cup Snow Peas, trimmed, and 3 Scallions, thinly sliced. Cover and simmer until snow peas are bright green, about 2 minutes. Add cornstarch mixture; heat through until sauce thickens slightly. Serve immediately over noodle nests. Top with Toasted Pumpkin Seeds.

Nutrition per serving; 420 calories; 11gm protein; 69gm carbo.; 5mg fiber; 11 gm total fats; 0mg cholester.; 101mg calcium; 4mg iron; 5mg magnesium; 207mg potassium; 1140mg sodium; Vit. C 67mg; Vit. E 1 IU.

THAI NOODLES

This recipe works for: Circulatory Health, Waste Management, Good Digestion
Makes 4 servings: Bring it all together in a wok.

Cook 4 oz. Japanese Udon or Ramen Noodles according to package directions, only 2 to 4 minutes. Don't let them get mushy. Drain and toss with a little Toasted Sesame Oil. Turn out on a large serving plate.

—Whisk together sauce ingredients in a saucepan: $^1/_4$ cup Dry Sherry, $^1/_4$ cup Water, 1 teasp. Miso Paste, 1 TB chopped Fresh Ginger Root, 1 TB minced Fresh Garlic, 1 TB Tamari, 1 TB Crunchy Peanut Butter, 1 tsp. Kuzu Powder or Arrowroot Powder, $^1/_2$ tsp. Sambal Hot Chili Sauce. Bring to a boil over medium-high heat. Reduce heat; simmer 2 minutes, stirring, until sauce thickens slightly. Set aside.

—In a wok over high heat, bring $^1/_4$ cup Water, 1 teasp. Miso Paste to a boil. Add 1 cup peeled, sliced Cucumber and $^1/_2$ cup diced Red Bell Pepper. Cook 1 to 2 minutes, stirring. Stir in 1 cup fresh Mung Bean Sprouts and one 7-oz. can sliced Water Chestnuts. Heat through, tossing to coat. Remove from heat.

—Arrange vegetables on top of noodles. Cover with sauce and serve hot.

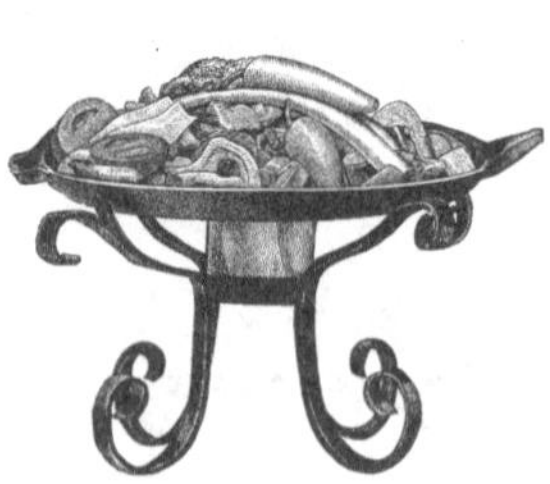

Asian One-Dish Healing Meals

Asian cultures are famous for one-pot cooking. Far more than just throwing in yesterday's leftovers, or a helter-skelter ingredient mix, Asian "hot-pots" are carefully crafted for taste, nourishment.... and healing. They're also easy to fit right in with busy American lifestyles.

VEGETABLE NABE A Japanese Hot Pot

This recipe works for: Circulatory Health, Waste Management, Good Digestion
For about 6 people (use about 2 cups fresh vegetables per person):

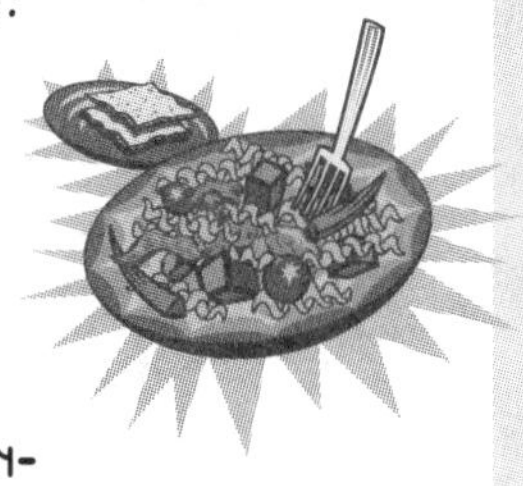

If you don't have a sectioned Nabe Pot, use a large wok and simply remove each vegetable to a serving platter as it is cooked.

—Slice a good mix of greens, like Spinach, Endive, Kale, Chinese Cabbage, Red and Green Cabbage, Leeks, Mustard Greens, Scallions, Dandelion Greens, Broccoli, Green Beans, Celery, Peas and Snowpeas, Bok Choy, Sunflower Sprouts, or Cauliflower. Place each vegetable in a pile on a large platter.

—Slice a good mix of roots and place in piles on the platter, like Daikon Radish, Carrots, fresh Shiitake and other Mushrooms, and Red Radishes.

—Cube 1 LB Firm Tofu. Have ready 1 LB fresh Egg or Udon Noodles.

—Pour 2" of water into the nabe pot. Add a 2"x 3" strip of dry kombu. Bring to a rapid boil and cook until the kombu softens. No other seasoning is needed.

—Begin to add the vegetables in separate sections to the rapidly boiling broth, starting with the denser vegetables which require the longest cooking time; boil until tender crisp. Most require only 1-2 minutes of boiling. End with the sprouts, scallions, and greens that require only several seconds of cooking. If you're using a wok, remove each vegetable with a slotted spoon as soon as it is finished. Add the tofu and noodles to the broth and boil 2 to 3 minutes. (Add more water during cooking as the bubbling broth evaporates.)

—This dish yields a large sectioned nabe pot of green, fresh and light vegetables. Serve immediately. (If you use an electric wok, cook at the table, so vegetables may be eaten continuously and new ones added to the pot.)

—Mix a dipping broth in a bowl then pour into small individual dishes, about $^1/_2$ cup for each person: use the Nabe Cooking Broth as the sauce base. Add Miso Paste to taste. Add Umeboshi Plum Paste or Plum Sauce to taste. Add grated Fresh or Crystallized Ginger to taste. Snip in with scissors very thin Toasted Nori strips. Add pinches of Stevia Herb to sweeten sauce. Add freshly chopped Scallions and serve hot.

CHICKEN STEW JAPANESE-STYLE

Makes 4 servings: Use a large wok.

Soak 6 dried Shiitake Mushrooms in water until soft and remove stems; sliver tops. Cut 1 small can Bamboo Shoots into matchsticks. Thinly slice 2 Carrots.

—Put 3 TBS Sake, 3 TBS Tamari and 1 TB Fructose in a wok and bring to boil. Cut 4 organic Chicken Breast halves in bite size pieces. Remove chicken and set aside.

—Add 2 TBS Canola Oil, 2 TB Sake, 2 TB Tamari, 2 TBS Fructose to chicken liquid in wok and heat. Add boiled bamboo shoots, carrot slices, shiitake mushrooms, the chicken and 1 cup sliced Water Chestnuts. Add enough water to barely cover the ingredients. Bubble until liquid is almost gone. Remove from heat, cover and top with $^1/_4$ cup frozen Green Peas.

ASIAN BROWN RICE and GREENS

This recipe works for: Circulatory Health, Waste Management, Good Digestion
For 6 main dish servings:

Have everything ready before you start to cook this dish. It goes together fast.

—Have ready 4 cups cooked Brown Rice. Preheat a large wok.

—Toast $^1/_2$ cup chopped Walnuts and 2 TBS Sesame Seeds. Remove and set aside.

—Shred 2 cups Baby Bok Choy, 1 cup Nappa Cabbage, 1 cup Baby Spinach.

—Slice thinly 1 Onion. Dice 1 Carrot. Dice 1 large head Broccoli.

—Heat until fragrant 4 TBS Canola Oil, 1 teasp. minced Crystallized Ginger and 1 minced Clove Garlic. Add carrots, onion and broccoli; sauté about 5 minutes. Add the greens and toss just until color changes, about 1 minute. Add 2 cups Bean Sprouts or Sunflower Sprouts. Toss to coat. Add brown rice and mix all together.

—Turn off heat. Make a well in the center and add 2 Eggs. Toss for 3 minutes until hot and set. Turn onto large serving platter.

—Mix a sauce in a small bowl and pour over top: 2 TBS Hoisin Sauce, 2 TBS Tamari, 2 tsp. Toasted Sesame Oil and 2 tsp. Fructose. Top with walnuts and sesame seeds.

TRADITIONAL SHABU - SHABU STEW

This recipe works for: Respiratory Health, Women's Health, Sugar Imbalances
For 8 servings:

Press a 1 LB. Block Tofu between 2 plates with a weight on top. Let stand for 30 minutes to press out excess fluid. Drain, slice in thin strips and set aside. —Soak an 8-oz. package dried Bean Threads in water til soft. —Cut 1 LB organic Chicken Breasts into bite size slices, or use 1 LB Shrimp.

—Slice 1 large Onion in half rings. Shred 1 small head Chinese Nappa Cabbage. Soak 8 large dry Shiitake Mushrooms. When soft, discard woody stems, and slice caps. Save soaking water. Chop 1 small bag Baby Spinach, and mix with 4-oz. Bean Sprouts.

—Assemble the stew. Bring 4 cups Miso Soup to a boil. Add mushroom soaking water and 2 TBS Sake. Add tofu strips, and chicken or seafood. Cook for 5 minutes.

—Remove tofu and meat with a slotted spoon and divide in shallow soup bowls. Add onions; simmer 5 minutes. Add cabbage and mushrooms; simmer 5 more minutes. Ladle into soup bowls. Add sprouts and spinach for 30 seconds just to wilt. Ladle into soup bowls. Add bean threads and heat through. Divide the liquid and threads between bowls, and serve with dipping sauces.

—Make up a dipping sauce and put in small individual bowls near each person's plate. Serve with chopsticks so pieces of the stew can be easily picked up and dipped into the sauces.

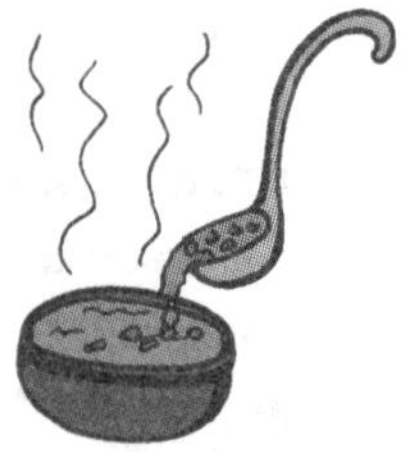

—ORANGE TAMARI DIPPING SAUCE: Squeeze 1 Orange into a measuring cup. Add an equal amount of Tamari and 1 teasp. Ground Ginger.

Nutrition per serving; 305 calories; 21gm protein; 7gm carbo.; 4mg fiber; 9gm total fats; 35mg cholester.; 121mg calcium; 5mg iron; 112mg magnesium; 494mg potassium; 524mg sodium; Vit. C 24mg; Vit. E 3 IU.

Stir-Frys Unlimited

A stir fry is a healthy cooking technique for every cuisine. It's one of the easiest ways to fit healthy meals into your busy life. You can: 1) use your own fresh garden harvest; 2) use up leftovers in a new way; 3) suit your individual tastes.

—Have all ingredients prepared before you start. The key to perfection is quick, hot cooking, and keeping the food constantly moving.

—Use a large heavy-bottom wok or high side skillet, that can conduct heat evenly.

—Cut all ingredients as uniformly as possible. Pat all food dry before you stir-fry or it will stew. Dust moist poultry with flour for browning.

—Heat wok over medium high heat first, then add oil or your liquid of choice; then add spices and heat until fragrant; then add the stir-fry ingredients.

—Don't crowd the pan. Too many ingredients stews, rather than sears in the valuable juices and flavor.

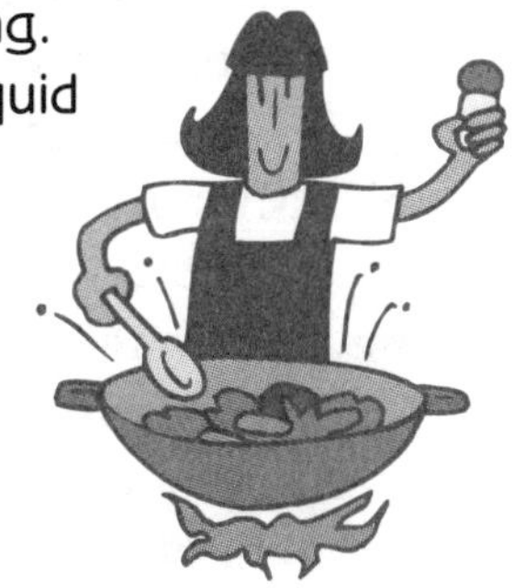

Step-by-step to the perfect stir-fry:

1: Heat wok alone for 1 minute over medium high heat.

2: Add oil and spices to coat pan bottom. Heat for 1 to 2 minutes until aromatic.

3: Add onions if you are using them, and heat for 1 to 2 minutes until fragrant.

4: Add dense vegetables first: cauliflower, broccoli, thin potato slices, carrots, celery, cabbage, etc. Toss for about 2 minutes.

5: Add lighter vegetables next: mushrooms, daikon radish slices, squash or zucchini slices, bell peppers, nappa cabbage, etc. Toss for 1 minute.

6: Add even lighter vegetables next: water chestnuts, black mushrooms, bok choy, tofu chunks, scallions, etc. Toss for 1 more minute.

7: Add seasoning sauce and stir through for 1 minute to let bubble.

8: Top with green leafy veggies, sprouts, cooked noodles or toasted nuts. **Do not stir in**. Just cover and steam 1 minute. Serve over rice, pasta or crisp Chinese noodles.

SPICY SZECHUAN STIR-FRY on JASMINE RICE

This recipe works for: Circulatory Health, Waste Management, Good Digestion
Makes 4 servings: Use a large wok.

Have ready 2 cups cooked Jasmine Rice.

In a wok heat 1/2 cup Miso Broth to bubbling. Add 1 cup Broccoli Florets and 1/2 cup shredded Carrots; stir-fry 1 minute. Add 2 Green Onions, sliced; stir-fry 1 minute.

—Add 2 TBS chopped Pickled Ginger, 1/2 tsp. Honey, and 1/2 tsp. Sambal Hot Chili Sauce. Cover and cook 2 minutes, until vegetables are crisp-tender. Mix 2 TBS Water and 2 TBS Hoisin Sauce; add to stir-fry and heat. Serve over Jasmine rice.

Nutrition per serving; 176 calories; 4gm protein; 37gm carbo.; 2mg fiber; 1 gm total fats; 0mg cholester.; 37mg calcium; 2mg iron; 25mg magnesium; 208mg potassium; 143mg sodium; Vit. C 25mg; Vit. E 1 IU.

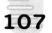

INDONESIAN STIR FRY VEGGIES

This recipe works for: Men's Health, Sports Nutrition, Good Digestion
Makes 8 servings: Use a large wok.

Toss hot, cooked Rice with $^1/_2$ teasp. Sambal Hot Chili Sauce. Spoon onto a platter.

—Cook 2 sliced Red Potatoes in boiling water until tender. Drain; spoon over rice.

—Make a sauce in a small saucepan. Sauté 1 minced Clove Garlic, 1 TB Canola Oil, and 1 small minced Onion for a few minutes until fragrant.

—Add 1 cup Crunchy Peanut Butter, 1 cup Piña Colada Yogurt and 2 TBS Water for consistency; stir until smooth and set aside.

—Heat a large wok for 1 minute. Add 2 TBS Canola Oil, and $^1/_4$ teasp. Turmeric Powder and heat until fragrant. Add 1 LB peeled Shrimp and stir-fry 1 minute just until pink. Remove with a slotted spoon and arrange on top of rice and potatoes.

—Add a 16-oz package frozen, French-Cut Green Beans and 1 small head Cauliflower in halved flowerettes. Steam/sauté until tender crisp, about 8 minutes

—Remove from heat and add 8-oz. Bean Sprouts. Cover and steam 2 minutes.

—Arrange veggies attractively around prawns and rice. Keep warm

—Heat wok again to hot and add 1 TB. Canola Oil and 1 sliced Onion; stir-fry until very brown. Add 1 cup Pineapple Chunks and toss to coat. Remove with a slotted spoon, and top veggies and rice. Pour any remaining liquid into Peanut Butter Sauce, stir to blend and drizzle over top. Crumble on a Hard Boiled Egg for a Dutch touch.

SNOW PEAS with BLACK MUSHROOMS

This recipe works for: Cancer Prevention, Fatigue Syndromes, Immune Health
Makes 8 servings:

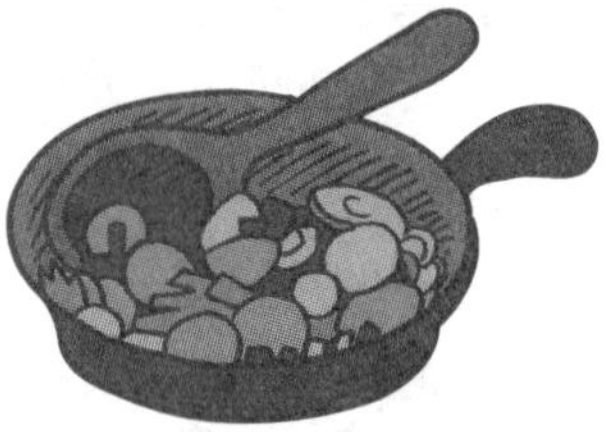

—Soak 15 dry Shiitake Mushrooms in 1 cup Water til soft; sliver and discard stems. Save soaking water. Mix 2 TBS Miso Paste with $1^1/_2$ cups Water and the mushroom soaking liquid. Set aside.

—Mix sauce ingredients in a bowl: 1 teasp. Arrowroot Powder, $^1/_2$ teasp. Sesame Salt, 1 teasp. Fructose, 2 teasp. Tamari. Add slivered mushrooms; toss to coat, and set aside.

—Trim 8-oz. fresh Snow Peas. Slice 4 Scallions. Shred a 2-inch slice Fresh Ginger.

—Heat wok for 1 minute over medium heat. Add 2 TBS Peanut Oil and sizzle the ginger until aromatic, about 1 minute. Add mushrooms and green onions and simmer 1 minute.

—Add miso sauce, and bring to a boil, cover and simmer for 5 minutes.

—Add 3 TBS Oyster Sauce and the arrowroot mixture. Stir to thicken and blend. Turn stir fry onto a serving platter.

—Add 2 teasp. Peanut Oil to the wok, heat; then add the snow peas and $^1/_2$ teasp. Sesame Salt. Toss and sauté until color changes to bright green, about 2 minutes. Spoon over the mushroom mix and serve.

SESAME TOFU STIR-FRY Loaded with essential fatty acids

This recipe works for: Cancer Prevention, Fatigue Syndromes, Women's Health
Makes 6 servings: Use a large wok.

Marinate 1 LB Firm Tofu cubes in 4 TBS Tamari, 1/2 tsp. Garlic Granules, 1/2 tsp. Sesame Salt, and 1 tsp. Ginger Powder for 15 minutes. Drain tofu, set aside and whisk 1 tsp. Arrowroot Powder into the marinade.

—In another bowl combine 1 Egg and 1 TB Arrowroot Powder. Dip tofu cubes into egg mix, then crust with a mix of 1/4 cup each: Black, Brown and White Sesame Seeds.

—Heat a wok for 1 minute over high heat. Heat 3 TBS Canola Oil and brown crusted tofu cubes. Remove cubes and set aside.

—Add 1 TB Canola Oil to wok and heat. Stir fry 2 small Onions sliced, 2 Carrots sliced, 1 cup Asparagus Tips and 1 can (8-oz.) sliced Water Chestnuts, drained. Stir-fry 3 minutes. Stir in marinade until thickened, about 1 minute. Stir in tofu. Serve hot.

Nutrition per serving; 300 calories; 15gm protein; 16gm carbo.; 5mg fiber; 21 gm total fats; 41mg cholester.; 130mg calcium; 6mg iron; 160mg magnesium; 435mg potassium; 314mg sodium; Vit. C 8mg; Vit. E 5 IU.

MONK FISH and BLACK MUSHROOM STIR FRY

This recipe works for: Cancer Prevention, Fatigue Syndromes, Immune Health
Makes 4 servings:

Soak 8 dry Shiitake Mushrooms in 1 cup water til soft; then sliver and discard stems. Save soaking water for sauce.

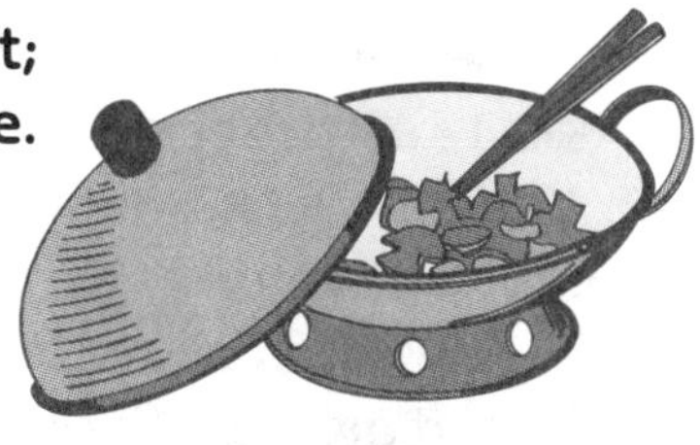

—Skin and cube about 1 LB thick Monkfish Fillets. Julienne 1 Carrot. Slice 1 Zucchini in thin rounds. Trim 4-oz. fresh Snow Peas. Thinly slice 1 small Red Bell Pepper.

—Heat wok over high heat for 1 minute. Add 2 TBS Canola Oil and 1 teasp. shredded fresh Ginger Root and heat until aromatic, 3 minutes.

—Add Monk fish, carrots, shiitake mushrooms and zucchini; stir-fry for 4 minutes. —Add snow peas, bell pepper, and 2 TBS White Wine; stir-fry til fish is opaque. Remove from heat.

—Make a SPICY OYSTER SAUCE: Pan roast 1/2 teasp. grated Ginger Root, 1/4 teasp. 5-Spice Powder, 1/4 teasp. Chili Powder, and 1/2 teasp. Sesame Salt until fragrant. Add 2 TBS Dry Sherry, 2 TBS Oyster Sauce, 1 teasp. Fructose, dashes Sambal Hot Chili Sauce, and 2 teasp. Arrowroot dissolved in 1/2 cup saved mushroom broth.

—Return to a fast bubble and cook until sauce thickens, 3 minutes.

—Turn onto a large serving platter and sprinkle with Sesame Seeds.

Nutrition per serving; 267 calories; 25gm protein; 16gm carbo.; 3mg fiber; 11 gm total fats; 36mg cholester.; 51mg calcium; 2mg iron; 64mg magnesium; 928mg potassium; 203mg sodium; Vit. C 29mg; Vit. E 1 IU.

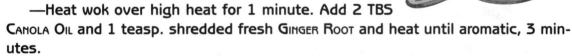

SWEET and SOUR SHRIMP

This recipe works for: Brain Health, Fatigue Syndromes, Female Balance
Makes 8 servings: Use a large wok

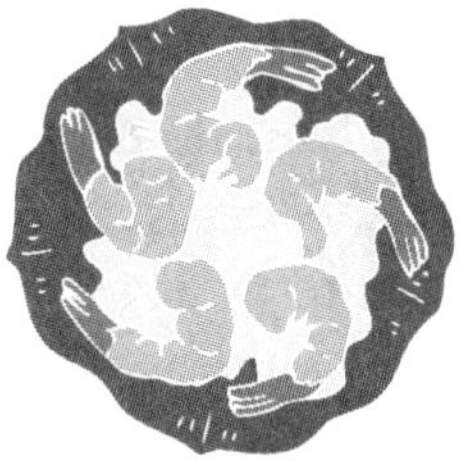

Heat wok. Add 2 TBS Canola Oil; stir-fry 2 cups cooked Rice for 10 minutes until almost dry. Turn on a serving platter and set aside.

—Add to wok, 1 1/2 LB peeled, deveined Shrimp; cook until just pink, 5 minutes. Turn out on rice and keep warm. —Add 2 TBS Canola Oil to hot wok. Stir fry 16-oz Broccoli Florets, 2 sliced Carrots, 1/2 cup sliced Celery, 1/2 cup sliced Water Chestnuts, 1 small can Bamboo Shoots, drained, and 16-oz. fresh, trimmed Peapods, until green veggies turn bright green. Snip over top 2 Green Onions. Spoon stir fry onto hot rice.

—In a saucepan make 1 cup SWEET and SOUR SAUCE: Sauté 2 teasp. Toasted Sesame Oil, 2 TBS Fructose, 1 Clove Garlic minced, and 1 TB fresh, grated Ginger Root until fragrant. Add 4 TBS Tamari, 1/2 cup Pineapple Juice, and 2 TBS Arrowroot Powder dissolved into 2 TBS Sherry. Stir briefly and pour over stir-fry.

HOT GINGER and GREENS

This recipe works for: Heart Health, Bone Building, Immune Breakdown
Makes 6 servings: Use a large wok.

Make the sauce: 4 TBS Sake or Dry Sherry, 1 TB Balsamic Vinegar, 2 TBS Oyster Sauce, 1 teasp. Toasted Sesame Oil, and teasp. Honey.

Heat the wok briefly, then add 3 TBS Peanut Oil, 1 Clove Garlic minced, and 1 teasp. Crystallized Ginger minced; sizzle until fragrant.

—Add 1 can sliced Water Chestnuts and toss to heat through, about 1 minute.

—Add greens. Wash, pat dry and slice: 2 cups Nappa Cabbage, 2 cups Bok Choy, 3 cups Baby Spinach, 2 cups Chard Leaves (or Baby Asian Greens), and 1 cup Celery. Toss just to coat with oil and turn bright green, 1 minute. Serve on cooked Basmati Rice.

Nutrition per serving; 270 calories; 8gm protein; 42gm carbo.; 7mg fiber; 9 gm total fats; 0mg cholesterol.; 173mg calcium; 4mg iron; 86mg magnesium; 616mg potassium; 172mg sodium; Vit. C 51mg; Vit. E 3 IU.

STIR-FRIED RICE with EGGS, PEAS and PARMESAN

This recipe works for: Sugar Imbalances, Fatigue Syndromes, Recovery
Makes 4 servings:

Have ready 2 cups cooked Basmati Rice.

—Cook 2 chopped Carrots in small pot of boiling water for 5 minutes. Drain.

—In a bowl, whisk 3 Eggs and 2 Egg Whites until frothy. Add 1 TB Parmesan Cheese

and season with Lemon-Pepper.

—Heat 1 TB. Olive Oil in a wok over medium heat. Add 2 Garlic Cloves, minced and 1/2 cup chopped Red Onion and stir-fry for 4 minutes. Add carrots, 1/2 cup frozen Peas and 2 TBS minced Red Bell Pepper. Stir-fry until hot, about 1 minute. Add rice and 2 TBS snipped Fresh Basil. —Add Egg mixture. Stir and fold until eggs are just set, about 2 minutes. Season with more Lemon-Pepper. Spoon into serving platter. Sprinkle with 2 TBS toasted Pine Nuts, and 1 TB Parmesan Cheese and serve.

Nutrition per serving; 330 calories; 13gm protein; 34gm carbo.; 5mg fiber; 13gm total fats; 162mg cholester.; 97mg calcium; 2mg iron; 82mg magnesium; 396mg potassium; 139mg sodium; Vit. C 15mg; Vit. E 3 IU.

5-SPICE CHICKEN STIR FRY

This recipe works for: Women's and Men's Health, Respiratory and Lung Health
For 4 servings: Use a heavy bottomed wok.

Make a marinade: 1 cup organic Chicken Broth, 2 teasp. Toasted Sesame Oil, 2 TBS. Arrowroot Powder dissolved in 2 TBS Tamari, 1 teasp. 5-Spice Powder, 2 TBS Oyster Sauce and 2 TBS Sherry. Marinate 4 organic Chicken Breast Halves in bite size chunks.

—Heat wok on high heat for 1 minute. Add 2 teasp. shredded fresh Ginger Root, 2 Cloves Garlic, minced, and 1/2 teasp. Sambal Hot Chili Sauce and heat 1 minute.

—Add in order given, and stir-fry 1 minute: 3 Ribs Celery, diagonally sliced, 2 cups Baby Bok Choy, 1 small Jicama, sliced thin, 1 cup thin-sliced Green Onions.

—Add Chicken and Marinade and stir until sauce bubbles. Serve over Crispy Chinese Noodles.

Nutrition per serving; 230 calories; 20gm protein; 15gm carbo.; 4mg fiber; 10 gm total fats; 46mg cholester.; 96mg calcium; 2mg iron; 47mg magnesium; 644mg potassium; 339mg sodium; Vit. C 34mg; Vit. E 6 IU.

TURKEY TERIYAKI STIR-FRY

This recipe works for: Children's Health, Sugar Imbalances, Women's Health
Makes 6 servings: Use a large wok for best results.

Cube 1 LB Turkey Breast Meat. Sprinkle with 1/2 tsp. Chinese 5-Spice Powder.

—Soak 10 dry Shiitake Mushrooms in 1/2 cup water til soft; sliver caps, discard stems.

—Have ready 2 cups hot, cooked Brown Rice.

—Heat 1 TB Canola Oil in a wok. Add turkey and stir-fry 2-3 minutes only until meat is no longer pink. Don't over cook! Sprinkle with 1 TB bottled Teriyaki Sauce and remove from wok. Set aside.

—Add 1 TB Canola Oil to wok and heat. Add 1 Yellow Onion cut in strips and sizzle 3 minutes. Add mushrooms and soaking water; simmer 5 minutes. Add 1 Red Bell Pepper and 1 Yellow Bell Pepper, cut into strips and sizzle 3 minutes. Add 1 cup Snow Pea Pods; simmer 2 minutes. Add 6 sliced Green Onions. Remove from heat.

—Add turkey and 1 TB Teriyaki Sauce. Heat and serve over the hot cooked rice.

Healthy Asian Style Desserts

Sweets that don't ruin your diet but do give you energy and satisfaction.

ASIAN RICE PUDDING

This recipe works for: Children's Health, Sugar Imbalances, Women's Health
Enough for 4 people:

Put 2 cups cooked JASMINE RICE, 3 TBS RAISINS, 1 pinch SALT and 2 pinches CINNAMON in a large saucepan. Add $^{3}/_{4}$ cup APPLE JUICE or PEAR JUICE, $^{3}/_{4}$ cup WATER, 2 tsp. SESAME TAHINI, 2 teasp. LEMON JUICE and 2 TBS RICE SYRUP. Simmer on low heat for 25 minutes.
—Dissolve 1 TB KUZU or ARROWROOT POWDER in 3 TBS cold WATER; add to other ingredients and stir so it will thicken the mixture - just a few minutes. Spoon into dessert dishes and let sit until ready to serve. Top with toasted, slivered ALMONDS.

Nutrition per serving; 262 calories; 5gm protein; 52gm carbo.; 2mg fiber; 5 gm total fats; 0mg cholester.; 38mg calcium; 2mg iron; 43mg magnesium; 201mg potassium; 16mg sodium; Vit. C 2mg; Vit. E 3 IU.

CHINESE 5-SPICE DESSERT NOODLES Unusual but delicious.

This recipe works for: Low Energy, Food for Men, Circulation
Enough for 4 people: Preheat oven to 350°.

Bring 1 cup HONEY and 1 cup WATER to a boil and simmer til slightly thickened.
—Toast 3 cups crisp CHINESE CHOW MEIN NOODLES in 2 TBS CANOLA OIL in a skillet.
—Pour honey syrup over noodles and simmer for 8 to 10 minutes, stirring.
—Spread the sweet noodles on a baking sheet and sprinkle with $^{1}/_{2}$ teasp. CHINESE 5-SPICE POWDER. Bake for 10 minutes until all liquid is absorbed and noodles are crisp and brown. Serve warm if possible.

VANILLA SCENTED GINGER PEARS

This recipe works for: Low Energy, Food for Men, Circulation
Makes 4 servings:

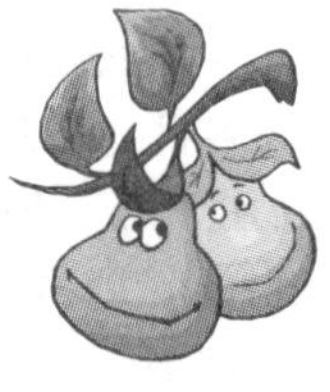

Scrape seeds from 1 WHOLE VANILLA BEAN into 2 TBS FRUCTOSE in a bowl. Set aside.
—In a skillet, bring the scraped VANILLA POD, 6 TBS FRUCTOSE and 1 cup WATER to a boil. Let boil about 5 minutes.
—Slice in 2 LBS peeled, cored, firm PEARS, the VANILLA SUGAR and 1 TB LEMON JUICE.
—Add 3 TBS minced CRYSTALLIZED GINGER. Bubble 5 minutes. Serve warm or cool.

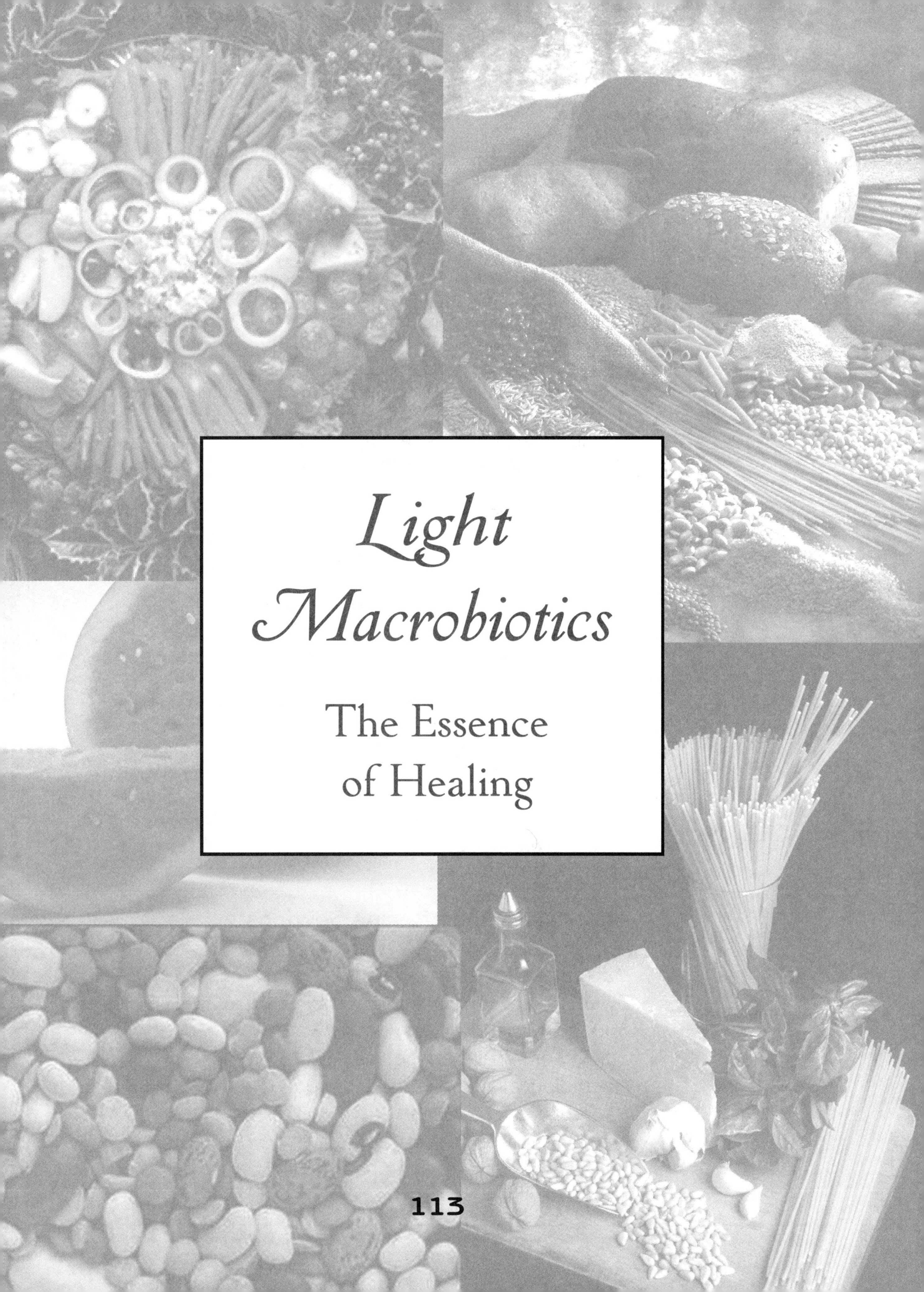

Light Macrobiotics

The Essence of Healing

Macrobiotics

A Healing Way of Life

An Asian way of eating for long life and health, macrobiotics is a 4000 year old philosophy based on the ancient principles of traditional Oriental medicine. It is popular in the West today for its success in combating serious degenerative disease like cancer, diabetes and heart disease. People who have given up on drugs often find healing success in the macrobiotic way of life.

Macrobiotic adherents believe that our health is intimately tied to our environment, social ties and the foods we eat. Macrobiotics views illness as the body's natural attempt to regain balance in both our internal and external worlds. While a strict macrobiotic diet is usually too rigid to work with today's lifestyles, macrobiotics can be tailored to meet your individual needs.

After an initial macrobiotic detox diet, I believe in a light, modified macrobiotic diet for longer term health, one that does not follow a set pattern, but rather emphasizes the principles of macrobiotics with the flexibility of individual needs.

For most people, this means a non-mucous forming diet, low in the types of fats that can alter body chemistry or enhance cancer potential, and high in vegetable fiber and protein.

Such a diet stimulates the heart and circulatory system through emphasis on foods like miso, green tea, and shiitake mushrooms. It balances body chemistry with rich minerals from sea greens and soy foods. Its greatest benefit is that it is cleansing and strengthening at the same time.

Light Macrobiotic Recipe Sections

Try this **Modified Macrobiotic Diet For Cancer**, a step-by-step three to seven day nutrition plan especially effective for cancer.

The night before you begin....

—Have a green leafy salad for dinner to give your bowels a good sweeping.

—Before each meal (wait 20 minutes before eating), and before bed: take a glass of aloe vera juice.

The next day....

—**On rising:** take 2 fresh squeezed lemons, 1 TB maple syrup and 8-oz. of water; or a ginseng based restorative herbal tea.

—**Breakfast:** have a green drink: 6 carrots, 1 beet, 8 spinach leaves and 1/4 cup fresh parsley; or have a mixed fresh fruit salad.

—**Mid-morning:** take an herbal cleansing and purifying tea.

—**Lunch:** have a veggie drink like this: 2 carrots, 2 tomatoes, handful each of spinach and parsley, 2 celery ribs, 1/2 cucumber, 1/2 green bell pepper. Add 1 TB of a green superfood like Chlorella or Spirulina. Or have steamed broccoli or cauliflower with brown rice; or have a big fresh green salad.

—**Mid-afternoon:** have a fresh carrot juice; or a recovery broth like a green vegetable drink with Chlorella.

—**Dinner:** have brown rice and steamed vegetables with maitake or shiitake mushrooms. Maitake's unique natural killer cells are powerful against tumors and boost interleukin, an immune protein that fights cancer. Snip on dry sea greens, sprinkle with 1 TB flax or olive oil, and nutritional yeast.

—**Before Bed:** have a cup of green tea. Green tea exhibits anticancer and cancer chemoprotective effects.

Note: In order for the macrobiotic balance to work correctly with your body, avoid the following foods and food types:

—Red meat, poultry, preserved, smoked or cured meats of all kinds, and dairy products, except occasional eggs.

—Coffee and carbonated drinks. All refined, frozen, canned, processed foods; white vinegar, and table salt.

—Nightshade plants: tomatoes, potatoes, peppers, eggplant; and hot spices. (Modified macrobiotic diets may use these foods sparingly.)

—Sugars, corn syrup, artificial sweeteners; tropical sweet fruits.

Cooking with Tea for Healing

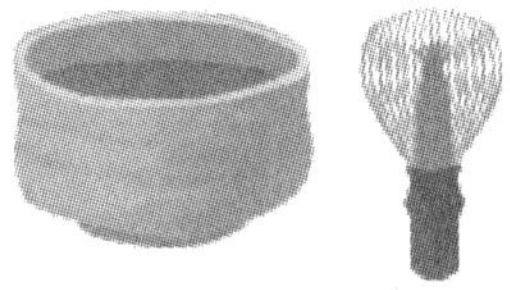

The hottest new cuisine in the gourmet world is cooking with tea. Using healing teas as a basis for drinks, juices, soups, sauces and flavoring has its "roots" in macrobiotics. Teas can add exotic, different flavors to any recipe; it's a wonderful way to incorporate herbal benefits into your meals.

Be careful though. Realize that cooking herbs neutralizes many of their subtle medicinal functions. It almost certainly kills the plant enzymes. Sometimes it's okay in the case of roots and barks, but it's the reason I'm so careful to pour boiling water over herbs and steep them rather than boil them when I'm making a medicinal tea.

The problem is easy to solve. Pick your favorite healing tea, and add it to your recipe **after** the cooking is done.... at the end of the recipe. The hot ingredients will warm the tea (but not cook it). You'll get the healing benefits and the flavor benefits.

Here are some important medicinal qualities a few common herbal teas provide. Add them freely as part of the liquid in your recipe:

—**Mint teas:** aid digestion and help purify the system

—**Citrus teas:** offer high amounts vitamin C and assist liver cleansing

—**Berry teas**: rich in anti-cancer carotenes and bioflavonoids, ellagic acid and potassium for body balancing

—**Spice teas** (licorice, cinnamon): help lower cholesterol and boost digestion.

—**Green and black teas**: offer a clean energy boost and antioxidant flavonoids.

—**Nettles, dandelion and yellow dock teas**: are diuretic and blood purifying.

—**St. John's wort, rosemary, ginkgo biloba, gotu kola teas**: for mood enhancement and mental focus.

—**Astragalus and echinacea teas**: for immune boosting, lymph cleansing action.

—**Ginseng root tea**: an antioxidant energizer with anti-stress action.

—**Alfalfa, spirulina, sea greens (green "superfood" teas)**: have concentrated nutrients for body building and foundation strength.

—**Lavender-Peppermint tea**: made with 2 tsp. dried lavender flowers, and a pinch of dried peppermint to 1 cup water, offers digestive, relaxing qualities.

ICY GRANITA made with green tea, honey and mint is a delicious dessert by itself or perfect over plain fruit for a fat-free healthy dessert that works with macrobiotics.

—Simply mix 3 TBS Honey and 12 fresh Mint Leaves in a bowl; lightly crush leaves with a wooden spoon. Pour 3 cups boiling water over 6 teaspoons Green Tea in a warm teapot or pitcher, add mint leaves and honey; allow to steep about 4-5 minutes. Strain. Freeze in ice trays 2-3 hours.

—Grind 1 tsp. green tea leaves to a powder in a food processor. Add a few tea cubes at a time and process on high until broken into granules. Serve immediately in chilled glasses or spoon on fruit, garnish with a sprig of mint.

Light Macrobiotic Grazers

I call the light, small serving, pick-up foods in this chapter "grazers." The macrobiotic way sees food and diet more as fuel and healing nutrition than as formal meals..... more a series of small grazings throughout the day, rather than large meals at pre-set times. In a macrobiotic diet, appetizers or hors d'oeuvres aren't starters to a meal, they may be the meal.

MACROBIOTIC MUSHROOM PATÉ

This recipe works for: Cancer and Illness Recovery, Immune Breakdown Diseases
For 16 grazer servings: Preheat oven to 400°.

Sizzle 1 TB Canola Oil, 6 chopped Scallions and 1 chopped Celery Rib in a hot skillet. Add 1 cup Whole Grain Bread Crumbs, 1 cup chopped Walnuts and 1 Cake Tofu cubed. Toss together to coat and remove from heat.

—Add 5 cups sliced mixed Mushrooms (I like button, cremini, and shiitake); sauté until fragrant. Season with 1/2 teasp. dry Basil (or 1 TB fresh), 1/4 teasp. dry Thyme, 1/2 teasp. dry Tarragon, 1/4 teasp. Rosemary, 1/4 teasp. Paprika.

—Make a sauce and add to mushrooms: 1/4 cup Sesame Tahini, 2 TBS Tamari, 2 TB White Wine, and Black Pepper to taste

—Mix all ingredients together. Oil a loaf pan with lecithin spray, and line it with oiled waxed paper. Spoon in paté, and fold extra waxed paper over top. Bake about 1 hour and 15 minutes until a toothpick comes out clean. Cool in pan. Invert on a plate, peel off paper and surround with greens. Serve with rice crackers.

Nutrition per serving: 120 calories; 5gm protein; 8gm carbohydrate; 2gm fiber; 8g fat; 0 choles.; 44mg calcium; 2mg iron; 45mg magnesium; 208mg potass.; 94mg sodium; Vit. C 5mg; Vit. E 1 IU.

SWEET HOT ORIENTAL MUSHROOMS

This recipe works for: Circulation and Heart Health, Immune Power
Enough for 4 people: Use a large wok.

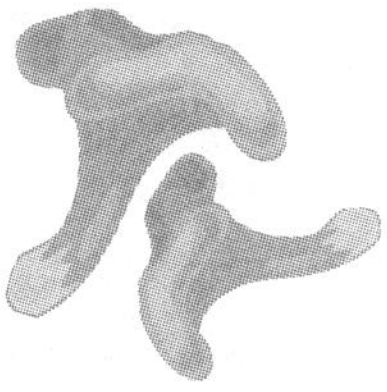

Soak 6 dry Shiitake Mushrooms in water til soft; sliver caps and discard stems.

—Heat wok alone 1 minute. Then sauté 3 cups whole Button Mushrooms and the slivered Shiitake Mushrooms in 10 drops Sambal Hot Chili Sauce and 2 TBS Canola Oil for 5 minutes. Add and toss until hot: 1 minced Clove Garlic, 1 teasp. minced Crystallized Ginger, 4 TBS Tamari, 1 TB Honey, 1 teasp. Mirin or Sherry. Add a few more drops Hot Chili Sauce. Serve hot. Mound on a plate, surround them with chopped greens, and offer a cup of toothpicks.

Nutrition per serving: 120 calories; 3gm protein; 12gm carbohydrate; 2gm fiber; 7g fat; 0 choles.; 8mg calcium; 1mg iron; 20mg magnesium; 339mg potass.; 284mg sodium; Vit. C 3mg; Vit. E 3 IU.

TAHINI DIP and SPREAD

This recipe works for: Allergies, Immune Breakdown Diseases, Sugar Imbalances
For about 1 cup:

Mix together $^1/_4$ cup Sesame Tahini, $^1/_2$ cup Plain Yogurt, $^1/_4$ cup Brewer's Yeast Flakes, 2 TBS Toasted Sesame Oil, 2 or 3 TBS Tamari or Bragg's Liquid Aminos.
—Cover and chill to let flavors bloom before serving with raw veggies.

FAMOUS SOY BEAN SPREAD

This recipe works for: Anti-Aging, Immune Breakdown Diseases, Women's Health
Enough for 12 people:

Cook 1-LB Soy Beans (2 $^1/_2$ cups dry) well until very soft; mash.
—Mix the sauce: $^1/_2$ cup Olive Oil, $^3/_8$ cup Lemon Juice, $^3/_8$ cup Tamari, 2 TBS minced Fresh Parsley, $^3/_8$ teasp. Onion Powder, $^3/_8$ teasp. Garlic Powder, $^3/_8$ teasp. Paprika, $^1/_4$ teasp. Cumin Powder.
—Combine the sauce with the cooked beans and chill until flavors bloom. Use for raw veggies, crackers, chips, or dip up with Romaine or Belgian Endive Leaves.

Nutrition per serving: 244 calories; 15gm protein; 13gm carbohydrate; 6gm fiber; 16g fat; 0 choles.; 108mg calcium; 6mg iron; 110mg magnesium; 712mg potass.; 142mg sodium; Vit. A 45 IU, Vit. C 7mg; Vit. E 5 IU.

GINGER SHRIMP MUSHROOMS

This recipe works for: Circulation and Heart Health, Immune Power
For 24 appetizers: Use a wok with a steamer rack. Bamboo steamers work great.

Stem 24 large Stuffing Mushrooms; mince stems.
—Blend the SHRIMP PATÉ in the blender: 8-oz. small cooked Shrimp, minced mushroom stems, 1 TB shredded fresh Ginger, 1 TB Sake, 2 Egg Whites, 1 teasp. Garlic-Lemon Seasoning, 1 teasp. Fructose, $^1/_2$ teasp. Sesame Salt, $^1/_2$ teasp. Toasted Sesame Oil, $^1/_2$ teasp. Paprika.
—Stuff mushrooms with the paté, and place filled side up on the steamer rack. Press Frozen Peas into the tops. Chill briefly to set. Steam over simmering water until paté feels firm when pressed.
—While mushrooms are steaming, mix the DIPPING SAUCE: 2 TBS Tamari, 1 TB minced Crystallized Ginger, 1 teasp. Honey, 1 teasp. Sambal Hot Chili Oil, 1 minced Green Onion.
—Place mushrooms on crisp greens. Put a small dish of dipping sauce in the center and serve.

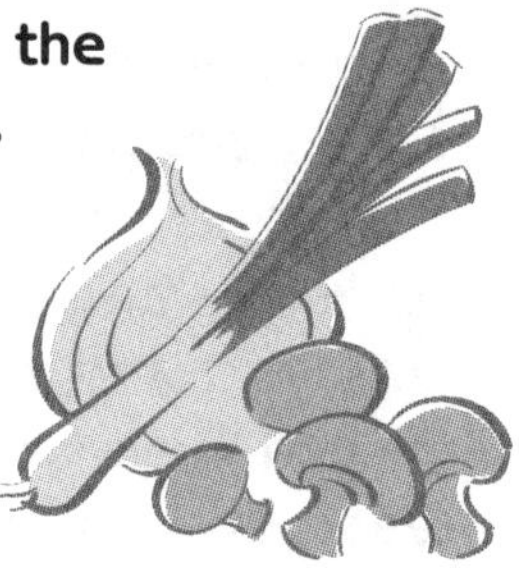

Nutrition per each: 29 calories; 4gm protein; 3gm carbohydrate; 1gm fiber; 1g fat; 19mg choles.; 9mg calcium; 1mg iron; 11mg magnesium; 188mg potass.; 66mg sodium; Vit. A 47 IU, Vit. C 9mg; Vit. E 1 IU.

AUTHENTIC TABOULI

This recipe works for: Circulation and Heart Health, Allergies and Asthma
For 6 appetizer servings:

Combine 1 cup raw Bulgur and $1^{1}/_{2}$ cups Hot Water in a bowl and allow to sit til soft, about 30 minutes to 1 hour. Drain off excess water.

Combine with rest of ingredients: 1 cup finely chopped Green Onions, $^{1}/_{4}$ cup Olive Oil, 1 cup minced fresh Parsley, 2 minced Tomatoes or 1 minced Red Bell Pepper, 1 teasp. Lemon-Garlic Seasoning, 1 teasp. dry Mint. Toss well and chill 1 hour. Top liberally with Ground Pepper at serving.

Nutrition per serving: 178 calories; 4gm protein; 21gm carbohydrate; 6gm fiber; 9g fat; 0mg choles.; 38mg calcium; 2mg iron; 52mg magnesium; 294mg potass.; 16mg sodium; Vit. A 430 IU, Vit. C 24mg; Vit. E 3 IU.

DOUG'S POPCORN

This recipe works for: Men's, Women's, Senior's and Kid's Health
For 6 appetizer servings:

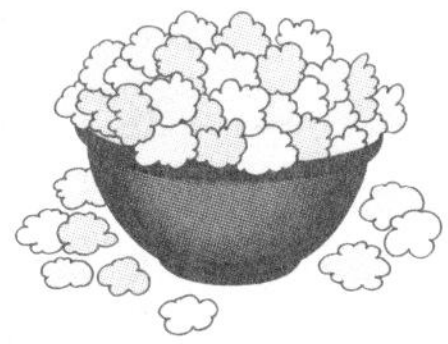

First make up a batch of hot air popcorn.

—Mix and pour over top: 2 TBS Canola Oil, 1 teasp Cumin Powder, 2 TBS Bragg's Liquid Aminos, 1 teasp. Chili Powder. Sprinkle on Nutritional Yeast Flakes to taste and toss. Top with a little Spike Seasoning if desired.

CHINESE STUFFED MUSHROOMS

This recipe works for: Anti-Aging, Cancer Recovery, Immune Power
For 20 large fresh Shiitake mushrooms: Preheat oven to 350°.

Stem fresh Shiitake Mushrooms and wipe clean. Sprinkle a little Arrowroot Powder on the open side of each mushroom cap.

—Mix filling in a bowl: 1 TB Seasoned Rice Vinegar, 1 teasp. Arrowroot Powder, 1 TB Sherry, $^{1}/_{2}$ teasp. Fructose, 8 minced Water Chestnuts and $^{1}/_{4}$ cup <u>each</u>: minced Scallions, Bok Choy, Bean Sprouts and Watercress or Cilantro.

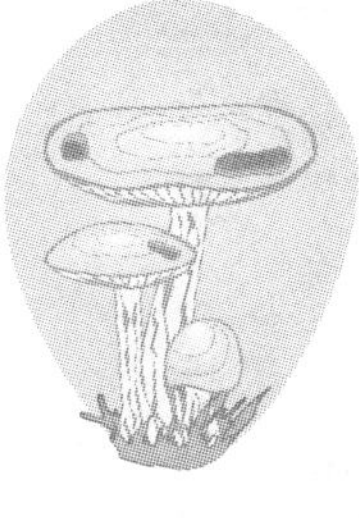

—Fill caps. Press a Cilantro or Watercress Leaf on top. Coat a round baking pan with Lecithin Spray and arrange mushrooms in a layer. Mix $^{1}/_{4}$ cup Onion Stock with 2 TBS Oyster Sauce and pour around mushrooms. Cover with foil and bake 15-20 minutes. Remove foil. Baste and heat again briefly. Remove with slotted spoon to serving plate.

Nutrition per each: 22 calories; 1gm protein; 4gm carbohydrate; 1gm fiber; 0g fat; 0mg choles.; 5mg calcium; 1mg iron; 4mg magnesium; 49mg potass.; 12mg sodium; Vit. A 30 IU, Vit. C 1mg; Vit. E trace.

BROCCOLI PUREE Dip onto toasted pita or chapati pieces.

This recipe works for: Immune Breakdown, Cancer Control, Women's Health
For 12 servings:

Sauté in a hot skillet until fragrant: 2 TBS Canola Oil, 2 cups chopped Onions, $^1/_2$ teasp. Sesame Salt or Herb Salt, $^1/_4$ teasp. coarse ground Pepper, $^1/_2$ teasp. dry Basil (or 1 TB fresh), $^1/_2$ teasp. Lemon-Garlic Seasoning. Add 2 cups diced Broccoli, 1 cup diced Zucchini, 1 diced Bell Pepper any color, 2 TBS Balsamic Vinegar, $^1/_4$ teasp. dry Thyme. Steam and braise covered for about 5 minutes. Let cool in pan. Puree in the blender.

—Turn puree into a shallow serving bowl and top with roasted Pumpkin Seeds or toasted Sunflower Seeds, chopped Black Olives and Black Pepper sprinkles. Serve hot.

Nutrition per each: 58 calories; 2gm protein; 5gm carbohydrate; 2gm fiber; 4g fat; 0mg choles.; 22mg calcium; 1mg iron; 21mg magnesium; 161mg potass.; 44mg sodium; Vit. A 315 IU, Vit. C 29mg; Vit. E 3 IU.

APPETIZER RELISH

This recipe works for: Men's, Women's, Senior's and Kid's Health
Enough for 6 appetizer servings:

Sauté 2 shredded Carrots, 2 shredded Zucchini and 1 slivered Red Bell Pepper, seeded and slivered in 1 TB Canola Oil for 3 minutes until aromatic.

—Add $^1/_3$ cup raw Bulgur, 1 cup Onion or Vegetable Broth, and 2 TBS Tamari and sauté for 5 more minutes. Bring to a boil, cover and remove from heat. Let stand until liquid is absorbed and bulgur is tender - about 20 minutes.

—Chill overnight if serving as an appetizer. Serve like a tabouli with chapatis or roll in romaine leaves. Or use as a side dish for broiled fish.

Sweet Treats for a Macrobiotic Diet

Satisfying, yet healing and energizing.

NUT BUTTER HONEY BALLS

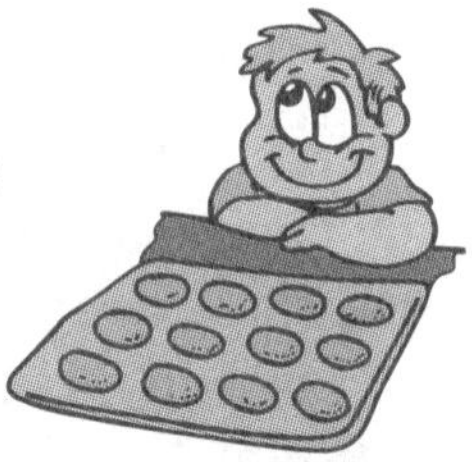

This recipe works for: Men's, Women's, Senior's and Kid's Health
For about 8 balls:

Toast until brown in the oven: 3 TBS Sunflower Seeds, 3 TBS Sesame Seeds, $^1/_2$ cup chopped Almonds.

—Blender blend: 3 TBS Sesame Tahini, 3 TBS Honey and 1 TB Peanut Butter. Toast $^1/_2$ cup shredded Coconut in the oven until gold and roll balls in it. Chill.

CASHEW DELIGHT

This recipe works for: Sports Nutrition, Men's and Kid's Health
For 12 servings: Use one 8 x 8" square pan:

Oven toast 2 cups Cashew Pieces, 1/2 cup Sunflower Seeds, 1/2 cup chopped Almonds, 1/2 cup Coconut Shreds. Blend with 2 to 3 TBS Honey, 1/4 cup Date Pieces and 1 teasp. Vanilla Extract to candy consistency. Press into pan. Cut and chill.

OATMEAL-PUMPKIN SPOONBREAD

This recipe works for: Sports Nutrition, Men's Health, Waste Management
Makes 3-4 servings: Preheat the oven to 350°F.

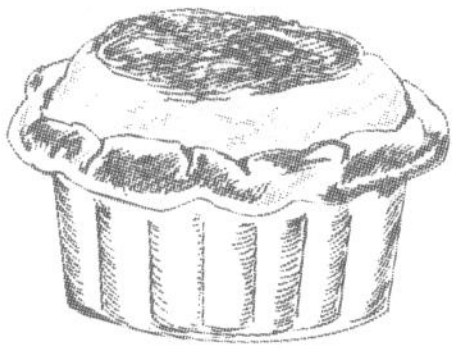

In a mixing bowl, mix 1 1/2 cup Quick Oats with 1 cup Plain or Vanilla Yogurt and 3/4 cup Water. Let mixture rest 15 minutes, then stir in 1 TB Canola Oil, 2 TBS Honey, 2 Eggs, and 3/4 cup canned Pumpkin.

—Whisk dry ingredients: 1/2 cup unbleached Whole Wheat Flour, 1/2 tsp. non-aluminum Baking Powder, 2 tsp. ground Ginger, 1/2 teasp. Nutmeg. Lightly stir dry ingredients into oatmeal mix. Pour batter into a Lecithin-sprayed 2-quart casserole dish dusted with flour. Bake in top half of the oven for 45 minutes.

Nutrition per serving: 326 calories; 14gm protein; 49gm carbohydrate; 7gm fiber; 9g fat; 110mg choles.; 202mg calc.; 1mg iron; 93mg magnes.; 459mg potass.; 125mg sod.; Vit. A 5390 IU, Vit. C 3mg; Vit. E 3 IU.

FIG and HONEY BARS

This recipe works for: Hair and Skin Health, Waste Management, Energy
For 24 bars: Use a square 8 x 8" baking pan.

Toast 4 TBS Sesame Seeds in the oven. Scatter over bottom of baking pan.

—Cook and stir 1/2 cup Honey, 1/2 cup Almond Butter and 4 TBS Butter over low heat until smooth and melted, about 5 minutes. Remove from heat; mix in 2 1/2 cups Granola and 1/2 cup chopped dried Figs. Press into pan. Cool 1 hour before cutting.

CRANBERRY CUBES

This recipe works for: Women's Health, Bladder-Kidney Problems, Weight Loss
Makes 12 to 14 cubes: Store cubes for up to one month.

Put 1 bag (12 ounces) Fresh Cranberries in a saucepan with 1 cup water and 3 TBS Fructose or 4 TBS Honey. Heat until the berries pop. Cool and puree in a blender. Scoop into ice trays and freeze. When solid, remove and use or store in an air-tight freezer-proof container. Pop 1 to 2 cubes into a cup for a healing sweet dessert.

Sandwiches

In our fast moving world, sandwiches have gotten a reputation as unhealthy fast foods.... even junk foods. The truth is they can be healthy convenience foods. With a macrobiotic influence, like those in this section, they can be healing mini-meals.

HOT ZUCCHINI POCKET PIZZAS

This recipe works for: Men's Health, Waste Management, Heart Health
For 2 sandwiches: Use a heavy-bottom skillet.

Sauté 2 small, thin-sliced Zucchini in 2 TBS Canola Oil or Miso Broth 3 minutes.
—Add and heat: 1 Tomato, chopped, 1 TB Tamari, one pinch Oregano, one pinch Basil. Grate a little Low-Fat Cheese, Parmesan or Soy Cheese on top. Cover pan, remove from heat and leave a few minutes to melt. Stuff into hot pita pockets.

Nutrition: 145 calories; 2gm protein; 4gm carbohydrate; 1gm fiber; 14g fat; 0mg cholesterol; 25mg calcium; 1mg iron; 15mg magnesium; 225mg potass.; 146mg sodium; Vit. A 230 IU; Vit. C 17mg; Vit. E 6 IU.

HOT CLOUD

This recipe works for: Men's Health, Waste Management, Heart Health
For 2 sandwiches:

Split one Extra Large Pita Bread horizontally, so you have 2 circles (clouds). Lay each circle flat, and spread with Hummus (or my Seed-Y Hummus spread, page 419), or Tabouli, or Famous Soy Bean Spread (page 118).
—Top each cloud with 2 TBS each: chopped Green Onions, sliced Black Olives, thin-sliced Cucumbers, thin-sliced Mushrooms or Tofu slices, sliced Tomatoes and grated Parmesan Reggiano Cheese. Broil to bubble slightly and top with Alfalfa Sprouts.

THE WEDGE

This recipe works for: Men's Health, Sports Nutrition, Heart Health
For 2 sandwiches: Good hot or cold.

Cut 1 Pita Bread in half. Line each pocket with Alfalfa or Sunflower Sprouts. Stuff each side with 1 TB each: shredded Carrot, sliced Cucumber, chopped Red Bell Pepper, chopped Tomato, toasted Sunflower Seeds, and 1 slice Red Onion. Top with grated Soy Parmesan Cheese or light Lemon-Mayonnaise.

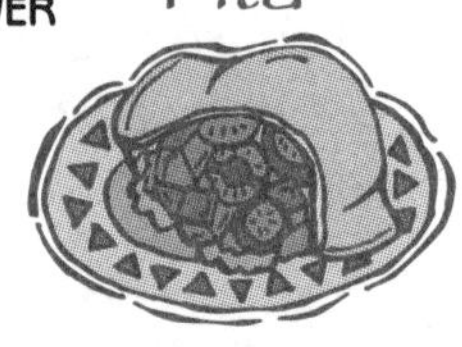

Nutrition per each: 126 calories; 5gm protein; 17gm carbohydrate; 3gm fiber; 5g fat; 0mg cholesterol; 22mg calcium; 2mg iron; 54mg magnes.; 202mg potass.; 124mg sodium; Vit. A 1185 IU; Vit. C 19mg; Vit. E 7 IU.

TERIYAKI MUSHROOM MELT

This recipe works for: Men's Health, Sports Nutrition, Heart Health
For 2 open-faced sandwiches: Use a large skillet.

Stem 1 cup fresh cleaned Shiitake Mushrooms. Sizzle with $^1/_4$ teasp. Garlic-Lemon Seasoning and $^1/_4$ teasp. Ginger Powder in 1 TB hot Canola Oil until aromatic.

—Add 2 teasp. Tamari, 1 teasp. snipped Sea Greens (like dry Wakame or Dulse), and 1 teasp. Honey. Reduce heat to low and simmer for 2 minutes.

—Pile onto 2 pieces of Whole Grain Toast. Sprinkle with 2 chopped Scallions, and some grated Parmesan or Soy Cheese. Run briefly under broiler to melt. Serve hot.

Nutrition per serving: 209 calories; 6gm protein; 31gm carbohydrate; 4gm fiber; 9g fat; 0mg choles.; 65mg calcium; 2mg iron; 47mg magnesium; 266mg potass.; 275mg sodium; Vit. A 55 IU; Vit. C 6mg; Vit. E 3 IU.

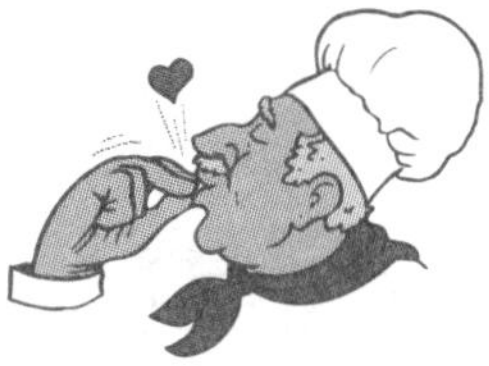

Soups for a Macrobiotic Diet

Soups are a very important part of a macrobiotic diet. They're used as healing teas by an herbalist - for quick energy and nourishment with little cost or drag on system resources. Macrobiotic influenced soups are generally simple, full of vegetables and seasoned with healing spices and herbs.

GREEN GINGER SOUP

Making this delicate healing broth from scratch takes a little time, but it makes all the difference, and the soup is so delicious.

This recipe works for: Detoxification, Heart and Circulation, Arthritis
For 10 bowls: Use a large soup pot.

Make the ginger broth: sizzle 6 minced Cloves Garlic, 1 large chopped Onion and 6 slices fresh Ginger minced, and 1 teasp. Sesame Salt in 2 TBS Canola Oil. Add 7 cups Water, 2 to 3 TBS Miso Paste; and 8 dry Shiitake Mushroom Caps (break off and discard woody stems). Partially cover and simmer about 45 minutes until aromatic.

—Add 1 small can sliced Water Chestnuts, 2 cakes Firm Tofu (8-oz.) in cubes and 2 TBS Tamari and 1 bunch Baby Bok Choy sliced. Partially cover and simmer 5 minutes.

—Add 4 chopped Scallions, 4-oz. fresh, trimmed Snow Peas, and 1 cup frozen Peas. Simmer briefly until everything is hot, and fragrant. Put in individual soup bowls. Drizzle drops of Brown Rice Vinegar and Toasted Sesame Oil over top of each bowl, and snip on some Green Onion tops.

Nutrition: 125 calories; 7gm protein; 12gm carbohydrate; 3gm fiber; 6g fat; 0mg choles.; 93mg calcium; 3mg iron; 40mg magnesium; 281mg potass.; 323mg sodium; Vit. A 370 IU; Vit. C 15mg; Vit. E 1 IU.

NOURISHING LENTIL SOUP with DEEP GREENS

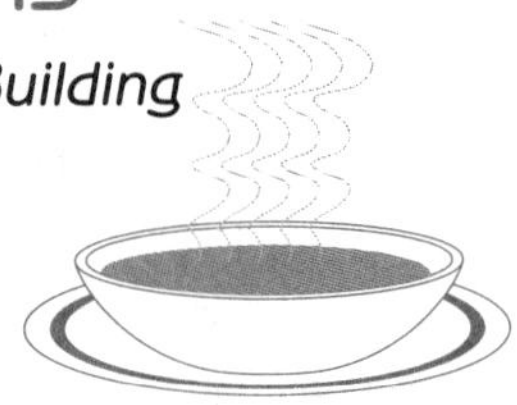

This recipe works for: *Cancer Protection, Sports Nutrition, Bone Building*
For 6 bowls: Use a heavy-bottomed soup pot.

Heat 2 TBS Canola Oil. Sizzle 1 Onion, chopped, 3 Garlic Cloves, minced, and 1 large Carrot, sliced, until soft, about 10 minutes.

—Add 6 cups Miso Broth, 1 cup Lentils, 2 large fresh Tomatoes, chopped (or one 14-oz. can Corn), 3 Sprigs Fresh Thyme, and 1 Bay Leaf and bring to boil. Reduce heat to low and simmer, partially covered, for 20 minutes.

—Stir in 3 cups sliced deep Greens, like Kale, Spinach, Endive or Collards. Cook until greens are wilted and lentils are tender. Remove thyme branches and bay leaf. Season with Herb Salt to taste and dashes of Balsamic Vinegar. Serve immediately.

Nutrition per serving: 230 calories; 14gm protein; 33gm carbohydrate; 8gm fiber; 6g fat; 0mg choles.; 101mg calcium; 4mg iron; 65mg magnes.; 684mg potass.; 367mg sodium; Vit. A 3400 IU, Vit. C 62mg; Vit. E 3 IU.

CARROT and LEMON SOUP Loaded with vitamin A.

This recipe works for: *Hair, Skin and Nails, Respiratory Infections, Liver Health*
For 6 to 8 servings:

Sizzle 1 chopped Onion and 1 Clove Garlic minced, in 4 TBS Onion Broth for 5 minutes. Add 2 TBS Canola Oil and stir fry $1\frac{1}{2}$ LBS thin sliced Carrots, 1 Crookneck Squash, 3 sliced Tomatoes, $\frac{1}{4}$ cup fresh snipped Basil Leaves (or 2 TBS dry), 2 teasp. Lemon-Pepper and 1 teasp. snipped fresh Lemon Mint (or $\frac{1}{2}$ teasp. dry).

—Add 4 cups Vegetable Stock; bring to a boil, reduce heat and simmer for 30 minutes. Remove from heat. Puree soup in the blender. Add back to the pot with 1 cup Plain Yogurt and $\frac{1}{4}$ teasp. Sambal Hot Chili Sauce. Heat 5 minutes and ladle in $\frac{1}{4}$ cup Lemon Juice. Top with snipped Cilantro Leaves and thin Lemon Slices. Serve hot.

SPRING-TONIC GARLIC BROTH

This recipe works for: *Heart Health, Respiratory Infections, Liver and Organ Health*
Makes 4 servings: Use a heavy saucepan.

Mince cloves of 2 Heads Garlic. Sizzle in the pot for 5 minutes with 2 TBS Olive Oil, 1 chopped Onion, $\frac{1}{2}$ tsp. dried Sage, $\frac{1}{2}$ tsp. Curry Powder, and a pinch of Saffron.

—Add 6 cups Water and bring to a boil. Add 1 Bay Leaf, 2 stalks Celery, chopped, and 2 fresh Sage Sprigs. Lower heat and simmer 20 minutes. Remove bay leaf and sage sprigs. Remove from heat and let cool slightly. Purée broth and vegetables in a blender or food processor. Season with Herb Salt. Snip in 8 sprigs Fresh Parsley.

Nutrition per serving: 108 calories; 3gm protein; 13gm carbohydrate; 2gm fiber; 5g fat; 0mg choles.; 92mg calcium; 1mg iron; 20mg magnes.; 244mg potass.; 158mg sodium; Vit. A 105 IU, Vit. C 15mg; Vit. E 1 IU.

HOT and SOUR SOUP

This recipe works for: Cancer Protection, Immune Breakdown Diseases, Liver Health
For 6 servings: Use a heavy soup pot.

Soak 6 Shiitake Mushrooms in 1/2 cup water. Reserve soaking water. Sliver mushroom caps and discard woody stems. Set aside.

—In the soup pot, sizzle for 5 minutes 1 teasp Garlic Granules, 1 teasp. Honey, 1 teasp. Toasted Sesame Oil, 1 TB Canola Oil, 2 TBS Brown Rice Vinegar, 2 TBS Teriyaki Sauce, 1/2 teasp. Sesame Salt and 1/2 teasp. Pepper. Add 4 cups Water, 4 TBS Miso Paste and the mushroom soaking liquid. Bring to boil, reduce heat and add 2 cakes cubed Tofu (8-oz.), the shiitake mushrooms, and 1 teasp. Arrowroot Powder dissolved in 1 TB Water. Simmer 5 minutes. Add 3 Green Onions, chopped. Serve hot.

Nutrition per serving: 107 calories; 5gm protein; 11gm carbohydrate; 2gm fiber; 5g fat; 0mg choles.; 61mg calcium; 3mg iron; 55mg magnesium; 183mg potass.; 294mg sodium; Vit. A 47 IU, Vit. C 3mg; Vit. E 1 IU.

LENTILSTRONE

This recipe works for: Men's Health, Immune Power, Overcoming Addictions
For 8 servings:

Sizzle in the soup pot for 5 minutes: 2 TBS Olive Oil, 12 minced Cloves Garlic, 2 TBS. Light Miso, 1/2 teasp. Cumin Seeds, 1/2 teasp. dry Thyme, 1/2 teasp. Lemon-Pepper, 1 teasp. GREAT 28 MIX (pg. 487) or Herb Seasoning Salt.

—Bring 8 cups Water or Vegetable Stock to a boil in a large soup pot. Add 1 cup rinsed Lentils and 1 large Red Onion, chopped. Cook for 30 minutes.

—Add 3 Carrots diced, 2 Zucchini diced, 2 Stalks Celery diced, 2 cups chopped Cabbage, 2 cups chopped Bok Choy and 1 cup sliced Swiss Chard. Simmer 5 minutes. Add 4 chopped Green Onions, 1 cup frozen Peas, 1 cup frozen Corn, and 1 chopped Tomato (optional). Remove from heat. Add 1/3 cup minced fresh Basil (or 3 teasp. dry), 2 teasp. Dill Weed and 3 TBS snipped fresh Parsley. Cover 5 minutes. Serve hot.

Nutrition: 194 calories; 11gm protein; 31gm carbohydrate; 7gm fiber; 4g fat; 0mg choles.; 96mg calcium; 2mg iron; 52mg magnesium; 643mg potass.; 135mg sodium; Vit. A 4400 IU, Vit. C 36mg; Vit. E 1 IU.

HERBAL IMMUNE SOUP Good for chemotherapy-radiation recovery

This recipe works for: Cancer Protection, Immune Power, Women's Problems
For 8 servings: May be taken hot or cold.

Simmer for 1 hour: 8 cups Water, 8 TBS Miso Paste, 2-oz. Astragalus Bark pieces, 1-oz. dried Shiitake Mushroom Caps, 1-oz. Dioscorea pieces (Wild Yam), 1 sliced Carrot, 1 sliced Yam, 1/2 cup Brown Rice. Discard herb pieces.

—Add 1 teasp. Toasted Sesame Oil, 2 TBS Tamari.

BEAN and VEGETABLE SOUP

Soak beans overnight before you start.

This recipe works for: Men's Problems, Recovery, Energy

For 6 servings: Use a big soup pot. Serve hot

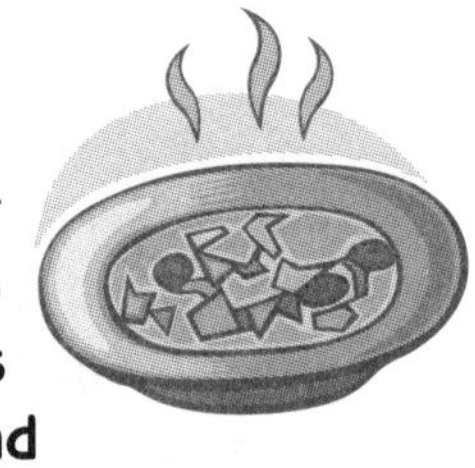

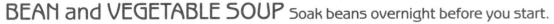

For best digestibilty, soak 1 cup dried mixed Beans, (like Split Peas, Small White Beans, Black Turtle Beans, Pinto Beans and Garbanzos) in water to cover. Drain off soaking liquid. Add fresh water to beans to cover by 1/2" to 1". Add 1 chopped Onion. Bring to a quick boil and simmer covered for one hour. Drain excess cooking water into a measuring cup and add fresh water to make 3 cups.

—Put 1 cup of the liquid into soup pot. Add 1 diced Carrot, 1 diced Zucchini, 1 bunch Broccoli diced, 2 stalks Celery with leaves, diced, 1 teasp. dry Oregano. Bring to a boil. Reduce heat. Cover and cook 10 minutes. Add beans and rest of reserved water. Bring to a boil again. Stir in 2 TBS Lemon Juice, 1 TB Molasses, 1/4 teasp. Cayenne. Add more water if needed; adjust seasoning. Stir in 1/2 cup minced Parsley.

Nutrition per serving: 141 calories; 8gm protein; 28gm carbohydrate; 9gm fiber; 1g fat; 0mg choles.; 114mg calcium; 4mg iron; 73mg magnesium; 788mg potass.; 36mg sodium; Vit. A 2260 IU, Vit. C 60mg; Vit. E 1 IU.

MILLET and LENTIL SOUP

This recipe works for: Fatigue Syndromes, Immune Breakdown, Allergy-Asthma

For 8 servings: Use a big soup pot.

Sauté in 2 TBS Olive Oil: 4 Cloves Garlic minced, 2 Onions chopped, 1 teasp. Sesame Salt, 1 teasp. Lemon-Pepper, 1/2 teasp. Cumin Powder, 1/2 teasp. ground Coriander, 1/4 teasp. Lemon Peel Powder and 1 teasp. Sambal Hot Chili Sauce for 10 minutes.

—Add 7 cups Water and 1 cup White Wine (or 8 cups Water), 2 TBS. fresh chopped Cilantro Leaves and 1/2 cup Lentils. Simmer for 20 minutes. Add 1/2 cup Millet. Cover and cook 30 minutes until tender. Top each serving with more chopped Cilantro.

Nutrition per serving: 158 calories; 5gm protein; 21gm carbohydrate; 3gm fiber; 3gm fat; 0mg choles.; 22mg calcium; 2mg iron; 40mg magnesium; 218mg potass.; 138mg sodium; Vit. A 70 IU, Vit. C 4mg; Vit. E 1 IU.

ONION GINGER BROTH

This recipe works for: Detoxification, Respiratory Infections, Allergy-Asthma

For 6 servings: Use a big soup pot.

Sizzle for 3 minutes: 1 TB Canola Oil, 1 teasp. Toasted Sesame Oil, 3 TBS Onion Broth, 1/2 cup minced Scallions, 2 TBS minced, fresh Ginger, 1/2 cup minced Shallots.

—Add 2 teasp. ground Coriander, 1 TB Honey, 4 cups Onion Broth and bring to a boil. Remove from heat, and stir in 1/2 cup fresh Cilantro, 1/4 cup minced Green Onions and 1/2 teasp. Lemon-Pepper. Puree in the blender. Return to heat briefly just to warm.

Sea Greens

CORNERSTONES OF A HEALING DIET

Sea plant chemical composition is so close to human plasma, that it can help balance your body at the cellular level. Sea greens purify the blood from the effects of an unhealthy lifestyle. They strengthen your body against environmental toxins. They reduce stores of excess fluid and fat, and work to transform toxic metals, including radiation, into harmless salts that your body can eliminate. Sea greens rival the healing powers of their land-based cousins broccoli and cabbage. Just two tablespoons of chopped dried sea vegetables go a long way toward fulfilling the healing requirements for many nutrient deficiencies.

Sea greens are a veritable medicine chest of proteins, complex carbohydrates, minerals (especially iron, calcium, potassium, and iodine) and all forty-four trace minerals. They contain vitamins A, C, E, and B Complex and the only vegetarian source of measureable B-12. Ounce for ounce, sea greens are higher in vitamins and minerals than any other food group. They are one of Nature's richest sources of carotenes, chlorophyll, enzymes and fiber.

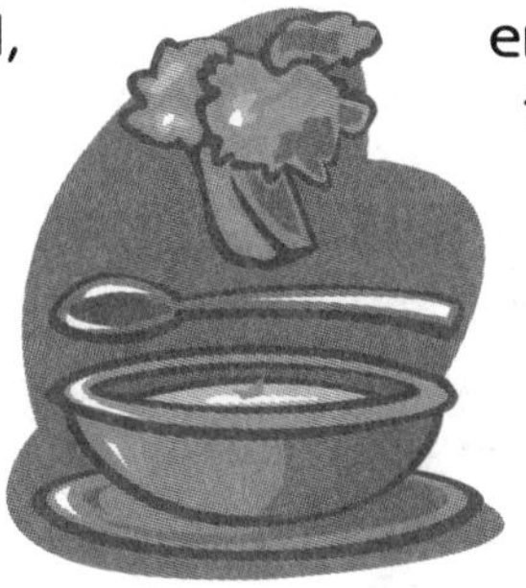

Sea greens build strong teeth, bones, nails and hair. They strengthen nerves synapses, and digestive, circulatory and nervous systems. They help reduce cholesterol and regulate blood sugar levels. (See the DIET BOOK pages 102-107 for more about sea greens benefits.)

Since today's oceans are polluted, the question about purity is valid. My research with Ocean Harvest Company and Maine Coast Sea Vegetables, small companies that hand-gather and dry their sea weeds on wind-swept northern coasts, shows that the alginic acids in sea greens perform a dual miracle. "First, they bind with the ions of toxic heavy metals which are then converted to harmless salts. These salts are insoluble in human intestines, and are excreted. Second, they actually chelate radioactive matter already present in the human body and bind it for elimination via the large intestine." In other words, the sea greens purify the ocean, themselves and you of harmful toxins.

SEA GREENS SUPREME

A flavor enhancer and nutritional booster. The sea greens expand in any recipe with liquid, and when heated, return to the beautiful green color they had in the ocean. Use freely as a seasoning on salads, soups, pizzas and rice. No salt is needed.

Crumble into a bowl; then just whirl for a second in the blender, so that there are still sizeable chunks of the different greens: **$^3/_4$ cup crumbled dry Dulse, $^1/_4$ cup crumbled dry Wakame, $^1/_4$ cup crumbled dry Kombu. $^3/_4$ cup crumbled dry Nori, $^1/_4$ cup crumbled dry Sea Palm, $^1/_2$ cup Toasted Sesame Seeds.**

DELICIOUS SEA GREENS and MISO SOUP

This recipe works for: Hair, Skin and Nails, Weight Control, Women's Health
For about 4 bowls:

Bring 4 cups Water to a boil. Reduce to a simmer. Add 4 TBS Light Miso Paste.
—Add 2 Green Onions, chopped 2 cakes Firm Tofu (8-oz) in small cubes, and $^1/_4$ cup Dry Wakame snipped into tiny bits (it expands to 10 times its dry size).
—Simmer for 2 minutes. Remove from heat and add $^1/_2$ cup Low Fat Mozzarella Cheese in small cubes. Sprinkle on 3 teasp. Nutritional Yeast. Let cheese melt 30 seconds and serve.

Nutrition per serving: 168 calories; 17gm protein; 9gm carbohydrate; 2gm fiber; 8g fat; 8mg choles.; 235mg calcium; 8mg iron; 75mg magnesium; 277mg potass.; 312mg sodium; Vit. A 210 IU; Vit. C 4mg; Vit. E 1 IU.

HIGH PROTEIN SPROUTED NORI ROLLS

This recipe works for: Strong Bones, Weight Control, Immune Power
Makes enough for 6 to 10 rolls:

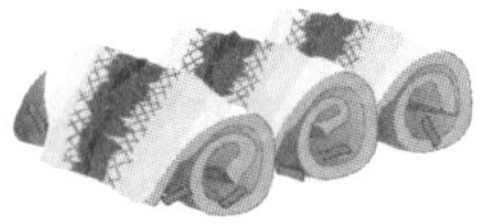

Blender blend a nut-seed mixture: 2 cups Almonds and 1 cup Sunflower or Sesame Seeds, $^1/_2$ teasp. Toasted Sesame Oil, 1 Lemon peeled, 1 TB. fresh chopped Ginger (or Pickled Sushi Ginger), and 3 TBS. Tamari. Add a little water if needed to blend.
—Lay out 6 to 10 Toasted Nori Sheets. Spread nut-seed mixture over sheets. Use 3 cups Alfalfa or Sunflower Sprouts, forming a line down the edge of each sheet.
—Cut 1 Carrot, 1 Avocado and 1 Cucumber into long thin sticks and place lengthwise across nori. Roll up like a burrito. Then eat like a burrito, or cut in 2" thick slices and decorate with fresh Basil Leaves, Sweet-Hot Mustard or a dab of Wasabi Paste.

FRIED RICE with SEA GREENS Excellent protein complementarity.

This recipe works for: Hair, Skin and Nails, Weight Control, Women's Health
For 3 to 4 servings:

Sauté 1 cup diced Red Onions and 1 TB shredded fresh Ginger in 2 teasp. Toasted Sesame Oil or 1 TB Onion Broth until soft and fragrant.
—Add $^1/_2$ cup Carrots, cut in thin matchsticks, and 1 cup dry crumbled Toasted Nori or snipped dry Wakame. Toss and stir-fry for 5 minutes. —Add and toss 3 minutes: $^1/_2$ cup diced Celery, $^1/_2$ cup diced Bok Choy, 2 TBS Tamari and 1 TB Seasoned Brown Rice Vinegar. Add and toss 3 minutes: 2 cups cooked Brown Rice, 1 TB Sake, 3 TBS Water. Top with 3 TBS toasted slivered Almonds and serve hot.

Nutrition per serving: 199 calories; 7gm protein; 31gm carbohydrate; 4gm fiber; 6gm fat; 0mg choles.; 55mg calcium; 2mg iron; 77mg magnesium; 357mg potass.; 206mg sodium; Vit. A 2095 IU; Vit. C 9mg; Vit. E 3 IU.

SESAME NORI NO-OIL SALAD DRESSING

This recipe works for: Hair and Skin Health, Cancer Protection, Building Bones
For about 2 cups:

Combine in a jar and shake vigorously to blend: 1 cup toasted, crumbled Nori, 4 TBS Brown Rice Vinegar, 3 TBS pan-roasted Sesame Seeds, 1 cup Water or Miso Broth, 1 teasp. Tamari or Bragg's Liquid Aminos, and 1 teasp. Fructose.

—Serve over vegetable salads or cooked veggies, ramen noodles, or rice blends or rice salads.

Nutrition per serving: 38 calories; 3gm protein; 3gm carbohydrate; 1gm fiber; 2g fat; 0mg choles.; 48mg calcium; 1mg iron; 21mg magnesium; 222mg potass.; 78mg sodium; Vit. A 12 IU; Vit. C 1mg; Vit. E 1 IU.

SEA PALM and TOFU CASSEROLE

This recipe works for: Hair, Skin and Nails, Women's Health, Liver Health
For 6 servings:

Soak 1-oz. dried Sea Palm slices in water. Drain and sliver into 2-inch lengths. Place in a pan with a little water, cover and simmer for 20 minutes until tender.

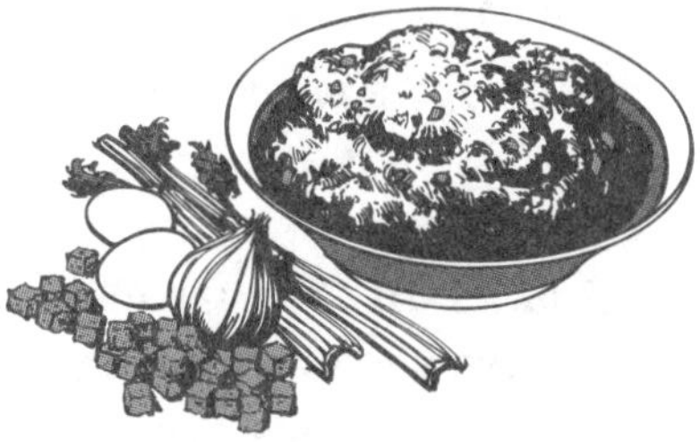

—Mash 1 LB Tofu with the tender sea greens and toss with 1 teasp. dry Basil and 1 teasp. dry Oregano.

—Make the sauce: dice 1 large Onion and 1 1/2 LBS Carrots. Sauté in 2 TBS Canola Oil or Onion Broth for 10 minutes. Remove from heat and puree in the blender with 3 TBS bottled Sweet and Sour Sauce. Toss with palm fronds; mix in a skillet to heat.

—Make the topping: puree 1/3 cup pan-toasted Sesame Seeds in the blender with 1 teasp. Tamari, 6 Sprigs Fresh Parsley and enough Water to make a thick sauce. Spread on tofu mixture in the skillet, and cook for 5 more minutes to heat. Serve hot.

WAKAME SUCCOTASH

This recipe works for: Hair and Skin Health, Cancer Protection, Immune Power
For 4 servings:

Soak 1-oz. dried Wakame in water for 30 minutes. Drain and steam for 10 minutes until tender. Snip into 1-inch pieces, removing the tough stems. Cook a 10-oz. package of frozen Succotash Vegetables and 1 Cake Tofu cubed in a pan according to package directions.

—Sauté 1 thin-sliced Red Onion in 2 teasp. Canola Oil until fragrant. Toss with vegetables and wakame. Add and toss 2 TBS minced Green Onions and 2 TBS Seasoned Brown Rice Vinegar, and let marinate for 3 to 4 hours before serving.

SHRIMP and SEA GREENS with VINEGAR SAUCE

This recipe works for: Liver and Organ Health, Cancer Protection, Immune Power
For 4 salads:

Cut about 2-oz. Wakame or Kombu into 1-inch lengths. Soak for 1 hour in $^1/_4$ cup Lemon Juice and $^1/_4$ cup Water (acidity tenderizes sea greens). Rinse, drain, set aside.

—Peel and halve 1 small European type Cucumber lengthwise; cut into matchsticks. Sprinkle with 1 teasp. Sea Salt and put in a colander to drain for 30 minutes. Squeeze out remaining excess water and set aside. Rinse 8-oz. cooked Shrimp and set aside.

Make the VINEGAR SAUCE: Mix together 1 TB Brown Rice Vinegar, 1 teasp. Chili Powder or 2 dashes Sambal Hot Chili Sauce, 1 crushed Clove Garlic, 1 TB Honey, 1 TB pan-roasted Sesame Seeds, and $^1/_2$ bunch Green Onions with tops, finely chopped.

—Toss all ingredients together and serve on tiny appetizer plates.

Nutrition per serving: 143 calories; 22gm protein; 12gm carbo.; 2gm fiber; 3g fat; 111mg choles.; 81mg calcium; 7mg iron; 65mg magnes.; 437mg potass.; 482mg sodium; Vit. A 405 IU; Vit. C 15mg; Vit. E 3 IU.

BLACK BEAN and DULSE CHILI

This recipe works for: Men's Health, Detoxification, Immune Breakdown
For 6 bowls:

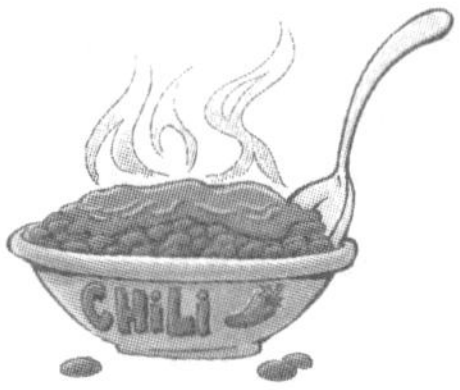

Soak 1-oz. Shiitake Mushrooms, and $^1/_2$-oz. dry Dulse in water to cover. Drain, save soaking water; sliver mushrooms and dulse. Chop finely 2-inch piece Daikon Radish, mince 1 Clove Garlic, and shred a 1-inch piece Fresh Ginger.

—Simmer $^1/_2$ cup Black Beans, 6 cups Vegetable Stock, the mushrooms, dulse and herbs, 2 TBS ground Pasilli Chili, 1 teasp. ground Chili Negro and 1 teasp. Herb Salt for 1 hour. —Add 1 cup fresh String Beans until bubbly and fragrant.

—Top with $^1/_2$ cup toasted Pumpkin Seeds and $^1/_2$ cup fresh minced Cilantro.

SUSHI MAIN DISH SALAD California maki in a bowl.

This recipe works for: Bone-Building, Women's and Men's Health, Immune Power
For 4 salads:

Toast 1 cup Brown Rice, or mixed Wild and Brown Rice in a dry pan til fragrant.

—Add 2 cups Water or Light Miso Broth. Bring to a boil, cover and simmer 30 minutes until all liquid is absorbed. Remove from heat.

—Mix and toss in a bowl: 1 Avocado chopped, 3 Scallions minced, 1 cup King Crab pieces, 2 TBS. Brown Rice Vinegar and a pinch Wasabi Powder or $^1/_2$ teasp Wasabi Paste. Crumble a toasted Nori Sheet over the top.

—Serve with a dab of HOT MUSTARD DRESSING: Mix 4 teasp. Chinese Hot Mustard, 1 TB Tamari, $^1/_4$ teasp. Wasabi Paste, 2 teasp. Toasted Sesame Oil.

KELP and HONEY BITS SNACK

Sea greens are good for snacks and munchies on a strict macrobiotic diet.
This recipe works for: Hair and Skin Health, Cancer Protection, Immune Power

Soak dried Kelp or Kombu pieces in water until soft. Drain and snip into bite size pieces to fill $\frac{1}{2}$ cup. Bring $\frac{1}{4}$ cup Honey and $\frac{1}{2}$ cup Water to a boil. Reduce heat, add sea greens and simmer until liquid is evaporated, about an hour.

—Spread 1 cup Sesame Seeds or Ground Almonds on a baking sheet and arrange sea green pieces on top, turning with tongs to coat. Bake at 300°F in oven 30 mins.

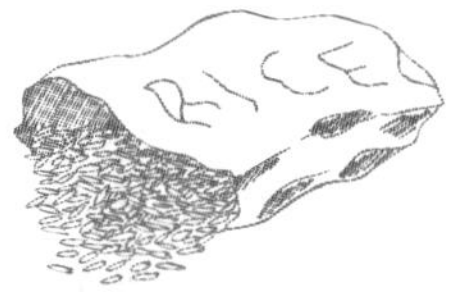

Macrobiotic Rice Meals

BASIC MACROBIOTIC VINEGAR RICE

This recipe works for: Allergies and Asthma, Cancer Protection, Immune Power
For 6 cups of cooked rice:

Soak 2 cups Short-Grain Brown or Brown Basmati Rice in 4 $\frac{1}{2}$ cups cold Water in a large pan for about 30 minutes. Add a 2-inch square dry Kombu or Wakame. Bring to a rapid boil. Cover, reduce heat and cook for 10 minutes until water is absorbed.

—Reduce heat; simmer for 5 minutes to dry and separate grains. Let rest for 5 minutes. Remove cover. Discard sea vegetable.

—Make and pour on VINEGAR DRESSING: Combine in a pan, and bring to a boil, $\frac{1}{3}$ cup Brown Rice Vinegar, 2 TBS Fructose, 2 teasp. Sea Salt, 2 TBS Mirin.

BROWN RICE PILAF PLUS

This recipe works for: Hair, Skin and Nails, Respiratory Infections, Liver Health
For 4 main course servings:

Pan roast $\frac{1}{2}$ cup sliced Almonds and 2 TBS Sesame Seeds in an oven ready skillet until golden, about 5 minutes. Remove and set aside.

—Add 2 TBS Canola Oil to the skillet. Sauté 1 small Onion, sliced, 2 Shallots, minced, and 1 TB Soy Bacon Bits about 5 minutes. Add 1 Stalk Celery, $1\frac{1}{4}$ cups Short Grain Brown Rice. Toss until shiny. —Add spices: $\frac{1}{4}$ teasp. ground Ginger, $\frac{1}{2}$ teasp. Lemon Peel, $\frac{1}{2}$ teasp. Sesame Salt, $\frac{1}{4}$ teasp. Pepper. Add $2\frac{1}{4}$ cups Water or Miso Broth.

—Bring to a boil. Cover and simmer on the range top (or bake at 350° for 1 hour) until liquid is absorbed. Top with reserved nuts, seeds, snipped Parsley and Paprika.

Nutrition: 400 calories; 11gm protein; 52gm carbohydrate; 5gm fiber; 17g total fat; 0mg choles.; 79mg calcium; 2mg iron; 154mg magnes.; 42mg potass.; 153mg sodium; Vit. A 56 IU; Vit. C 6mg; Vit. E 8 IU.

RICE BALLS

This recipe works for: Fatigue Syndromes, Stress and Exhaustion, Recovery
Easy to make.... use up leftovers... portable health food.

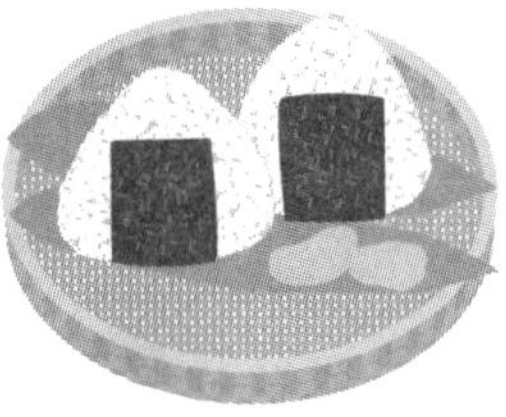

—Use 1 sheet Toasted Nori for every 2 rice balls. Fold each toasted nori sheet in half and tear along the fold. Then fold in half again and tear so that you have 4 equal-sized pieces about 3-inches square.

—Use 1/2 Umeboshi Plum, or a small cube of seasoned, baked Tofu or Tempeh, or a small cooked Shrimp as the stuffing "surprise" for each rice ball.

—Use 1 handful cooked Brown Rice for each ball. Wet your hands slightly in a dish of water. Take a handful of cooked rice and form into a ball, as if you were making a snowball. Pack the rice to make it solid. Using your index finger, press a hole into the center of the ball; place half a umeboshi plum, tofu or tempeh cube or a shrimp inside. Then pack the rice again to close the hole. Place 1 square of the toasted nori on top of the rice ball. Wet your hands slightly and press the nori around half the ball. Place the other, uncovered side on another nori square. Wet your fingers and press the nori around the ball so it covers and sticks. Repeat until the rice, nori and umeboshi are used up.

—Have Tamari available for dipping the balls.

Cooking brown rice with beans creates a rich, satisfying, nutritionally complete dish. But beans usually require longer to cook than grains, so advance preparation is a good idea. Soak them for several hours, roast them briefly in a dry-skillet, or parboil them for several minutes prior to combining them with brown rice.

1) Soaking beans prior to cooking makes them easier to digest. Rinse in cold water, first, then place beans in a bowl and add enough cold water to cover. Let stand 6 to 8 hours. Drain and discard water.

2) Pre-roasting beans like soybeans and garbanzos in a dry skillet stops foaming and beans stay firmer during cooking. Pre-roasting also yields a tempting sweet dish.

3) Parboiling beans for 20 minutes before mixing them with brown rice, and using the cooking water as part of the liquid measurement, produces a bright-colored dish.

BROWN RICE with LENTILS

This recipe works for: Sugar Imbalances, Stress and Exhaustion, Arthritis
Serves 6 people: Use a large covered pot

Place 2 1/2 cups organic Brown Rice, 1/2 cup organic Green or Brown Lentils, 1/4 teasp. Sea Salt and 4 1/2 cup Water in a large pot and mix thoroughly. Bring to a boil and cook for 45 to 50 minutes until all water is absorbed. Remove lid and allow the rice and lentils to sit for 5 minutes before placing in a wooden serving bowl.

CURRIED BASMATI RICE

This recipe works for: Healing Infections, Better Digestion, Heart Health
For 6 servings:

In a pan, soak 2 cups Basmati Rice and 2 TBS dry minced Onion in 2 cups Vegetable Broth for 1 hour. Mix 2 TBS Curry Powder in 2 TBS Water to a paste. Set aside.

—Heat 2 teasp. Canola Oil for 1 minute. Add 1 TB Crystallized Ginger, and 1 Clove Garlic minced and cook 1 minute until golden. Add the curry paste, simmer 15 minutes and remove from heat. Set aside, covered.

—Heat 2 TBS Canola Oil and sauté 2 chopped Onions for 10 minutes until brown and aromatic. Season with 1 TB Balsamic Vinegar and add to rice. Bring to a boil and cook for 3 minutes. Reduce heat to low and cook until tender, 10 minutes.

—While rice is cooking, add 1 TB Canola Oil to a skillet and quickly sauté 1/2 cup each: Red, Green and Orange Bell Pepper, and 1/4 cup minced Cilantro.

—Toss curry mix with rice and serve with tender-crisp vegetables.

BAKED STUFFED ACORN SQUASH

This recipe works for: Weight Control, Sports Nutrition, Immune Breakdown
Serves 2 people: Have cooked brown rice ready. Preheat oven to 450°.

Heat 2 TBS Canola Oil in a skillet. Sizzle 1/4 cup diced Onion for 1 minute. Add 1/4 cup diced Celery, 1/4 cup minced Mushrooms, and sauté for another 2 minutes. Sprinkle 6 drops of Tamari over veggies. Turn vegetables into a large bowl.

—Add to the skillet: 1/2 cup cooked Brown Short Grain Rice, 1/2 cup Whole Wheat Bread, cubed , and 1/4 cup Water. Stir to heat and blend. Then mix with veggies.

—Cut 1 Acorn Squash and remove seeds. Fill each squash half with stuffing. Place in a baking dish. Cover with foil and bake for 35 to 40 minutes or until done. Poke with a fork to test. Remove to a serving platter.

BROWN RICE and HEALING MUSHROOMS

This recipe works for: Cancer Control, Fatigue Syndromes, Immune Breakdown
For 6 people:

Soak 6 large dry Shiitake Mushrooms in water until soft. Sliver caps; discard stems. Save soaking water. Snip 2 TBS dried Wakame or Dulse in soaking water to soften.

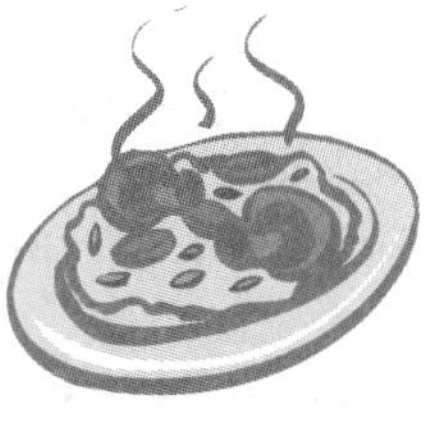

—Dry roast 1 cup Brown Rice in a pan for 5 minutes. Add 2 cups Miso Broth and mushroom-sea greens soaking water. Cook covered until liquid is absorbed. Fluff.

—Slice 1 cup Button Mushrooms. Sauté in 2 TBS Canola Oil for 5 to 7 minutes.

—Add to rice with 2 cups chopped Tomatoes, 4 minced Green Onions, 2 teasp. Lemon Juice and 1/4 teasp. Pepper. Toss to mix.

Macrobiotic Salads

High fiber, high protein, high complex carbohydrates, low-fat, low sodium, low cholesterol, dairy free, great taste. What more could you ask?

SUMMER GRAIN SALAD

This recipe works for: Stress Control, Waste Management, Men's Health
For 4 large salads:

Soak 1/2 cup Bulgar grain in Vegetable Broth for 15 minutes. Drain; press out excess liquid. Slice 1/2 cup Jicama, 1/2 cup Green Onions and 1/4 cup fresh Daikon Radish.

—Sauté bulgar, jicama and scallions briefly in 2 teasp. Olive Oil until aromatic, about 5 minutes. Remove from heat and set aside to cool.

—Mix the DRESSING: 3 TBS Olive Oil, 3 TBS Lemon Juice, 1/2 teasp. dry Thyme, 1/2 teasp. Sesame Salt or GREAT 28 (page 487), and 1/4 teasp. Lemon-Pepper (page 485).

—Before serving, add 1 cubed European-type Cucumber and 1 Tomato, cubed to grain blend. Toss with dressing to coat grain and vegetables. Snip fresh Mint Leaves on top. Chill before serving.

Nutrition: 191 calories; 4gm protein; 23gm carbohydrate; 7gm fiber; 7g total fat; 0mg choles.; 40mg calcium; 2mg iron; 54mg magnesium; 380mg potass.; 148mg sodium; Vit. A 225 IU; Vit. C 28mg; Vit. E 4 IU.

WILD RICE WINTER SALAD

This recipe works for: Immune Health and Recovery, Sports Nutrition, Men's Health
For 4 salads: Use a large salad bowl.

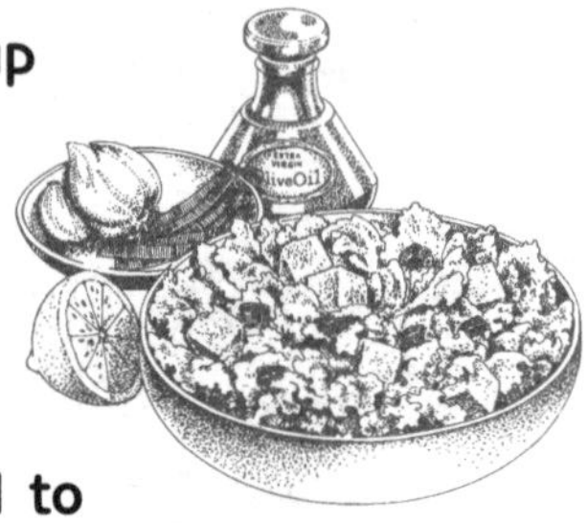

Toast in a dry pan until fragrant: 3/4 cup Wild Rice, 1/4 cup Brown Rice. Add 2 cups Water. Cover and cook on low heat until liquid is absorbed. Put in salad bowl.

—Heat pan again, add 1/2 cup chopped Walnuts, and 1/2 teasp. Herb Seasoning. Toast for 10 minutes until fragrant. Set aside

—Soak in the 1/2 cup Orange Juice: 1/3 cup Raisins, 1 Fuji Apple, 1 Fennel Bulb, chopped and 1 Celery Rib, chopped. Add to rice.

—Make a LEMON-ORANGE VINAIGRETTE: mix the grated peel of 1 Orange, 4 TBS Orange Juice, 5 minced Scallions, 5 TBS Olive Oil, 2 TBS Lemon Juice, 1 TB fresh Cilantro, minced, 2 teasp. Balsamic Vinegar, 1 TB Toasted Sesame Oil, 1 teasp. Tarragon, 1/2 teasp. Herb Seasoning or GREAT 28 MIX (page 487), 1/4 teasp. ground Anise. Toss with rice mixture. Top salad with toasted nuts and serve.

Nutrition: 458 calories; 9gm protein; 51gm carbohydrate; 6gm fiber; 27g total fat; 0mg choles.; 76mg calcium; 2mg iron; 94mg magnesium; 707mg potass.; 99mg sodium; Vit. A 150 IU; Vit. C 42mg; Vit. E 5 IU.

MILLET SALAD with DULSE

This recipe works for: Allergies and Asthma, Fatigue Syndromes, Women's Health
For 4 salads:

Roast 1 cup Millet in a dry pan until aromatic. Add 2 $^1/_2$ cups Water and cover. Cook 25 minutes. Remove from heat and fluff.

—Snip $^1/_2$ cup Dulse pieces into hot water. Blanch 3 minutes. Remove with a slotted spoon; set aside. Keep water hot and dice in $^1/_2$ cup Carrots, $^1/_4$ cup Celery, $^1/_3$ cup Daikon or Red Radish. Blanch 5 minutes and drain. Season with Lemon-Pepper.

—Add $^1/_2$ cup snipped fresh Parsley, $^1/_2$ cup diced Cucumber, $^1/_2$ cup Dry-Roasted Peanuts. Toss all together with millet, and serve on Spinach Leaves.

—Make a SESAME MISO DRESSING: blender blend $^1/_4$ cup Canola Oil, 1 teasp. Miso Paste, 1 teasp. Toasted Sesame Oil, 1 TB Brown Rice Vinegar, 1 teasp. Lemon Juice, 2 TBS toasted Sesame Seeds, $^1/_4$ teasp. Veggie Salt or SPIKE, and 3 dashes Cayenne. Pour over top.

SPRING BITTERS SALAD

This recipe works for: Female Health, Digestive Disorders, Liver and Organ Health
Use about 2 cups greens per salad:

Gather a blend of unsprayed fresh Spring greens - young Dandelion Leaves, fresh Parsley, fresh Baby Spinach, young Violet Leaves if available, mixed tips of Chives, Fennel, Lemon Mint, Tarragon, and 4 cups Red Leaf Lettuce. Rinse greens, then gently tear them into bite-size pieces and place in a salad bowl.

—Make a light dressing so the greens tastes really come through: whisk 2 TBS cold-pressed Olive Oil, 1 Clove Garlic, pressed, 2 teasp. fresh Lemon Juice, 1 TB minced Scallions, 1 TB Black Sesame Seeds, 1 TB White Sesame Seeds, Salt and freshly ground Pepper to taste. Serve with the Lemon Wedges and young Nasturtium Flowers.

LEEKS and DAIKON in BROWN SAUCE Tasty over brown rice.

This recipe works for: Heart Health, Waste Management, Allergies-Asthma
Makes 6 servings: Use a large wok.

Slice white parts of 2 large Leeks and 1 Daikon Radish. Cube 2 cakes Firm Tofu.

—Heat wok alone for 1 minute. Add 1 TB Canola Oil and sizzle. Add 1 sliced Onion and sizzle 3 minutes. Add leeks, daikon and tofu. Toss 5 minutes. Season with 2 TBS Tamari, 1 TB Lemon Juice and 2 teasp. Fructose. Add 1 $^1/_2$ cups Water. Reduce heat, cover, and simmer 15 minutes, stirring occasionally. Serve warm over rice.

Nutrition: 98 calories; 5gm protein; 12gm carbohydrate; 3gm fiber; 4g total fat; 0mg choles.; 83mg calcium; 3mg iron; 62mg magnesium; 28mg potass.; 117mg sodium; Vit. A 430 IU; Vit. C 20mg; Vit. E 1 IU.

HOT BASMATI-WILD RICE SALAD

This recipe works for: Immune Power, Recovery, Anti-Aging, Stress Reactions
For 6 large salads: Preheat oven to 375°.

Cook 1 cup Wild Rice in 2 cups Water with 2 teasp. Sea Salt for 1 hour. Set aside.
—Sauté 1 chopped Red Onion in 2 TBS Canola Oil and 2 TBS Tamari until fragrant.
—Put in a 2-qt. baking dish: 2 cups Basmati Rice, 1 Green Bell Pepper chopped, 1 Red Bell Pepper chopped, and the red onions. Pour 4 cups Vegetable Stock over. Cover, bake for 25 minutes; stir in the cooked wild rice. Fluff.
—Serve warm on Spinach Leaves with HONEY ITALIAN DRESSING: Whisk 1/2 cup Olive Oil, 3 TBS Lemon Juice, 1 tsp. Honey, 1/2 tsp. Italian Seasoning and 1 tsp. Sesame Salt.

Nutrition: 546 calories; 9gm protein; 75gm carbohydrate; 6gm fiber; 25g total fat; 0mg choles.; 26mg calcium; 2mg iron; 30mg magnes.; 189mg potass.; 409mg sod.; Vit. A 630 IU; Vit. C 44mg; Vit. E 6 IU.

COUSCOUS SALAD

This recipe works for: Healthy Pregnancy, Women's Health, Weight Control
For 6 salads:

Toast 1/4 cup <u>each</u>: Pine Nuts, Sunflower Seeds and sliced Almonds in the oven until golden. Soak 1/2 cup Raisins in water to cover for 10 minutes. Drain, and set aside.
—Pour 1 cup Boiling Water over 1 cup Couscous in a bowl. Add 1 teasp. Sea Salt, and let steam until water is absorbed, about 15 minutes. Fluff with a fork. Add 2 TBS Olive Oil and toss with rice, nuts and seeds.
—Heat 1/4 cup Miso Broth in a skillet. Add 2 cups sliced Celery, 2 cups diced Carrots, 1/2 teasp ground Ginger, 1 teasp. dried Mint (or 1 TB fresh). Simmer for 5 to 7 minutes. Toss with couscous blend, and let rest for 30 minutes before serving.

GOURMET GRAINS and VEGETABLES SALAD

This recipe works for: Weight Control, Detoxification, Cancer Protection
For 4 salads:

Dry roast 1/4 cup <u>each</u> in a pan until fragrant: Brown Short-Grain Rice, Brown Basmati Rice, Buckwheat Berries and White Sesame Seeds. Bring 2 cups Water to a boil, add grains, cover, reduce heat and steam for 25-30 minutes until liquid is absorbed. Fluff and chill.
—Sauté in 1 TB Canola Oil 1/2 cup <u>each</u>: sliced Mushrooms, cubed Firm Tofu, chopped Bell Pepper, chopped Zucchini, minced Scallions. Add 1 small can sliced Water Chestnuts, 1/2 cup diced Celery, and 1/4 cup minced Parsley. Remove from heat and let cool.
—Toss and serve with a HONEY-DIJON DRESSING: Whisk together 4 TBS Olive Oil, 2 TBS Honey, 3 TBS Balsamic Vinegar, 4 TBS Tamari, 2 teasp. Dijon Mustard and Lemon-Pepper to taste. Place on shredded greens.

HOT QUINOA and WILD RICE SALAD

This recipe works for: Men's Health, Sports Nutrition, Overcoming Addictions
For 6 salads:

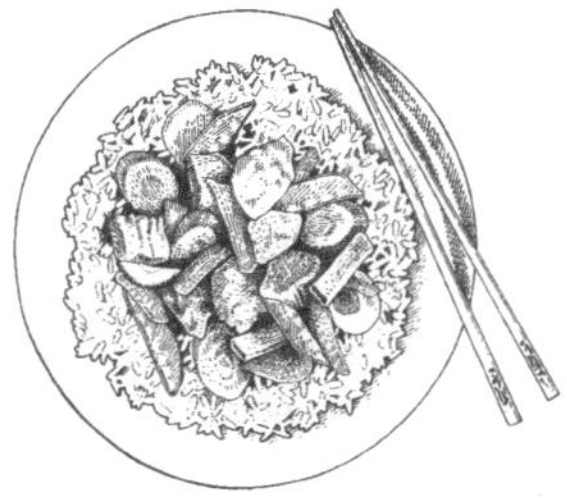

Toast 1 cup Wild Rice in a dry pan until aromatic. Add 3$^1/_2$ cups Boiling Water. Cover and simmer for 30 minutes. Add $^1/_2$ cup Quinoa. Cover and simmer 10 to 15 minutes. Drain and fluff with fork. Chill while you make the rest of the salad.

—Dry toast $^1/_2$ cup Walnuts in a skillet until brown. Remove and set aside.

—Heat 2 TBS Canola Oil in the skillet and sauté 1 chopped Onion for 5 minutes.

—Add 1 chopped Fuji Apple and sauté until lightly fragrant, about 3 minutes.

—Add chilled wild rice mix to skillet and toss to heat and coat. Remove from heat, place in salad bowl and sprinkle with walnuts.

—Serve with PINEAPPLE-ORANGE DRESSING: Whisk together $^1/_4$ cup Orange Juice, $^1/_2$ cup Pineapple Juice, 6 TBS Currants, 5 TBS Canola Oil, $^1/_2$ teasp. crushed Anise Seed, $^1/_4$ teasp. powdered Ginger and 1 teasp. Lemon Zest.

Nutrition: 374 calories; 7gm protein; 38gm carbohydrate; 4gm fiber; 23g total fat; 0mg choles.; 34mg calcium; 2mg iron; 79mg magnesium; 391mg potass.; 95mg sodium; Vit. A 41 IU; Vit. C 10mg; Vit. E 8 IU.

Macrobiotic Grains and Pastas

The essence of macrobiotic eating is based on cooked whole grains as the way of life to health. Originally this was interpreted almost entirely in terms of brown rice, but today other grains are also recognized for their efficient protein, high complex carbohydrates and fiber as primary health supports. Today's wide variety of whole grains and pastas are wonderful in salads, both cold and hot, (where raw veggies are added and heated by hot grains), baked casseroles, pasta mixes, and hearty soups.

In fact, a whole grain blend is much more interesting and flavorful than any single grain alone. A blend of grains and seeds tastes nuttier, and chewier. It cooks easier, with more definition and less stickiness. I make up a large batch of mixed grains, (see page 489 for recipe) and keep it in a cannister for ready use.

Note: For the best flavor, dry roast whole grains in the cooking pan for about 5 minutes until fragrant, before adding water or stock. It makes a delicious difference.

The key to perfect vegetable pastas? the less you can cook them the better. Cook just to al dente. Have your sauce ready, then cook the pasta at the last minute so it won't be sticky and starchy. Especially with delicate Asian pastas - you must stay with them the entire few minutes of cooking. Keep testing for perfect doneness. Then drain, and immediately coat with a little oil or your sauce.

RAISIN NUT BULGAR

This recipe works for: Fatigue Syndromes, Respiratory Infections, Allergy-Asthma
Makes 6 servings: Serve at room temperature.

In large saucepan bring 1 $^1/_2$ cups organic Chicken Broth to boil; add 2 cups Bulgar gradually, stirring; cook covered over very low heat for 10-15 minutes until liquid is absorbed. Fluff with fork; add $^1/_3$ cup Raisins. Remove from heat; let stand, covered 5 minutes. Stir in $^1/_2$ cup minced Scallions.

—Make a sauce: whisk 6 TBS fresh Lemon Juice, 6 TBS Canola Oil, $^1/_4$ tsp. Cinnamon, $^1/_2$ cup mixed chopped Nuts, and Lemon-Pepper to taste. Transfer bulgar mixture to large bowl, drizzle dressing over.

FOUR RICES HOT PILAF SALAD

This recipe works for: Fatigue Syndromes, Cancer Protection, Sports Nutrition
For 4 salads:

Toast in a large skillet until aromatic $^1/_4$ cup <u>each</u>: Brown Short-Grain Rice, Wild Rice, Basmati Rice and Jasmine Rice. Set aside.

—Sizzle in 2 TBS Canola Oil for 5 minutes: 1 Onion, chopped, 1 Clove Garlic, minced, 1 Carrot, chopped, 1 teasp. Dry Basil (1 TB fresh), $^3/_4$ teasp. Dry Oregano, $^1/_2$ teasp. Sesame Salt and $^1/_2$ teasp. Pepper. Mix in grains.

—Bring 2 cups Miso Broth or Vegetable Broth and $^1/_4$ cup White Wine to a boil.

—Add broth to grain mix. Cover, reduce heat and simmer 25 minutes. Drain.

—Make a simple VINAIGRETTE DRESSING. Mix 5 TBS Canola Oil, 5 TBS Balsamic or Tarragon Vinegar, 1 TB Dijon Mustard, $^1/_2$ teasp. Dry Tarragon or Savory. Pour over and serve salad plates heaped with Spinach Leaves.

Nutrition: 406 calories; 7gm protein; 46gm carbohydrate; 4gm fiber; 22g fat; 0mg choles.; 97mg calcium; 3mg iron; 77mg magnesium; 495mg potass.; 290mg sodium; Vit. A 4450 IU; Vit. C 20mg; Vit. E 9 IU.

RICE PASTA with ROAST PEPPERS

This recipe works for: Allergies-Asthma, Respiratory Infections, Immune Health
For 4 servings:

Bring a large pot of water to a rapid boil. Add 1 teasp. Sea Salt and 16-oz. Orzo (rice pasta). Cook stirring for 6 minutes. Drain and set aside.

—Sauté in 6 TBS. Olive Oil until soft, about three minutes, 3 Cloves Garlic minced, 6 chopped Shallots. Add $^1/_4$ cup slivered Sun-Dried Tomatoes, $1^1/_2$ cups Organic Chicken Broth, 1 teasp. Sea Salt and 1 teasp. Black Pepper. Add 1 cup chopped fresh Basil. Add orzo and stir til stock is absorbed. Add 1 jar Roasted Red Bell Peppers, chopped. Increase heat to high and boil until reduced by half, 3 to 5 minutes. Remove from heat, put in serving dish, and top with 1 cup Soy Parmesan.

POLENTA SQUARES with VEGGIES and SAUCE

This recipe works for: Fatigue Syndromes, Recovery, Men's Health, Stress
Makes 6 servings: Use a heavy 2-quart saucepan.

Bring 3 cups Water to a boil with 1 TB Butter and 2 pinches Salt. In a bowl, combine 1 cup Stoneground Yellow Cornmeal with 1 cup cold Water. Slowly pour cornmeal mixture into boiling water, stirring constantly. When mixture begins to "pop," reduce heat. Cook, uncovered, stirring frequently, for about 10 minutes, until mixture begins to mound onto itself when dropped from spoon.

—Line bottom and sides of a 9-by-9-by-2-inch baking pan with foil. Spoon in polenta; cover and chill. When ready to serve, remove from pan using foil. Cut in half, then cut each half cross-wise in thirds. Place polenta squares on a broiler pan. Brush tops and sides lightly with melted Butter. Broil 4 inches from heat for 8 to 10 minutes on each side, or until browned and crisp, brushing again after turning.

—Make the LEMON SAUCE: Combine in a bowl, 2 tsp. minced Lemon Zest, 1 tsp. minced Garlic, 2 TBS minced Cilantro or Parsley and $^1/_2$ teasp. Lemon-Pepper. Set aside.

—Fix the VEGETABLE TOPPING: Heat 2 TBS Olive Oil over medium-high heat in a large skillet. Add half an Onion, sliced and cook 3 minutes til fragrant. Add 2 Carrots, cut in matchsticks, 2 small Zucchini, cut in matchsticks, 2 small Yellow Squash, cut in thick matchsticks, $^1/_2$ cup sliced Brown Cremini Mushrooms, and 1 Red Bell Pepper, cut in thin strips. Cook, stirring about 4 to 5 minutes. Sprinkle with 2 tsp. Lemon Juice and LEMON SAUCE; toss gently to combine. Spoon over polenta squares.

—Briefly steam 1 bunch Asparagus Spears and lay on top.

Nutrition: 191 calories; 7gm protein; 23gm carbo.; 8gm fiber; 11g total fat; 8mg choles.; 40mg calcium; 2mg iron; 51mg magnesium; 380mg potass.; 148mg sodium; Vit. A 235 IU; Vit. C 28mg; Vit. E 8 IU.

COUSCOUS and RED LENTILS Delicious, low fat, high protein.

For 6 servings: Use a large pot.

Bring $1^1/_4$ cups Water to a boil. Add 1 cup Cous-cous, 2 TBS Butter and $^1/_2$ teasp. Sea Salt. Stir, cover and remove from heat. Let stand for 5 minutes. Fluff with a fork.

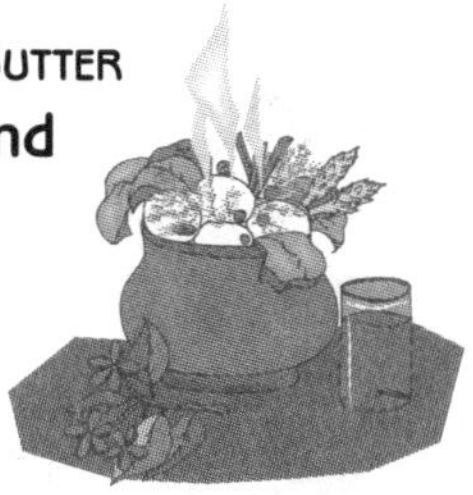

—Sizzle 1 TB Canola Oil, 1 teasp. Garlic-Lemon Seasoning and 1 TB Red Wine in a skillet for 1 minute. Add and sauté $^1/_2$ cup chopped Leeks (white parts only), and $^1/_4$ cup chopped Celery.

—Add and stir in 2 cups Water with 2 Vegetable Bouillon Cubes or 2 cups Miso Broth, 1 cup Red Lentils, 2 pinches Cayenne Pepper, 1 teasp. Tamari, 1 small chopped Tomato (or 1 TB Sun-dried Tomatoes), and teasp. Red Wine Vinegar. Reduce heat, cover and simmer 20 minutes. Let stand a few minutes before serving.

Nutrition: 242 calories; 12gm protein; 35gm carbohydrate; 6gm fiber; 6g total fat; 11mg choles.; 32mg calcium; 4mg iron; 45mg magnesium; 398mg potass.; 208mg sodium; Vit. A 246 IU; Vit. C 7mg; Vit. E 2 IU.

COUSCOUS with STEAMED VEGGIES and SPROUTS

This recipe works for: Women's Health, Detoxification, Weight Loss and Control
For 4 meal-size servings:

Steam together until tender 2 cups frozen or fresh Corn Kernels and 2 cups diced Carrots. Remove from heat and add 2 cups frozen Peas. Cover to steam.

—Bring 3 cups organic Chicken Broth to a boil with 1 teasp. Sea Salt. Add 2 cups Couscous. Remove from heat. Cover and let stand for 5 minutes. Fluff with fork.

—Stir in $^1/_4$ cup chopped Green Onions, 1 cup chopped fresh Watercress.

—Put couscous mix on a serving platter. Surround with vegetables. Sprinkle with 2 TBS Parmesan or Soy Parmesan, and 2 handfulls Sunflower Sprouts.

BULGUR SHEPHERDS PIE

This recipe works for: Men's Health, Sports Nutrition, Sugar Imbalances
For 8 serving size squares: Use a 9 x 13" pan. Bake at 400°.

Soak 1$^1/_2$ cups Bulgar in Water to cover for 15 minutes. Drain well; set aside.

—Boil 4 to 5 Potatoes (enough for 3 cups mashed) until soft. Mash potatoes. Mix 3 TBS fresh chopped Parsley and 3 TBS chopped Scallions into mashed potatoes.

—Sauté 3 cups chopped Onion and 2 Cloves Garlic minced in 2 TBS Canola Oil or White Wine. Add 1 teasp. dry Basil, $^1/_2$ teasp. Nutmeg, $^1/_2$ teasp. ground Cumin, 1 teasp. Sesame Salt, $^1/_2$ teasp. Pepper. Stir to blend. Sprinkle on 3 TBS Whole Wheat Flour.

—Mix bulgur and potatoes. Spray the baking pan with Canola Spray and spread on half the bulgar-potato mixture. Top with onion blend. Sprinkle on $^1/_2$ cup toasted chopped Pine Nuts. Cover with rest of bulgar-potatoes. Sprinkle with 1 TB ITALIAN VINAIGRETTE to moisten the top. Bake for 45 minutes until edges turn golden.

Nutrition: 219 calories; 7gm protein; 42gm carbohydrate; 7gm fiber; 3g total fat; 2mg choles.; 58mg calcium; 2mg iron; 74mg magnesium; 516mg potass.; 227mg sodium; Vit. A 118 IU; Vit. C 8mg; Vit. E 1 IU.

MOCK TUNA-NOODLE CASSEROLE High protein, great taste.

This recipe works for: Women's Health, Stress Reduction, Men's and Kid's Health
For 6 servings: Use a large soup pot. Preheat oven to 350°

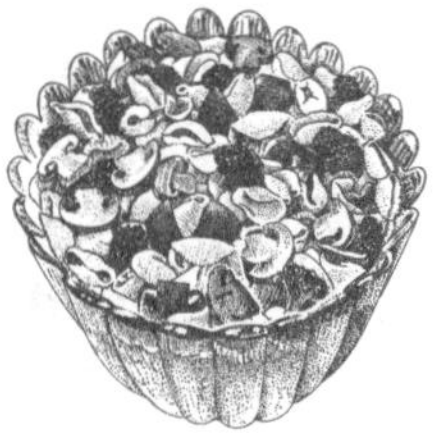

Bring a large pot of Lightly Salted Water to a boil. Add 10-oz. Spinach or Artichoke Noodles or Spinach Tortellini, and 1 TB Olive Oil. Cook according to package directions until just tender. Drain; rinse under cool water and drain again. Put into a large baking-serving dish.

—Finely dice 2 large Ribs Celery, 2 cups frozen Peas, 2 Scallions, and $^1/_3$ cup chopped Black Olives. Toss with $^1/_2$ cup Soy Mayonnaise. Season with $^1/_4$ teasp. Lemon Pepper. Add 8-oz. package baked marinated Tofu (any flavor), finely diced. Bake in oven just to heat through, about 20 minutes. Serve hot.

Balancing Your System Type

Check out your system type. Over the years, I have seen and heard from literally thousands of people with individual nutritionally related health problems. It has gradually become clear to me that people with similar food preferences and similar eating habits, fall prey to the same type of disease conditions.

Congestive diseases, like arthritis, constipation, eczema, bursitis, respiratory problems, gallbladder and kidney stones, blood pressure and heart problems, arteriosclериosis, hemorrhoids, overweight, candida and vaginal yeasts, diverticular disease, varicose veins, and hypoglycemia, seem to afflict people who like soft, creamy foods.

Ice cream and other creamy desserts, potatoes and squashes, chocolate, pastas with creamy sauces, macaroni and cheese, dairy products, especially milk and cheeses, soft breads and sandwiches, cakes and pastries, Italian foods, and creamy fruits are good examples of these kinds of foods.

Corrosive diseases, like staph and strep infections, virus infections like Epstein Barr virus and chronic fatigue syndrome, liver problems, mononucleosis; degenerative diseases like cancer, leukemia, fybromyalgia, multiple sclerosis and muscular dystrophy; digestive problems, colitis and spastic colon, hiatal hernia, herpes, hepatitis, toxic shock, ulcers, and skin cancers, seem to affect people who eat lots of hard, brittle, crunchy foods.

Crackers, sodas, cookies, celery, carrots and broccoli, Chinese and Mexican foods, spicy and condiment seasoning foods, hard candies, coffee, crunchy fruits, etc. are good examples of these kinds of foods.

I have noticed this phenomenon so many times, it is worth consideration as part of identifying an individual imbalance for yourself.

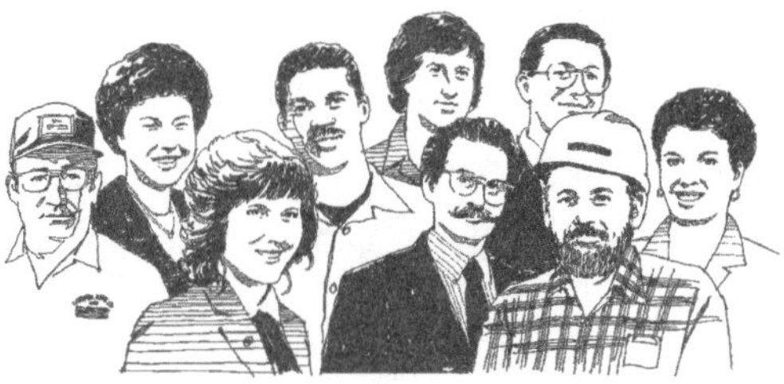

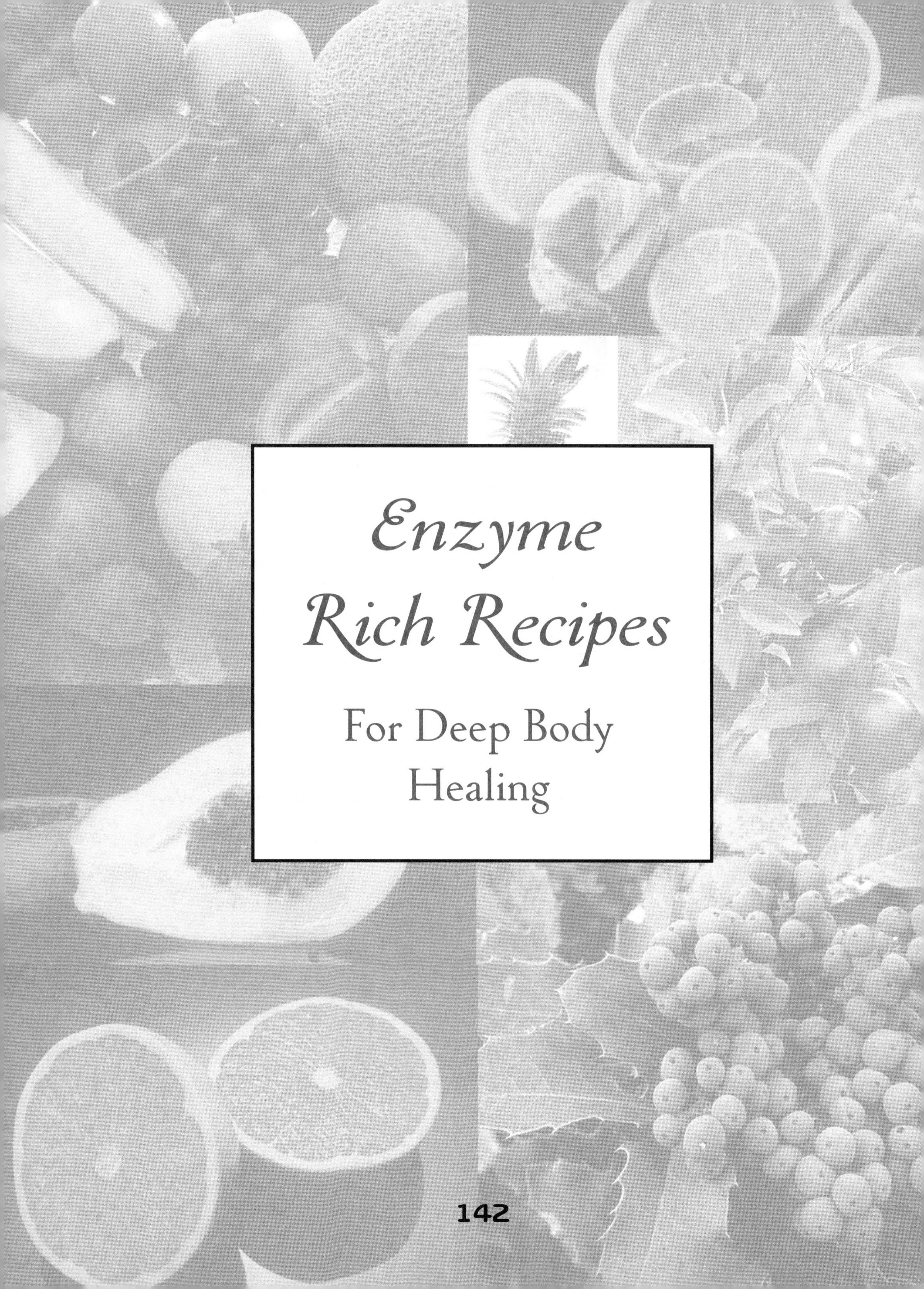

Enzyme Rich Recipes

For Deep Body Healing

Enzymes are Excellent!

Enzyme therapy is critical to healing. Enzyme-rich foods are the key to healing with your diet. Enzymes are the catalysts for literally every body process. Even when you're not in a healing mode, none of your body's vitamins, minerals or hormones can work without the right enzymes. Yet we often overlook the importance of enzyme-rich foods as we try to focus on what a healing diet should be. But enzymes are so complex and their work is so interactive it's hard to target enzyme functions.

Each of us is born with a battery charge of enzymes at birth; as we age our internal enzyme stores are naturally depleted. A 60-year-old has 50% fewer enzymes than a 30-year-old. Eating enzyme-rich foods is critical as we age.

Where have all the enzymes gone?

Most of us are enzyme deficient today regardless of age. Our food undergoes processing and alterations that deplete enzymes. Almost every food we buy has been heated to destroy bacteria (including those like juices that we think are fresh). Enzymes are highly sensitive to heat. Heat above 120 F. destroys them. Environmental stresses like tobacco smoke, chlorine and fluoride in drinking water, chemical additives and air pollutants sap our enzymes. Many prescription drugs, caffeine and alcohol deplete enzymes. The result: An inadequate enzyme supply burdens our digestive and metabolic systems, often leading to fatigue, weight gain, skin disorders, degenerative disease and accelerated aging.

I'm a firm believer in adding more enzymes to our diets. Fresh foods contain the highest amount of enzymes to work with your own. But do you have to eat only raw foods to get them? Some enzyme enthusiasts say a raw foods diet is the only way to really reap the benefits of enzyme therapy, but I find adding enzyme booster foods to lightly cooked foods works very well for most people. It's especially beneficial for people with cancer, AIDS or immune breakdown diseases whose digestive systems can't tolerate a completely raw foods diet. Some nutrients like lycopene (a carotenoid in tomatoes) are actually absorbed better by the body when they're slightly cooked.

What can enzyme therapy do for your healing program?

1) Improve digestive problems like heartburn, gas, indigestion.
2) Speed healing from injuries or surgery. Enzyme therapy especially promotes recovery from common sports' injury.
3) Reduce pain and inflammation of arthritis and colitis. Some patients have been able to completely avoid surgery.
4) Relieve sinusitis. In one study, the pineapple enzyme bromelain resolved sinus infection in 85% of patients after 9 days.
5) Help shingles. Enzymes reduce neuralgia reoccurrence.
6) Boost weight loss. Animals who are fed high enzyme foods lose significantly more weight than those fed cooked foods.
7) Enhance sexuality. Enzymes are high in pheromones linked to sexual attraction and arousal. A sperm enzyme dissolves a spot on the female egg so the sperm can enter and fertilize it.

The enzyme protease is remarkable. Protease boosts immune response, fights infections, reduces scarring from radiation burns, unclogs arteries and even shrinks tumors. Transformation *Purezyme* is a protease supplement I've used with excellent results.

High enzyme foods to include in your healing diet:
—fresh fruit and vegetable juices, and sprouts
—fermented foods like miso, yogurt, kefir, cultured vegetables
—cruciferous vegetables like broccoli, cabbage and cauliflower
—fruits like pineapple, papaya, bananas, mangos, avocados
—superfoods like barley grass, alfalfa and chlorella

Include a plant enzyme supplement to boost your enzyme-rich diet. Transformation's *DigestZyme* is a good broad spectrum formula.

To learn more about the healing power of enzymes, I recommend *The Complete Book of Enzyme Therapy*, a valuable enzyme resource written by my esteemed colleague, Anthony J. Cichoke M.A., D.C., D.A.C.B.N.

Enzyme Rich Recipe Sections

Enzyme Booster Recipes, pg. 145-148
High Enzyme Salads, pg. 149-152
Food Combinations for Enzyme Action, pg. 152-155

Enzyme Booster Foods

Get the most from your body's enzymes.... and the enzymes in your foods with these recipes. They add extra food enzymes, and help focus enzyme activity and enzyme pathways.

DOUBLE GINGER DESSERT

This recipe works for: Heart and Artery Health, Women's Health, Arthritis
Makes 4 servings:

Slightly soften 5 cups VANILLA RICE DREAM frozen dessert by letting it stand at room temperature about 10 minutes. Scoop into a large bowl. Add $^1/_4$ cup diced CRYSTALLIZED GINGER, $^3/_4$ tsp. CARDAMON POWDER, and $^1/_2$ tsp. CINNAMON; swirl ingredients together. Place bowl in freezer until dessert is firm enough to scoop.... about $1^1/_2$ hours; if storing up to 1 week, cover air-tight.

—Divide into 4 large water goblets. Slowly fill glasses with icy GINGER ALE, and serve immediately.

Nutrition: 147 calories; 9gm protein; 17gm carbohydrate; 1gm fiber; 6gm total fat; 0mg choles.; 21mg calcium; 2mg iron; 60mg magnesium; 438mg potass.; 44mg sodium; Vit. A 48 IU; Vit. C 1mg; Vit. E trace.

SIZZLING LEMONADE

This recipe works for: Heart and Artery Health, Hair and Skin, Arthritis
Makes 8 cups:

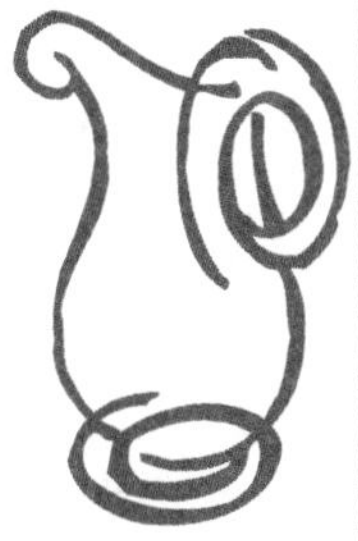

Stir in a pitcher: 8 cups SPARKLING WATER, $^1/_2$ cup FRESH LIME JUICE, $^2/_3$ cup FRESH LEMON JUICE, $1^1/_3$ cups MAPLE SYRUP, 2 teasp. CRYSTALLIZED GINGER, and 2 pinches CAYENNE PEPPER. Serve hot or chilled.

Nutrition: 149 calories; trace protein; 39gm carbohydrate; trace fiber; 0g total fat; 0mg choles.; 39mg calcium; 1mg iron; 10mg magnesium; 152mg potass.; 5mg sodium; Vit. A 10 IU; Vit. C 14mg; Vit. E 1 IU.

PAPAYA FROSTY

This recipe works for: Digestive Health, Waste Management, Liver-Organ Health
Makes 6 servings:

Blender blend: 2 cups frozen PAPAYA CHUNKS, $^1/_4$ cup LEMON JUICE and 1 cup WATER.

—Add $^1/_2$ cup BROWN RICE SYRUP, 12 ICE CUBES and 1 TB GINGER SYRUP; continue blending until very smooth. Pour into a large pitcher; add 4 cups WATER.

Nutrition: 90 calories; 1gm protein; 23gm carbohydrate; 1gm fiber; trace fat; 0mg choles.; 30mg calcium; 2mg iron; 9mg magnesium; 188mg potass.; 4mg sodium; Vit. A 65 IU; Vit. C 33mg; Vit. E 1IU.

TOMATO HAMMER

This recipe works for: Detoxification, Men's Health, Allergies, Addictions
Makes 4 servings:

Stir in a pitcher: 3 cups Tomato Juice, 2 TBS Lime Juice, 2 tsp. Worcestershire Sauce, 1 tsp. bottled Horseradish, 1/2 tsp. Celery Salt, 1/4 tsp. Hot Pepper Sauce. Cover and chill thoroughly. Serve with a short Celery Spear with leafy top.

Nutrition: 39 calories; 2gm protein; 10gm carbohydrate; 2gm fiber; 0g total fat; 0mg choles.; 38mg calcium; 1mg iron; 24mg magnesium; 499mg potass.; 198mg sodium; Vit. A 540 IU; Vit. C 38mg; Vit. E 1 IU.

ORANGE-CARROT SOUP with GINGER

This recipe works for: Heart and Artery Health, Men's Health, Candida Control
Makes 4 servings:

Have ready 1/3 cup sliced toasted Almonds.

Sizzle in a large pot: 2 TBS Balsamic Vinegar, 1 TB minced Crystallized Ginger, 4 minced Cloves Garlic, and 1 cup chopped Onions until fragrant, about 5 minutes.

—Add 4 cups water, 1 cup chopped Carrots, and 1 cup diced Red Potatoes. Bring to a boil, reduce heat, and simmer 20 minutes. Cover pan. Let cool slightly, then purée in a blender. Add 1/4 cup Orange Juice and 1 TB Honey.

HERBAL ENZYME PUNCH

This recipe works for: Digestive Health, Women's Health, Recovery from Illness
Makes 12 cups:

Steep 12 tea bags Hibiscus or Hibiscus Tea blend in 3 cups boiling Water 10 minutes. Transfer to a large pitcher. Stir in 1/2 cup Orange Honey, 1 cup frozen Pineapple Juice Concentrate, and 2 quarts cold Sparkling Lemonade or Sparkling Lemon-Lime Juice.

BUBBLING BANANAS in LIME JUICE

This recipe works for: Digestive Health, Kid's and Women's Health
Makes 8 servings:

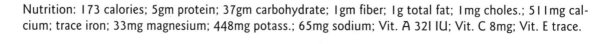

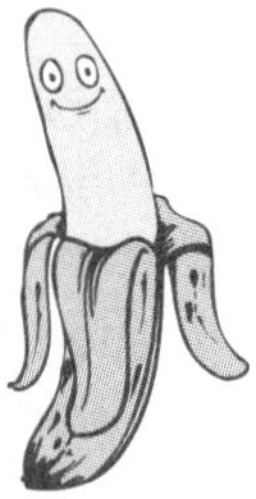

Sizzle 4 ripe but firm Bananas, thick sliced in 1 tsp. Canola Oil. Sprinkle with 3 TBS Fructose. Heat gently until fructose dissolves. Remove from heat; sprinkle with 4 TBS Lime Juice. Put on small dessert plates.

—Divide 4 cups Nonfat Vanilla Frozen Yogurt over top of bananas.

Nutrition: 173 calories; 5gm protein; 37gm carbohydrate; 1gm fiber; 1g total fat; 1mg choles.; 511mg calcium; trace iron; 33mg magnesium; 448mg potass.; 65mg sodium; Vit. A 321 IU; Vit. C 8mg; Vit. E trace.

BAKED APPLES with LEMON and TOFU

This recipe works for: Men's Health, Women's Health, Arthritis
Makes 8 servings: Preheat oven to 375°F.

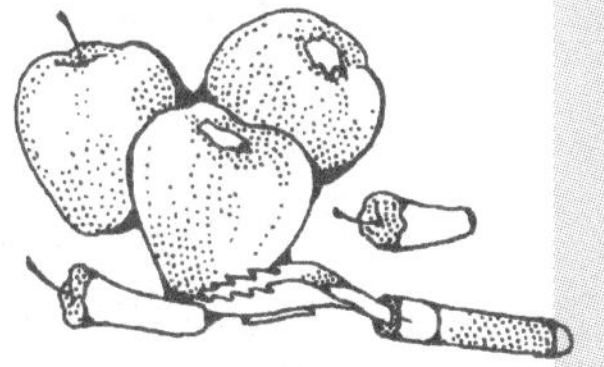

Partially core 4 Granny Smith Apples; remove the top 3/4 of the core but leave the base intact. Drop into cavity of each apple: 1 teasp. Raisins, 1 teasp. minced Walnuts and 1 teasp. dried Cranberries. Fill cavities to the top with Water.

—Pour boiling Water into a glass baking dish, and put the apples in. Bake uncovered for 35 minutes rotating the apples after 20 minutes to expose each inner half to the heat. While apples bake, whisk 8-oz. Soft Silken Tofu in a bowl with 1 1/2 TBS Maple Syrup, 2 TBS finely minced Fresh Lemon Zest, and 1/2 tsp. Cinnamon.

—When the apples are done (they'll turn yellow), cut each in half vertically and top each half with tofu mixture. Sprinkle with Lemon Peel, Raisins and Dry Cranberries.

Nutrition: 105 calories; 3gm protein; 18gm carbohydrate; 3gm fiber; 3g total fat; 0mg choles.; 47mg calcium; 2mg iron; 41mg magnesium; 201mg potass.; 4mg sodium; Vit. A 21 IU; Vit. C 9mg; Vit. E 1 IU.

ENZYME BOOSTER GREEN SOUP

This recipe works for: Detoxification, Liver and Organ Health, Arthritis, Recovery
Makes 6 servings:

Sizzle in 1 TB Olive Oil til aromatic, about 5 minutes: 2 Cloves Garlic minced, 1/4 cup minced Leeks, 1/2 cup minced Green Onions, 2 TBS minced Shallots, 1/4 cup minced Celery. Sprinkle with 1 TB Wheat Germ and toss to coat.

—Remove from heat and toss in: 1 cup finely chopped Leafy Greens (Spinach, Chard, Endive, Romaine, etc.), 1/4 cup minced Fresh Parsley, 1/4 cup minced Watercress.

—Heat 4 cups Miso Soup briefly. Add vegetables, 1 TB Lemon Juice, 1/2 tsp. Herb Salt, 1/4 tsp. White Pepper. Heat just through; top with slivers of Daikon White Radish.

COTTAGE CHEESE PANCAKES

This recipe works for: Waste Management, Digestive Health, Women's Health
Makes 4 servings:

—Make the batter: 1 LB Low-Fat Cottage Cheese, 6 Eggs, 2/3 cup Whole Wheat Pastry Flour, 1/3 cup Oatmeal, 3 TBS Honey, 2 TBS Vanilla Rice Milk, 1/2 tsp. Vanilla Extract, 1/4 tsp. ground Cardamom.

—Heat a non-stick skillet until a drop of water bounces. Spray lightly with a lecithin cooking spray, and ladle in 2 to 3 pancakes at a time. Cook until bubbles burst on the surface. Flip and cook until golden. Oil cooking surface between each batch. Serve with maple syrup or honey.

CRANBERRY-RAISIN SAUCE for TURKEY or SALMON

This recipe works for: Waste Management, Digestive Health, Women's Health
Makes $1^1/_2$ cups:

In a saucepan, sizzle 2 teasp. Canola Oil and 1 Sweet Onion minced 3 minutes. Add $^1/_2$ teasp. Garlic-Lemon Seasoning, 2 teasp. Crystallized Ginger and stir 30 seconds.

—Stir in $1^1/_2$ cups Cranberries, 1 cup Orange Juice and $^1/_2$ cup Raisins. Cover; simmer 10 minutes, stirring occasionally. Add 1 teasp. Maple Syrup. Serve hot or cold.

PIQUANT SAUCE for STEAMED VEGGIES

This recipe works for: Allergies, Immune Breakdown Diseases, Women's Health
Makes 4 servings:

Make a BROWN MISO SAUCE in a hot skillet: Stir 2 TBS Canola Oil, 1 minced Shallot and 2 TBS Whole Wheat Pastry Flour until well combined. Add 2 TBS Miso Paste, 2 cups Water and $^1/_2$ teasp. Lemon-Pepper. Stir until slightly thickened. Remove from heat.

—Add 3 TBS Balsamic Vinegar, 2 teasp. snipped Fresh Parsley, and 2 TBS Sweet Pickle Relish. It's ready to serve.

CHILLED CUCUMBER-YOGURT SOUP

This recipe works for: Digestive Health, Skin Health, Bladder-Kidney Health
Makes 6 servings:

Blender blend until smooth: $2^1/_4$ cups Plain Low Fat Yogurt, $1^1/_4$ pounds Lemon Cucumbers peeled and sliced, 2 teasp. Garlic-Lemon Seasoning, $1^1/_2$ tsp. ground Cumin, 2 teasp. Crystallized Ginger. Strain through fine sieve into large bowl. Refrigerate until well chilled, about 2 hours. Top with slivers of Daikon White Radish at serving.

SIZZLING GINGER STIR-FRY

This recipe works for: Digestive Health, Skin Health, Bladder-Kidney Health
Makes 4 servings:

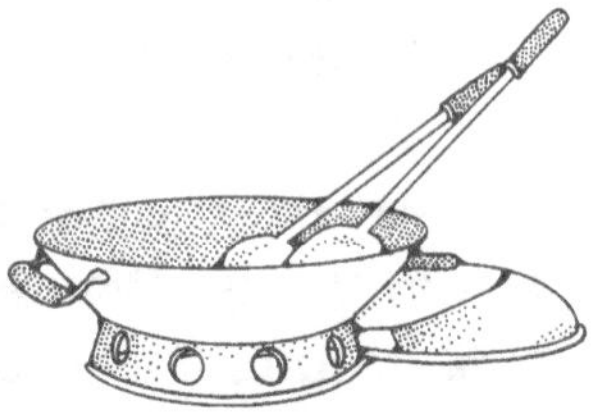

In a hot wok, sizzle in 1 TB Canola Oil over medium heat, 3 TBS Fresh Ginger, peeled and minced, 4 Cloves Garlic, minced for 10 minutes. Add 1 package Firm Tofu, drained and cut into $^1/_2$-inch chunks, 6 drops Toasted Sesame Oil, 1 teasp. Honey and 2 TBS Hoisin Sauce; gently turn until cooked through, about 10 minutes longer. Top with 2 TBS snipped Chives and 2 TBS Toasted Sesame Seeds and serve.

Nutrition: 190 calories; 14gm protein; 10gm carbohydrate; 1gm fiber; 12g total fat; 0mg choles.; 159mg calcium; 8mg iron; 86mg magnesium; 223mg potass.; 138mg sodium; Vit. A 95 IU; Vit. C 3mg; Vit. E 1 IU.

High Enzyme Salads

Salads can be your body's chief source of enzymes during a healing diet. Fresh food enzymes are the most easily available to your body. Both fruit and vegetable salads work equally well.

ROASTED RED PEPPER SALAD

This recipe works for: Men's Health, Digestive Health, Skin and Hair Health
Makes 4 servings:

Combine in a bowl: 2 Roasted Red Bell Peppers from a jar, slivered, 1 TB Balasmic Vinegar, 2 TBS Olive Oil and 3 pinches Garlic-Lemon Seasoning. Let stand for 15 minutes. Add 2 TBS Balasmic Vinegar, 4 TBS Olive Oil, pinches Sea Salt and Pepper to taste.

—Divide 1 small bag Arugula and 1 small bag Baby Spinach on 4 salad plates. Divide roasted red pepper mix over top.

LOTS O' GREENS SALAD

This recipe works for: Bone Building, Cancer Protection, Liver and Organ Health
Makes 6 servings:

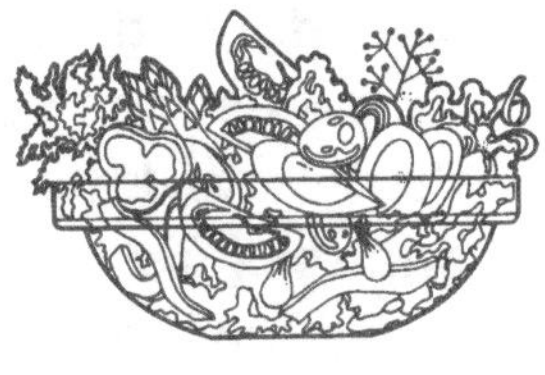

Make the salad. Thinly slice 1 cup Romaine, 1 cup Chinese Nappa Cabbage, 1/2 cup Cucumber, 1/2 cup Green Pepper, 1/2 cup Carrots, and 1/2 cup Celery. Add 1 cup Sunflower Sprouts and 1 cup trimmed Snow Peas, and toss in a large bowl.

—Shake the dressing in a jar and pour over greens: 3 TBS Tamari Sauce, 3 TBS Brown Rice Vinegar, 2 TBS Water or Sake, 1/4 tsp. minced Clove Garlic, 1/4 tsp. minced Lemon Peel, 1/4 tsp. minced Fresh Ginger.

Nutrition: 43 calories; 4gm protein; 7gm carbohydrate; 2gm fiber; 1g total fat; 0mg choles.; 40mg calcium; 1mg iron; 21mg magnesium; 228mg potass.; 424mg sodium; Vit. A 1565 IU; Vit. C 20mg; Vit. E 1 IU.

MANGO TRIFLE LAYERED SALAD

This recipe works for: Weight Control, Waste Management, Hair, Skin and Nails
For 10 servings: Use a clear glass bowl. Make ahead and chill for best results:

Have ready 2 cups sliced Strawberries, 3 sliced Bananas, 4 sliced Kiwi, and 1 Asian Pear or Jicama, peeled and sliced in matchsticks. Peel and cut 2 ripe Mangoes into cubes. Reserve 1/4 cup cubes. Whirl rest of mangoes in a blender with 2 TBS minced Crystallized Ginger and 4 TBS Lime Juice. Pour into bottom of glass serving bowl.

—Make layers: arrange sliced strawberries on mango sauce; top with banana slices; cover with kiwi slices. Mound pear or jicama sticks and reserved mango cubes on top. Sprinkle with ground Nutmeg or Coriander Powder.

THAI LEMON GRASS ENZYME SOUP

This recipe works for: Heart Health, Sugar Imbalances, Overcoming Addictions
Makes 4 servings: Check out Asian markets for authentic ingredients.

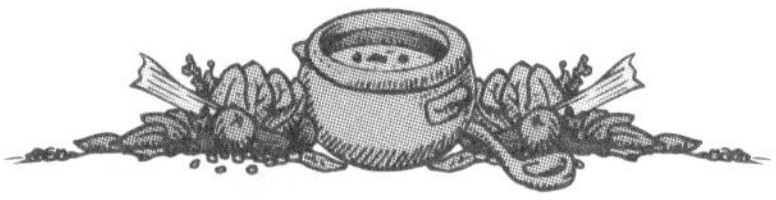

In a pan, simmer for 5 minutes: 4 cups VEGETABLE BROTH, 2 large LEMON GRASS STALKS and 3 or 4 dried LIME LEAVES. Discard stalks and leaves.

—Sizzle 1 teasp CANOLA OIL, 2 tsp. minced GARLIC and 2 tsp. minced GINGER in a skillet. Add and stir about 30 seconds. Add to broth; return to a boil and stir in 2 tsp. Thai roasted CHILI PASTE and $1^1/_2$ cups fresh slivered OYSTER or SHIITAKE MUSHROOMS. Simmer for 30 seconds until mushrooms wilt.

—Stir in 2 TBS LIME JUICE and 2 TBS TAMARI. Remove from heat and ladle soup into small bowls. Divide topping over bowls: finely chopped TOMATOES, FRESH CILANTRO LEAVES, and slivered, seeded GREEN CHILIES.

ORANGE, FENNEL and ARUGULA SALAD

This recipe works for: Cancer Protection, Arthritis, Men's Health
Makes 8 servings:

Make a Vinaigrette: Whisk 2 TBS BALSAMIC VINEGAR, and 2 tsp. DIJON MUSTARD. Gradually add 2 TBS OLIVE OIL, and season to taste with SEA SALT and BLACK PEPPER.

—Peel and section 4 NAVEL ORANGES into a bowl. Add 2 cups thinly sliced FENNEL BULB, 1 cup thinly sliced RED ONION, 2 TBS snipped FRESH BASIL. Add vinaigrette to bowl and toss gently to combine. Let stand 1 hour.

—Wash and tear 4 bunches ARUGULA (8 cups). Pile arugula onto individual salad plates; top with orange mix; sprinkle each salad with 2 TBS toasted PUMPKIN SEEDS.

Nutrition: 136 calories; 4gm protein; 15gm carbohydrate; 4gm fiber; 8g total fat; 0mg choles.; 86mg calcium; 2mg iron; 69mg magnesium; 400mg potass.; 169mg sodium; Vit. A 340 IU; Vit. C 48mg; Vit. E 1 IU.

PERFECT BALANCE SALAD

This recipe works for: Weight Control, Women's and Men's Health, Heart Health
For 6 salads:

Mix: 1 cup PLAIN LOW FAT YOGURT, 2 TBS SOY MAYONNAISE, 3 TBS LEMON JUICE, $1^1/_2$ teasp. CURRY POWDER, 1 teasp. grated FRESH GINGER, $^1/_2$ cup RAISINS, pinches LEMON PEPPER.

—Combine in a large bowl: 1 thinly sliced EUROPEAN CUCUMBER, 2 GREEN ONIONS, thin sliced, 1 FUJI APPLE diced. Stir in Yogurt mixture and chill all day if possible.

—Divide 1 quart BABY SPINACH LEAVES on salad plates. Mound with salad mix.

Nutrition: 137 calories; 5gm protein; 22gm carbohydrate; 3gm fiber; 4g total fat; 2mg choles.; 139mg calcium; 2mg iron; 54mg magnesium; 576mg potass.; 87mg sodium; Vit. A 1395 IU; Vit. C 23mg; Vit. E 1IU.

SUSHI SALAD

This recipe works for: Liver and Organ Health, Cancer Control, Hair and Skin Health
Makes 6 servings:

In a saucepan with a tight-fitting lid, combine 1 cup Short-grain Sushi Rice, 1 cup mixed Brown and Wild Rice, and 4 cups Cold Water. Bring to a boil, stirring occasionally. Reduce heat to low, stir, then cover and cook for 15 minutes, lifting the lid to stir only once. Remove pan from heat, stir, cover again, and set aside for 20 minutes. Brown and wild rices should be chewy in texture. Cool in a large bowl.

—Blanch 2 cups diced Broccoli, 1 diced Red Bell Pepper and 2 diced Carrots in boiling water for 1 minute. Drain and rinse with cold water to stop cooking; set aside. When rice is cool, toss with blanched vegetables, 1 Rib Celery, diced, 4 thin sliced Scallions, 2 TBS Pickled Sushi Ginger minced, 1/2 cup slivered Almonds, and 2 sheets Toasted Nori, snipped into small squares with scissors.

—Make a dressing: whisk together 1/2 cup Brown Rice Vinegar, 2 TBS Tamari, and 2 teasp. Wasabi Paste to make a dressing. Toss with salad and serve.

Nutrition: 195 calories; 7gm protein; 32gm carbohydrate; 4gm fiber; 5g total fat; 0mg choles.; 68mg calcium; 2mg iron; 86mg magnesium; 390mg potass.; 308mg sodium; Vit. A 792 IU; Vit. C 57mg; Vit. E 5 IU.

RED and GREEN SALAD with CRANBERRY DRESSING

This recipe works for: Bladder-Kidney Problems, Women's Health, Heart Health
Makes 8 servings:

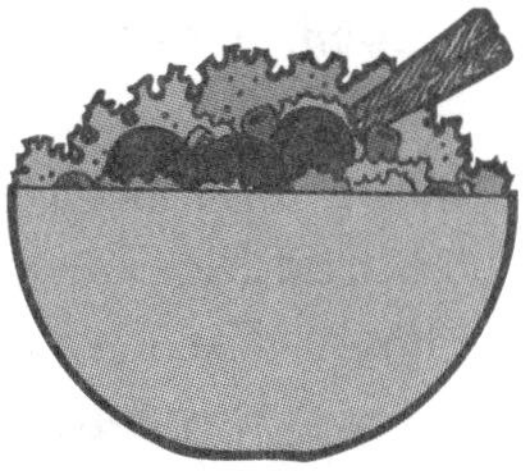

Blender blend 1/4 cup Fresh Cilantro, 1 Shallot chopped, 1/3 cup Balsamic Vinegar, 1/3 cup Cranberry Juice Blend, 1 TB Honey, 1 tsp. Dijon Mustard, and Herb Seasoning Salt to taste. Turn into a bowl and stir in 1/3 cup Dried Cranberries.

—Toss in a large bowl: 10 cups Baby Green Salad Leaves, 1 cup shredded Red Cabbage, 1 cup Radicchio Leaves, 1/3 cup thinly sliced Red Onion, 1 Red Bell Pepper, thinly sliced, and cranberry dressing.

FRESH VEGETABLE SALAD with SAFFRON and GINGER

This recipe works for: Cancer Control, Liver and Organ Health, Colon Health
For 4 salads:

Mix together in a bowl: 1/2 LB. Carrots, shredded, 1 small head Green Cabbage, shredded, 1 Yellow Bell Pepper in thin slivers.

—Make the SAFFRON/GINGER SAUCE in a bowl. Mix 1/4 teasp. Saffron Threads and 1 teasp. Curry Powder in 1 TB Water until it turns orange. Add 4 TBS Olive Oil, 3 TBS minced Ginger Root, 4 TBS White Wine Vinegar, 1 Jalapeno Chili, seeded and minced, 1/2 teasp. Sea Salt, 1/4 teasp. Pepper. Pour on vegetables. Toss and chill until serving.

THAI PAPAYA SALAD

This recipe works for: Anti-Aging, Liver and Organ Health, Digestive Health
For 6 salads:

Roast $^3/_4$ cup Pine Nuts in the oven or a dry skillet until golden. Set aside. In a hot skillet, sauté 1 minced Clove Garlic and 2 teasp. minced Crystallized Ginger in 2 TBS Olive Oil until fragrant. Add 1 LB bite size Scallops and toss until opaque, about 2 minutes. Remove to a plate and cool.

—Shake vigorously in a jar to combine, and chill while you assemble the salad: 3 TBS Lime Juice, 2 TBS Honey, 2 minced Scallions, 1 TB Tamari, 1 TB minced Cilantro, $^1/_2$ teasp. Hot Thai Chili Sauce.

—Peel and thin-slice 2 small Papayas and 1 Kiwi Fruit. Peel and dice 1 Cucumber. Toss together fruits and scallops, and all but 2 TBS of the pine nuts. Divide onto 6 greens covered salad plates, spoon on dressing, and sprinkle with rest of pine nuts.

Nutrition: 283 calories; 19gm protein; 24gm carbohydrate; 4gm fiber; 15g total fat; 25mg choles.; 73mg calcium; 3mg iron; 113mg magnes.; 836mg potass.; 265mg sodium; Vit. A 525 IU; Vit. C 72mg; Vit. E 6 IU.

THE SUPER BOWL

This recipe works for: Anti-Aging, Women's and Men's Health, Immune Recovery
For 10 servings:

Rub a large salad bowl with the cut side of a Garlic Clove. Slice and add to the bowl: 1 cup Spinach Leaves washed and dried, 1 cup Celery, 1 head Boston or Butter Lettuce, 1 small head Romaine Lettuce, 1 bunch Arugula, 1 peeled Cucumber, 3 Red Radishes and 4 large Tomatoes. Toss and top with 1 small head Cauliflower in florets, 2 shredded Carrots, 1 Bell Pepper in rings, 2 cups mixed Sprouts and $^1/_4$ cup snipped Fresh Parsley. Toss and top with 1 chopped Hard Boiled Egg, Toasted Croutons, and Toasted Sunflower Seeds.

—Make a NATURAL FRENCH DRESSING: Mix and shake in a jar, 1 cup Tomato Juice, 1 minced Scallion, $^1/_2$ cup White Wine Vinegar, 6 TBS Olive Oil, 2 TBS Honey, 1 teasp. Sea Salt, 1 teasp. Herbs de Provence (optional) and $^1/_2$ teasp. Cracked Pepper.

Good Food Combining Enhances Enzyme Activity

Combining certain foods boosts enzyme activity even more than using the foods alone. The recipes in the following section offer enzyme synergy for the best results in your healing diet.

HIJIKI NOODLES

This recipe works for: Detoxification, Illness Recovery, Hair, Skin and Nails
Makes 6 servings:

Combine all ingredients: 1 LB Spinach Noodles, cooked and drained, 1 package Hijiki Seaweed, soaked in water, rinsed and cut into strips, 1 cup grated Carrots, $^1/_2$ cup chopped Celery, $^1/_2$ cup fresh snipped Parsley, $^1/_2$ cup minced Scallions, 1 clove Garlic, minced. Toss with 6 TBS. Olive Oil. Let stand a half hour before serving.

SEA VEGGIE PIZZA

This recipe works for: Immune Breakdown, Illness Recovery, Women's Health

Have ready dried Laver (Nori) circles found at Asian Markets.

—Mash 2 Avocados. Blender blend 2 Carrots, mix with avos and spread on the laver. Sprinkle dulse flakes to completely cover the avocado mixture.

Top with your choice of toppings: diced Tomatoes, Red Onions, Red Bell Peppers, Zucchini slices, Arugula, Baby Spinach Leaves, snipped Cilantro, sliced Cucumbers.

—Make the sauce: mix Sun-dried Tomatoes, Fresh Tomatoes and Toasted Walnuts with Rice Mozarrella Cheese and spread on.

SCRAMBLED EGGS with WATERCRESS

This recipe works for: Illness Recovery, Men's and Women's Health, Strong Bones
Makes 4 servings:

Beat 4 eggs; season with Sea Salt and Cracked Pepper to taste. Sizzle 1 TB Canola Oil in a skillet. Add 2 TBS White Wine and 2 small, thinly sliced Leeks (white part only). Sizzle 5 minutes. Add 4 small grated Carrots; cover and cook until softened, 5 more minutes. Remove veggies to a plate and set aside. Add to skillet: 1 TB Canola Oil, and the eggs. Scramble and heat until just cooked. Stir in the sautéed vegetables and $^1/_2$ cup chopped Watercress. Serve immediately, sprinkled with drops Hot Sauce.

MARINATED TOFU A basic, very simple way to fix tofu.

This recipe works for: Immune Breakdown Diseases, Recovery, Weight Loss
Makes 4 servings:

Cube 1 LB Tofu. Blanch in boiling water for a few minutes to firm.

Mix the marinade: 1 TB Fresh Grated Ginger, 1 TB Toasted Sesame Oil, 2 TBS Sherry, $^1/_2$ teasp. Fructose, $^1/_4$ cup Tamari, 2 teasp. toasted Sesame Seeds, 2 TBS Brown Rice Vinegar, $^1/_2$ teasp. granulated Dulse, 2 TBS toasted diced Walnuts, dashes Hot Pepper Sauce or Herb Seasoning Salt. Marinate tofu cubes for 1 hour or longer in the fridge.

BLACK BEAN SOUP with VEGGIES

This recipe works for: Immune Breakdown Diseases, Illness Recovery, Allergies
For 8 servings:

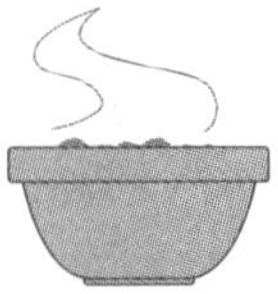

Bring to a boil in a kettle: $1^{1}/_{2}$ cups Black Turtle Beans, $1^{1}/_{2}$-qts. Vegetable Broth, 2 tsp. Soy Bacon Bits and 1 TB Olive Oil. Cover; simmer $2^{1}/_{2}$ hours until beans are soft.

—Heat 1 TB Olive Oil in a skillet. Add and sizzle until aromatic: 1 sliced Carrot, 1 diced Onion, 1 diced Potato, 2 diced Stalks Celery, 2 teasp. Lemon-Pepper or Herbal Seasoning Salt, 2 teasp. Honey Mustard, 1 teasp. dry Oregano, and $^{1}/_{4}$ teasp. dry Savory. Remove from heat. Add to beans in the last hour of cooking.

—At serving, add 2 TBS Red Wine, juice of 1 Lemon and thin Lemon Slices on top.

Nutrition: 148 calories; 7gm protein; 23gm carbohydrate; 5gm fiber; 3g total fat; 0mg choles.; 38mg calcium; 1mg iron; 44mg magnesium; 387mg potass.; 305mg sodium; Vit. A 1710 IU; Vit. C 15mg; Vit. E 1 IU.

POTATO-PEPPER RATATOUILLE

This recipe works for: Sports Nutrition, Men's Health, Liver and Organ Health
Makes 4 servings:

Cook 2 Cloves Garlic minced, and 2 large Yellow Onions diced, in a large pot with $^{1}/_{4}$ cup water; stir for about 3 minutes. Add 2 large potatoes, peeled and chopped, 4 small Zucchini sliced, 4 cups peeled, diced Tomatoes, and 1 Red, 1 Yellow and 1 Green Bell Pepper diced. Sprinkle with 2 tsp. snipped Fresh Basil (or $^{1}/_{2}$ tsp. dried), 2 tsp. snipped Fresh Oregano (or $^{1}/_{2}$ tsp. dried) and 2 TBS snipped Fresh Parsley (or 1 TB dried). Cover and cook over medium heat for 30 minutes, stirring occasionally. Season with Cracked Pepper at serving.

Nutrition: 177 calories; 6gm protein; 40gm carbohydrate; 7gm fiber; 1g total fat; 0mg choles.; 79mg calcium; 2mg iron; 83mg magnesium; 1250mg potass.; 29mg sodium; Vit. A 1040 IU; Vit. C 113mg; Vit. E 5 IU.

GINGER-CARDAMOM BREAD

This recipe works for: Digestive Health, Liver and Organ Health, Heart Health
Makes 16 servings: Preheat oven to 350°F. Use an eight-inch square baking pan.

Combine dry ingredients: 2 cups Unbleached White Flour, $1^{1}/_{2}$ tsp. Baking Soda, 2 tsp. Crystallized Ginger, $^{3}/_{4}$ tsp. Cinnamon, 1 tsp. Cardamom Powder and $^{1}/_{2}$ tsp. Sea Salt.

—In a separate bowl, combine 3 Eggs, $^{1}/_{2}$ cup Honey, $^{1}/_{2}$ cup Unsulphured Molasses, 2 TBS Grated Ginger, 3 TBS Water and $^{1}/_{4}$ cup Canola Oil.

—Fold wet mixture into dry mixture, and mix until just blended. Pour batter into pan and bake for 30 minutes until an inserted toothpick comes clean. Let cool completely before removing from pan. Cut into 16 squares to serve.

ENZYME RICH COLD KEY LIME PIE

This recipe works for: Cancer Protection, Immune Breakdown, Women's Health

Preheat oven to 350°F. Lecithin-spray an 11-inch pie pan.

Blend crust in a food processor, 5 to 10 seconds, until about half way cut: 4 cups Granola, 2 TBS Canola Oil, 2 TBS Maple Syrup, 2 TBS Orange Juice. Pat mixture into the prepared pie pan, pressing firmly. Bake crust for 7 minutes. Do not over-bake. Remove and place on a wire rack to cool.

—Make the filling in a pan: Squeeze in $^1/_4$ cup fresh Lime Juice. Grate in Lime Rind from the juiced limes. Add 2 cups Vanilla Rice Milk, 2 cups Apple Juice or Orange Juice, $^3/_4$ cup Rice Syrup, $^3/_4$ cup Maple Syrup, $^1/_2$ tsp. Sea Salt and 1 TB Vanilla Extract. Bring to a boil and simmer briefly. Add 6 TBS Arrowroot Powder mixed with $^3/_4$ cup Lime Juice Simmer, stirring until well combined. Set aside and wait 15 minutes to cool down. Pour filling into pie shell. Place in the refrigerator and allow to set.

—Make the topping: Blender blend 1 cup Kefir Cheese, 1 teasp. Vanilla, 2 TBS Honey, and 1 TB Lime Juice. Pour over pie, smooth with a spatula and chill until ready to serve. Decorate by thinly slicing a Lime and cutting slices into half-moons. Arrange the moons over top. Store in the refrigerator and serve cold.

SWEET and SOUR TOFU with VEGGIES

This recipe works for: Heart and Artery Health, Recovery, Men's Health

For 6 people:

Cube 2 cakes Tofu into a bowl. Mix the marinade: 2 TBS Brown Sugar, 3 TBS Tamari, 6 TBS Brown Rice Vinegar, 4 TBS Ketchup, 1 TB minced Crystallized Ginger, dashes Hot Chili Oil. Pour over tofu and let sit for 20 minutes.

—Heat 2 TBS Canola Oil and 1 TB grated Ginger in a wok. Add and sizzle until aromatic: 2 cups thin sliced Yellow Onions, 1 cup thin sliced Red Onions for 3 minutes. Add 1 sliced Green Bell Pepper, 2 Carrots sliced in matchsticks, 4 cups Zucchini, sliced in thin rounds and 8-oz. French-cut Green Beans. Toss briefly to coat. Turn down heat. Cover wok, and simmer until just tender crisp, about 5 minutes.

—Add $^3/_4$ cup Pineapple Chunks and the drained marinated Tofu, and toss.

—Dissolve 1 TB Arrowroot Powder into $^1/_2$ cup Pineapple Juice. Add to veggie/tofu mix. Toss until glossy for 4 minutes. Shake on drops of Hot Chili Oil and serve.

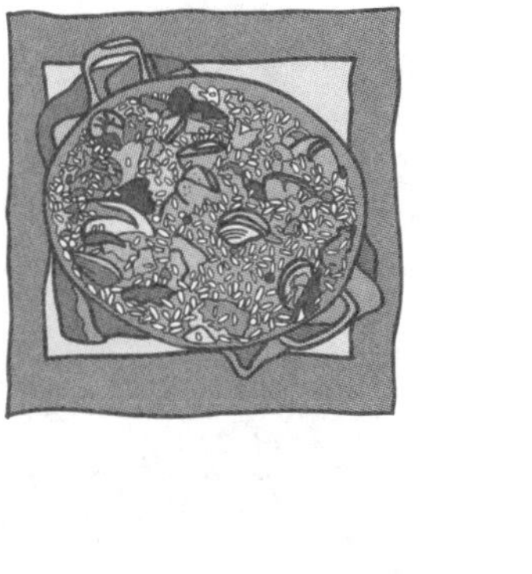

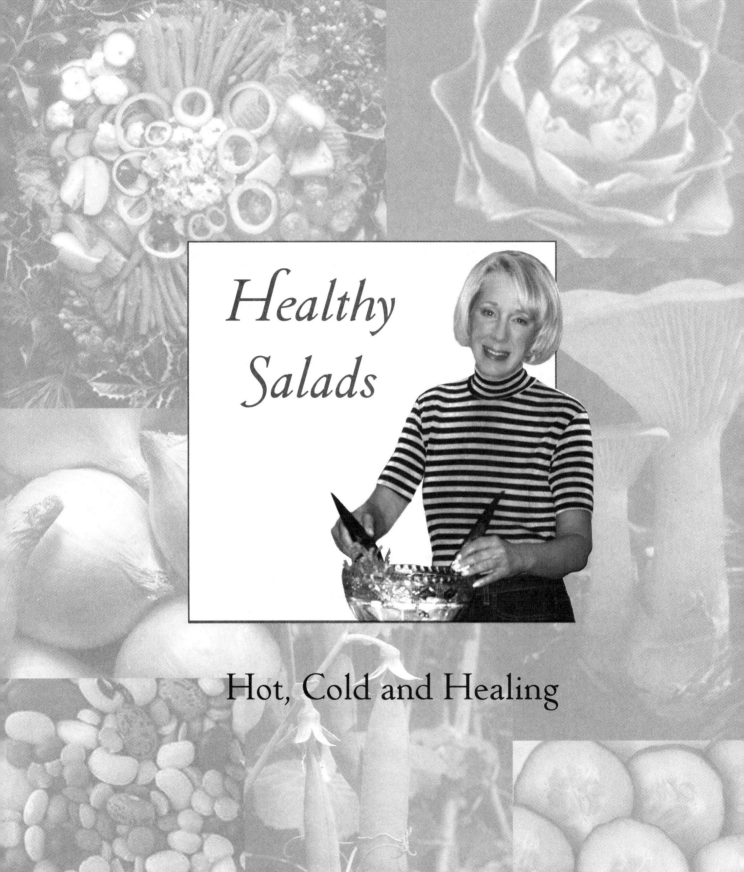

Healthy Salads

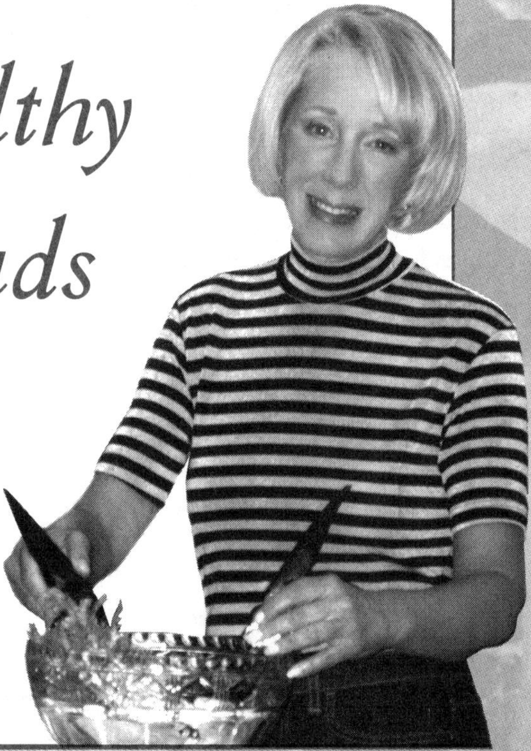

Hot, Cold and Healing

Salads
Cardinal Points for Health

If you do only one thing for your health, have a green salad every day. A fresh salad is a vital requisite for body cleansing and healing. Even when you're on an all-liquid diet, you can have a daily salad in liquid form.

What's a salad?

A salad can be almost any dish you like as long as it's full of greens and vegetables or fruits. Salads can be anything from snacks to meal starters to whole meals to desserts. Salads can be hot or cold. Healthy salads can have healthy meats, cheeses, grains, pastas or beans.

Salads are almost unlimited combinations of healthy foods that provide high fiber, protein, and complex carbohydrates for energy. Salads can supply almost every nutritional need.

Salads are full of water for good body elimination. High liquid content means light, but satisfying eating, perfect for weight loss. Rich chlorophyll from greens has proven healing properties, and as fresh food, the nutrients, vitamins and minerals in a salad are easily absorbed.

Salads and all fresh foods take a longer time to eat than cooked foods... a plus for anyone concerned with weight control. Many of us eat on the run and under stress today. We give our bodies no time to register a feeling of fullness to our brains..... so many of us overeat before we know it. Fresh foods give your body time to signal satisfaction before you overeat.

You can do just about anything with a salad. The recipe selection in this chapter is extensive, (good salads are included in almost every other recipe section of this book, too) because I believe that salads are the basis of healthful eating.

Search out the freshest foods you can and fix them in the healthiest way possible.... that's a salad!

Almost any fresh food combination can be made into a successful salad with the invigorating bite of a fresh dressing.

A healthy salad can be all too unhealthy if the dressing is loaded with high fats and salty condiments. All the salads in this book are made with low-fat, low salt contents in mind. What's more, salad dressings are a perfect way to use healing herbs and herbal teas.

<u>For a healthy, low-fat, low salt dressing</u>:

—Use only unsaturated vegetable oils, like canola, olive or rich Omega-3 flax oil. Sesame oil is wonderful for your skin, loaded with EFA's. Keep opened bottles refrigerated to avoid rancidity.

—Use a good vinegar, like brown rice vinegar, balsamic, cider, wine or tarragon vinegar. Apple cider vinegar is especially good for cleansing and alkalizing.

—Use sesame salt, herb salt, sea greens salt, or a vegetable seasoning instead of table salt.

—Dress your salads with a light touch. One to 3 tablespoons of dressing per salad, to keep fats, sodium and cholesterol low.

Salad Recipe Sections

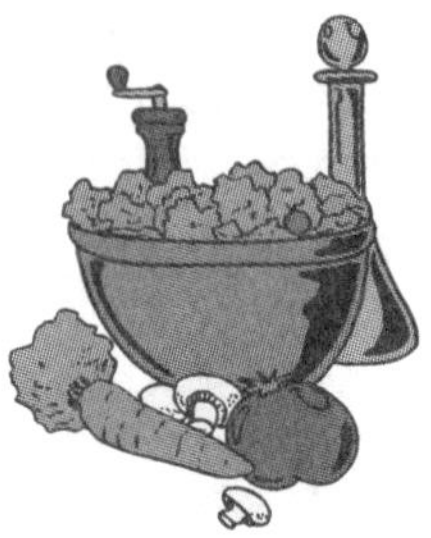

Snacks and Appetizer Salads

Bright, zippy, light refreshing.... use these small salads for body cleansing, for between meal snacks, for meal starters or for when you just want to eat less food.

FIREBIRD A good salad to eat while you watch a sunset..... or a sunrise.

This recipe works for: Cancer Recovery, Detoxification, Immune Power
For 2 appetizer salads:

Toss together 1 cup fresh Alfalfa Sprouts or Sunflower Sprouts, 2 cups grated Carrots, 1 cup minced Celery.

—Make the dressing: Mix 2 TBS Canola Oil, 3 TBS Tomato Juice Blend (like Knudsen's VERY VEGGIE-SPICY), 2 TBS Lime Juice, 1 teasp. Sesame Salt. Pour over salad just before eating.

Nutrition: 190 calories; 3gm protein; 16gm carbohydrate; 5gm fiber; 14gm total fat; 0mg choles.; 63mg calcium; 1mg iron; 31mg magnesium; 608mg potass.; 305mg sodium; Vit. A 15,590 IU; Vit. C 25mg; Vit. E 6 IU.

KIWI CARPACCIO with LEMON-LIME DRESSING

This recipe works for: Respiratory Healing, Detoxification, Weight Loss
For 4 appetizer salads:

Warm 3 TBS Honey, 3 TBS Lemon Juice and 2 TBS Lime Juice in a saucepan; stir until combined. Set aside to cool.

—Thinly slice 6 peeled Kiwi and arrange in a spiral to cover four chilled salad plates. Scatter $^1/_2$ pint Raspberries over each plate and pour dressing over fruit.

HYDRATING-CLEANSING SALAD

This recipe works for: Bladder Problems, Detoxification, Liver and Organ Healing
For 6 salads:

Toss together: 1 large European Cucumber, sliced thin, 4 fresh Tomatoes, cut in wedges, 4 Green Onions, sliced thin, $^1/_3$ cup chopped fresh Mint Leaves.

—Make the dressing: mix $^1/_4$ cup Olive Oil, $^1/_4$ cup Lime Juice, 2 TBS Tarragon Vinegar or Balsamic Vinegar. Pour over salad. Stir gently; cover. Let chill in the fridge to blend flavors.

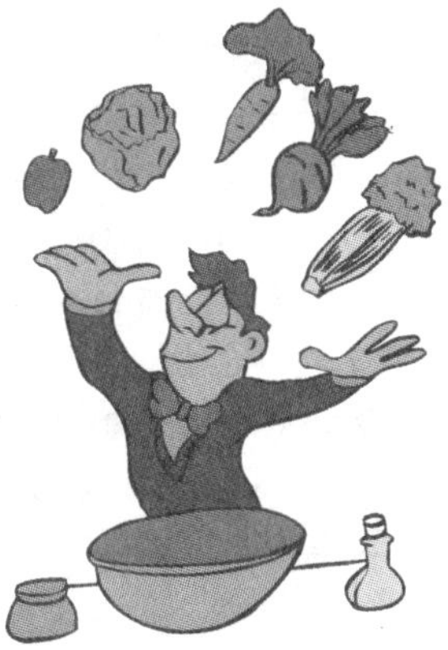

Nutrition: 119 calories; 2gm protein; 9gm carbohydrate; 2gm fiber; 9gm total fat; 0mg choles.; 29mg calcium; 1mg iron; 19mg magnesium; 327mg potass.; 13mg sodium; Vit. A 78 IU; Vit. C 26mg; Vit. E 3 IU.

APPLE, SPROUT and CARROT SALAD

This recipe works for: Arthritis, Illness Recovery, Immune Power, Bone Building
For 4 appetizer salads:

Combine in a bowl: 2 cups fresh Alfalfa Sprouts or Sunflower Sprouts, 2 Carrots, shredded, 1 Rib Celery, diced, 1 Granny Smith Apple, cored and diced.
—Mix the dressing and pour over: 2 TBS Lime Juice, $^{1}/_{4}$ teasp. Garlic-Lemon Seasoning, 1 TB Toasted Sesame Oil, $^{1}/_{2}$ TB Tamari. Top salad with 1 TB Toasted Sesame Seeds

EARLY SPRING GREENS, HERBS and FLOWERS

This recipe works for: Detoxification, Liver Health, Immune Power, Skin and Hair
Makes 4 servings: Use a large, wide salad bowl.

In a small skillet over low heat, sizzle $^{1}/_{4}$ cup Pine Nuts or Sesame Seeds in 1 TB Olive Oil until golden, 3 to 4 minutes. Add $^{1}/_{4}$ cup Balsamic Vinegar. Let cool.
—Pour nut mixture into a wide bowl. Add to the wide salad bowl: $^{1}/_{2}$ cup Arugula Leaves, $^{1}/_{4}$ cup organic Dandelion Leaves, picked before flowering, $^{1}/_{4}$ cup unsprayed Sweet Violet Flowers (*Viola spp.*, the common wild perennial), $^{1}/_{3}$ cup unsprayed Sweet Violet Leaves, stems removed, 12 tips each: Dill, Mint and Lemon Balm, and $^{1}/_{4}$ cup chopped fresh Basil Leaves (or 2 tsp. dried Basil) and 2 quarts rinsed, crisped Baby Lettuces and Greens (like red leaf, green leaf, endive, escarole, chicory, etc.).
—Mix in nuts. Sprinkle with drops of Olive Oil and Balsamic Vinegar to glisten. Season with Lemon-Pepper to taste.

Nutrition: 123 calories; 5gm protein; 6gm carbohydrate; 3gm fiber; 11g total fat; 0mg choles.; 72mg calcium; 2mg iron; 53mg magnesium; 428mg potass.; 16mg sodium; Vit. A 239 IU; Vit. C 15mg; Vit. E 5 IU.

HEALING MUSHROOM SALAD

This recipe works for: Weight Control, Liver Health, Immune Power, Recovery
Makes 6 servings:

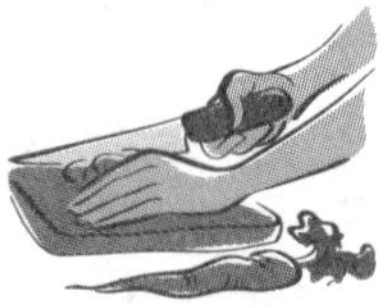

Soak 12 dry Shiitake Mushrooms and 2 or 3 dry Chinese Tree Fungus Mushrooms in water to cover. When soft, drain mushrooms, sliver caps, and discard woody stems.
—Stir-fry mushrooms over medium-high heat in 2 TBS Canola Oil until liquid evaporates and mushrooms are well browned, 15 to 20 minutes.
—Add 2 TBS Canola Oil, 2 teasp. Sweet-Hot Mustard, and $^{1}/_{4}$ cup Brown Rice Vinegar. Simmer to blend flavors.
—Rinse and crisp about $^{1}/_{2}$ LB mixed Baby Asian or Spring Greens. Place salad in wide bowl. Toss mushrooms with greens. Dash on dry Tarragon or Thyme.

Nutrition: 106 calories; 3gm protein; 9gm carbohydrate; 2gm fiber; 7g total fat; 0mg choles.; 17mg calcium; 1mg iron; 15mg magnesium; 216mg potassium; 19mg sodium; Vit. A 37 IU; Vit. C 4mg; Vit. E 3 IU.

LIGHT, CRUNCHY, CRISP SALAD

This recipe works for: Weight Control, Sexuality, Liver Health, Respiratory Healing
Enough for 10 appetizer salads:

Cook 2 $^1/_2$ LBS French-cut Green Beans gently in a large pot of boiling salted water until crisp-tender, 5 minutes. Drain beans; rinse in cold water. Drain again; pat dry.
—Whisk together: $^1/_4$ cup fresh Lemon Juice, 2 TBS Balsamic Vinegar, 4 tsp. Dijon Mustard, $^1/_2$ cup Olive Oil and $^1/_2$ cup fat-free organic Chicken Broth.
—Add 1 bunch chopped Watercress, 1 Jicama diced, and 1$^1/_2$ cups thinly sliced Radishes. Toss with beans. Season with Lemon-Pepper.

ZUCCHINI CARPACCIO an authentic Italian appetizer salad.

This recipe works for: Bone Building, Liver and Organ Health, Arthritis, Skin, Hair
Makes 4 servings: make the paper-thin slices of zucchini with a food processor.

Cover small salad plates with tart garden greens, like Arugula, Endive or Radicchio.
—Pile on Sunflower Sprouts or Watercress Leaves to cover. Slice 4 small Zucchini paper thin and divide between salad plates.
—Sprinkle a few drops of Olive Oil and squeeze fresh Lemon Juice drops over each salad, grate on some Reggio-Parmesan Cheese and Lemon-Pepper.

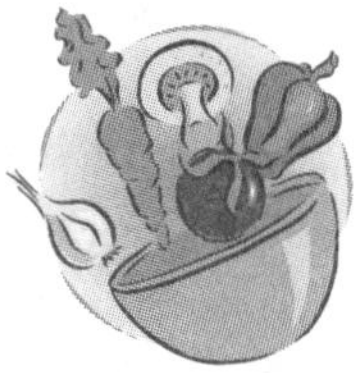

ROASTED WALNUTS with FETA CHEESE

This recipe works for: Bone Building, Allergies and Asthma
For 2 appetizer salads:

Pan roast $^3/_4$ cup Walnut Pieces in 2 teasp. Canola Oil until fragrant; (or oven roast at 275° for 45 minutes). Whisk the dressing in a bowl: 1 TB Red Wine Vinegar, 1 TB Dijon Mustard, $^1/_4$ teasp. Sea Salt and 2 pinches of Pepper.
—Divide 1 quart loosely packed tender Greens onto two salad plates. Sprinkle with $^1/_3$ cup crumbled Feta Cheese. Top with dressing and walnuts.

VERY LOW FAT CARROT-RAISIN SALAD

This recipe works for: Weight Control, Bone Building, Respiratory Health
For 8 appetizer salads: Make it all in a large salad bowl.

Toss: 4 large Carrots, shredded, $^1/_2$ small Jicama, peeled and shredded, 1 cup Raisins, $^1/_2$ cup Celery, finely diced, and $^1/_4$ cup Sesame Seeds. Mix $^1/_4$ cup fresh Lemon Juice, 1 TB Olive Oil, 2 TBS Honey, and $^1/_2$ tsp. ground Cardamom and toss with salad.

Nutrition: 137 calories; 3gm protein; 25gm carbohydrate; 3gm fiber; 4g total fat; 0mg choles.; 32mg calcium; 1mg iron; 31mg magnesium; 387mg potass.; 24mg sodium; Vit. A 1014 IU; Vit. C 12mg; Vit. E 1 IU.

Focused Fruit Salads

Consider good food combining when using fruit salads in a healing diet. Serve fruit salads as appetizers before a meal, for breakfast or brunch or as a full meal lunch. Fruits at the end of a meal make a satisfying, healthy sweet closure.

SWEET WALDORF SALAD

This recipe works for: Waste Management, Bone Building, Arthritis
For 4 salads: Serve on chilled plates.

Toss together: 2 diced Fuji Apples, 1 cup diced Celery, 1 cup halved Red Flame Seedless Grapes, $^{1}/_{2}$ cup oven toasted Walnuts, $^{1}/_{4}$ cup Lemon Yogurt, 2 TBS Low-Fat Mayonnaise, $^{1}/_{2}$ teasp. Sweet-Hot Mustard, 2 TBS Lemon Juice, $^{1}/_{2}$ teasp. Honey.

Nutrition: 218 calories; 5gm protein; 29gm carbohydrate; 3gm fiber; 11g total fat; 0mg cholesterol; 58mg calcium; 1mg iron; 44mg magnesium; 394mg potass.; 50mg sodium; Vit. A 19 IU; Vit. C 16mg; Vit. E 3 IU.

TROPICAL FRUIT SALAD

This recipe works for: Weight Control, Detoxification, Sugar Imbalances
For 6 salads:

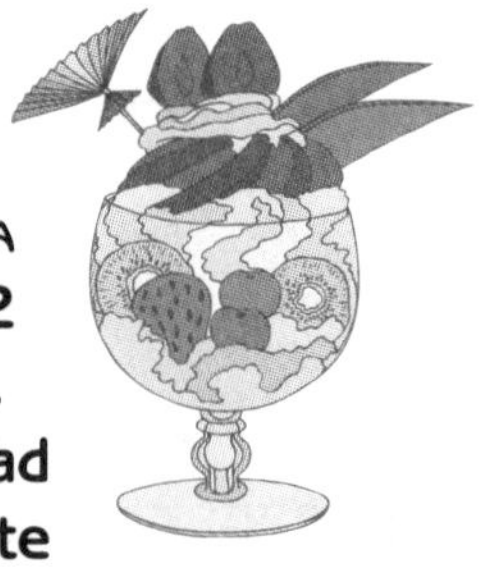

Whisk together in a bowl: 2 TBS Lime Juice, 1 TB Honey, 1 TB Raspberry Vinegar, 1 minced Shallot, 3 TBS Olive Oil, pinch Cayenne Pepper.
—Toss together in a large bowl: 1 Cantaloupe cubed, 1 small Papaya cubed, 1 Star Fruit, peeled and sliced, 2 Mangoes, peeled and cubed, 2 Kiwi Fruits, peeled and sliced, grated zest each of 1 Lemon and 1 Lime.
—Pour dressing over fruit and stir gently. Divide among chilled salad plates and squeeze over juices of the Lemon and Lime you used to grate the zest.

HAWAIIAN SALAD

This recipe works for: Stress Management, Respiratory Health, Anti-Aging
For 4 salads:

Combine: $^{1}/_{4}$ fresh Pineapple, peeled, cored and chunked, 1 Mango, peeled and diced, $^{1}/_{2}$ Papaya, peeled, seeded and diced, 2 large Oranges, peeled and chopped, 2 TBS Brown Sugar, $^{1}/_{3}$ cup fresh Orange Juice, $^{1}/_{4}$ cup chopped Mint Leaves.
—Line four salad bowls with large Bibb Lettuce cups. Spoon in salad and serve.

Nutrition: 128 calories; 2gm protein; 32gm carbohydrate; 4gm fiber; 0g total fat; 0mg choles.; 58mg calcium; 1mg iron; 25mg magnesium; 423mg potassium; 5mg sodium; Vit. A 244 IU; Vit. C 98mg; Vit. E 1 IU.

CALIFORNIA FRUIT SALAD

This recipe works for: Hair and Skin, Anti-Aging, Fatigue Syndromes, Recovery
Makes 8 servings: Make in a large bowl. Serve in individual bowls.

Pan roast $^1/_4$ cup Pine Nuts or slivered Almonds over medium heat until golden, 3 to 5 minutes. Remove from pan and set aside.

—Put into large bowl: 2 large Navel Oranges, 2 Kiwi Fruit, peeled and sliced and 2 Ruby Grapefruit, peeled and sectioned. Add 2 Avocados and 1 firm-ripe Papaya, peeled and sliced. Toss fruits to coat slices with the citrus juice from the bowl.

—Line 8 salad bowls with Bibb Lettuce Leaves, rinsed and crisped. Spoon fruits on leaves. Sprinkle with nuts. Drizzle on POPPY SEED DRESSING: Blend $^1/_4$ cup Canola Oil, $^1/_4$ cup Olive Oil, $^1/_4$ cup Raspberry Vinegar, 1 $^1/_2$ TBS Dijon Mustard, 1 $^1/_2$ TBS Lemon Juice, 1 $^1/_2$ TBS Honey, 2 teasp. Poppy Seeds, $^1/_2$ teasp. Lemon Pepper.

Nutrition: 295 calories; 4gm protein; 26gm carbohydrate; 6gm fiber; 22g total fat; 0mg choles.; 78mg calcium; 1mg iron; 49mg magnes.; 785mg potass.; 33mg sodium; Vit. A 125 IU; Vit. C 100mg; Vit. E 7 IU.

TROPICANA with WASABI-HONEY SAUCE

This recipe works for: Digestive Problems, Waste Management, Liver Health
Makes 4 servings:

Toast $^1/_3$ cup dry Coconut Strips in the oven til golden

—Combine 1 ripe Mango, peeled and cubed, and 4 cups fresh Pineapple, cubed, and 1 Orange sectioned in a bowl. Toss with $^1/_4$ cup Lime Juice. Divide salad on 4 plates. —Sprinkle with $^1/_2$ pint fresh Raspberries and Coconut. Make a YOGURT SAUCE: Mix 1 cup Lemon-Lime Yogurt, 2 TBS Honey and $^1/_2$ tsp. Wasabi Paste. Dollop on salads.

Nutrition: 282 calories; 5gm protein; 59gm carbohydrate; 6gm fiber; 6gm total fat; 0mg choles.; 133mg calcium; 1mg iron; 51mg magnesium; 540mg potass.; 42mg sodium; Vit. A 222 IU; Vit. C 69mg; Vit. E 1 IU.

RED and GREEN SALAD

This recipe works for: Illness Recovery, Healthy Pregnancy, Weight Control
Makes 6 servings:

Pan roast 1 cup Walnut Pieces in 2 tsp. Canola Oil until fragrant. Toss 1 Fuji Apple and 1 Granny Smith Apple, chunked, in a large bowl. Add 1 head shredded Lettuce, 2 ribs Celery, sliced, and 2 Green Onions, sliced. Mix a HONEY-YOGURT DRESSING: $^1/_3$ cup Low-Fat Yogurt, 2 TBS Honey, $^1/_4$ teasp. Sesame Salt and Pepper, and top salad. Sprinkle with walnuts.

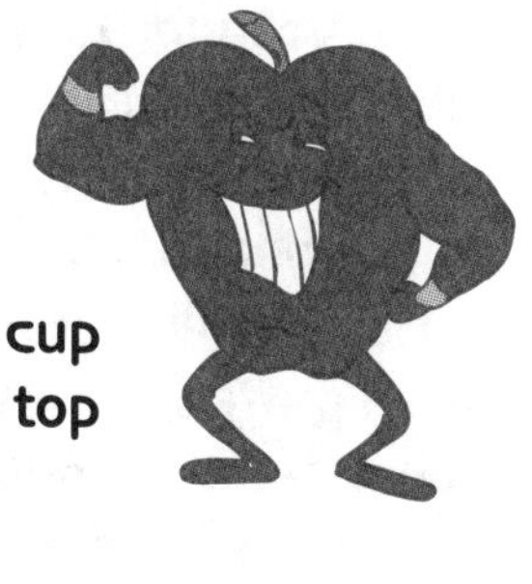

Nutrition: 221 calories; 7gm protein; 19gm carbohydrate; 3gm fiber; 14g total fat; 0mg choles.; 70mg calcium; 1mg iron; 59mg magnesium; 405mg potass.; 74mg sodium; Vit. A 46 IU; Vit. C 10mg; Vit. E 3 IU.

PEARS and CHEVRE SALAD with TOASTED WALNUTS

This recipe works for: Respiratory Recovery, Healthy Pregnancy, Digestive Health
Makes 8 salads: Make in a large salad bowl.

Pan roast 1/2 cup WALNUT PIECES in 1 tsp. CANOLA OIL until fragrant.

—Whisk the dressing together: 1/2 cup WALNUT OIL, 1 TB RED WINE VINEGAR, 1/2 teasp GARLIC-LEMON SEASONING and 2 pinches WHITE PEPPER. Stir in walnuts.

—Tear 2 heads BOSTON or BIBB LETTUCE, 1 bunch ARUGULA and 1 bunch WATERCRESS and toss together in a large bowl. Divide onto salad plates. Chunk 8-oz. mild GOAT CHEESE (CHEVRE), or FETA CHEESE and divide in mounds over greens.

—Peel and thin slice 3 ripe PEARS and place around cheese. Pour dressing over.

ROSE PETAL FRUIT SALAD

This recipe works for: Weight Loss, Illness Recovery, Detoxification
Makes 6 servings:

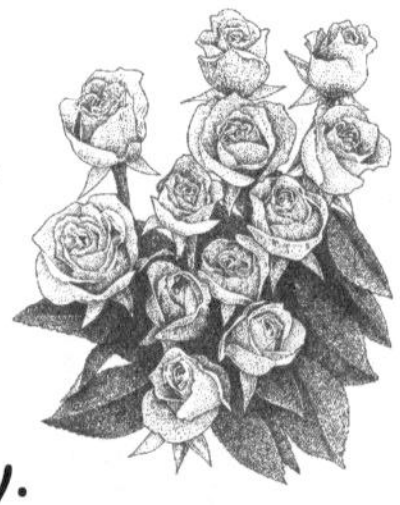

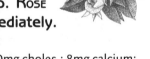

Artfully arrange 1 1/2 cup rinsed BLUEBERRIES and 3 1/2 cups sliced NECTARINES on a platter. Sprinkle fruit with 1/2 cup ROSE PETALS and 1/4 cup VIOLETS or NASTURTIUMS.

—In a small bowl, whisk 2 TBS RASPBERRY VINEGAR, 1 1/2 tsp. ROSE FLOWER WATER and 2 pinches FRUCTOSE. Pour over salad. Serve immediately.

Nutrition: 62 calories; 1gm protein; 15gm carbohydrate; 3gm fiber; 1gm total fat; 0mg choles.; 8mg calcium; 1mg iron; 9mg magnesium; 210mg potass.; 2mg sodium; Vit. A 71 IU; Vit. C 10mg; Vit. E 1 IU.

STAR FRUIT SALAD With CRISPY RICE NOODLES

This recipe works for: Weight Control, Hair and Skin, Arthritis, Anti-Aging
Makes 4 servings:

Whisk SESAME-LIME VINAIGRETTE ingredients in a bowl: 2 TBS OLIVE OIL, 2 TBS LIME JUICE, 1/2 teasp. STEVIA LEAVES, 2 tsp. TOASTED SESAME OIL, 1 teasp. GARLIC-LEMON SEASONING, 1 teasp. GINGER ROOT POWDER, 2 TBS TAMARI. Set aside.

—Arrange 5 cups BABY SPRING GREENS or BABY ASIAN GREENS on 4 plates. Peel and cube 1 large MANGO and thinly slice 2 STAR FRUITS. Arrange over greens.

—In a bag, break up 1-oz. RICE STICK NOODLES into 2 to 3-inch lengths. In a shallow skillet, heat 1 TB. CANOLA OIL until hot but not smoking. Add a thin layer of noodles ..... they will instantly puff up and turn white. Turn noodles over with a spatula. When puffed, remove to paper towels; drain. Repeat with remaining noodles. Do not crowd pan or noodles will not cook properly.

—Top salads with crispy noodles. Drizzle with SESAME-LIME VINAIGRETTE.

Nutrition: 214 calories; 3gm protein; 23gm carbohydrate; 5gm fiber; 13g total fat; 0mg choles.; 35mg calcium; 1mg iron; 24mg magnesium; 399mg potass.; 238mg sodium; Vit. A 301 IU; Vit. C 45mg; Vit. E 5 IU.

Marinated Salads

Far more than just a "3-Bean" tradition, marinated salads mean cultured vegetables, and that means they have a digestive health bonus in every bite. Marinades "cold cook" and tenderize the vegetables. They are a boon to time-pressed, busy people, because they keep food so beautifully. Just make these salads when you have some time, and chill them for later.

ONION MARINATED MUSHROOMS and GREEN BEANS

This recipe works for: Stress Control, Hair, Skin and Nails, Arthritis
For 4 salads, about 3/4 cup each:

Slice 8-oz. Button Mushrooms; trim 8-oz. French-cut or Italian Green Beans.
—Whisk the marinade. 1 TB Dijon Mustard, 2 TBS each chopped Green Onion and chopped Red Onion, 3 TBS Tarragon Vinegar, 6 TBS Olive Oil, 1 TB chopped fresh Basil or 1 teasp. dry Basil. Toss with mushrooms and beans. Chill overnight.

Nutrition: 224 calories; 3gm protein; 8gm carbohydrate; 3gm fiber; 21g total fat; 0mg choles.; 47mg calcium; 1mg iron; 22mg magnesium; 366mg potass.; 39mg sodium; Vit. A 34 IU; Vit. C 11mg; Vit. E 5 IU.

LEMON MUSHROOMS These mushrooms are absolutely delectable.

This recipe works for: Immune Power, Cancer Protection, Fatigue Syndromes
For 4 salads:

Use a blend of 20 to 24 gourmet mushrooms: Chanterelles, fresh Shiitakes, Enokis, and Buttons. Brush clean, then halve or slice them. Add 1 small, sliced Red Onion.
—Mix the marinade: 1 cup Olive Oil, 1 minced Shallot, 1 TB fresh Oregano or 1 teasp. dry Oregano, 1/2 cup White Wine, 1/4 cup Lemon Juice, 1/2 teasp. Lemon-Pepper. Toss marinade with mushroom mix. Chill, covered overnight. Top with 1/3 cup Watercress Leaves or Sunflower Sprouts.

BALSAMIC ONIONS

This recipe works for: Respiratory Infections, Allergies and Asthma, Arthritis
For 4 to 6 servings:

Sizzle 2 sliced Red Onions and 2 sliced Yellow Onions in 4 TBS Olive Oil or Organic Chicken Broth until aromatic, about 5 minutes. Add 2 to 3 TBS Balsamic Vinegar, 1 teasp. dry Thyme, and 1/2 teasp. Pepper. Chill for at least an hour. Serve over very tart greens like Escarole, Frisee or Arugula.

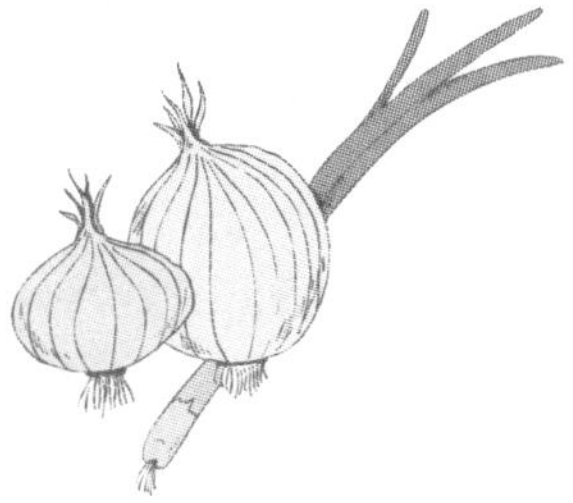

SIX BEAN MEXI-SALAD

This recipe works for: Sports Nutrition, Men's Health, Fatigue Syndromes
Makes 6 servings:

In a large bowl, whisk 2 TBS Olive Oil, 1 TB Balsamic Vinegar, 1 teasp. <u>each</u> Whole Cumin Seeds and Mustard Seeds, pan toasted until fragrant, and $^1/_2$ tsp. Sea Salt.

—Stir in 1 grated Carrot, 1 Habañero Pepper, seeded and minced. Toss to coat.

—Add 1 cup <u>each</u> canned Pinto Beans, Black Beans, Garbanzos, Red Kidney Beans and Small White Beans, drained and rinsed. Add 1 cup frozen Lima Beans, thawed. Mix in 4 TBS minced Cilantro Leaves; add $^1/_4$ teasp. dry Coriander Powder if desired.

Nutrition: 284 calories; 14gm protein; 44gm carbohydrate; 13gm fiber; 6g total fat; 0mg choles.; 103mg calcium; 5mg iron; 79mg magnes.; 695mg potass.; 692mg sodium; Vit. A 352 IU; Vit. C 24mg; Vit. E 1 IU.

FIESTA BEAN SALAD

This recipe works for: Sports Nutrition, Men's Health, Healing and Recovery
Makes 8 salads:

Thaw, rinse and drain 2 16-oz packages frozen French-cut Green Beans. Place in a large bowl. Add 1 can Small White Beans, rinsed and drained, and <u>either</u> 1 can Dark Red Kidney Beans, rinsed and drained, or 1 jar roasted Red Bell Peppers, slivered. Snip in 4 Scallions and 4 TBS fresh Cilantro. Season with Lemon-Pepper to taste.

—Make a LEMON MARINADE: Whisk together until thickened, 6 TBS Olive Oil, 3 TBS Lemon Juice, 1 $^1/_2$ tsp. grated Lemon Zest, 1 $^1/_2$ tsp. Dijon Mustard, 1 $^1/_2$ tsp. Honey, and Black Pepper to taste. Toss with bean mix. Let stand overnight. Snip on Cilantro.

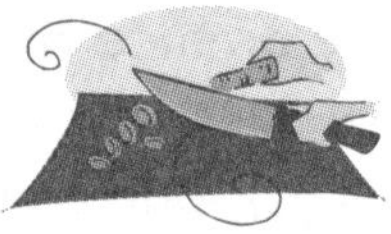

Pasta, Rice and Whole Grain Salads

Check pasta ingredients carefully if you are on a healing or restricted diet. I recommend using one of the many fine vegetable or whole grain pastas available.

HOT CORN SALAD

This recipe works for: Fatigue Syndromes, Arthritis, Hair, Skin and Nails
Makes 6 salads:

In a skillet over medium heat, sizzle 1 diced Onion in the liquid from a small jar of Artichoke Hearts. Add 4 cups Corn Kernels and sizzle for 5 minutes. Add $^1/_4$ cup Yellow Bell Pepper, chopped, $^1/_4$ cup Red Bell Pepper, chopped, Tarragon Leaves from 2 sprigs, and Garlic-Lemon Seasoning to taste. Serve on Baby Spinach or Radicchio Leaves.

ADVANTAGE SALAD

This recipe works for: Sports Nutrition, Men's and Women's Health, Anti-Aging
For 4 salads:

Cook 2 cups Vegetable Pasta Elbows in 2-qts. boiling salted water with 1 TB Olive Oil added to prevent boiling over. Cook uncovered, stirring occasionally for 10 minutes until tender. Drain and toss. Put pasta into a large marinating bowl.

—Add $^1/_2$ cup chopped Celery, 1 grated Carrot, $^1/_2$ cup frozen Green Peas, $^1/_4$ cup Soy Bacon Bits, and $^1/_4$ cup Sweet Pickle Relish.

—Make the HONEY MUSTARD DRESSING: Mix 2 chopped Scallions, 1 teasp. Sweet-Hot Mustard, 2 TBS Olive Oil, $^1/_2$ teasp. dry Basil, $^1/_4$ teasp. dry Tarragon, $^1/_4$ teasp. dry Thyme, $^1/_4$ cup Tarragon Vinegar, 2 teasp. Honey. Chill to blend flavors. Pour over salad.

ARTICHOKES and LINGUINE MONTEREY

This recipe works for: Arthritis, Men's Health, Anti-Aging
For 4 salads:

Sizzle in 2 TBS Olive Oil until fragrant: 1 clove minced Garlic, $^1/_2$ cup chopped Red Onion, 2 TBS sliced Black Olives, $^1/_2$ cup chopped Mushrooms, $^3/_4$ cup chopped Tomato. Remove from heat; toss with 1 TB Lemon Juice and $^1/_2$ cup White Wine. Put in a bowl.

—Bring 3 to 4-qts. salted water to a boil. Add contents of an 11-oz. jar water-packed Artichoke Hearts, and simmer 4 minutes. Remove artichokes with a slotted spoon, and add to salad bowl. Set aside.

Add 6-oz. dry Linguine to boiling artichoke water. Cook just to al dente, 5 to 7 minutes. Drain, and toss with salad ingredients. Turn onto a platter. Slice on top, 1 ripe Avocado. Sprinkle with Parmesan-Reggiano Cheese and chill until ready to serve.

KASHA SPINACH SALAD

This recipe works for: Arthritis, Men's Health, Anti-Aging
For 6 salads:

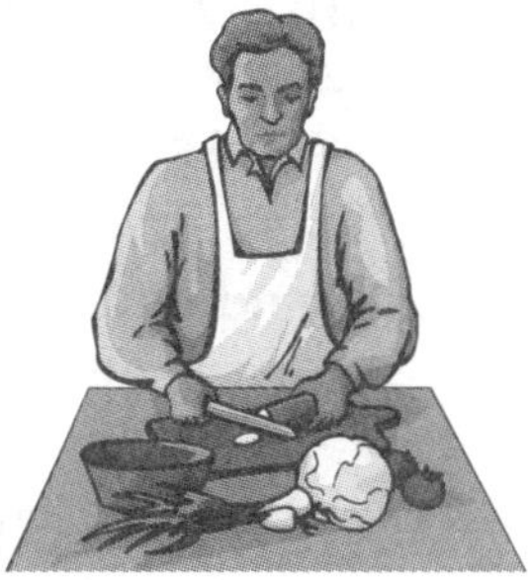

Sizzle in a skillet until aromatic, 1 minute: 1 TB Olive Oil, 2 chopped Shallots and 1 teasp. Garlic-Lemon Seasoning.

—Add $^1/_2$ cup Kasha (cracked wheat); sauté for 1 more minute. Sprinkle with Lemon-Pepper. Add 1 cup Water. Cover, reduce heat and cook until water is absorbed, about 10 to 12 minutes. Remove from heat and fluff with a fork. Toss with Kasha: 4-oz. sliced Mushrooms, 4 diced Plum Tomatoes, 6 chopped Scallions, $^1/_3$ cup Walnut Pieces, 3 TBS Raisins.

—Whisk the simple dressing together: $^1/_3$ cup Olive Oil, 1 TB Dijon Mustard, 2 TBS Tarragon Vinegar, $^1/_4$ teasp. Black Pepper.

Divide 1 bag Baby Spinach between individual salad plates and top with mounds of salad. Drizzle with dressing and serve.

CREAMY RICE SALAD

This recipe works for: Stress Management, Fatigue Syndromes, Immune Power
For 6 salads:

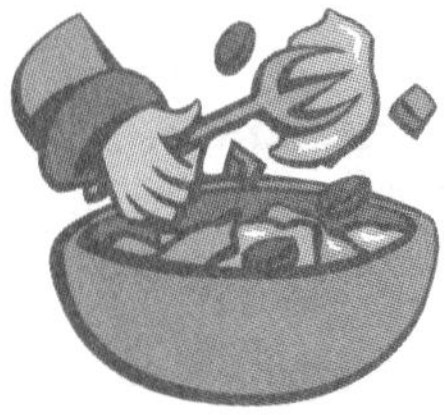

Bring 1 1/2 cups Salted Water to boil. Add 6-oz. White Basmati Rice or Golden Rose Rice. Add rice and return to boil. Cover and cook over low heat until water is absorbed and rice is tender, about 40 minutes. Remove from heat, add 1 cup frozen Green Peas, fluff; set aside.

—Mix the dressing: 1/2 cup Low-fat Mayonnaise, 1/2 cup Lemon-Lime Yogurt, 1/2 cup thinly sliced Green Onions, 1/4 cup snipped Parsley, 1/4 teasp. Lemon-Pepper, 1/2 teasp. Sesame Salt. Let sit to bloom. Stir into dressing: 1 cup Cocktail Tomatoes, halved, 1 cup diced Hothouse Cucumber, 1/2 cup diced Celery. Add dressing and veggies to rice blend; toss to mix. Serve at room temperature in a large bowl lined with Bibb Lettuce Leaves.

Nutrition: 169 calories; 6gm protein; 35gm carbohydrate; 3gm fiber; 1g total fat; 1mg choles.; 65mg calcium; 1mg iron; 22mg magnesium; 314mg potass.; 268mg sodium; Vit. A 88 IU; Vit. C 20mg; Vit. E 1 IU.

MOROCCO SALAD

This recipe works for: Digestive Disorders, Weight Control, Liver and Organ Health
For 4 salads:

Pour 1 1/4 cups Boiling Water over 1 1/2 cup Dry Couscous. Cover; let sit for 10-15 minutes until water is absorbed. Remove cover and fluff. Add 1 teasp. Sesame Salt and a pinch Saffron Threads OR 4 TBS fresh chopped Mint. Set aside.

—Toast 1/2 cup slivered Almonds in the oven until golden. Set aside.

—Steam until tender crisp: 1 cup diced Carrots, 1 diced Bell Pepper (any color), 1 cup frozen French-cut Green Beans, 1/3 cup diced Red Onion. Drain when done; toss with the almonds and 1/3 cup Currants. Mix with couscous and set aside.

—Make the dressing. Whisk 6 TBS Olive Oil, 4 TBS Lemon Juice, 3 TBS Orange Juice, 1/2 teasp. Lemon-Pepper, 1/4 teasp. Cinnamon, 1/4 teasp. Paprika. Toss with salad ingredients and couscous, and chill to blend flavors.

CORNY RICE SALAD A great way to use leftover rice. Lots of EFA's.

This recipe works for: Fatigue Syndromes, Hair, Skin, Nails, Brain Boosting
For 6 salads:

Have ready 4 cups cooked Brown Rice. In large bowl, combine rice with 2 cups thawed frozen Corn Kernels, 2 cups finely shredded Spinach Leaves, 1/3 cup chopped Black Olives, 2 Scallions, minced, 1/4 cup snipped fresh Parsley, 2 TBS Olive Oil, 2 TBS fresh Lemon Juice, 2 TB Sesame Seeds, 1 tsp. Sesame Salt, 1/2 tsp. White Pepper. Toss until well mixed and serve at room temperature.

INCA CHILI GRAINS SALAD

This recipe works for: Fatigue Syndromes, Women's Health, Sports Nutrition
For 4 salads:

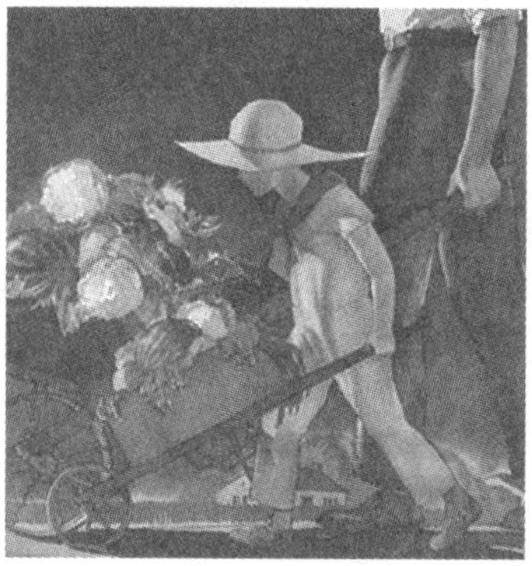

Sizzle 1 Clove Garlic minced, 1 Onion finely chopped, and $^1/_4$ teasp. dried Chili Flakes in 2 teasp. Olive Oil until browned, 5 minutes. Add $^1/_3$ cup Amaranth and $^1/_3$ cup Quinoa; stir until slightly toasted, 3 minutes. Add 1 cup canned Corn Kernels, and 1 cup organic Chicken Broth. Bring to a boil; cover and simmer over medium heat until liquid is absorbed, about 15 minutes.

—Let cool to room temperature. Mix 2 TBS Lime Juice, $^1/_3$ cup chopped Green Chilies, $^1/_4$ cup minced fresh Cilantro. Spoon into salad bowls lined with 4 large Butter Lettuce Leaves, rinsed and crisped. Add Sea Salt and fresh-ground Pepper to taste.

Nutrition: 193 calories; 7gm protein; 33gm carbohydrate; 5gm fiber; 5g total fat; 0mg choles.; 74mg calcium; 3mg iron; 44mg magnesium; 376mg potassium; 238mg sodium; Vit. A 54 IU; Vit. C 13mg; Vit. E 5 IU,

High Protein Salads without Meat

Vegetarians can get plenty of protein for healing without meat or dairy foods. Diet scientists tell us that our bodies need an average of 2.5% calories from protein in a healthy meal… potatoes supply 10%, broccoli provides 43%, oranges offer 9%. These salads almost ensure a drop in high cholesterol.

QUINOA SALAD Quinoa is higher in protein than any other grain.

This recipe works for: Immune Breakdown, Illness Recovery, Heart Health
For 4 salads:

Rinse 1 cup Quinoa in a strainer to remove bitter edge. Bring 2 cups Water to a boil with 1 teasp. Sea Salt. Add Quinoa and cook over low heat until slightly chewy, about 10 minutes. Drain off any excess water. Put in a large mixing bowl and mix in $^1/_2$ cup Raisins, 2 TBS chopped Chives, $^1/_4$ cup minced Celery, and $^1/_4$ cup diced Carrots.

—Roast 4 TBS Pine Nuts in a dry skillet or the oven until golden; set aside.

—Make the dressing: whisk $^1/_4$ cup Canola Oil, 1 TB Lemon Juice, 1 teasp. grated Lemon Zest, $^1/_4$ teasp. Paprika, $^1/_4$ teasp. ground Cumin and $^1/_4$ teasp. ground Coriander. Add pine nuts and toss. Cover individual plates with Baby Spinach Leaves and mound salad on them. Pour dressing over and serve.

Nutrition: 420 calories; 11gm protein; 48gm carbohydrate; 5gm fiber; 23g total fat; 0mg choles.; 77mg calcium; 7mg iron; 154mg magnes.; 754mg potass.; 310mg sodium; Vit. A 400 IU; Vit. C 15mg; Vit. E 11 IU.

NUTS and BOLTS

This recipe works for: Stress and Fatigue, Men's Health, Sports Nutrition, Arthritis
For 4 salads:

Toast in a 375°F oven for 10 minutes until brown: 1/2 cup each, chopped Almonds and chopped Cashews. Let cool 5 minutes. Mix with 1 cup diced Celery, and 1/4 cup each, diced Carrots, snipped Parsley, diced Red Bell Pepper and snipped Green Onions.

—Make the protein-rich ALMOND BUTTER DRESSING: Blend 1/2 cup Almond Butter, 2 TBS Tamari, 1 TB Soy Bacon Bits, 1 TB Canola Oil, 1/2 teasp. Black Pepper, 1/2 teasp. dry Sweet Basil. Pour over salad and sprinkle on Toasted Pumpkin Seeds and Alfalfa Sprouts.

EGG SALAD LIGHT

An excellent protein source and very nutritious food, egg yolk cholesterol which got such a bad "rap" for years is balanced by the egg white lecithin phosphatides.

This recipe works for: Hair, Skin and Nails, Women's Health, Arthritis
For 4 servings:

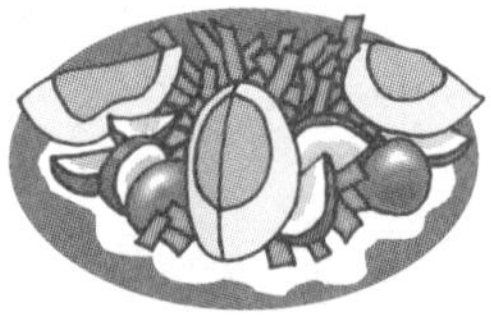

Hard boil 6 Eggs the foolproof way. Put eggs in a pan of cold water. Bring to a boil. Immediately turn off heat and cover pan. Let eggs sit exactly 6 minutes. Pour off water and cover with cold water. Let sit til ready to peel.

—Mash together in a bowl: the hard boiled Eggs, 2 TBS Low-Fat Mayonnaise, 2 ribs Celery minced, 2 teasp. Dijon Mustard, 2 TBS snipped Parsley, 2 TBS Low-Fat Plain Yogurt, 1/4 teasp. Curry Powder, juice of 1 small Lemon, 1/4 teasp. Lemon-Pepper.

—Mound on individual Boston Lettuce Cups and top mounds with dashes of Paprika.

Nutrition: 136 calories; 10gm protein; 4gm carbohydrate; 1gm fiber; 8g total fat; 318mg choles.; 67mg calcium; 1mg iron; 13mg magnesium; 201mg potass.; 150mg sodium; Vit. A 140 IU; Vit. C 8mg; Vit. E 1 IU.

CHERRY TOMS and BOW TIES

This recipe works for: Fatigue Syndromes, Men's Health, Sports Nutrition
For 4 small salads:

Halve 2 pints Cherry Tomatoes into a large bowl. Snip in 1 whole bunch Scallions and 1 cup fresh Parsley. Toss and chill while pasta is cooking. Bring 2-qts. Water and 1 teasp. Canola Oil to a boil; cook 2 cups Bow Tie Pasta to al dente. Drain, and toss with tomato blend. —Divide salad onto Spinach heaped salad plates. Sprinkle with Parmesan, cubes of Mozzarella, and drizzles of Olive Oil and Balsamic Vinegar.

—Top each salad with 2 TBS DILL MAYONNAISE SAUCE: Mix 1/2 cup Low-Fat Mayonnaise, 1/2 cup Low-Fat Yogurt, 1 TB fresh snipped Dill Weed (or 1 teasp. dry), 2 teasp. Lemon Juice, 1/2 teasp. GREAT 28 MIX (Pg. 487) or Herb-Vegetable Seasoning Salt.

PROTEIN VEGGIE BURGERS with MANGO SALSA SALAD

This recipe works for: Heart Health, Men's and Kid's Health, Sports Nutrition
Makes 4 salads: Preheat oven to 400°F.

Toss in a bowl: 2 Mangoes peeled, pitted and diced, $^1/_2$ small Red Onion minced, 4 TBS Orange Juice, 1 small Jalapeño Chile seeded and minced (wear rubber gloves), 2 TBS minced fresh Cilantro Leaves and Herb Seasoning Salt to taste. Set aside.

—Bake 4 frozen Veggie Burgers until hot, turning once, about 10 minutes.

—Place 2 QTS Baby Greens rinsed and dried in a large bowl. Drizzle with 1 TB Olive Oil and mango mixture; toss and coat. Divide salad among four plates. Place one hot burger on top of each portion. Serve immediately.

SZECHUAN TOFU SALAD

This recipe works for: Fatigue Syndromes, Women's Health, Bone Building
For 6 salads:

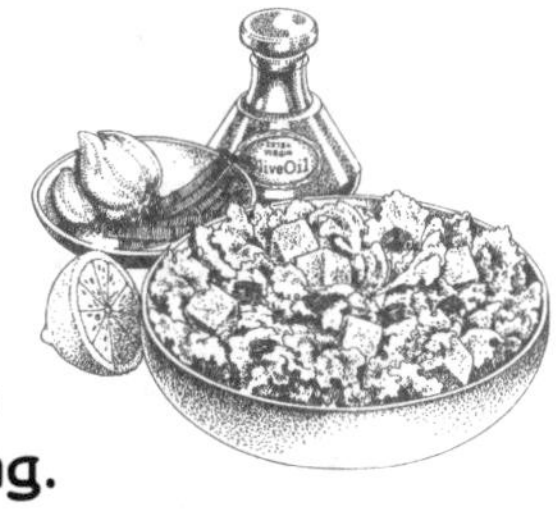

Make the marinade in the blender: 6 fresh Basil Leaves (or $^1/_2$ teasp. dried), $^1/_2$ teasp. dried crushed Hot Pepper (or $^1/_8$ teasp. Sambal Hot Chili Sauce), $^1/_4$ cup grated Ginger, $^1/_4$ cup Tamari, $^1/_4$ cup Brown Rice Vinegar, $^1/_4$ cup Toasted Sesame Oil and 3 TBS Honey.

—Marinate 1 LB firm Tofu Cubes in a skillet. Then brown cubes in the marinade. Pour $^1/_2$ cup marinade into a bowl for the dressing.

—Leave the rest in the skillet with the tofu and add $1^1/_2$ cups shredded Green Cabbage, $1^1/_2$ cups grated Carrots, 6 chopped Scallions. Toss to blend.

—Thinly slice 1 head Romaine. Divide on 6 salad plates. Mound on tofu and cabbage mix. Top with crunchy Chinese Noodles, and pour remaining marinade over.

Nutritional analysis per serving: 278 calories; 15gm. protein; 22gm. carbohydrate; 3gm. fiber; 14gm. fat; 0 cholesterol; 213mg. calcium; 10mg. iron; 96mg.magnesium; 581mg. potassium; 233mg. sodium; 2mg. zinc.

BLACK BEAN and CELERY SALAD

This recipe works for: Arthritis, Healthy Pregnancy, Recovery from Illness
For 6 salads: Use a heavy cooking pot for beans.

Cover 8-oz. Black Beans with cold water and soak overnight. Drain, add cold water to cover by 2"; bring to a rapid boil. Reduce heat to low and simmer 45 minutes. Add $^1/_2$ teasp. Sea Salt and cook for 45 minutes more. Drain and chill.

—Sizzle 1 sliced Red Onion in 2 TBS Olive Oil until aromatic. Turn cooked beans into a large bowl and add 3 ribs diced Celery and $^1/_2$ diced Red Bell Pepper; toss to mix.

—Make the dressing: $^1/_3$ cup Canola Oil, 3 TBS Lime Juice, grated Zest of 1 Lime, $^1/_2$ teasp. Lemon-Pepper, $^1/_2$ teasp. Cumin Seeds. Toss gently with the salad.

Nutrition: 251 calories; 7gm protein; 21gm carbohydrate; 8gm fiber; 15g total fat; 0mg choles.; 38mg calcium; 2mg iron; 59mg magnesium; 383mg potass.; 197mg sodium; Vit. A 39 IU; Vit. C 19mg; Vit. E 35 IU.

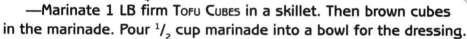

SESAME NOODLE SALAD

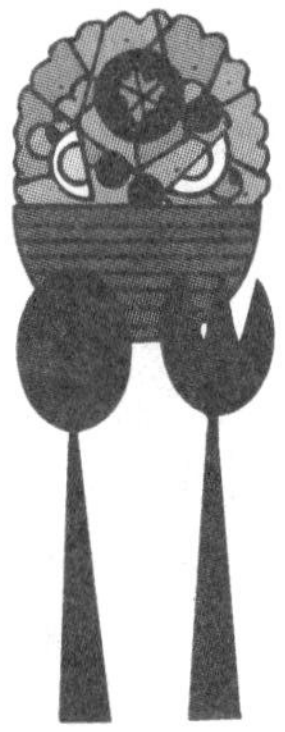

This recipe works for: Cancer Control, Women's Health
For 6 salads:

Dry roast 1/4 cup Sesame Seeds in a skillet until golden. Set aside.

—Soak 10 dry Shiitake Mushrooms in Water until soft. Sliver and set aside. Reserve mushroom soaking water.

—Bring 3-qts. of Salted Water to boil in a large pot. Add mushroom soaking water. Blanch 1 bunch Broccoli, diced (stems) and sliced (florets) 3 minutes only. Remove with slotted spoon to a bowl of ice water.

—Bring water to boil again and drop in 1 LB Asparagus in 1" pieces, and 1 cup Mung Bean Sprouts. Blanch for 1 minute until asparagus is bright green. Remove with slotted spoon and add to broccoli ice water. Chill briefly.

—Bring water to boil again, and cook 8-oz dry Chinese Spaghetti Noodles for 2 1/2 minutes, just to al dente. Drain and toss with 2 teasp. Toasted Sesame Oil. Set aside.

—Make the dressing. Bring 1/2 cup organic Chicken Broth to a boil in a saucepan. Add and stir until smooth and aromatic: 1/2 cup Peanut Butter, 1/4 cup Brown Rice Vinegar, 1/4 cup minced Scallions, 2 TBS Tamari, 2 TBS minced fresh Ginger, 1 TB Toasted Sesame Oil, 1 TB Sherry, 1 teasp. Sambal Chili Sauce, 1/2 teasp. Garlic-Lemon Seasoning, and the reserved sesame seeds.

—Toss the sauce with vegetables and noodles. Top with 2 TBS minced Cilantro Leaves, and slivers of Red Bell Pepper.

Seafood, Chicken and Turkey Salads

Chicken and turkey are low fat meats; they make any salad a satisfying protein-rich meal. Make sure they are organic for healing to avoid hormones and anti-biotics.

TUNA NOODLE SALAD

This recipe works for: Fatigue Syndromes, Weight Control, Men's-Kid's Health
For 4 large salads:

Have ready 2 cups lightly cooked Egg Noodles drizzled with a little Olive Oil.

—Steam 1 cup Green Peas and 1 cup thinly sliced Scallions in a steamer until bright green. Dump peas and onions into a salad bowl. Set aside.

—Add to steamer 2 cups French-cut Green Beans; cook covered until bright green. Add to salad bowl with peas and onions. Add 2 cups cubed Tomatoes and one 7-oz. can water-packed Tuna. Mix together: Juice of 1 Lemon, 2 TBS Olive Oil, 2 TBS each fresh minced Parsley and Basil. Mix and toss all. Serve on Spinach mounds.

Nutrition: 351 calories; 22gm protein; 47gm carbohydrate; 9gm fiber; 9g total fat; 58mg choles.; 134mg calcium; 6mg iron; 115mg magnes.; 930mg potass.; 286mg sodium; Vit. A 531 IU; Vit. C 68mg; Vit. E 5 IU.

FANCY CHICKEN - COUSCOUS SALADS in BUTTER CUPS

This recipe works for: Respiratory Health, Weight Control, Women's Health
Makes 16 appetizer salads:

Have ready 4 cups skinned cooked Chicken Breasts, diced.

—Make the CUMIN ONIONS: Thinly sliver 1 large Red Onion. In a 3-qt pan, bring 6 cups water and 1/4 cup Brown Rice Vinegar to a boil. Add onion and 1 tsp. Cumin Seed. and 1 teasp. Fructose. Return to boil; pour onion and seed in a strainer to drain.

—Make the SPICY COUSCOUS: in a 4-qt. pan, bring 3 cups Organic, Low-Fat Chicken Broth to a boil. Add 2 TBS Mustard Seed, 1 1/2 tsp. Coriander Seed, 1 tsp. Cumin Seed, 1 tsp. Tarragon Leaves, 1 tsp. Curry Powder, and 1/2 teasp. Hulled Cardamom Seed. Simmer 5 minutes, then add 2 cups Couscous and 1 teasp. Sea Salt. Stir, remove from heat, and cover. Let stand until cool. Fluff with a fork, cover and chill.

—Make the ORANGE-LIME DRESSING. Combine 1 1/2 cups Orange Juice and 1 cup Lime Juice with 1/4 cup minced fresh Ginger, and 1 tsp. crushed dried Red Chilies (or 1/8 teasp. Sambal Hot Chili Paste). Let stand 15 minutes to blend flavors.

—In a large bowl, mix chicken breasts, Cumin Onions, 1 1/2 cups chopped Orange Segments, 3/4 cup fresh minced Cilantro, and 1/2 the Orange-Lime Dressing. Mix remaining dressing with Spicy Couscous.

—To serve, mound chicken salad and couscous salad in separate mounds on a serving platter. Sprinkle 2 TBS minced Cilantro over the chicken mound; grate the Zest of 1 Orange over the the couscous mound. Separate the leaves of 1 head Butter Lettuce. Arrange around the salad mounds. Alternate the slices of 2 Oranges and 2 Limes between lettuce leaves. Spoon bite-size portions of salad onto leaves.

Nutrition: 170 calories; 20gm protein; 16gm carbohydrate; 2gm fiber; 3g total fat; 48mg choles.; 51mg calcium; 1mg iron; 34mg magnes.; 368mg potass.; 180mg sodium; Vit. A 29 IU; Vit. C 39mg; Vit. E 1 IU.

EASY TURKEY COBB SALAD

This recipe works for: Arthritis, Stress Control, Women's and Men's Health
For 4 meal size salads:

Shred 1 head Romaine Lettuce and 1 cup Watercress Leaves into a big bowl.

—Mix together: 1/3 cup oven-toasted, sliced Almonds, 8-oz. cooked Turkey in matchstick slices, 2 sliced hard boiled Eggs, 1 cup Sunflower Sprouts, 4-oz. grated Low-Fat Cheddar Cheese, and 2 large Tomatoes, chopped.

—Top with a CREAMY MUSTARD DRESSING: whisk together 2 TBS Dijon Mustard, 4 TBS Plain Low-Fat Yogurt, 1/4 cup White Wine, 1/2 teasp. Lemon-Pepper, 1/2 cup Olive Oil 1/4 teasp. Rosemary.

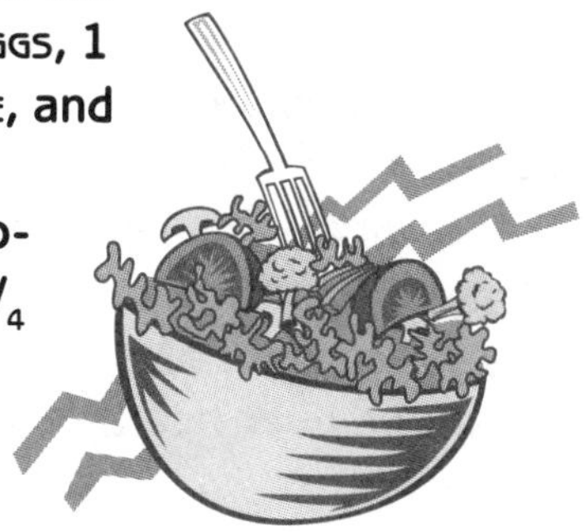

—Spoon over salad. Sprinkle with crisp Chinese Noodles.

SESAME CHICKEN SALAD WITH PEA PODS

This recipe works for: Respiratory Health, Illness Recovery, Women's Health
For 6 small salads:

Blanch 8-oz. trimmed Snow Peas and $^1/_4$ cup thin sliced Green Onions in boiling water for 1 minute only. Rinse under cold water to set color. Set aside.

—Dry toast 2 TBS Sesame Seeds in a skillet until golden. Toss 2 teasp. of the seeds with the snow peas. Add 4 TBS Olive Oil to remaining sesame seeds and sauté until fragrant with 2 Cloves Garlic minced, 3 TBS Lemon Juice, $1^1/_2$ TBS Tamari, 1 TB fresh minced Ginger and $1^1/_2$ TBS Brown Rice Vinegar.

—Add to sauce and toss: 3 cups shredded cooked Organic Chicken Breast, 1 cup diced Celery and $^1/_3$ cup fresh chopped Cilantro Leaves. Chill and serve on greens.

Nutrition: 294 calories; 35gm protein; 13gm carbohydrate; 3gm fiber; 12g total fat; 80mg choles.; 47mg calcium; 2mg iron; 65mg magnes.; 497mg potass.; 168mg sodium; Vit. A 19 IU; Vit. C 11mg; Vit. E 1 IU.

HOT TURKEY and SPICE SALAD

This recipe works for: Stress and Exhaustion, Illness Recovery, Circulatory Health
Makes 8 large servings: Use a large stew pot.

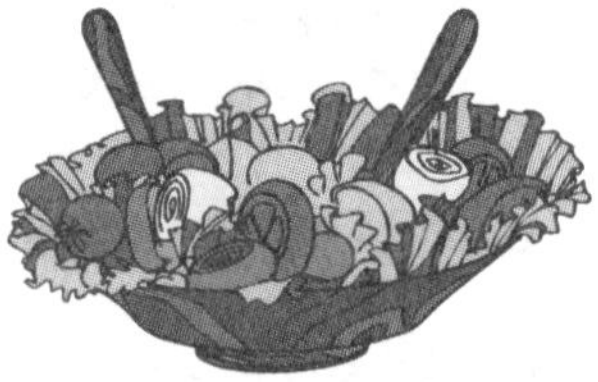

Have ready 4 cups hot cooked Brown Rice.

—Make the TURKEY MEATBALLS: In a bowl, mix 1 LB ground Lean Turkey, 1 Egg, 4 TBS dry Bread Crumbs, 1 tsp. ground Coriander, $^1/_3$ cup chopped Onion, and 1 tsp. Sea Salt until well blended. Shape meatball mixture into 1-inch balls.

—Sizzle in 1 TB Canola Oil: 1 cup chopped Onion, $1^1/_2$ TB minced Crystallized Ginger, and 2 minced Cloves Garlic about 8 minutes. Add 2 TBS Curry Powder, $^1/_2$ tsp. ground Cumin, $^1/_4$ tsp. Rosemary and $^1/_2$ tsp. Honey; stir until spices are fragrant, for 1 minute. Add 3 cups organic Low-Fat Chicken Broth and bring to a boil. Drop Turkey Meatballs into boiling broth. Simmer until meatballs are no longer pink (8 minutes).

—In a small bowl, mix 3 TBS Arrowroot Powder and $^1/_3$ cup organic Low-Fat Chicken Broth. Add to pot, stirring until sauce boils, about 2 minutes. Season to taste.

—Make the CHUTNEY SAUCE: Pare yellow skin from 1 Lemon with a vegetable peeler, and finely chop. With a knife, cut off and discard white pith from Lemon. Coarsely chop lemon; discard seeds. In a pan, bring to a boil 1 cup Water, the Lemon Peel, the chopped Lemon, 1 cup dried or fresh chopped Apricots, 5 TBS Fructose, 1 TB each minced fresh Ginger, Coriander Seed, Mustard Seed, and $^1/_2$ tsp. Hot Chili Sauce. Reduce heat, and simmer stirring often, until most of the liquid is absorbed, 10 to 12 minutes. Sprinkle with Herbal Seasoning Salt and 2 TBS Lemon Juice, to taste.

—Mound rice on plates; surround with $^1/_2$ LB. Baby Spinach Leaves. Spoon meatballs and sauce over rice and spinach. Top with Chutney and Low-fat Yogurt dollops.

Nutrition: 347 calories; 22gm protein; 47gm carbohydrate; 5gm fiber; 8g total fat; 41mg choles.; 310mg calcium; 3mg iron; 100mg magnes.; 587mg potass.; 361mg sodium; Vit. A 247 IU; Vit. C 15mg; Vit. E 1 IU.

TURKEY ALMOND SALAD the taste of a holiday turkey in a salad.

This recipe works for: Heart Health, Arthritis, Women's and Men's Health
For 4 salads:

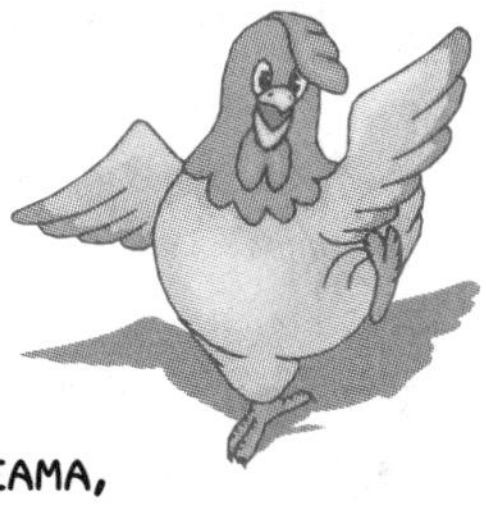

Toast in a 350°F oven until golden: 1 TB minced Shallots, $^1/_2$ cup slivered Almonds, $^1/_2$ cup Whole Wheat Bread cubes.

—Mix dressing: 4 tsp. Tamari, $^1/_3$ cup Brown Rice Vinegar, $^1/_3$ cup Canola Oil, 1 TB Soy Bacon Bits, $^1/_2$ tsp. Black Pepper. Mix salad ingredients: 2 cups cooked diced Turkey, 1 cup sliced Celery, $^1/_2$ cup Jicama, diced. Toss with roasted mixture, and with dressing; serve on chopped Spinach Leaves.

Nutrition: 441 calories; 31gm protein; 11gm carbohydrate; 4gm fiber; 27g total fat; 60mg choles.; 86mg calcium; 3mg iron; 85mg magnes.; 562mg potass.; 194mg sodium; Vit. A 5 IU; Vit. C 5mg; Vit. E trace.

LOW FAT CHICKEN and MUSHROOM SALAD

This recipe works for: Respiratory Infections, Arthritis, Immune Strength
For 8 salads:

Make the marinade: 6 TBS Olive Oil, 4 thinly sliced Scallions, 2 TBS Lemon Juice, 2 TBS minced Cilantro, 1 teasp. Seseame Salt, $^1/_4$ teasp. Black Pepper. Pour over 4-oz. Button Mushrooms, sliced, 4-oz. Shiitake Mushrooms, sliced, 6 cups cooked Organic Chicken Breasts, sliced, and 1 small head Chinese Nappa Cabbage, shredded. Let sit 1 hour.

—Mound on salad plates heaped with Watercress. Sprinkle with Sesame Seeds.

OLD FASHIONED SOUTHERN CHICKEN SALAD

This recipe works for: Respiratory Health, Illness Recovery, Women's Health
For 6 salads:

Put stock ingredients into a large pot: 1 small chunked Onion, 1 small chopped Carrot, $^1/_2$ cup Celery Leaves, $^1/_4$ cup fresh Parsley, 1 tsp. Sea Salt, 10 Peppercorns. Cover with water by 2 inches and bring to a boil. Add 2 whole Organic Chicken Breasts; simmer for 30 to 40 minutes until tender. Remove skin and bones; cube meat. Put in a bowl with 2 sliced hard boiled Eggs, $^1/_2$ cup chopped Green Onions, $^1/_2$ cup chopped Celery and 2 TBS Lemon Juice. Chill.

—Make the DRESSING: Heat 2 tsp. Canola Oil in a pan. Add 2 tsp. Unbleached Flour and stir until bubbly. Add $^1/_4$ cup Tarragon Vinegar, 2 TBS Sherry, 2 TBS Water, $1^1/_2$ TBS Honey, $^1/_2$ tsp. Herbal Seasoning Salt, $^1/_2$ tsp. Dry Mustard, $^1/_4$ tsp. Black Pepper. Whisk until mixture boils and thickens; remove from heat. Stir 1 TB dressing into 1 beaten Egg to warm it, then pour back into the dressing and whisk smooth. Let cool. Toss with the salad to coat. Serve warm on torn greens.

Nutrition: 186 calories; 22gm protein; 10gm carb; 2gm fiber; 5g total fat; 150mg choles.; 55mg calcium; 2mg iron; 35mg magnes.; 382mg potass.; 457mg sodium; Vit. A 266 IU; Vit. C 17mg; Vit. E 1 IU.

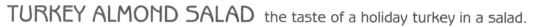

VERY LOW-FAT CHINESE CHICKEN SALAD

This recipe works for: High Blood Pressure, Weight Control, Sugar Imbalances
For 6 salads: Mix salad in a large mixing bowl.

Simmer 2 whole Organic Chicken Breasts in Organic Vegetable Broth for 1 hour until tender. Skin, bone; cut into bite size pieces.

—Mix the marinade: 2 TBS Brown Rice Vinegar, 2 TBS Tamari, 2 TBS sliced Green Onions, 1 TB Soy Bacon Bits, 1 TB Red Star Nutritional Yeast, 1/2 teasp. Black Pepper, 1/4 teasp. dry Mustard, 1 teasp. grated Orange Zest, 1/2 cup Olive Oil. Pour over chicken.

—Chop 1 bunch Broccoli in Chinese Restaurant style. (Cut off ends of each stalk to make 5" stems. Slit lengthwise.) Cook in boiling salted water until broccoli turns a bright green. Drain, add to chicken pieces and chill.

—Mix in a salad serving bowl: 3 cups mixed Baby Asian Greens, 1/2 cup diced Celery, 2 TBS thin-sliced White Daikon Radish, 2 thin-sliced Scallions. Remove chicken and broccoli from the marinade with a slotted spoon, and pour remaining liquid over greens. Toss to mix.

—Arrange broccoli with stems to the center in a ring over the top of the greens. Fill the ring with the chicken. Sprinkle with crumbled Hard Boiled Egg.

Nutrition: 227 calories; 25gm protein; 6gm carbohydrate; 3gm fiber; 12g total fat; 117mg choles.; 71mg calcium; 2mg iron; 54mg magnes.; 571mg potass.; 190mg sodium; Vit. A 128 IU; Vit. C 42mg; Vit. E 3 IU.

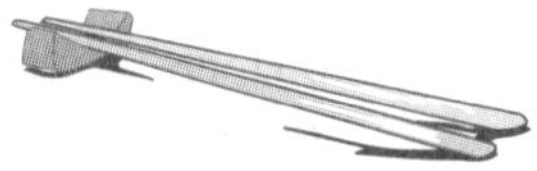

Layered Salads

These salads are delicious to look at and to eat. Make them in a large clear straight-sided bowl for the best effect, allowing the multicolored layers to show through.

BROWN RICE and BAKED TOFU LAYERED SALAD

This recipe works for: Women's Health, Sports Nutrition, Heart Health
For 4 servings: Use a glass salad bowl.

Have ready a 16-oz. package Baked Marinated Tofu.

—Have ready 2 cups cooked Brown Rice. Stir with 1/2 teasp. Granulated Dulse.

—Toast 1/2 cup sliced Almonds in a 350° oven for 10 minutes. Remove; set aside.

—Build the salad layers: Cover bottom of serving bowl with half the rice. Cover rice with Baby Spinach Leaves. Crumble half the baked tofu slices on top of spinach. Cover tofu with a layer of diced Red Bell Pepper, then a layer of diced Celery. Cover celery with rest of the brown rice. Cover rice with a layer of fresh Cilantro Leaves (or Baby Spinach Leaves). Crumble rest of tofu slices on top. Cover tofu with diced Red Bell Pepper, the toasted almonds and drizzle with 2 TBS Balsamic Vinegar.

SUNDAY SALAD

This recipe works for: Waste Management, Weight Control, Men's Health
For 6 to 8 servings: Use a big glass bowl.

Shred Head Lettuce to completely cover the bottom of the bowl.

—Cover lettuce with 3/4 cup chopped Celery. Cover celery with 1/2 Jicama, peeled and diced. Cover jicama with 8-oz. cooked Salad Shrimp or 1/2 diced Red Onion. Cover shrimp or onion with 1/2 cup chopped Bell Pepper.

Parboil for 1 minute, a 10-oz. package frozen Peas until bright green. Layer over bell pepper. Sprinkle on 2 tsp. Fructose. Frost with Low-Fat Mayonnaise to cover. Top with a thick layer of Parmesan Reggiano Cheese. Sprinkle on 2 crumbled hard-boiled Eggs. Arrange a circle of Tomato Wedges on top; sprinkle with snipped Parsley. Chill.

LAYERED SPINACH SALAD

This recipe works for: Hair, Skin and Nails, Liver-Organ Health, Men's Health
Makes 6 servings:

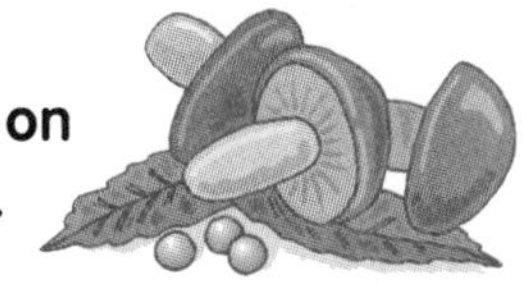

Cover a large rimmed platter with Baby Spinach Leaves. Layer on top 2 thinly sliced Tomatoes, 1 small Red Onion, thinly sliced and 1 cup thinly sliced Button Mushrooms.

—Make the dressing in small bowl: mix 3 TBS Olive Oil, 2 TBS Red Wine, 2 TBS Balsamic Vinegar, 1/4 cup fresh Watercress or Cilantro Leaves, 1 TB minced Chives, Lemon-Pepper to taste. Drizzle over vegetables. Sprinkle on 3 TBS grated Mozzarella.

Nutrition: 101 calories; 3gm protein; 6gm carbohydrate; 2gm fiber; 8g total fat; 2mg choles.; 73mg calcium; 2mg iron; 40mg magnesium; 390mg potassium; 43mg sodium; Vit. A 295 IU; Vit. C 21mg; Vit. E 3 IU.

LAYERED CHICKEN SALAD

This recipe works for: Illness Recovery, Men's Health, Overcoming Addictions
For 6 servings:

Shake dressing in a jar: 1/3 cup Olive Oil, 1/4 cup Tarragon Vinegar, 1/2 teasp. ground Cumin, 1 teasp. Chili Powder, pinches of Sesame Salt, Black Pepper and Nutmeg.

—Shave 1 head Romaine Lettuce; cover bottom of a large clear salad bowl. Cover lettuce with 1 small bunch Spinach washed and torn. Cover spinach with 2 large Beefsteak Tomatoes, thinly sliced. Cover Tomatoes with 1 1/2 cups diced cooked Organic Chicken Breast. Cover chicken with 1/2 cup grated Low-Fat Soy Cheddar or Swiss Cheese.

—Sprinkle with 1/3 cup fresh chopped Parsley, 1/2 cup steamed Green Peas, and 3 minced Green Onions. Cover with 1/3 cup toasted chopped Pecans. Pour dressing over.

Nutrition: 265 calories; 22gm protein; 10gm carbohydrate; 4gm fiber; 16g total fat; 48mg choles.; 93mg calcium; 3mg iron; 66mg magnes.; 665mg potass.; 129mg sodium; Vit. A 377 IU; Vit. C 38mg; Vit. E 5 IU.

SEVEN LAYER TOFU SALAD

This recipe works for: Arthritis, Women's and Men's Health, Liver and Organ Health
For 10 servings: Serve in a 3-qt. clear salad bowl.

Heat the TOFU MARINADE in a saucepan. 1/3 cup Canola Oil, 2/3 cup Tarragon Vinegar, 1 TB Soy Bacon Bits, 1 TB Sherry, 2 teasp. dry Basil (or 1 TB fresh Basil), 1 teasp. dry Thyme, 1/2 teasp. dry Tarragon, 2 teasp. dry Parsley, 1 teasp. Black Pepper.

—Put in a large skillet, 1-lb. Extra Firm Tofu cut in strips, and 1/2 cup thin-sliced Red Onion. Pour on marinade; let sit for 1 hour. Sauté in the marinade until aromatic.

—Assemble the layers: Cover bottom of bowl with 3 cups Baby Spinach Leaves. Cover spinach with chopped Watercress Leaves or Arugula Leaves. Cover leaves with 2 cups halved Cocktail Tomatoes. Cover tomatoes with 1 Hothouse Cucumber, thinly sliced. Cover cucumber with the tofu and onions. Cover tofu with 2 cups diced Carrots. Cover carrots with 1/2 cup sliced Black Olives. Cover the top with crunchy Chinese Noodles or Mozarrella Cheese cubes.

Nutrition: 156 calories; 9gm protein; 10gm carbohydrate; 2gm fiber; 10g total fat; 0mg choles.; 139mg calcium; 6mg iron; 70mg magnes.; 431mg potass.; 120mg sodium; Vit. A 792 IU; Vit. C 18mg; Vit. E 3 IU.

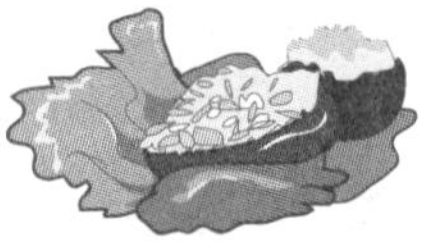

Hot Salads

Hot salads impart more intense flavor and texture to vegetables and other ingredients. Try them good for your winter diet, side dishes, brunches or lunches.

HOT POTATO SALAD

This recipe works for: Men's Health, Weight Control, Sugar Imbalances
For 6 salads:

Cube 3 large Red Potatoes in bite size pieces. Steam until tender. Put into a large salad bowl.

—Hard boil 4 Eggs. Peel under cool running water.

—Sizzle 1 chopped Onion, 1/4 cup Soy Bacon Bits, 1 teasp. Sea Salt, and 1/2 teasp. Pepper in 2 TBS Canola Oil until aromatic. Remove from heat; turn into salad bowl and toss with potatoes. Add 1/2 cup Low-Fat Cheddar and toss.

—Mound dark greens like Spinach or Arugula or Endive in individual salad plates. Divide salad among plates. Crumble hard boiled eggs and sprinkle over top. Dash each salad with Nutmeg. Serve right away.

Nutrition: 181 calories; 14gm protein; 14gm carbohydrate; 3gm fiber; 8g total fat; 152mg choles.; 196mg calcium; 3mg iron; 54mg magnes.; 501mg potass.; 537mg sodium; Vit. A 295 IU; Vit. C 13mg; Vit. E 1 IU.

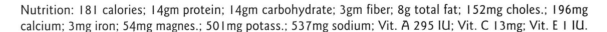

MUSHROOM MELT WITH HERBS

This recipe works for: Cancer Control, Weight Control, Sugar Imbalances
For 4 servings:

Soak 8 Shiitake Mushrooms and 1 sprig fresh Rosemary Leaves in water to cover. When soft, sliver mushroom caps; discard woody stems; save soaking water.

—Sauté for 5 minutes: 1 minced Clove Garlic, $^1/_2$ cup sliced Onion, $^1/_2$ teasp. dry Oregano and $^1/_2$ teasp. dry Thyme in 1 TB Olive Oil and 3 TBS Rosemary-Mushroom soaking water. Add 1 cup Button Mushrooms sliced, the Shiitake Mushrooms, and rest of the Rosemary water. Simmer for 5 minutes until liquid is absorbed.

—Stir in $^1/_4$ cup White Wine. Remove from heat, and cover mushrooms with grated, Low-fat Mozarrella. Cover pan and let melt slightly. Serve on individual salad plates on a bed of chopped Arugula greens.

SPINACH SALAD with HOT "BACON" DRESSING

This recipe works for: High Blood Pressure, Men's Health, Heart/Artery Health
For 4 servings:

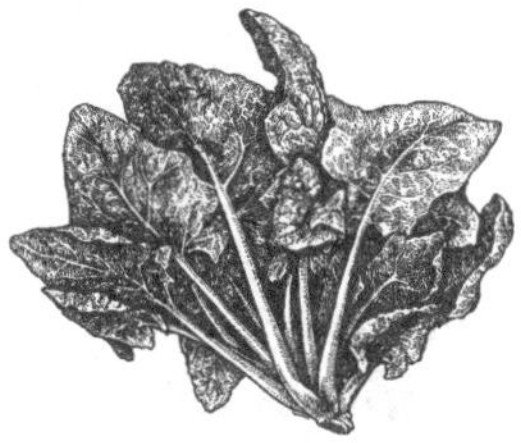

Divide 1 package Baby Spinach Leaves between 4 salad plates.

—Dry roast 3 TBS Soy Bacon Bits in a skillet until fragrant. Add and simmer briefly: 4 TBS Canola Oil, 4 TBS Balsamic Vinegar, 2 TBS Lemon Juice, $^1/_2$ teasp. Honey, 1 teasp. Sesame Salt and $^1/_2$ teasp. Lemon Pepper. Pour over spinach and toss to coat.

HOT DEVILED EGG SALAD

This recipe works for: Sports Nutrition, Men's Health, Hair, Skin and Nails
For 6 salads:

Sauté $^1/_2$ cup thinly sliced Red Onion and 2 thinly sliced Red Potatoes in 3 TBS Butter for 5 minutes. Add 8-oz. Button Mushrooms thinly sliced, and 1 large Stalk Broccoli, chopped; sauté briefly, tossing to coat about 5 minutes.

—Mix in a bowl: 2 chopped hard boiled Eggs, $^1/_2$ cup Sweet Relish, $1^1/_2$ cups grated Low-Fat Cheddar, 1 teasp. Dry Mustard, $^1/_2$ teasp. Dill Weed, $^1/_2$ teasp. Lemon-Pepper and $^1/_2$ teasp. Hot Pepper Sauce.

—Make the YOGURT-WHITE WINE SAUCE: $^1/_4$ cup Plain Low-fat Yogurt, 2 TBS White Wine, 2 TBS Water, $^1/_4$ cup Low-Fat Mayonnaise.

—Assemble the salad. Spread half of the vegetable mix in a heat-proof serving dish. Top with half of the egg mix. Repeat layers. Top with Yogurt-Wine Sauce.

—Dust with Paprika. Cover; heat for 30 minutes. Serve warm on Arugula greens.

Nutrition: 245 calories; 12gm protein; 24gm carbohydrate; 3gm fiber; 11g total fat; 101mg choles.; 240mg calcium; 2mg iron; 38mg magnes.; 614mg potass.; 356mg sodium; Vit. A 237 IU; Vit. C 45mg; Vit. E 1 IU.

HOT BROCCOLI SALAD

This recipe works for: Cancer Control, Immune Breakdown, Women's Health
For 4 servings:

Steam two bunches fresh Broccoli for 5 minutes. Trim woody ends. Slice in 5-inch lengths. Make the LEMON-OIL DRESSING: whisk together 2 TBS Lemon Juice, $^3/_4$ teasp. Sea Salt, $^1/_2$ teasp. Dry Mustard, $^1/_4$ teasp. Lemon-Pepper, 2 TBS Olive Oil, 4 dashes Hot Pepper Sauce. Toss with broccoli to coat.

—Skillet toast 4 TBS Pine Nuts or slivered Almonds until brown. Toss with broccoli.

—Heat 2 TBS Canola Oil in the skillet; sauté $^1/_2$ small Red Onion until very brown.

—Toss with broccoli and serve over a bed of Romaine Lettuce.

Nutrition: 169 calories; 5gm protein; 9gm carbohydrate; 4gm fiber; 14g total fat; 0mg choles.; 76mg calcium; 1mg iron; 48mg magnes.; 447mg potass.; 298mg sodium; Vit. A 182 IU; Vit. C 110mg; Vit. E 6 IU.

RADICCHIO POOLS

This recipe works for: Hair, Skin and Nails, Illness Recovery, Men's Health
Makes 6 salads: Preheat oven to 350°. Use a 9 by 13-inch baking dish.

Mix 1 TB Olive Oil and 2 TBS Lemon Juice; brush liberally over 2 heads Radicchio Leaves. Separate leaves and set cupped side up in baking dish. Divide 3-oz. Low Fat Mozarrella or Havarti Cheese, cut in $^1/_4$-inch thick cubes, between radicchio cups. Sprinkle with Lemon-Pepper. Bake just until the cheese melts, 5 minutes. Serve warm.

Nutrition: 69 calories; 4gm protein; 2gm carbohydrate; trace fiber; 5g total fat; 7mg choles.; 112mg calcium; 1mg iron; 9mg magnesium; 135mg potass.; 39mg sodium; Vit. A 28 IU; Vit. C 5mg; Vit. E 1 IU.

WARM WINTER BEAN SALAD Loaded with protein and EFA's.

This recipe works for: Immune Power, Illness Recovery, Sports Nutrition
Makes 6 salads:

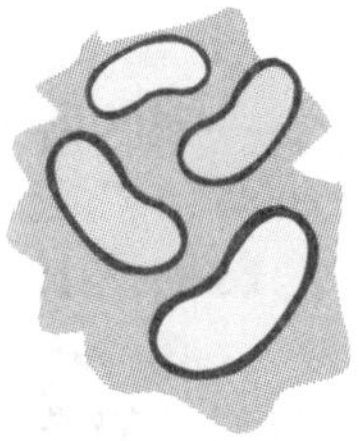

In large pot, cover 2 cups dried Cannellini Beans or Small White Beans with cold water. Cover and let stand overnight. Drain beans and return to pot. Add 5 cups Vegetable Broth, 1 cup White Wine and 1 Onion diced; bring to a boil. Reduce heat to low and simmer until beans are tender, about 2 hours. Drain beans and place in serving bowl.

—Stir in $^1/_4$ cup Balsamic Vinegar, 4 Shallots minced, 2 TBS Lemon Juice, 1 TB Honey, 1 diced Red Bell Pepper, 1 cup canned Corn Kernels, 1 Rib Celery diced, $^1/_2$ cup chopped fresh Cilantro and $^1/_2$ teasp. Dulse Granules. Season with Bragg's LIQUID AMINOS if desired and serve warm over tart, dark greens like Arugula.

Nutrition: 328 calories; 17gm protein; 65gm carbohydrate; 2gm fiber; 1g total fat; 0mg choles.; 115mg calcium; 5mg iron; 155mg magnes.; 2295mg potass.; 247mg sodium; Vit. A 106 IU; Vit. C 33mg; Vit. E 1 IU.

WARM ARTICHOKE - FENNEL SALAD

This recipe works for: Arthritis, Liver and Organ Health, Weight Control
Makes 6 salads:

Wash $2\frac{1}{2}$ lbs Baby Artichokes under cold running water. Bend back outer leaves and snap off near base. Snap off and discard leaves until central green cone is reached. Cut stem close to bottom. Cut off green top. Pare green layer from bottom. Slice in quarters. Place in Water to cover with 1 TB Lemon Juice to set color. Drain artichoke slices just before cooking.

—Thinly slice 4-oz. Brown Crimini Mushrooms. Trim a Fennel Bulb (about 1 lb.) and slice thinly. Thinly slice white parts only of 1 large Leek.

—Sauté 2 Garlic Cloves minced, the artichokes, mushrooms, fennel and leeks and in 4 TBS Olive Oil until lightly browned, about 20 minutes. Stir in 2 chopped Plum Tomatoes, 4 TBS chopped Cilantro, 4 TBS fresh chopped Basil, 4 TBS fresh Lemon Juice, 2 TBS snipped Chives, $\frac{1}{2}$ teasp Sea Salt and $\frac{1}{4}$ teasp Lemon-Pepper.

—Mound Baby Asian Greens onto salad plates and top with warm salad.

Meal Size Salads

Meal-size salads give you lots of nutrition packed into one bowl. They are perfect for meals-in-a-hurry and outdoor eating. (Why does food taste better outside?) So get a big bowl and a fork, pour on a little dressing, prop your feet up, and enjoy a delicious sunset, or a midday break with a salad.

CHICKEN SALAD in a BOAT A good company starter salad

This recipe works for: Respiratory Health, Illness Recovery, Heart Health
Makes 6 salads: or 12 appetizer salads: Pre-heat oven to 325°.

Serve in a round Whole Wheat Sourdough Bread Shell. Slice off the top, scoop out the middle, leaving about $\frac{1}{2}$-inch crust on bottom and sides. (Cube the middle for croutons and save.) Put on a baking pan and toast to crisp, about 10 minutes; remove and set aside.

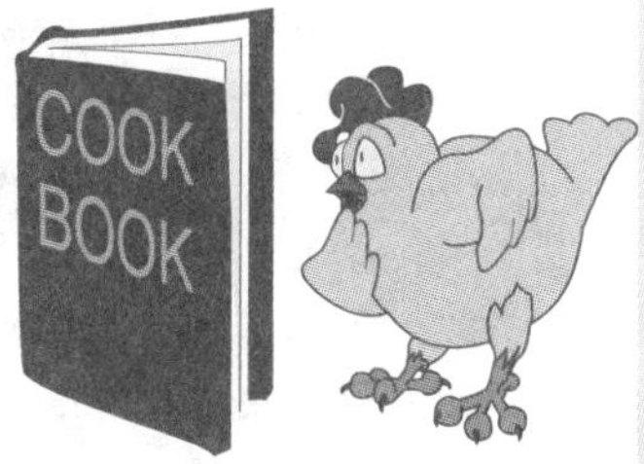

—Mix the filling: 3 cups cubed, cooked Organic Chicken Breast, 1 peeled diced Jicama, 2 teasp. minced fresh Cilantro, 2 teasp. minced fresh Ginger, 2 teasp. Curry Powder, $\frac{1}{4}$ cup White Wine, $\frac{1}{2}$ cup Low Fat Cream Cheese, 4 TBS Low Fat Mayonnaise, 2 TBS Lemon Juice, $\frac{1}{2}$ cup chopped Green Onions, Sea Salt and Pepper to taste. Cover and chill for several hours.

—Blanch 8-oz. Green Peas in rapidly boiling water until bright green, 1 minute. Drain; rinse with cold water to set color. Cover bottom of bread shell with peas. Pile salad on top. Garnish with more Cilantro leaves.

THAI VEGGIE RICE SALAD

This recipe works for: Women's Health, Digestive Problems, Heart and Artery Health
Makes 6 salads:

Have ready one 8-oz. package Baked Marinated Tofu sliced (or marinate Extra Firm Tofu in $^1/_4$ cup Tamari, $^1/_2$ tsp. Wasabi Paste and 2 TBS Toasted Sesame Oil).

—Have ready 3 cups cooked Basmati Rice in a large bowl. Whisk together 3 TBS Brown Rice Vinegar, $^1/_2$ teasp. Sea Salt and 1 TB Sake. Mix with rice. Set aside.

—Add to rice: 1 cup Corn Kernels, 1 cup thinly sliced Brown Cremini Mushrooms, 4 Radishes and 3 small Carrots cut in matchsticks, and Tofu slices. Toss to blend.

—Trim off stems from 3 bunches Watercress, or use 1 large package Baby Spinach Leaves. Rinse, then dry thoroughly in salad spinner or with paper towels.

—Toss greens with PEANUT-MISO DRESSING: blend $^1/_4$ cup Organic Peanut Butter, $^1/_2$ cup Water, 1 TB Yellow Miso Paste, 1 tsp. minced Crystallized Ginger and $^1/_8$ tsp. Cayenne Pepper. Blend until smooth.

—Cover individual serving plates with greeens. Top greens with rice salad. Sprinkle on 1 cup shredded White Daikon Radish.

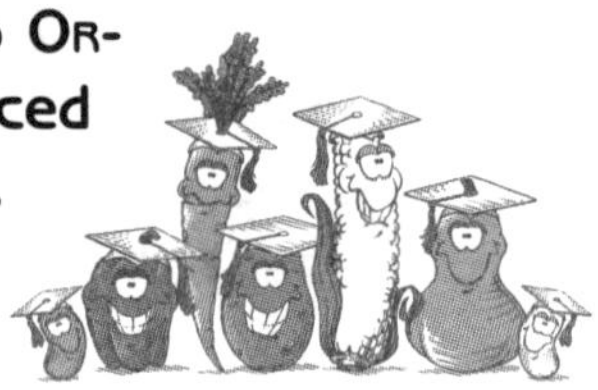

Nutrition: 397 calories; 16gm protein; 60gm carbohydrate; 4gm fiber; 12g total fat; 0mg choles.; 159mg calcium; 5mg iron; 85mg magnes.; 564mg potass.; 366mg sodium; Vit. A 912 IU; Vit. C 29mg; Vit. E 3 IU.

GARDEN HARVEST with SHARP VINAIGRETTE

This recipe works for: Arthritis, Detoxification, Boosting Sexuality, Recovery
For 6 salads:

Mix the vinaigrette, and let chill: $^1/_2$ cup Olive Oil, $^1/_4$ cup Tarragon Vinegar, $^1/_4$ teasp. Hot Pepper Sauce, 2 minced Shallots, 2 TBS Dijon Mustard, 1 TB Sesame Seeds, $^1/_2$ teasp. Sea Salt, $^1/_4$ teasp. Pepper.

—Make the salad. For half the salad, choose about 2 quarts from a mix of the following greens, or whatever is available in your garden at the moment: Lettuces like Romaine, Red Leaf, Green Leaf, Butter, Bibb and Boston; greens like Arugula, Endive, Radicchio, Spinach, Watercress, Baby Spring or Asian Greens; cabbages like Bok Choy, Red and Green, Nappa and Savoy.

—For the other half of the salad, choose about 4 cups from a mix of the following: sliced Button or fresh Shiitake Mushrooms, sliced Avocado, sliced Artichoke Hearts, sliced Green Onions, halved Cocktail Tomatoes, sliced Hothouse Cucumber, thin-sliced Daikon or Red Radishes.

—For the toppings, choose about 2 mixed cups from the following: grated Low Fat Cheese, Soy Bacon Bits, trimmed fresh Pea Pods, Sunflower or Alfalfa Sprouts, toasted Sunflower or Pumpkin Seeds, toasted Pine Nuts, toasted Walnut Pieces or sliced Almonds.

—Pour dressing over. Toss and enjoy.

Nutrition: 280 calories; 9gm protein; 13gm carbohydrate; 3gm fiber; 22g total fat; 10mg choles.; 206mg calcium; 3mg iron; 47mg magnes.; 519mg potass.; 294mg sodium; Vit. A 309 IU; Vit. C 32mg; Vit. E 5 IU.

MEAL SIZE GRILLED VEGETABLE SALAD

This recipe works for: Men's and Kid's Health, Immune Power, Addiction Control
Makes 4 servings: Preheat the grill to high.

Mix 1 TB Garlic Granules with 3 TBS Olive Oil; infuse for 10 minutes. Cut a French Bread Loaf in half horizontally, save half; cut the other into 4 diagonal slices. Lightly brush with 1 TB Garlic Oil; grill slices for 30 seconds until golden brown. Cool.

—Cut 2 Zucchini into diagonal slices; cut 1 Onion into wedges; cut 4 Plum Tomatoes, 2 Large Mushrooms and 2 Red Bell Peppers in quarters. Lightly brush rest of the garlic oil on veggies and grill for 2 minutes per side until a golden brown. Combine the vegetables in a large bowl with 1 TB Olive Oil, 1 TB Lemon Juice, 2 TBS Balsamic Vinegar, 2 TBS chopped Fresh Basil, and Sea Salt and Lemon-Pepper to taste. Toss well.

Place one grilled bread slice in the center of each of four salad plates and spoon grilled vegetables on top. Garnish each salad with Basil Leaves and serve at once.

MEAL SIZE GREENS and GRAINS SALAD

This recipe works for: Weight Control, Allergy-Asthma, Liver-Organ Health
For 6 salads:

Dry roast 1 cup Brown Basmati Rice in a large skillet, stirring often. When grains are fragrant, add 2 cups Organic Chicken Broth. Bring to a boil, cover, reduce heat and steam for 25 minutes until water is absorbed. Remove from heat, fluff and cool.

—Sizzle for 2 to 4 minutes in 2 TBS Canola Oil and 4 TBS Organic Chicken Broth: 2 Ribs Celery diced, 1 Zucchini sliced, 1 stalk Broccoli chopped, 1 Green Bell Pepper sliced, 1 cup edible Pea Pods trimmed, 1 cup sliced Button Mushrooms, 1 can sliced Water Chestnuts and 1 cup Green Onions thin sliced. Remove from heat and toss veggies with 3 TBS Tamari, 1 TB Honey, 1 teasp. Sesame Salt, $^1/_2$ teasp. Pepper. Combine sauced vegetables with the rice. Serve cold in Bibb Lettuce cups.

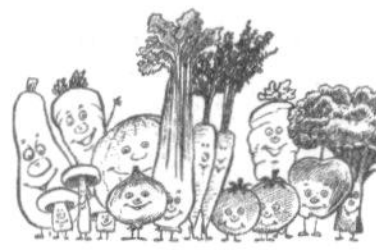

Dressings and Salad Sauces

Are they dressings? Are they dips? Are they sauces? I just call them toppings. You can use them with confidence for their health benefits on salads and a lot more.

RASPBERRY VINAIGRETTE

This recipe works for: Hair, Skin and Nail Health, Women's Health, Liver and Organ
For $1^1/_2$ cups:

Whisk: 6 TBS Raspberry Vinegar, $^1/_2$ cup Canola Oil, 1 teasp. Dijon Mustard, 1 teasp. Honey, 3 toasted Shallots, minced, $^1/_4$ teasp. Black Pepper and 1 pinch Paprika.

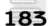

LOW FAT, NON-DAIRY THOUSAND ISLAND DRESSING

This recipe works for: Men's Health, Hormone Related Problems, Weight Loss
For 6 salads: Use a food processor for extra nice results.

Process 3 Shallots, halved, and Pickle Relish until finely minced. Add 1 cup Ketchup, $^1/_2$ teasp. Lemon-Pepper and 6-oz. Low-fat Soft Tofu, 2 TBS Sherry and $^1/_2$ cup Water; process until blended. Store in a glass jar in the refrigerator.

Nutrition: 80 calories; 3gm protein; 15gm carbohydrate; 1gm fiber; 2g total fat; 0mg choles.; 44mg calcium; 2mg iron; 41mg magnes.; 284mg potass.; 30mg sodium; Vit. A 27 IU; Vit. C 8mg; Vit. E 1 IU.

HAWAIIAN GUACAMOLE

This recipe works for: Anti-Aging, Hair, Skin, Nails, Allergy-Asthma
For about $1^1/_2$ to 2 cups:

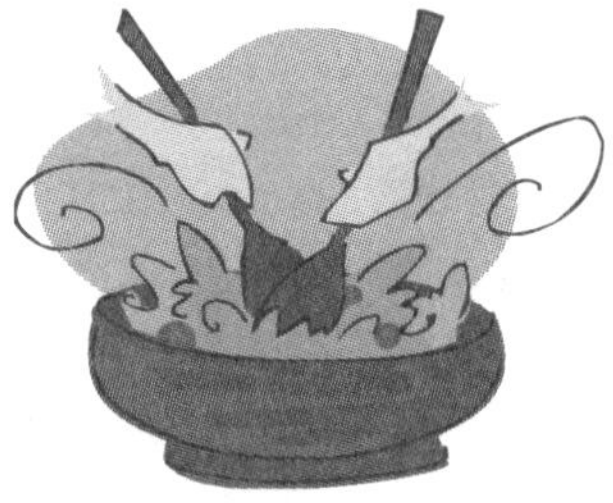

Amounts vary depending on size of the avocado. Taste as you add seasonings.

—Mash and mix: 1 large Avocado, $^1/_2$ cup Plain Low-Fat Yogurt, 1 to 2 TBS Chunky Salsa or Picante Sauce, 1 to 2 teasp. Lemon Juice, 2 to 3 teasp. Bragg's LIQUID AMINOS or Tamari, 2 dashes SPIKE or other herbal seasoning salt.

LIGHT BALSAMIC DRESSING especially nice over edible flowers

This recipe works for: Digestive Problems, Immune Breakdown, Women's Health
Makes $1^1/_2$ cups: Make in a blender; store in refrigerator.

Combine $^1/_4$ cup Balsamic Vinegar, $1^1/_2$ TBS Honey, 1 TB each Dijon Mustard and Lemon Juice, 1 $^1/_2$ TB. Shallots, finely chopped, $^1/_8$ teasp. Hot Pepper Sauce, $^1/_2$ teasp. Italian Herbs, $^1/_3$ cup each Olive Oil and Canola Oil, 1 pinch each Sea Salt and White Pepper, $^1/_2$ peeled Kiwi Fruit.

SESAME DRESSING

This recipe works for: Cancer Control, Digestion, Arthritis, Anti-Aging
For 6 salads:

Whisk in small bowl: $^1/_4$ cup Canola Oil, $^1/_4$ cup Toasted Sesame Oil, $^1/_4$ cup Lime Juice 1 TB Brown Rice Vinegar, 1 teasp. Honey, 1 teasp. Curry Powder, 1 teasp. Oyster Sauce $^1/_8$ tsp. Cayenne Pepper.

Nutrition: 169 calories; 1gm protein; 2gm carbohydrate; 0gm fiber; 18g total fat; 0mg choles.; 3mg calcium; 3mg iron; 2mg magnes.; 24mg potass.; 4mg sodium; Vit. A 3 IU; Vit. C 3mg; Vit. E 5 IU.

HEALING LEMON-OIL DRESSING

During your healing program you may use this as the basis for all French Dressings, as a marinade for fish or vegetables, or as a sauce for any dish.

This recipe works for: Detoxification, Immune Breakdown, Fatigue Syndromes
Makes 1 cup:

Shake in a covered jar: 6 TBS Olive Oil, 3 TBS Lemon Juice, 1 minced Scallion, 1 TB minced Parsley, 1 tsp. minced dry Sea Greens (like Dulse, Arame, Kelp, Kombu or Wakame).

FRESH ORANGE JUICE DRESSING

This recipe works for: Heart and Artery Health, Women's Health, Arthritis
Makes 8 servings:

In a small bowl, whisk: $^1/_4$ cup Raspberry Vinegar, 1 TB Orange Zest, juice of 1 large, fresh Orange, 1 TB chopped fresh Parsley, 1 tsp. Honey, $^1/_2$ tsp. Paprika, $^1/_4$ tsp. Sea Salt. Gradually whisk in $^1/_2$ cup Canola Oil until well blended.

Nutrition: 134 calories; 1gm protein; 3gm carbohydrate; 0gm fiber; 13g total fat; 0mg choles.; 4mg calcium; 0mg iron; 3mg magnesium; 51mg potass.; 67mg sodium; Vit. A 16 IU; Vit. C 12mg; Vit. E 5 IU.

TOASTED ALMOND MAYONNAISE

This recipe works for: Fatigue Syndromes, Women's Health, Sports Nutrition
For 2 cups:

Toast 1 cup Whole Almonds in a 350° oven til browned, about 15 minutes. Coarse chop briefly in the blender and set aside.

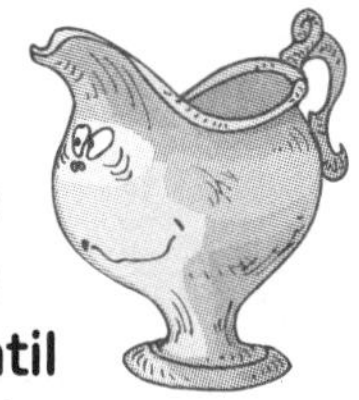

—Add to the blender: 1 Egg, 2 teasp. Dijon Mustard, 1 TB White Wine Vinegar, $^1/_2$ teasp. Sea Salt. Whirl briefly, then add in a thin stream while whirling 1 cup Canola Oil (or $^1/_2$ cup Canola Oil and $^1/_2$ cup Olive Oil) until mayonnaise thickens. Combine with almonds, chill, and dollop over salads.

GOOD FAT DRESSING

This recipe works for: Brain Boosting, Heart Health, Hair, Skin, Nails, Arthritis
Makes 8 servings: Bring to room temperature and shake well before using.

Whisk $^1/_2$ cup Balsamic Vinegar, $^1/_4$ cup Olive Oil, $^1/_4$ cup Canola Oil, 2 TBS Sweet-Hot Mustard, 1 TB Honey, 1 tsp. dried Basil, 1 teasp. dried Parsley.

Nutrition: 146 calories; 1gm protein; 6gm carbohydrate; 1gm fiber; 14g total fat; 0mg choles.; 12mg calcium; 1mg iron; 1mg magnes.; 16mg potass.; 45mg sodium; Vit. A 3 IU; Vit. C 1mg; Vit. E 3 IU.

NO FAT VINAIGRETTE

This recipe works for: Weight Loss, Heart Health and High Blood Pressure
Makes 14 servings, 2 TBS each: Store in a covered glass jar in the refrigerator.

Blender blend: 1 cup Water, $^1/_2$ cup White Wine Vinegar, 1 TB Apple Juice Concentrate, 2 TBS Dijon Mustard, 1 teasp. <u>each</u> of the following dry herbs: Parsley, Tarragon, Thyme and Garlic Powder; $^1/_2$ teasp. each: Cracked Black Pepper and Rosemary.

Nutrition: 9 calories; 1gm protein; 2gm carbohydrate; 1gm fiber; 0 fat; 0mg choles.; 8mg calcium; trace iron; 2mg magnes.; 29mg potass.; 18mg sodium; Vit. A 2 IU; Vit. C 1mg; Vit. E trace.

OIL FREE PARMESAN DRESSING

This recipe works for: Men's Health, Digestive Health, Sports Nutrition
For 3 cups:

Blender blend until smooth: 6-oz. grated Parmesan Reggiano Cheese, 1 cup Plain Low-Fat Yogurt, 4 TBS Kefir Cheese or Low-Fat Cream Cheese, $^1/_3$ cup White Wine, 1 Egg, $^1/_2$ teasp. Garlic-Lemon Sesame Seasoning (pg. 487), $^1/_2$ teasp. Sesame Salt, and $^1/_2$ teasp. Pepper.

STRAWBERRY MAYONNAISE

This recipe works for: Fatigue Syndromes, Stress Reactions, Women's Health
For $1^1/_4$ cups: **This is also delicious with Kiwi instead of strawberries.**

Whirl in the blender: $^1/_2$ cup Low-Fat Mayonnaise, 2 TBS Honey, $^3/_4$ cup fresh sliced Strawberries, 1 teasp. Lemon Juice; chill before serving.

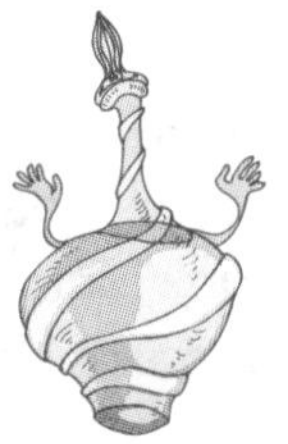

EGG DRESSING

This recipe works for: Brain Boosting, Hair, Skin and Nails
For 1 cup:

Stir together: 6 TBS Olive Oil, 2 hard boiled Eggs, crumbled fine, 2 TBS Lemon Juice, 1 TB minced Chives, $^1/_2$ teasp. Lemon-Pepper, pinch Sea Salt, pinch Paprika.

SWEET and SOUR FRENCH

This recipe works for: Arthritis, Colds and Flu Recovery, Sugar Imbalances
For $1^1/_2$ cups:

Blender blend: $^3/_4$ cup Olive Oil, $^1/_4$ cup Tarragon Vinegar, $^1/_4$ cup Sherry, 2 teasp. Stevia Leaves, 1 tsp. Onion Powder, $^1/_2$ tsp. dry Mustard, 1 tsp. dry Basil, 1 tsp. grated Lemon Zest, $^1/_2$ teasp. Celery Seed, 1 tsp. Lemon Garlic Seasoning, $^1/_2$ teasp. Paprika.

Lose the Fat!

Low Fat and Very Low Fat Recipes

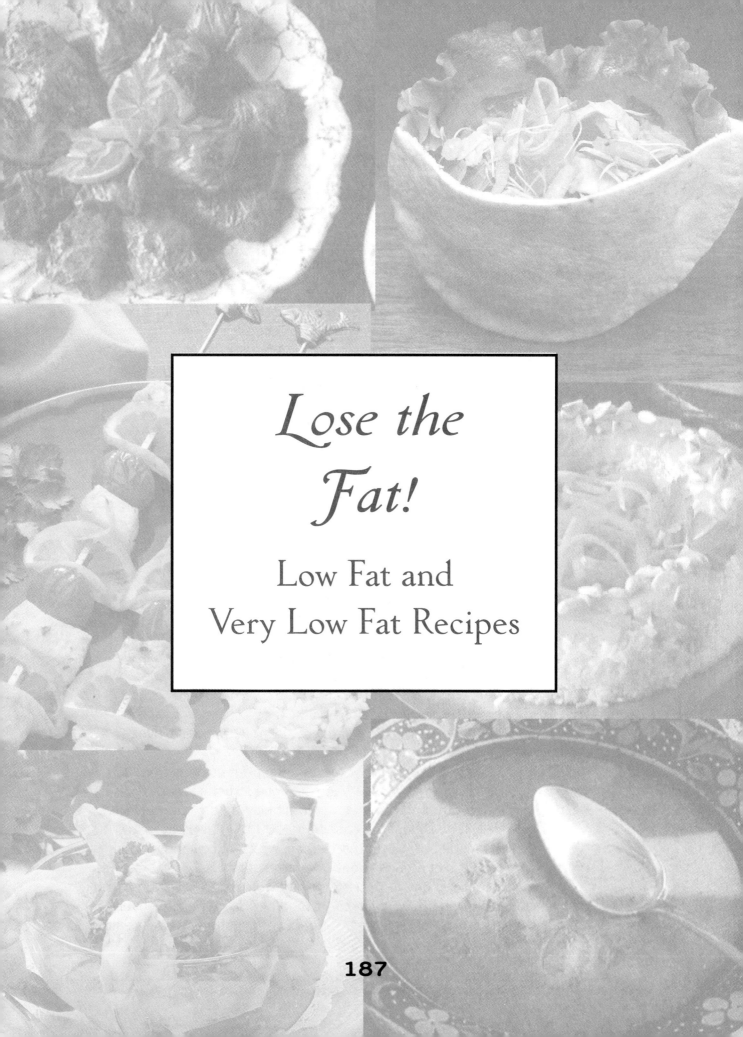

Low Fat and Very Low Fat!

No More Tasteless Remarks!

Keeping fats low in your diet and your bloodstream is the key to heart health, long life and weight control. We know this.... almost 60 percent of Americans say they are on a weight loss or health-related diet. We are earnestly trying to avoid fats, especially saturated fats, and empty calorie foods.

Even when we think we're avoiding fat, it is concealed in commercially processed, fat filled prepared foods, in hydrogenated oils and trans fats. Hidden fat in some of these foods is so high that it is easy to take in as many fat calories as a stick of butter a day!

A quick formula chart for estimating your percent body fat:

1) Divide your weight by 2.2.

   ______ ÷ 2.2 = ______ .

2) Multiply your height in inches by 2.54, then divide the result by 100.

   ______ x 2.54 = ______ ÷ 100 = ______ .

3) Multiply the result of step two by itself.

   ______ x ______ = ______ .

4) Divide the result of step one by the result of step three.

   ______ ÷ ______ = ______ .

Measure your results against the standards of body fat for adults:

Men: essential fat, 5%; healthy range depends on age, 10 to 25%; for fitness, 12 to 18%; athlete, 5 to 13%; obese, over 27%.

Women: essential fat, 8%; healthy range depends on age, 18 to 30%; for fitness, 16 to 25%; athlete, 12 to 22%; obese, over 33%.

For a low-fat to very low-fat diet, keep fat calories from 15 to 23% of total calorie intake. Sex, age, bone structure, activity level, metabolic rate, and general health all play a part in determining your daily fat calories, but based on 2000 calories a day, a low-fat diet means about 42 grams of fat, or 393 fat calories a day. A very low fat diet means about 30 grams of fat, or 284 fat calories a day. (Note: many weight-conscious women do not even come close to eating 2000 calories of food per day.) If you're over 45 consciously undereat from the diet of your youth for better health.

Fats are not all bad. Unsaturated, naturally occurring fats, like those in whole grains, fruits and vegetables, seafoods, beans, seeds and low-fat dairy products, are our greatest source of energy and fuel. They play an integral role in prostaglandin levels, hormones that regulate body functions at the molecular level. "Good" fats help us use B vitamins, transport fat soluble A, D, E, and K vitamins, elevate blood calcium levels, and activate digestive bile flow.

Too much saturated fat, like the fat in fried and fast foods, pasteurized dairy foods and processed foods, is at the heart of most health problems today. The biggest saturated fat culprits are over 90% fat: butter, oils, margarine, cream, mayonnaise, sausage, gravy, and prepared sandwich meats. Cream cheese, red meats, and salad dressings are over 80% fat. Hard cheeses, nuts, half-and-half, and potato chips are over 70% fat. Ice cream, eggs, cream soups and sweet pastries are over 60% fat. Pies, doughnuts, french fries, cakes, and corn chips are over 50% fat. Cookies, whole milk, most crackers and snack foods are over 40% fat.

All fried foods are high in fat. Frying raises fat calories in any food, often more than 100% greater than the fat in the food itself. For example, the 2 fat calories in potatoes become 219 fat calories in French Fries.

De-fat your lifestyle with flavor

Low-fat recipes contain less than 9 grams of fat per serving. Very low-fat recipes contain less than 5 grams per serving. Try these great-tasting, low fat choices instead of similar high fat dishes anytime you want great flavor without all the fat.

Low Fat Recipe Sections

Fat can hurt. Four reasons to lower the fat in your diet:

#1) **Dietary fat becomes body fat.** Overweight is not a result of total calorie intake. Fatter people actually tend to eat fewer calories. Saturated fat is a far more common cause of excess body fat than carbohydrates. And your body uses up more energy to convert carbohydrates to body fat than to convert dietary fat to body fat. Fatty foods actually do go straight from your mouth to your thighs.... and are likely to be stored there. Carbohydrate calories are hardly ever stored as fat (but sugary carbohydrates DO raise your insulin levels.... your body's signal to make fat).

#2) **Fat consumption is linked to cancer.** Ovarian, breast, cervical, and colon cancer are especially linked to a high-fat diet.

#3) **Saturated fat raises blood cholesterol levels.** Saturated fat has the strongest influence on blood cholesterol because it affects the way your liver works..... the liver is less able to remove it normally from the bloodstream, allowing it to accumulate on artery walls. Your body's own cholesterol occurs in conjunction with healthy fatty acids. Dietary cholesterol is found only in animal foods, including dairy products. Plant foods, except for tropical oils, do not contain dietary cholesterol.

#4) **Environmental toxins accumulate in body fat.** Recent UCLA pollution studies show that environmental poisons accumulate in our fatty tissues. Food animals were found to be "bio-concentraters" of pollutants.....pesticides, sprays and toxins could build up over an animal's lifetime. Vegetables and plant foods may contain these chemical toxins, but the levels are low compared to those in animals. The human body stores toxins in fatty tissue. Reducing anmal fat in your diet means you'll shed excess pounds AND get rid of many accumulated chemical poisons.

Techniques to lower the fat in your favorite dishes:

1) **Instead of pan frying:** braise food in water or stock, then deglaze the pan with wine or water to retain the flavorful bits for a sauce. Steam or sauté in a little oil, broth or wine. Steam or blanch vegetables to crunchy tenderness. Roast or poach poultry, fish and seafood in broth, wine, or an herb sauce. Oven bake small pieces of food like meatballs. Roll them in a healthy coating and arrange on a baking sheet with enough space between to let moisture evaporate quickly. Brown well in a 400° oven.

2) **Instead of deep fat frying:** broil one to two minutes in the oven to sear in juices, then bake for a nice crispy crust.

3) **Instead of milk:** use a yogurt, white wine and water blend, for a delicious gourmet flavor without the fat calories or dairy sensitivity.

4) **Instead of full fat cheeses:** use low-fat, no-fat, rice or soy cheese.

5) **Instead of sour cream, cream cheese or ricotta:** use yogurt cheese, kefir cheese, low-fat cottage cheese, or soy cheese, cream cheese style.

6) **Instead of butter and rich sauces:** season with herbs and spices.

7) **Instead of ice cream or sherbet, with up to 10% fat:** use plain or frozen yogurt.

8) **Instead of greasing baking pans:** use a Lecithin no-stick spray.

9) **Fill in with water instead of fat:** fat makes sauces and dressings taste smooth, but you can easily replace some or all of it with water and eliminate the fat calories.

Low Fat Snacks and Appetizers

Check these recipes out if your diet downfall is high fat snack foods (you're not alone). Keep plenty of them around for mini-meals, blood sugar drops and grazing.

VEGETABLE PICKLES

This recipe works for: Illness Recovery, Heart Health, Good Digestion
Makes 8 appetizers:

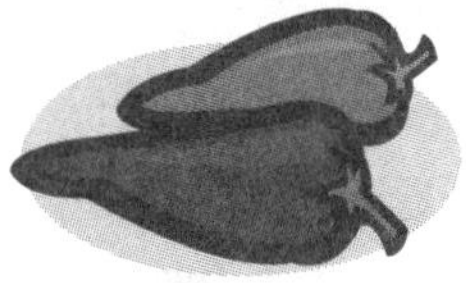

In a bowl, toss together 1 cup sliced Red or White Radishes, 1/2 cup thinly sliced English Cucumber, 1/2 cup thinly sliced Carrot and 1/2 tsp. Sea Salt. Let sit at room temperature for 2 hours. Press vegetables gently in a colander to drain off liquid, then return to bowl.

—In a pan, bring 2 TBS Umeboshi Vinegar or Seasoned Brown Rice Vinegar and 6 TBS Sake to a boil. Immediately remove from heat. Let cool; pour over veggies. Cover and chill for 24 hours. Serve in small lettuce cups that can be hand-held to eat.

LOW-FAT JALAPEÑO POPPERS

This recipe works for: Kid's and Men's Health, Heart Health, Weight Control
Makes 28 appetizers: Use a 12 by 15-inch baking sheet.

Blend in a bowl: 4-oz. Low Fat Cream Cheese, 2 tsp. Lemon-Garlic Seasoning, 1/4 cup minced Scallions, 2 TBS minced Green Olives, 3 TBS shredded Low Fat Cheddar Cheese, and 1 TB Lime Juice.

—Wearing rubber gloves, cut 14 fresh Jalapeño Chilies in half lengthwise. With a knife, cut seed lump from beneath the stem inside, leaving stem end in place to form a cup. Remove veins. Fill halves with cheese mixture, spreading smooth.

—In a bowl, whisk 2 large Egg Whites until slightly frothy. Put 1 cup Crumbled Dry Cornbread in another bowl. Dip filled chili halves, 1 at a time, in egg whites then roll in cornbread crumbs. Set chilies slightly apart on a baking sheet, and bake at 350°F until crumbs are brown and crisp, about 20 minutes. Serve hot or warm.

Nutrition each: 19 calories; 1gm protein; 1gm carbohydrate; 1gm fiber; 1g total fat; 3mg choles.; 15mg calcium; 0mg iron; 2mg magnes.; 17mg potass.; 33mg sodium; Vit. A 27 IU; Vit. C 6mg; Vit. E trace.

SPINACH DIP for RAW VEGGIE STRIPS

This recipe works for: Hair, Skin and Nails, Digestive Health, Weight Control
Makes 1 1/3 cups:

Blender blend until fine chopped: 1 bag fresh Baby Spinach chopped, 1 Green Onion chopped, 1 cup Plain Low Fat Yogurt, 1/2 teasp. Dill Weed.

CAPONATA

This recipe works for: Men's Health, Heart / High Blood Pressure, Weight Control
Makes 8 appetizers: Preheat grill or broiler.

Peel and slice 2 Eggplants; cut lengthwise into $^1/_2$" slices. Lay slices in single layer on paper towels. Sprinkle both sides with Sea Salt; let stand 1 hour to allow bitter juices to drain. Rinse slices and pat dry. Brush lightly with 2 TBS Olive Oil.

—Grill or broil eggplant until slightly charred, 3 minutes per side; set aside.

—Heat 1 TB Olive Oil in large sauté pan over low heat. Sauté 1 large minced Yellow Onion 1 minute. Add 2 Large Mushrooms diced; sauté about 10 minutes.

—Add $1^1/_2$ cups canned Italian Roma Tomatoes with juice, $^1/_4$ cup pitted Black Olives and 1 TB rinsed, drained Capers. Simmer, stirring until tomato liquid has been reduced, about 5 minutes. Chop cooked eggplant slices. Cook in sauté pan for 1 minute. Pour on $^1/_2$ cup Balsamic Vinegar and sprinkle on $^1/_2$ teasp. Stevia Leaves; simmer, stirring occasionally, until most liquid is evaporated, about 10 minutes. Remove from heat; stir in $^1/_4$ cup chopped fresh Basil Leaves and $^1/_4$ teasp. Tarragon.

Nutrition: 103 calories; 2gm protein; 16gm carbohydrate; 5gm fiber; 4g total fat; 0mg choles.; 23mg calcium; 1mg iron; 26mg magnes.; 491mg potass.; 347mg sodium; Vit. A 42 IU; Vit. C 12mg; Vit. E 1 IU.

APPETIZER ASPARAGUS

This recipe works for: Women's Health, Liver and Organ Health, Arthritis
Makes 8 appetizers:

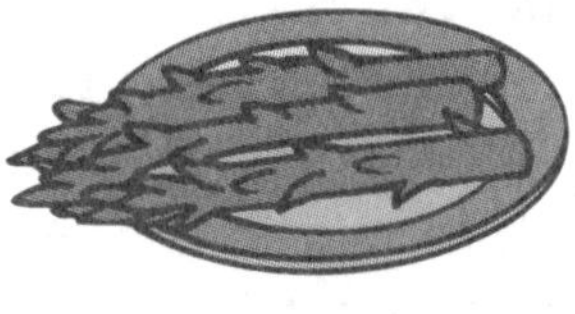

Steam 2 LBS fresh, trimmed Asparagus until bright green and tender-crisp, 4 minutes. Drain; put in a shallow dish. Whisk 4 TBS Lemon Juice and 4 tsp. Dijon Mustard and $^1/_2$ teasp. Lemon-Pepper; drizzle over asparagus. Cover and chill. Serve cold.

Nutrition: 31 calories; 3gm protein; 6gm carbohydrate; 3gm fiber; trace fat; 0mg choles.; 28mg calcium; 1mg iron; 21mg magnes.; 325mg potass.; 23mg sodium; Vit. A 66 IU; Vit. C 19mg; Vit. E 3 IU.

LOW-FAT HOT TUNA PATÉ

This recipe works for: Hair and Skin, Heart-Artery Health, Brain Boosting
Makes 8 servings: Good on hard-toasted rye cocktail rounds.

Mix in a bowl, and spoon into Lecithin-sprayed ramekins: 1 can water-packed, White Tuna, drained, 1 teasp. Lemon Juice, 1 TB Dijon Mustard, $^1/_4$ teasp. Lemon-Pepper, $1^1/_2$ TBS Sweet Relish, 1 TB minced Parsley. Heat at 325° for 40 minutes until browned.

Nutrition: 103 calories; 9gm protein; 16gm carbohydrate; 2gm fiber; 1g total fat; 0mg choles.; 159mg calcium; 2mg iron; 6mg magnesium; 60mg potassium; 375mg sodium; Vit. A 6 IU; Vit. C 11mg; Vit. E trace.

GARDEN SHRIMP DIP

This recipe works for: Hair and Skin, Liver and Organ Health, Waste Management
Makes 12 servings: Especially good on hard-toasted rye cocktail rounds.

Combine in a bowl: 3/4 cup Plain, Low Fat Yogurt, 8-oz. chopped cooked Shrimp, 2 TBS Lemon Juice, 1/2 cup Low Fat Mayonnaise, 1/4 cup minced Red Bell Pepper, 2 TBS minced Chives, 1/4 cup minced Cucumber. Chill to blend flavors.

Nutrition: 111 calories; 9gm protein; 17gm carbohydrate; 2gm fiber; 1g total fat; 38mg choles.; 64mg calcium; 2mg iron; 10mg magnes.; 90mg potass.; 320mg sodium; Vit. A 15 IU; Vit. C 6mg; Vit. E 1 IU.

SPICY PAPAYA SHRIMP

This recipe works for: Digestive Health, Liver and Organ Health, Brain Boosting
Makes 24 appetizers, for 8 people:

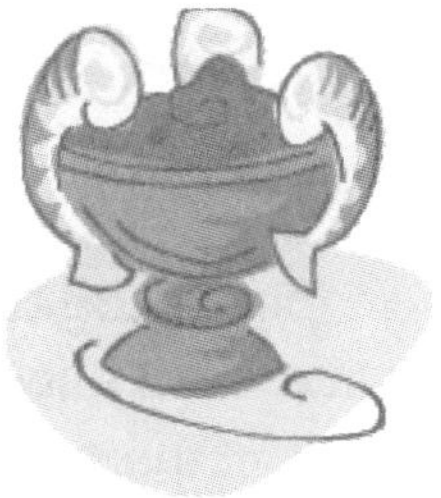

In a bowl, mix 1/3 cup Lime Juice, 1/4 cup minced fresh Cilantro, 1/4 cup thinly sliced Green Onions, 2 teasp. Chili Sauce and 1/2 teasp. Stevia Leaf or Fructose. Peel and seed 1 firm-ripe papaya; cut in 1/2-inch cubes and add to lime sauce. Add 8-oz. chopped cooked shrimp, and 1 TB Oyster Sauce. Pour into shallow dish and surround with lettuce leaves. Scoop papaya mixture into 24 Butter Lettuce Cups and hold to eat.

Nutrition: 55 calories; 7gm protein; 6gm carbohydrate; 1gm fiber; 1g total fat; 55mg choles.; 32mg calcium; 1mg iron; 18mg magnes.; 249mg potass.; 58mg sodium; Vit. A 58 IU; Vit. C 29mg; Vit. E 1 IU.

TWO DELICIOUS TOFU DIPS

This recipe works for: Women's - Men's Health, Weight Control, Sugar Imbalances
Each recipe makes about 8 servings:

Tofu Dip # 1:
Mash together: 2 cubes Tofu (8-oz.), 1/4 cup Plain, Low Fat Yogurt, 1 teasp. Tamari, 1/3 cup diced Celery, 1/2 teasp. Herbal Seasoning, 2 chopped Green Onions, 1/4 cup Toasted Sunflower Seeds.

Tofu Dip # 2:
Mash together: 2 cubes Tofu (8-oz.), 1/3 cup Plain, Low Fat Yogurt, 2 teasp. Mustard, 1/3 cup Sweet Pickle Relish, 1/2 teasp. Sesame Salt, 1/4 cup diced Tomato, 1/4 cup diced Celery, 2 TBS chopped Chives, 1 Hard Boiled Egg.

Nutrition: 49 calories; 4gm protein; 4gm carbohydrate; 1gm fiber; 2g total fat; 27mg choles.; 65mg calcium; 2mg iron; 35mg magnes.; 110mg potass.; 160mg sodium; Vit. A 21 IU; Vit. C 2mg; Vit. E trace.

HOT SALMON PATÉ

This recipe works for: Hair, Skin, Nails, Anti-Aging, Bone Health, Brain Boosting
For twelve 2-oz. servings: Preheat oven to 400°.

Blender blend: 8-oz. Low Fat Cream Cheese or Yogurt Cheese, 2 TBS fresh chopped Parsley, 2 chopped Green Onions, dashes of Worcestershire and Hot Pepper Sauce. one 7-oz. can Boneless Salmon, one 4-oz. can sliced Button Mushrooms.

—Spray a small oven-safe mold with Lecithin Spray. Line with waxed paper and spray the paper. Pack in the paté and bake til puffy and brown. Serve with toasted rye rounds or raw vegetables.

Nutrition: 73 calories; 6gm protein; 2gm carbohydrate; 1gm fiber; 4gm total fat; 18mg choles.; 66mg calcium; 1mg iron; 9mg magnes.; 145mg potass.; 80mg sodium; Vit. A 57 IU; Vit. C 2mg; Vit. E 1 IU.

LOW-FAT CLAM DIP

This recipe works for: Weight Control, Bone Health, Brain Boosting
For about $1^1/_2$ cups, 12 servings:

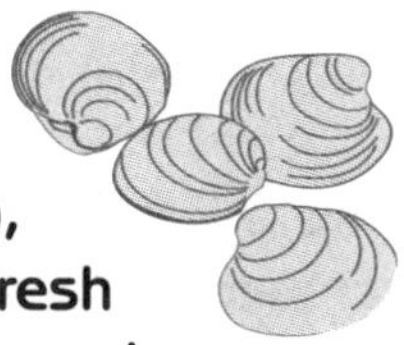

Mash together: one 7-oz. can minced Clams or Crab (drain and save clam juice), one 8-oz. carton Kefir Cheese (or Low Fat Cream Cheese), 2 TBS Lemon Juice, 1 teasp. Worcestershire Sauce or Hoisin Sauce, 2 TBS fresh chopped Parsley, $^1/_4$ teasp. Sesame Salt and $^1/_4$ teasp. Lemon-Pepper. Add enough reserved clam juice for good consistency.

—Chill to blend flavors and serve with crisp Pita Chips or Bagel Chips.

Nutrition: 97 calories; 7gm protein; 8gm carbohydrate; 1mg fiber; 4g total fat; 22mg choles.; 41mg calcium; 5mg iron; 17mg magnesium; 183mg potass.; 141mg sodium; Vit. A 74 IU; Vit. C 6mg; Vit. E 1 IU.

BAKED YAM CHIPS

This recipe works for: Women's Hormone Health, Weight Control
Enough for 8 people as an appetizer: Preheat oven to 250°.

Peel and slice 4 large Yams or Sweet Potatoes very thin. Rinse in cold water. Drain and dry on paper towels.

—Put in a large bowl and toss with $^1/_2$ teasp. Sea Salt, $^1/_2$ teasp. White Pepper, 2 teasp. Maple Syrup or Maple Sugar, and 3 TBS Canola Oil.

—Layer in a large oven-proof skillet. Mound slightly in center. Pour in any liquid from the mixing bowl. Cover with foil. Bake for 1 hour until tender.

—Serve right from the skillet, topped with thin strips of fresh Lemon Peel and snips of fresh Mint.

Nutrition: 123 calories; 2gm protein; 22gm carbohydrate; 3gm fiber; 3g total fat; 0mg choles.; 31mg calcium; 1mg iron; 18mg magnesium; 315mg potassium; 143mg sodium; Vit. A 1882 IU; Vit. C 23mg; Vit. E 1 IU.

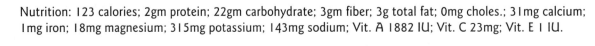

LOW-FAT STUFFED MUSHROOMS

This recipe works for: Men's and Women's Health, Immune Power
For 6 servings:

Remove stems from 8-oz. large Stuffing Mushrooms. Chop stems and sauté them briefly with 1 TB Butter with 2 TBS Soy Bacon Bits until aromatic. Remove from heat and add 1 Egg, 1/2 teasp. Celery Salt, 1 TB White Wine, 1/2 teasp. Caraway Seed, 2 teasp. dried minced Onions, 1/2 cup Whole Grain Bread Crumbs.

—Fill caps; bake in a shallow dish at 350° for 15 minutes until brown on top.

SMOKY EGG DIP

This recipe works for: Men's Health, Immune Power, Waste Management
Makes about 6 servings:

Mash with a fork to good dip consistency: 2 crumbled Hard Boiled Eggs, 1 cup Low Fat Cottage Cheese, 2 TBS Sweet Relish, 1/2 teasp. Dijon Mustard, 1/4 teasp. Natural Liquid Smoke, or 1 TB Soy Bacon Bits.

Nutrition: 60calories; 7gm protein; 3gm carbohydrate; 1gm fiber; 2gm total fat; 70mg choles.; 33mg calcium; trace iron; 4mg magnesium; 146mg potassium; 232mg sodium; Vit. A 37 IU; Vit. C trace; Vit. E 1 IU.

FRESH STRAWBERRIES and FIGS APPETIZERS

This recipe works for: Men's Health, Immune Power, Waste Management
For 2 people:

Toss gently 1 pint fresh Strawberries, halved, 3 fresh Figs, quartered 2 TBS minced fresh Basil Leaves, and 2 teasp. Balsamic Vinegar. Serve on small hors d'oeuvres plates with a decorative toothpick.

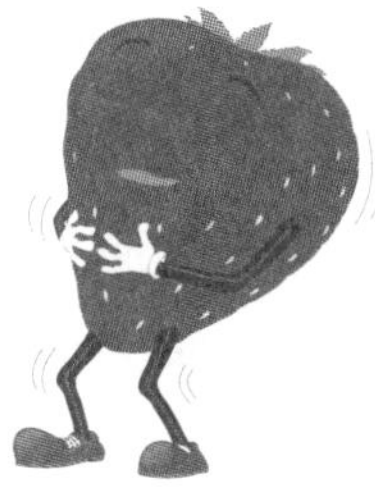

LOW-FAT SAVORY POPCORN TREATS

This recipe works for: Men's Health, Immune Power, Waste Management
For 8 servings: Make 4-qts. popcorn in an air popper for the lowest fat results.

Mix 4-qts. Popcorn with 1/4 cup grated Low Fat Parmesan, 1 TB Chicken Bouillion Granules or Paste, 1 teasp. Lemon-Garlic or Herbal Seasoning Salt.

—Quickly toss 1 Egg White, whipped to soft peaks with a pinch of Cream of Tarter, with popcorn so it doesn't deflate and pour into baking pans. Bake at 350° until crisp and dry, about 10 to 15 minutes, stirring often.

Nutrition: 78 calories; 4gm protein; 13gm carbohydrate; 3gm fiber; 1gm total fat; 2mg choles.; 45mg calcium; trace iron; 23mg magnesium; 60mg potassium; 21mg sodium; Vit. A 9 IU; Vit. C trace; Vit. E trace.

DEVILED CLAM TOASTS

This recipe works for: Heart Health, Boosting Sexuality, Waste Management
For 8 appetizer toasts: Preheat oven to 400°.

Cut 2 pieces Whole Grain Bread in quarters. Toast squares on a baking sheet.
—Sauté 1 Clove Garlic minced in 2 TBS Olive Oil until fragrant. Add 1 TB Wheat Germ and stir for a minute until frothy.
—Add 1 7-oz. can minced Clams with Juice, $^1/_2$ cup Seasoned Bread Crumbs, 1 teasp. Dijon Mustard, 2 teasp. Worcestershire Sauce or bottled Barbecue Sauce, $^1/_2$ teasp. Lemon-Pepper and 1 TB chopped fresh Parsley. Let bubble briefly, then pile on toast squares and bake until hot and bubbly. Sprinkle with pinches of parmesan if desired.

Nutrition: 103 calories; 8gm protein; 11gm carbohydrate; 1gm fiber; 3g total fat; 16mg choles.; 47mg calcium; 8mg iron; 18mg magnesium; 216mg potassium; 144mg sodium; Vit. A 45 IU; Vit. C 6mg; Vit. E 1 IU.

DILL FINGER CREPES with SPICY SHRIMP FILLING

This recipe works for: Hair, Skin and Nails, Brain Power, Digestive Health
For 8 crepe appetizers: Sparkling mineral water makes very light crepes.

Make the crepes. Mix: $^1/_2$ cup Unbleached Flour, 2 Egg Whites, beaten until foamy, $^1/_2$ cup Plain Sparkling Mineral Water, 2 TBS minced Chives, 2 teasp. Dill Weed, $^1/_4$ teasp. White Pepper. Let stand 20 minutes.
—Heat a griddle or teflon skillet. When a drop of water on the skillet sizzles, ladle on a small amount of crepe batter. Spread to make a thin crepe about 2 or 3" across. Cook until holes appear in the batter. Turn immediately and cook until golden. Stack between pieces of wax paper until all are done, and fill when cool. (Make crepes ahead if you like and freeze while still separated by waxed paper. Wrap tightly, and thaw while still wrapped so they won't dry out.)
—Make the filling: Sauté 8-oz. Salad Shrimp in 2 teasp. Canola Oil until just pink. Add 2 TBS White Wine; toss for 1 minute. Remove with a slotted spoon. Add 1 TB Canola Oil to the pan, and sauté 2 minced Mushrooms with 1 tsp. your favorite Marinade-Seasoning Sauce and 1 tsp. Dijon Mustard until aromatic, 3 minutes. Add pinches Ginger Powder, dry Tarragon, Chili Powder and Black Pepper. Toss shrimp with mushroom sauce. Divide between the 8 small crepes. Roll crepes. Put seam side down in a shallow baking dish and heat in a 350° oven until browned. Top each with snips of Parsley Leaves and a shake of Sea Salt.

Nutrition: 87 calories; 8gm protein; 7gm carbohydrate; 1gm fiber; 3gm total fat; 55mg choles.; 21mg calcium; 2mg iron; 15mg magnesium; 110mg potassium; 115mg sodium; Vit. A 22 IU; Vit. C 2mg; Vit. E 1 IU.

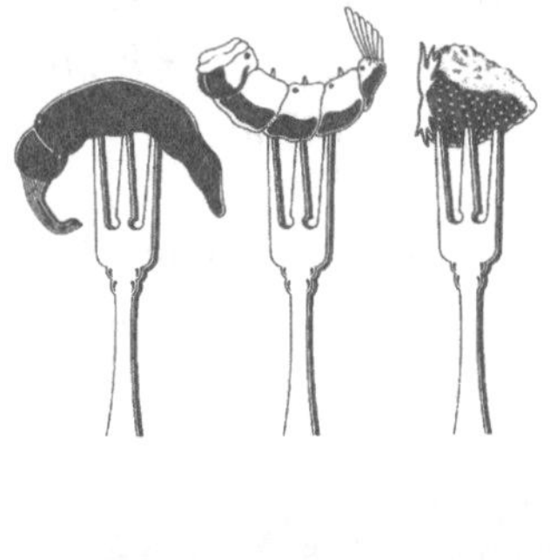

Low Fat Mexican Snacks

People love spicy Mexican snacks, but they have a reputation for being high in saturated fat and hard on digestion. Enjoy this healthy Mexican food guilt free.

AUTHENTIC LIME TORTILLAS Good tortillas are healthy food.

This recipe works for: Men's Health, Heart / High Blood Pressure, Weight Control
For 2-qts. tortilla chips:

Dip 12 Corn Tortillas in water and drain. Sprinkle with Sea Salt, Black Sesame Seeds and Lime Juice. Stack and cut into 8 wedges. Arrange in a single layer on 3 baking sheets. Bake at 500°F for 4 minutes. Turn with tongs and bake until brown and crispy, for 2 to 3 minutes.

SESAME CHILI CHIPS

This recipe works for: Digestive Health, Circulation, Weight Control
Makes 8 pieces: Use a 12 by 15 inch baking sheet

Brush 2 (10-inch) Fat-Free Flour Tortillas on 1 side with Lime Juice. Mix 1 teasp. Chili Powder, $^1/_2$ tsp. Ground Cumin, $^1/_2$ tsp. Sesame Seeds and $^1/_4$ tsp. Sea Salt. Sprinkle mixture over lime-moistened side of tortillas. Cut tortillas into quarters.

—Arrange pieces in a single layer, chili side up. Bake in a 400°F oven until chips are crisp and lightly browned, about 10 minutes.

Nutrition: 21 calories; 1gm protein; 5gm carbohydrate; 1gm fiber; trace fat; 0mg choles.; 7mg calcium; trace iron; 9mg magnesium; 31mg potassium; 86mg sodium; Vit. A 1 IU; Vit. C 7mg; Vit. E trace.

TOMATO and GREEN CHILE TOSTADAS

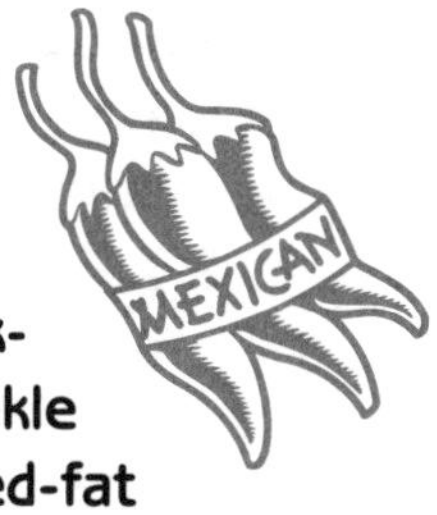

This recipe works for: Digestive Health, Circulation, Weight Control
Makes 6 servings: Preheat oven to 400°F.

Place 3 (8-inch) Low Fat Flour Tortillas flat on a large nonstick baking sheet. Arrange 3 thinly-sliced, firm Tomatoes on tortillas. Sprinkle with 2 (4-oz.) cans chopped Green Chilies, drained, 6-oz. grated reduced-fat Cheddar or Monterey Jack ($1^1/_2$ cups) and 2 TBS chopped fresh Cilantro and 2 TBS minced Green Onions.

—Bake until tortillas are lightly golden and crisp and cheese has melted, about 10 minutes. Alternatively, cook them on a nonstick griddle.
Cut each tostada into wedges, and serve hot.

Nutrition: 138 calories; 11gm protein; 14gm carbohydrate; 3gm fiber; 2g total fat; 20mg choles.; 314mg calcium; 1mg iron; 28mg magnes.; 200mg potass.; 288mg sodium; Vit. A 127 IU; Vit. C 21mg; Vit. E 1 IU.

FRESH CHERRY TOMATO SALSA

This recipe works for: Digestive Health, Circulation, Weight Control
For about 2 cups:

Pulse-chop all ingredients coarsely in the blender so there are still recognizeable chunks: 2 pints Cherry Tomatos, 1 chopped Shallot, 1 chopped Green Onion, 2 TBS fresh minced Cilantro, 1 TB Tarragon Vinegar, 2 teasp. Lime Juice, 2 Serrano Chilies seeded and minced (wear gloves), 1/2 teasp. Sea Salt, and Zest of 1/2 Lime.

LOW FAT HOT TACOS

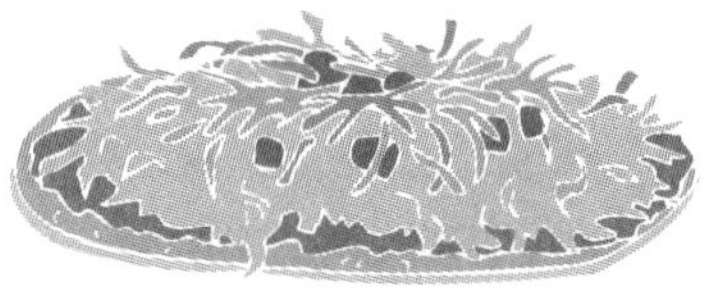

This recipe works for: Sports Nutrition, Kid's Health
For 6 tacos:

Toast 6 Taco Shells in 300° oven until crisp. Mix 1 Cube Tofu with 2 to 3 TBS Grain Burger or Tofu Burger mix. Sauté in 1 TB Olive Oil in a skillet until brown and crumbly. Line taco shells with Cilantro and spoon about 1 TB burger into each shell.

—Mix filling: 2 TBS chopped Green Olives, 1 chopped Tomato, 4 TBS grated Low Fat Cheddar, 1/2 minced Red Onion. Divide filling between tacos. Broil to melt cheese; top with shaved Head Lettuce or Sunflower Sprouts, and salsa drizzles (see above).

SOFT SEAFOOD TACOS with CITRUS SALSA

This recipe works for: Anti-Aging, Women's Health, Brain Boosting
For 6 people, 2 tacos each:

Sizzle 1 minced Clove Garlic and 1 minced Red Onion in 2 TBS Olive Oil. Add 1 large chopped Tomato and 1 LB cooked chopped Shellfish (Shrimp, Crab, Scallops). Sauté for 8 minutes until aromatic. While taco filling cooks, wrap 12 Corn Tortillas in foil and warm in a 350° oven for 10 minutes. Remove, and spoon in seafood filling.
—Top with CITRUS SALSA. Mix: 1/2 cup chopped Cucumber, 1 minced, seeded fresh Jalapeño Chili, 3 TBS Lime Juice, 1 teasp. grated Lime Zest, 1 cup canned Crushed Pineapple, 2 TBS minced fresh Cilantro, Sea Salt and Pepper to taste.

BABY SHRIMP TOSTADAS

This recipe works for: Anti-Aging, Women's Health, Illness Recovery
For 24 tostada chip rounds:

Have ready about 8-oz. cooked Salad Shrimp. Mix topping: 1/2 ripe Avocado, 1 TB minced Red Onion, 3 TBS Low Fat Mayonnaise or Kefir Cheese, 2 TBS Lemon Juice, 1 minced Green Jalapeño Chili, 1 TB. minced fresh Cilantro, 1 teasp. Lemon-Garlic Seasoning. Divide on 24 Tostada chip rounds. Top each with shrimp. Broil 1 minute. Serve hot.

BOCADILLOS CON QUESO

This recipe works for: Sports' Nutrition, Kid's Health, Sugar Imbalances
For about 24 nachos: Preheat oven to 375°.

Cut 3 large FRESH FLOUR TORTILLAS in 8 wedges each. Put on a baking sheet and drizzle a little OLIVE OIL over each wedge. Toast in the oven until light gold and crisp.

—Cut 4-oz. LOW FAT JALAPEÑO JACK CHEESE or into thin slices, and then into wedges the same size as the tortilla wedges. Top each wedge with a cheese wedge.

—Mix in a bowl: 1 chopped TOMATO, 6 sliced BLACK OLIVES, and 2 minced SCALLIONS. Divide over tortilla wedges. Bake about 8 minutes til cheese bubbles. Put on a serving plate and top each with a small dollop of LOW FAT YOGURT mixed with a little SALSA (see above), or a little drizzle of salsa by itself.

Nutrition per: 31 calories; 2gm protein; 3gm carbohydrate; 1gm fiber; 1g total fat; 3mg choles.; 55mg calcium; trace iron; 5mg magnesium; 42mg potassium; 59mg sodium; Vit. A 24 IU; Vit. C 2mg; Vit. E trace.

TOSTADA FIESTA

This recipe works for: Sports' Nutrition, Kid's and Men's Health, Sugar Imbalances
For 4 regular size corn tortillas:

Toast tortillas on a baking sheet til crisp. Mix topping: 1 cup Low Fat REFRIED BEANS (instant mix from your health food store is OK), 4 TBS SALSA (see previous page), 1 small sliced RED ONION, 3 TBS sliced GREEN OLIVES, 4 TBS grated LOW FAT JACK CHEESE or LOW FAT JALAPEÑO JACK CHEESE, 1 chopped TOMATO, and pinches CHILI POWDER to taste.

—Toast to melt cheese and heat beans. Top with SUNFLOWER SPROUTS.

Nutrition: 184 calories; 9gm protein; 30gm carbohydrate; 6gm fiber; 3g total fat; 5mg choles.; 157mg calcium; 2mg iron; 13mg magnes.; 500mg potass.; 344mg sodium; Vit. A 199 IU; Vit. C 16mg; Vit. E 1 IU.

Low Fat Baking and Pastries

Most people find it difficult to reduce fat in breads and pastries. Your favorite foods may fall into this category. You can still eat them and stay healthy. Just make a few changes in the way you bake. Make sure you are using only whole grain flours when you bake. It makes a big difference not only in metabolic activity and body assimilation, but in higher nutrition and fiber.

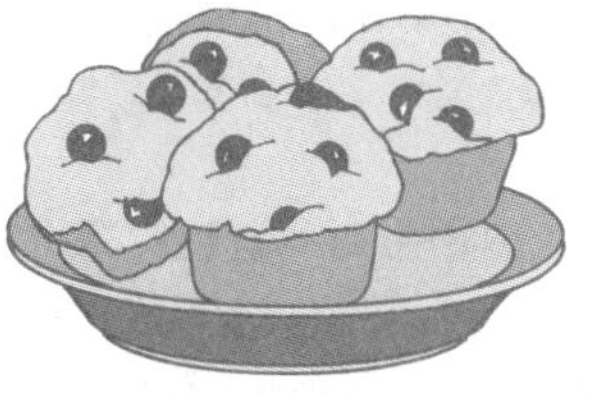

A mix of whole grain flours is lighter and more flavorful than whole wheat flour alone. See pg.489 for a light, nutty flour blend that may be used for the breads and muffins in this book. See the FOOD DIGEST in *The Healing Diets* for more on whole grains and flours.

VERY LIGHT POPOVERS Healthy little "carriers" for almost anything.

This recipe works for: Weight Control, Women's Health, Sugar Imbalances
For 6 popovers: Preheat oven to 425°.

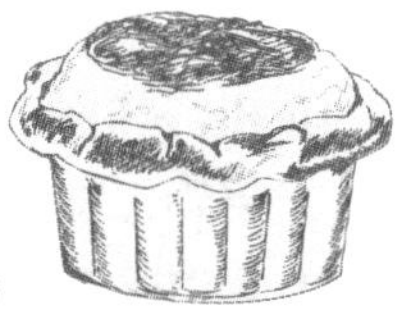

Preheat popover pan, or individual small pyrex custard cups that can take and hold high heat. Leave in the oven until just before use.

—Blend in the blender to the consistency of cream: 1 cup Unbleached Flour, pinch Sea Salt, 3 large Eggs, 1/2 cup Plain Low-Fat Yogurt, 1/2 cup Water.

—Fill hot popover cups half full. Bake 2 minutes. Reduce heat to 325° and bake 15 to 20 minutes more until golden and fully puffed.

Nutrition: 126 calories; 6gm protein; 18gm carbohydrate; 1gm fiber; 3gm total fat; 108mg choles.; 53mg calcium; 1mg iron; 11mg magnesium; 100mg potassium; 82mg sodium; Vit. A 51 IU; Vit. C trace; Vit. E 1 IU.

GINGER-SPICE BREAD

This recipe works for: Good Digestion, Men's Health, Heart Health
For 12 squares: Use a well-greased 8-inch square baking dish.

Combine all ingredients gently: 4 TBS Butter, 4 TBS Fructose, 1 Egg, 3/4 cup Maple Syrup, 3/4 cup Orange Juice, 2 cups sifted Unbleached Flour, 1 TB minced Crystallized Ginger, 1 tsp. Cinnamon, 1 tsp. Sea Salt, 1 tsp. Baking Soda, 1 TB grated Orange Peel, 2 cups Hot Water. Pour into baking pan. Bake at 350°F for 30 to 45 minutes, or until top springs back when lightly touched.

Nutrition: 192 calories; 3gm protein; 35gm carbohydrate; 1gm fiber; 4gm total fat; 028mg choles.; 25mg calcium; 1mg iron; 10mg magnes.; 103mg potassium; 291mg sodium; Vit. A 47 IU; Vit. C 8mg; Vit. E trace.

CRANBERRY-WALNUT BREAD

This recipe works for: Anti-Aging, Sugar Imbalances, Bladder-Kidney Problems
Makes 2 loaves (16 servings): Preheat oven to 350 F. Lightly oil and flour 2 loaf pans.

Have ready 3 cups Cranberries and 3/4 cups chopped toasted Walnuts.

—Sift together in a bowl: 2 cups Unbleached Flour, 1 1/2 cups Whole Wheat Pastry Flour, 1 1/2 tsp. Baking Powder (non-aluminum), 1 tsp. Baking Soda, 1/2 tsp. Sea Salt.

—In another bowl mix: 1/4 cup Canola Oil, 3/4 cup Date Sugar, 2 Eggs, 1 cup Orange Juice, 1 teasp. Orange Zest.

—Gently combine flour mixture and batter. Fold in walnuts and cranberries. Pour the batter into loaf pans and bake for 40 to 45 minutes, or until a toothpick inserted into the center comes out clean. Remove from pans and let cool.

Nutrition: 210 calories; 6gm protein; 31gm carbohydrate; 3gm fiber; 7g total fat; 26mg choles.; 51mg calcium; 2mg iron; 37mg magnesium; 190mg potassium; 189mg sodium; Vit. A 18 IU; Vit. C 11mg; Vit. E 1 IU.

NO-FAT MUFFINS

This recipe works for: Weight Control, Waste Management, Brain Power
For 12 muffins: Preheat oven to 400°.

Mix together: $1^1/_2$ cups Whole Wheat Pastry Flour, 2 Egg Whites beaten to foamy, 1 cup Oat Bran, 2 TBS Toasted Wheat Germ, $2^1/_2$ teasp. Baking Powder, $^1/_4$ teasp. Sea Salt.
—Stir in gently: 2 TBS Honey, $1^1/_2$ cups Apple Juice, $^1/_4$ teasp. Cinnamon.
—Line a 12 cup muffin tin with cupcake papers. Fill $^2/_3$ full and bake 30 minutes until a toothpick poked into the center comes out clean. Remove and cool.

LEMONADE BREAD

This recipe works for: Liver and Organ Health, Good Digestion, Bone Building
Serves 12: Preheat oven to 375°.

Mix gently: 5 TBS Honey, $^1/_2$ teasp. grated Lemon Zest, 3 TBS Butter, 2 cups Unbleached Flour, 1 cup Plain Low-Fat Yogurt, $^1/_2$ cup chopped Almonds, 1 Egg, 2 tsp. Baking Soda, $^1/_4$ cup Lemon Juice, $^1/_4$ tsp. Nutmeg. Fill lecithin-sprayed or paper-lined muffin cups; bake for 25 minutes until golden and a toothpick comes out clean.

LOW FAT SKILLET CORN BREAD Delicious.

This recipe works for: Weight Control, Men's Health, Bone Building
For 12 pieces: Preheat oven to 425° while you mix ingredients.

Mix in the blender: $^3/_4$ cup Water, 2 Eggs, $^1/_4$ cup Canola Oil, $^3/_4$ cup Plain Low-Fat Yogurt, 2 TBS Fructose or Honey. Gently combine just to moisten with: 1 cup Unbleached Flour, 2 TBS Toasted Wheat Germ, $1^1/_2$ cups Yellow Cornmeal, 4 teasp. Baking Powder, $^1/_2$ teasp. Sea Salt. Pour into a lecithin-sprayed 9 x 9" pan or cast iron skillet and bake 15 to 20 minutes until crusty.

GRANDMA'S CORN and RICE MUFFINS

This recipe works for: Weight Control, Women's Health, Sports' Nutrition
For 12 muffins: Preheat oven to 400°.

Mix everything just to moisten. Mixing too much toughens the batter: 1 cup Yellow Cornmeal, 1 TB Baking Powder (non-aluminum), 2 TBS Honey, $^3/_4$ teasp. Sea Salt, $1^1/_2$ TB Maple Syrup or Molasses, 1 cup cooked Short Grain Brown Rice, 2 Eggs, 2 TBS melted Butter, $^7/_8$ cup Low Fat Rice Milk. Pour into lecithin-sprayed muffin cups and bake for 20 minutes until a toothpick comes out clean.

Nutrition: 110 calories; 3gm protein; 18gm carbohydrate; 1gm fiber; 3g total fat; 40mg choles.; 123mg calcium; 1mg iron; 22mg magnesium; 61mg potass.; 196mg sodium; Vit. A 39 IU; Vit. C 1mg; Vit. E trace.

ORANGE GINGERBREAD

This recipe works for: Heart Health, Cancer Control, Women's Health
For 12 pieces: Preheat oven to 350°. Use a 9 x 9" lecithin-sprayed baking pan.

Combine wet ingredients: 3/4 cup Water, 1 Egg, 1/3 cup Orange Juice, 1 TB Orange Peel, 1/2 cup Unsulphured Molasses, 1/2 cup Maple Syrup, 5 TBS Canola Oil, 5 TBS melted Butter. Mix dry ingredients: 2 1/2 cups Whole Wheat Pastry Flour, 1 teasp. Baking Soda (non-aluminum), 2 teasp. minced Crystallized Ginger, 1 teasp. Cinnamon.

—Combine the two mixtures together just enough to moisten. Turn into baking pan, and bake for 35 to 40 minutes until a toothpick inserted in the center comes out clean. Center should still be moist. Serve warm or cool.

Nutrition: 216 calories; 4gm protein; 3gm carbohydrate; 3gm fiber; 9g total fat; 20mg choles.; 164mg calcium; 4mg iron; 68mg magnes.; 490mg potassium; 111mg sodium; Vit. A 63 IU; Vit. C 3mg; Vit. E 3 IU.

Low Fat Pasta

Whole grain and vegetable pastas are amazingly low in fat. Many are made only with the grain or vegetable and water. Fat content is minimal, usually only trace amounts. Ninety-nine percent of the fat in a pasta dish comes from the sauce. The tasty pasta sauces in this section have low fats. You can finally lose the guilt about pasta. Review the healthy pasta cooking techniques on pg.502 before you start.

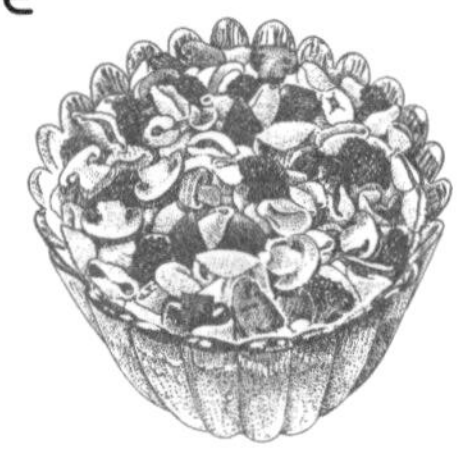

FRENCH PASTA SALAD

This recipe works for: Heart Health, Digestive Health, Men's and Women's Health
Makes 8 servings: Preheat oven to 325°F.

Have ready 1 frozen 16-oz. package French-cut Green Beans. Rinse in a bowl under warm water to thaw; drain immediately and set aside. Spread 1/2 cup chopped Hazelnuts in small baking pan and bake until fragrant, stirring once, about 15 minutes. Cool slightly; rub briskly in a kitchen towel to remove skins. Set aside.

—Make the FRESH VINAIGRETTE SAUCE; whisk together: 1/4 cup Olive Oil, 1/4 cup Balsamic Vinegar, 1 TB Dijon Mustard, 1 large Shallot, minced, 2 teasp. minced Fresh Tarragon, 2 teasp. minced Fresh Basil, 1 teasp. Sea Salt, 1/4 tsp. coarse Pepper.

—Have sauce completely ready. Then bring a large saucepan of water to a boil. Add 1 TB Olive Oil, 1 teasp. Sea Salt, and 1-LB dried Penne or Ziti Pasta. Cook 8 to 10 minutes, until al dente. (Test for doneness by biting into a piece.) Drain in a colander, then pour into a serving bowl, and toss with the FRESH VINAIGRETTE.

—Top pasta with green beans, toast nuts and 2/3 cup drained Roasted Red Peppers. Sprinkle with 1 crumbled Sprig Fresh Rosemary Leaves and 2 TBS snipped Parsley. Scatter on 1/2 cup crumbled Feta Cheese or Chevre. Serve at room temperature.

LOW FAT ITALIAN MACARONI and CHEESE

This recipe works for: Heart Health, Kid's and Men's Health, Allergies/Asthma
Makes 4 servings: Preheat oven at 325°F.

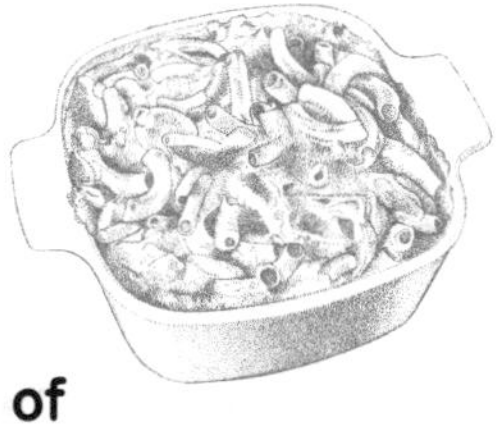

Make the sauce: Sauté 1 cup chopped Roma Tomatoes and $^1/_4$ cup chopped Onion in 1 TB Olive Oil for 5 minutes. Add 3 TBS Unbleached Flour and stir until blended. Mix in $^1/_2$ cup grated Low Fat Cheddar-style Rice Cheese.

—Have sauce completely ready. Then bring a large sauce pan of water to a boil. Add 1 TB Olive Oil, 1 teasp. Sea Salt and 8-oz. dry Macaroni. Cook 10 minutes, stirring occasionally, until al dente. (Test for doneness by biting into a piece.) Drain in a colander, run under cold water and drain again. Pour into a baking dish. Mix in the sauce. Bake until golden brown on top, about 20 minutes.

TUNISIAN PASTA SALAD

This recipe works for: Heart Health, Men's Health, Weight Control
Makes 4 servings:

—Mix veggies: 1 cup diced European Cucumber, $^1/_2$ cup sliced, pitted Black Olives, 2 sliced Scallions, 1 LB ripe Roma Tomatoes, slivered, 2 TBS snipped Fresh Parsley.

—Make a TUNISIAN DRESSING: combine 2 TBS Olive Oil, 5 TBS fresh Lemon Juice $^1/_2$ tsp. ground Cumin, 1 teasp. Black Sesame Seeds, pinch Cayenne, Black Pepper to taste.

—Have sauce completely ready. Then bring a large saucepan of water to a boil. Add 1 TB Olive Oil, 1 teasp. Sea Salt and 8-oz. dried Penne Pasta. Cook 10 minutes, stirring occasionally, until al dente. (Test for doneness by biting into a piece.) Drain in a colander, run under cold water and drain again. Pour into a serving bowl, and toss with the TUNISIAN DRESSING and veggie mix. Serve at room temperature.

Nutrition: 264 calories; 7gm protein; 38gm carbohydrate; 3gm fiber; 9g total fat; 0mg choles.; 56mg calcium; 3mg iron; 39mg magnesium; 260mg potassium; 265mg sodium; Vit. A 47 IU; Vit. C 21mg; Vit. E 3 IU.

PASTA with FRESH BASIL and TOMATOES

This recipe works for: Fatigue Syndromes, Women's and Men's Health
For 8 servings:

Heat 3 qts. Water with 1 teasp. Sea Salt. When you see a rolling boil, add 2 cups dry Egg Pasta Shells. Cook 12 to 15 minutes to al dente. (Test for doneness by biting into a piece.) Drain in a colander, run under cold water and drain again. Toss with 1 teasp. Olive Oil to separate. While pasta is cooking, sauté in a skillet until fragrant: 2 TBS Olive Oil, 2 LBS chopped Roma Tomatoes, $^1/_2$ cup sliced Scallions, and $1^1/_2$ cups Fresh Basil Leaves, minced. Toss with pasta. Top with grated Parmesan-Reggiano Cheese.

LOW-FAT CANNELLONI Heaven for an Italian food lover.

This recipe works for: Heart Health, Men's Health, Overcoming Stress
For 8 cannelloni rolls (2 per person): Preheat oven to 450°.

Combine 1 teasp. Olive Oil, 1 Clove Garlic minced, 1 Onion chopped in a 9 x 13" pan and bake until onion browns, about 15 minutes. Add 2 TBS Water, 2 TBS Balsamic Vinegar and 2 TBS Red Wine. Scrape browned bits free. Return to oven and bake 8 more minutes. Chunk 1$^1/_2$ LBS boneless Organic Chicken Breasts and scatter in the pan. Bake 10 minutes until white in the center. Remove and set aside.

—Whirl half of the chicken-onion mix in the blender with $^1/_2$ cup Parmesan Cheese and 4-oz. Low Fat Ricotta Cheese. Scrape into a bowl and repeat. Season with Nutmeg and Fennel Seed. Mix in 1 Egg, 2 TBS Bread Crumbs, and 2 TBS Red Wine. Cover and chill.

—Lay 8 Chinese Spring Roll Wrappers flat on a baking sheet; divide filling among them, placing it along one edge. Roll to enclose filling. Set seam side down.

—Make the YOGURT SAUCE: Melt 2 TBS Olive Oil in a saucepan. Add 1$^1/_2$ TBS Whole Wheat Flour and stir until toasted. Remove from heat and mix in 1 cup Plain Low Fat Yogurt and 1 cup Low Fat Organic Chicken Broth. Stir to a boil, and cook until sauce is reduced to 1$^1/_2$ cups, about 20 minutes.

—Make the TOMATO SAUCE: Lay 2 LBS halved Roma Tomatoes skin side down on a baking pan. Bake until juices evaporate, leaving a brown residue. Remove from oven; add to the pan, 1 cup Low Fat Organic Chicken Broth and 1 TB Balsamic Vinegar. Scrape up browned bits. Whirl in the blender until pureed. Then cook in a saucepan for 30 minutes to intensify flavors. Stir in $^1/_2$ cup minced Fresh Basil.

—Pour some of each sauce into two 7 x 10" baking pans. Swirl to make a marble effect. Set cannelloni onto the sauce, leaving $^1/_2$" between. Bake uncovered at 425° for 10 minutes.

PASTA MOLTO VERDE

This recipe works for: Liver and Organ Health, Immune Power, Hair, Skin and Nails
For 6 servings:

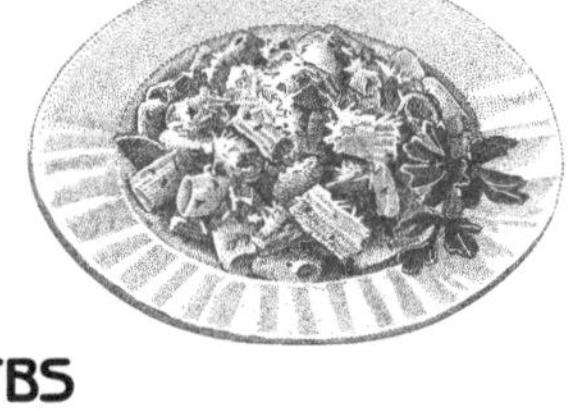

Heat 3 qts. Water with 1 teasp. Sea Salt. When you see a rolling boil, add 8-oz. dry Spinach Noodles and cook to al dente, about 5 to 7 minutes. (Test for doneness by biting into a piece.) Drain in a colander. Toss with 1 teasp. Olive Oil to separate.

—While noodles cook, sauté in a skillet until fragrant: 2 TBS Olive Oil, 8-oz. chopped Spinach or Chard Leaves, $^1/_4$ cup snipped Fresh Parsley, $^1/_3$ cup thin-sliced Scallions, and 1 cup Asparagus pieces or Green Peas. When color changes to bright green, remove from heat and toss with hot pasta.

—Mix the sauce: $^1/_2$ teasp. Garlic-Lemon Seasoning, $^1/_2$ teasp. dry Tarragon, $^1/_4$ cup grated Parmesan Cheese, $^3/_4$ cup Plain Low Fat Yogurt. Toss with pasta, and serve hot.

Nutrition: 217 calories; 10gm protein; 33gm carbohydrate; 6gm fiber; 4gm total fat; 5mg choles.; 188mg calcium; 2 iron; 110mg magnes.; 526mg potassium; 85mg sodium; Vit. A 313 IU; Vit. C 18mg; Vit. E 3 IU.

VERY LOW FAT MARINARA SAUCE for PASTA

This recipe works for: Respiratory Infections, Immune Power, Men's Health
For $2^1/_2$ cups:

Sauté 2 minced Cloves Garlic in 2 TBS Olive Oil until aromatic. Add 1 minced Onion, 1 minced Rib Celery, 1 minced Carrot, 1 minced Red Bell Pepper; sauté until color changes and vegetables soften, stirring. Remove from heat and add 2 chopped Roma Tomatoes, 1 cup chopped Fresh Cilantro, 2 TBS Tomato Paste, 1 teasp. Honey, $^1/_4$ teasp. crushed Fennel Seed, 1 teasp. dry Basil or 1 TB Fresh Basil.

VERY LOW FAT FRESH TOMATO-WINE SAUCE

This recipe works for: Weight Control, Digestive Health, Men's Health
For about 3 cups, 8 servings:

Sauté in 1 TB Olive Oil and 3 TBS Onion Broth until fragrant, about 7 minutes: 1 Clove Garlic minced, 1 small Onion chopped, $^1/_2$ Red Bell Pepper chopped, $^1/_2$ Carrot diced, 3 to 4 large Tomatoes chopped, $^1/_2$ teasp. dry Basil and $^1/_2$ teasp. dry Thyme.
—Add and simmer until stock reduces by about a third: 1 cup White Wine, 2 cups Water, 1 teasp. Honey, $^1/_2$ teasp. Garlic-Lemon Seasoning and $^1/_4$ teasp. Black Pepper.

Nutrition: 51 calories; 1gm protein; 6gm carbohydrate; 1gm fiber; 1g total fat; 0mg choles.; 14mg calcium; 1mg iron; 13mg magnesium; 199mg potassium; 9mg sodium; Vit. A 192 IU; Vit. C 22mg; Vit. E 2 IU.

Low Fat Pizzas

Real Italian cooking is light, low fat and easy - leagues apart from the greasy, heavy dishes we call Italian food in America. Italian pizzas are incredibly light, with thin, yeast-free semolina crusts, lightly strewn with buffalo milk mozarrella and aromatic vegetable soffrito toppings. In contrast American pizzas use heavily spiced meats, double cheese, few vegetables, and thick doughy crusts. Make pizza the way it should be - truly light, deliciously Italian - without the guilt or health problems.

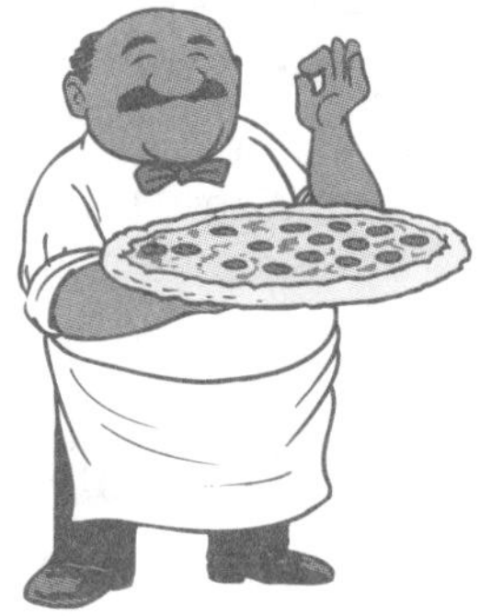

How to Make an Incredibly Light Pizza

<u>THE CRUST</u>: They don't come any better - quick and crisp. Make the dough ahead, freeze it, then thaw it when you're ready if you like. But it's so easy to make when you make the pizza. It only takes 5 minutes and you'll have it fresh.

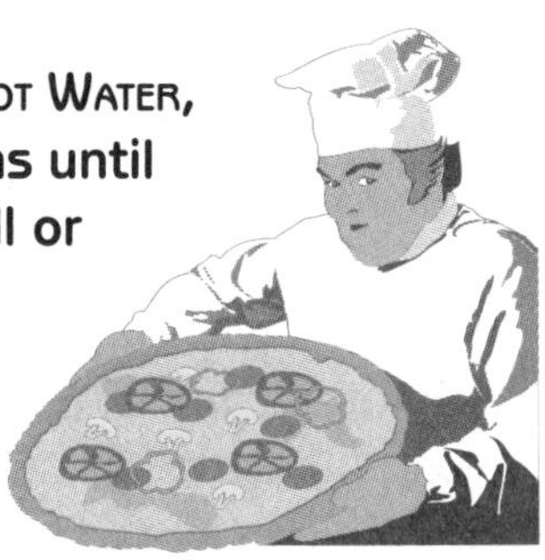

—Mix: 1 cup Semolina Flour, 1 tsp. Baking Powder, 1/3 cup Hot Water, 1/2 teasp. Sea Salt, and 1 TB Olive Oil. Knead dough a few turns until elastic. Let it sit, covered in plastic wrap for 15 minutes. Roll or pat out into a 7 or 8" circle.

—Heat a cast iron skillet. Test a tiny piece of dough in the skillet when it's hot. Bubbles should appear on the underside in 45 seconds. Lay in a dough circle, and cook on one side just until dark brown, about 3 minutes. Remove from skillet to a plate and strew on 1/3 cup Low Fat Mozarrella Chunks (or any soft low-fat melting cheese that lets the flavors of the veggies come through).

THE TOPPING: Try some of the delicious toppings on the next 2 pages. Each one makes enough for two crusts. Use about 1/2 cup topping per pizza. Drop dollops all over the pizza. Toppings go on top of the cheese for intense vegetable taste. Drizzle with Olive Oil and return pizza to hot iron skillet. Cover and cook for 2 minutes to melt cheese and heat veggies. Try it - almost fool proof - and low-fat too!

—For the best Low Fat Pizzas:

1) Make sure the vegetables aren't wet or heavy;

2) Be generous with seasonings, light on cheeses;

3) Keep sun-dried tomatoes, semolina flour, water-packed artichokes, and pesto-in-a-tube on hand;

4) Use the freshest low-fat mozarrella cheese and the best olive oil you can.

AUTHENTIC VERDE TOPPING

This recipe works for: Weight Control, Bone Building, Women's Health

Have ready 1 cup fresh chopped tangy Greens for each pizza. Use Spinach, Watercress, Endive, or Chard. Sauté in 2 TBS Olive Oil for 2 minutes: dashes Hot Sauce, 1/4 teasp. crushed Fennel Seed, 2 teasp. Pesto Paste, pinches Sea Salt and Pepper. Add greens to skillet, remove immediately from heat; let them wilt in the seasonings.

Nutrition: 93 calories; 2gm protein; 2gm carbohydrate; 1gm fiber; 8g total fat; 1mg choles.; 65mg calcium; 1mg iron; 26mg magnesium; 177mg potassium; 30mg sodium; Vit. A 195 IU; Vit. C 8mg; Vit. E 3 IU.

FRAGRANT ZUCCHINI - SUN-DRIED TOMATO TOPPING

This recipe works for: Weight Control, Respiratory Health, Men's Health

Slice 3 small Zucchini in thin rounds. Sprinkle with salt and let sit for 5 minutes in a colander to release moisture and bitterness. Drain and press out moisture.

—Sliver 4 oil-packed Sun Dried Tomatoes, or 2 Fresh Tomatoes. Pour packing oil from tomato jar in a skillet and sauté tomatoes with 1 minced Clove Garlic and 4 drops Hot Pepper Sauce. Add zucchini and sauté rapidly for 3 minutes. Remove from heat. Add 2 TBS Fresh Basil, chopped or 2 teasp. dry Basil, and 1/4 teasp. ground Fennel Seed.

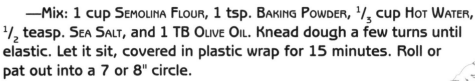

SCALLIONS and OLIVES SCENTED with ROSEMARY

This recipe works for: Liver and Organ Health, Heart and Circulatory Health

Top each Pizza with 3 TBS crumbled Feta Cheese, then with this sauce:
—Sauté in 2 TBS Olive Oil for 5 minutes until fragrant: 6 Scallion Whites (save chopped green parts for topping), 2 Sprigs Fresh Rosemary or 1 teasp. dry Rosemary, 1 Bay Leaf, 2 TBS Red Wine. Discard bay leaf and rosemary. Sprinkle with pinches Sea Salt, Pepper, reserved Scallion Tops, and 2 TBS chopped Black Olives.

ARTICHOKE HEARTS SAUCE

This recipe works for: Weight Control, Arthritis, Women's Health

Sauté in 2 TBS Olive Oil 5 minutes: $1^1/_2$ teasp. Garlic-Lemon Seasoning, $^1/_4$ teasp. Thyme, 8-oz. jar chopped Water-packed Artichoke Hearts, 1 TB Lemon Juice, 1 TB White Wine. Steam 3 minutes covered. Remove from heat; top with 4 TBS Fresh Parsley.

PESTO PIZZA

This recipe works for: Liver Health, Digestive Health, Men's Health

Toast 3 TBS Pine Nuts in the oven until golden. Blend them in the blender with 1 cup packed Fresh Basil Leaves, $^1/_2$ cup grated Parmesan-Reggiano Cheese, $^1/_4$ cup Olive Oil, pinches Sesame Seed, Sea Salt, Pepper and Oregano Leaves.

Low Fat Quiches

Most of us love quiches. They are perfect casual company food. But all the cream, butter and eggs weighs you and your circulation down. Traditional quiche recipes make it hard to stay away from fat. This section offers quiches with restructured recipes for low-fat eating. The good taste remains, the high fats don't. The recipes in this section serve around 8 people.

THE CRUST: Lots of fat comes from a traditional quiche crust. The three on the following page keep fats low. Another good choice: Grind up almost any vegetable casserole leftovers in the blender or food processor, re-season, and press the mixture into a quiche pan. Bake at 375° for 10 minutes to set the layer and you have an instant quiche crust. Even plain crackers layed in a single layer on the quiche pan make a lovely crust. Drizzle with oil, or spread lightly with butter if desired, and toast briefly before filling.

VEGETABLE QUICHE CRUST

This recipe works for: Bladder and Kidney Health, Digestive Health, Men's Health

Grate all vegetables in a blender or food processor; then combine: 2 cups diced Zucchini, $^1/_2$ cup diced Carrots, $^1/_2$ cup peeled diced Parsnips or fresh Daikon Radish. Salt vegetables, and let stand about 5 minutes. Squeeze out excess moisture.

—Mix vegetables with 2 TBS Olive Oil and $^1/_3$ cup Whole Wheat Pastry Flour or Light, Nutty Flour Blend (page 489.) Press into a lecithin-sprayed quiche pan. Brush with a little more oil, and bake for about 30 minutes at 375°. Cool and fill.

MASHED POTATO CRUST

This recipe works for: Fatigue Syndromes, Sports' Nutrition, Men's Health

Sauté $^1/_2$ cup chopped Onion in 2 TBS Olive Oil with pinches of Sea Salt and Pepper.

—Boil 2 large Potatoes until tender. Mash and mix with onions. Sculpt the mixture into a lecithin-sprayed quiche dish to form a high crust. Brush with Olive Oil and bake at 375° for 40 minutes until set and crusty. Remove, cool and fill.

WHOLE GRAIN and SEED CRUST

This recipe works for: Stress, Sugar Balance, Men's and Women's Health

Mix: 1 cup Whole Grain Bread Crumbs, $^1/_4$ cup Whole Wheat Pastry Flour, $^1/_2$ cup Toasted Wheat Germ, $^1/_2$ cup Toasted Sesame Seeds, 4 TBS Melted Butter, $^1/_4$ teasp. Sea Salt, pinches Mixed Italian Herbs to taste. Press into a lecithin-sprayed quiche pan and bake at 350° for 10 minutes. Cool and fill.

Nutrition: 94 calories; 3gm protein; 7gm carbohydrate; 2gm fiber; 6g total fat; 7mg choles.; 15mg calcium; 1mg iron; 38mg magnesium; 82mg potassium; 79mg sodium; Vit. A 27 IU; Vit. C 16mg; Vit. E 1 IU.

<u>THE FILLINGS</u>: The ones given here are low-fat, delicious and unusual. Cook quiches only enough to just set the filling; the interior keeps on cooking even after you remove it from the oven.

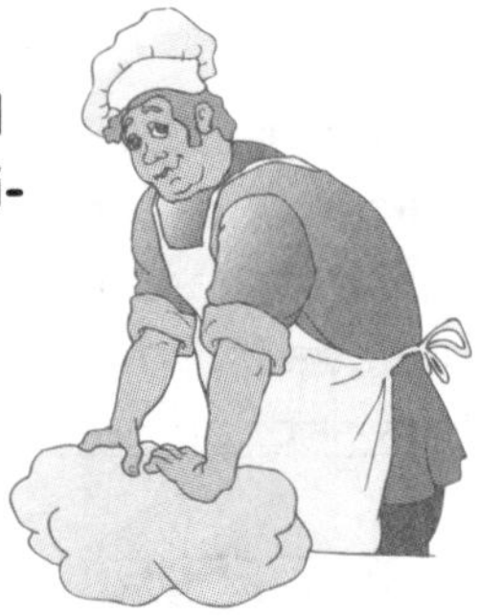

RUSSIAN SWEET CHEESE FILLING

This recipe works for: Kid's and Men's Health, Digestive Health

Mix: 16-oz. Low-Fat Cottage Cheese, 2 Eggs, 4 TBS Honey, $^1/_4$ cup Raisins, 2 TBS Low Fat Yogurt, $^1/_3$ cup chopped toasted Walnuts, 1 tsp. Cardamom, $^1/_4$ tsp. Nutmeg. Put in a whole grain crust, or thin unbaked crust. Bake at 375° for 10 to 20 minutes until crust browns.

ASIAN VEGETABLE FILLING

This recipe works for: Heart Health, Digestive Health, Cancer Protection

Soak 4 Shiitake Mushrooms until soft. Sliver and discard woody stems; reserve mushroom soaking water.

—Mix in the blender: 3 Eggs, 1 cup Plain Low Fat Yogurt, 1/2 cup Low Fat Cottage Cheese, 1/2 teasp. Sesame Salt, 1/4 teasp. Black Pepper, 1/2 teasp. Ground Ginger, 4 TBS mushroom soaking water, and 1 teasp. Tamari.

—Pour into a whole grain crust and add: One handful Sunflower Sprouts, the Shiitake Mushrooms, 1/2 cup sliced Water Chestnuts, 1/2 cup sliced Bok Choy.

—Bake at 450° for 10 minutes - then at 350° for 20 minutes, until filling is just set. Let sit for 5 minutes and serve hot.

Nutrition: 70 calories; 6gm protein; 5gm carbohydrate; 1gm fiber; 2g total fat; 80mg choles.; 81mg calcium; trace iron; 13mg magnesium; 162mg potassium; 185mg sodium; Vit. A 5 IU; Vit. C 3mg; Vit. E 1 IU.

FRESH TOMATO BASIL FILLING

This recipe works for: Bladder and Kidney Health, Digestive Health, Men's Health
Preheat oven to 400°.

Sprinkle 2 TBS Soy Bacon Bits onto a whole grain crust. Sauté in 2 TBS Olive Oil until aromatic: 1 Red Onion, chopped, 4 Tomatoes, chopped, 1/4 cup packed Fresh Basil, chopped, pinches Sea Salt and Pepper.

—Spoon into shell. Cover with grated Low Fat Mozarrella Cheese. Bake for 15 minutes until cheese melts and quiche is fragrant.

PROVENCE FILLING

This recipe works for: Recovery, Digestive Health, Skin, Hair and Nails
Preheat oven to 375°.

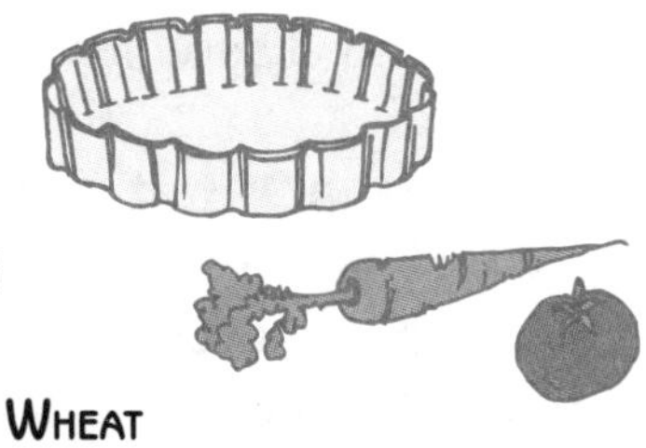

Sprinkle 3 TBS Parmesan Cheese onto a potato or vegetable crust. Then sauté in 2 TBS Olive Oil until aromatic: 1 clove Garlic, minced, 2 cups diced Onion, pinches Sea Salt and Pepper. Spread onion mix on quiche shell. Scatter 3 TBS chopped Black Olives on top.

—Mix together and pour over filling: 4 Eggs, 1 TB Toasted Wheat Germ, 1/2 cup Plain Low Fat Yogurt, 1/2 cup White Wine, 1/4 teasp. Dry Mustard. Sprinkle with 2 TBS Parmesan-Reggiano Cheese. Decorate with thin Tomato Slices on top. Bake for 40 minutes until just set.

Nutrition: 129 calories; 8gm protein; 7gm carbohydrate; 1gm fiber; 6gm total fat; 113mg choles.; 144mg calcium; 1mg iron; 19mg magnes.; 189mg potassium; 101mg sodium; Vit. A 74 IU; Vit. C 6mg; Vit. E 1 IU.

VERY LOW-FAT ITALIAN VEGETABLE FILLING

This recipe works for: Heart and High Blood Pressure, Liver and Organ Health
Preheat oven to 375°.

Use a pre-baked Potato Crust (or no shell). Sprinkle shell or quiche pan with 1 TB Soy Bacon Bits and Garlic-Lemon Seasoning. Sauté 1 Clove Garlic, minced and 1 Onion chopped in 1 TB Olive Oil until aromatic. Add and sauté 2 minutes: 1 Zucchini sliced thin, 1 Red Bell Pepper diced, pinches Italian Mixed Herbs and Black Pepper.

—Pour over vegetables: 2 Eggs, 2 TBS Plain Low-Fat Yogurt, 2 TBS snipped Fresh Parsley. Add mix to quiche shell or pan. Sprinkle with 2 TBS grated Parmesan Cheese. Bake until just set, about 30 minutes.

Nutrition: 58 calories; 5gm protein; 3gm carbohydrate; 1gm fiber; 2g total fat; 56mg choles.; 73mg calcium; 1mg iron; 17mg magnesium; 162mg potassium; 33mg sodium; Vit. A 95 IU; Vit. C 24mg; Vit. E 1 IU.

JAPANESE QUICHE

This recipe works for: Women's Health, Liver and Organ Health, Sexuality
Makes 8 servings:

Mix: 1 cup Sunflower Sprouts or Bean Sprouts, 1 cup grated Carrot, 1 cup French-cut Green Beans (if frozen, rinse in hot water first and drain), 4 chopped Green Onions, 2 TBS Tamari, $^1/_2$ minced Crystallized Ginger. Pour onto crust or bottom of baking dish.

—Mix 3 beaten Eggs to frothy, pour over filling. Bake at 350 F for 15 minutes, or top with toasted noodles and bake until set.

—Cook briefly in boiling water: Japanese Egg Noodles, Soba Buckwheat Noodles or Rice Stick Noodles. Coat with a little oil until shiny, and then sauté or bake until crispy. Line the bottom of a quiche dish with noodles and top with filling.

LEEK and MUSTARD TART

This recipe works for: Hair, Skin and Nails, Liver - Organ Health, Asthma-Allergies
Makes 8 servings: Preheat oven to 375°.

Cover a 9" tart or quiche pan with crushed Rye Crackers. Cover crackers with Low Fat Cheddar-type Rice Cheese. Sizzle 1 LB White Parts Leeks, sliced in rings, in 2 TBS Olive Oil for 5 minutes. Add $^1/_2$ cup White Wine, and simmer 10 minutes. Sprinkle with $^1/_2$ teasp. Sesame Salt and $^1/_4$ teasp. Pepper. Scrape into tart shell.

—Make the sauce; beat until smooth: $^1/_2$ cup Plain Low Fat Yogurt, $^1/_2$ cup Low Fat Cream Cheese, $2^1/_2$ TBS Dijon Mustard and 3-oz. crumbled Feta Cheese. Pour over quiche. Scatter on 2 TBS snipped Chives and 2 TBS Soy Bacon Bits. Bake until top is firm and golden, about 30 minutes. Let sit for 5 minutes and slice.

Nutrition: 178 calories; 8gm protein; 19gm carbohydrate; 3gm fiber; 7g total fat; 18mg choles.; 153mg calcium; 2mg iron; 45mg magnes.; 297mg potassium; 302mg sodium; Vit. A 55 IU; Vit. C 17mg; Vit. E 1 IU.

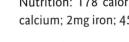

Turkey: Low Fat, Low Cholesterol Meat

Are you reducing the red meat in your diet? Turkey can be a good transition meat. It has plenty of flavor but is low in cholesterol and saturated fat. White meat from turkey (and chicken) contains less than half the fat, 20% less calories and 10% more protein than dark meat. Buy free-run turkeys, that have not been treated with hormones or antibiotics. Avoid pre-basted turkeys. Most are injected with partially hydrogenated oils which raise cholesterol levels, and treated with artificial coloring.

TURKEY in the STRAW A kids favorite... Turkey Sloppy Joes.

This recipe works for: Heart-Artery Health, Kid's Health, Hair, Stress Problems
For 6 servings:

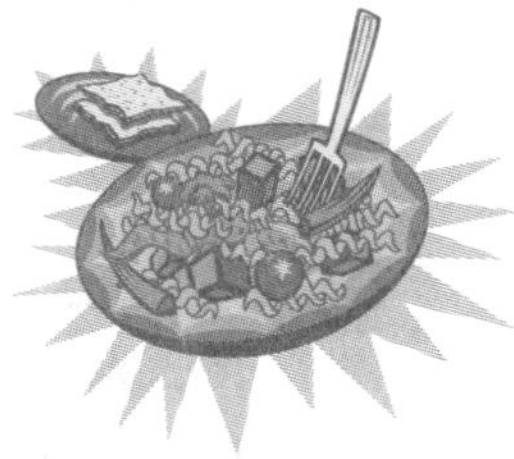

Sauté in a pot without oil or butter for 10 minutes: 1 LB ground TURKEY, 1 ONION, 1 RIB CELERY, minced, 1/2 RED BELL PEPPER minced, chopped, 1 teasp. SEA SALT and 1/4 teasp. BLACK PEPPER.

—Add and simmer uncovered for 1 hour: 1 cup WATER, one 6-oz can TOMATO PASTE, 4 TBS KETCHUP, 1 teasp. WORCESTERSHIRE SAUCE, and dashes HOT PEPPER SAUCE to taste.

—Spoon over crisp CORN CHIPS and top with grated LOW FAT CHEDDAR or SWISS CHEESE.

Nutrition: 260 calories; 21gm protein; 16gm carbohydrate; 2gm fiber; 12g total fat; 71mg choles.; 177mg calcium; 2mg iron; 45mg magnesium; 582mg potassium; 391mg sodium; Vit. A 160 IU; Vit. C 28mg; Vit. E 1 IU.

TURKEY SALAD with MAPLE-MUSTARD DRESSING

This recipe works for: Heart Health, Women's - Men's Health, Sugar Imbalances
Makes 6 large servings:

Place 2 large SWEET POTATOES diced in a steamer. Gently steam until a knife easily slides through a potato cube, about 6 minutes. Set aside.

—Heat a large nonstick skillet. Add 2 teasp. OLIVE OIL and 1 large ONION, thinly sliced; sauté 5 minutes. Reduce heat to low and cook 20 minutes until onion caramelizes. Add 2 cups shredded cooked TURKEY and heat briefly until warmed. Cover.

—Make the sauce: in a small saucepan over low heat, combine 1/2 cup DIJON MUSTARD and 1/2 cup real MAPLE SYRUP. Season with LEMON-PEPPER to taste.

—In a large salad bowl, mix 12 cups fresh BABY SPINACH LEAVES, 1/2 cup dried CRANBERRIES, 1 1/2 cups fat-free CROUTONS and sweet potatoes; toss with half of dressing. Divide mixture among 6 dinner plates. Top with turkey and onions; drizzle with remaining dressing. Sprinkle on 4 TBS SOY BACON BITS.

Nutrition: 318 calories; 26gm protein; 46gm carbohydrate; 8gm fiber; 5g total fat; 40mg choles.; 219mg calcium; 6 iron; 151mg magnes.; 1246mg potass.; 315mg sodium; Vit. A 1582 IU; Vit. C 45mg; Vit. E 5 IU.

TURKEY TACOS

This recipe works for: Heart and Artery Health, Kid's and Men's Health, Stress
For 12 tacos:

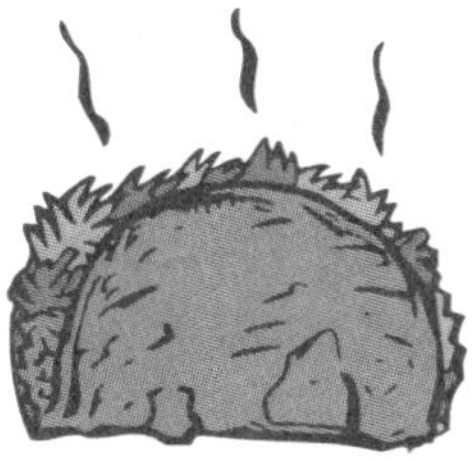

Sauté 1 Clove Garlic minced in 1 TB Canola Oil for 3 minutes. Add and sauté for 10 minutes: 1 diced Red Onion, 8-oz. uncooked Turkey Breast, cut in strips, 1/2 teasp. ground Cumin, 1/2 teasp. dry Oregano, seasoning pinches Sea Salt and Pepper.

—Remove from heat and add: 2 Tomatoes, diced, 1 cup shredded Lettuce, 1/3 cup Fresh Cilantro Leaves, chopped.

SPLIT PEA SOUP with TURKEY WEINERS

This recipe works for: Immune Power, Men's Health, Sports Nutrition
For 8 servings:

Bring 4 cups Water to a boil, and add 2 cups Quick-cooking Split Peas, 3 Ribs Celery, diced, 2 Yellow Onions in chunks, 4 cups Low-fat Organic Chicken Broth, 1 teasp. Sea Salt, 1/2 teasp. Black Pepper. Simmer, partially covered over low heat for 2 hours. Cool slightly. Purée in the blender until smooth. Return to the soup pot, and add 1 package Turkey Weiners, sliced in rounds. (Buy weiners from the natural food store that don't have fillers or preservatives.) Heat through for 5 minutes and serve.

Nutrition: 269calories; 22gm protein; 34gm carbohydrate; 5gm fiber; 5g total fat; 34mg choles.; 53mg calcium; 3mg iron; 75mg magnesium; 764mg potassium; 354mg sodium; Vit. A 9 IU; Vit. C 4mg; Vit. E 1 IU.

JAPANESE RICE BOWL with TURKEY

This recipe works for: Stress Reactions, Women's Health, Allergies and Asthma
Makes 6 servings:

In a medium saucepan, bring 3 cups Water to a boil. Add 2 cups Basmati Rice; reduce heat to low. Cover and cook 15 minutes. Let rice stand.

—In another saucepan, bring two 14-oz. cans Fat Free Organic Chicken Broth, 1/3 cup Tamari, and 1 TBS Fructose to a boil. Add 8-oz. Fresh Shiitake Mushroom Caps, slivered. Simmer, uncovered, 5 minutes. Stir in 1 1/2 cups shredded cooked Turkey, 6 Scallions, thinly sliced and 2 TBS minced Crystallized Ginger.

—In a small bowl, beat 3 large Eggs. Gently pour into hot stock. Let eggs spread naturally..... stirring will cause them to break apart. Cook eggs until they begin to ripple around edges, about 1 minute. Stir once; turn off heat. Divide rice among 6 deep soup bowls. Ladle broth mixture over rice.

Nutrition: 455 calories; 30gm protein; 74gm carbohydrate; 2gm fiber; 4g total fat; 155mg choles.; 46mg calcium; 2mg iron; 33mg magnes.; 368mg potassium; 321mg sodium; Vit. A 55 IU; Vit. C 4mg; Vit. E 1 IU.

EASY TURKEY TETRAZZINI Mmmm good.

This recipe works for: Heart Health, Kid's - Men's Health, Sugar Imbalances
For 4 people: Preheat oven to 350°.

Have ready 4 cups cooked Chinese Egg Noodles.
—Mix and put in a lecithin-sprayed baking dish: 1 diced Red Onion, 8-oz. sliced Mushrooms, 3 cups diced, cooked Turkey, 1 cup Organic Low Fat Chicken Broth, $^1/_2$ cup snipped Fresh Parsley, 1 cup Low Fat Cottage Cheese, 2 TBS Lemon Juice, $^1/_2$ cup grated Parmesan Cheese, and 2 Eggs. Season with $1^1/_2$ teasp. Lemon-Pepper. Sprinkle with Paprika, more Parmesan; top with crunchy Chinese Noodles. Bake for 40 minutes.

Good-Fat Seafood Fights Bad Fats

Good fats can fight bad fats. Seafoods are a delicious way to fight your high cholesterol, enhance the texture of your skin and hair with essential fatty acids, boost your brain power.... and lose weight.

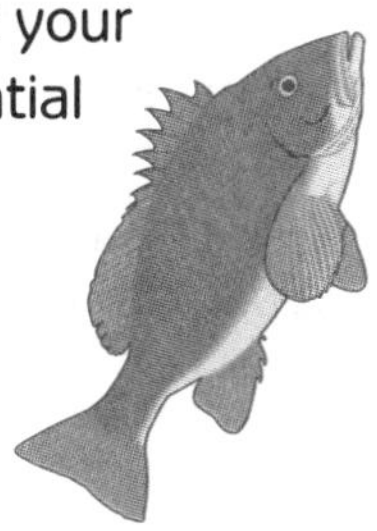

ASIAN STYLE STEAMED RED SNAPPER

This recipe works for: Cancer Protection, Weight Control

Place 1 whole Red Snapper or (Rockfish) in a baking dish. Soak 10 Shiitake Mushrooms until soft in water to cover. Then sliver caps and discard woody stems. Pour mushrooms and soaking water over fish.
—Make the ASIAN MARINADE and pour over fish: 1 TB Sherry, 1 teasp. toasted Sesame Oil, 2 TBS Tamari, $^1/_2$ tsp. Brown Sugar or Honey, $^1/_2$ tsp. Sea Salt, 1 tsp. minced Crystallized Ginger, 1 Scallion, sliced diagonally.
—Put baking dish with the fish into a large roasting pan that has a cover (baking dish may be placed on a rack inside larger pan). Pour boiling water into larger pan to a depth of 1-inch. Cover and steam on top of stove, about 30 minutes for a 2 $^1/_2$ pound fish, 15 minutes for a 1 pound fish. Serve immediately.

GARLIC-ROSEMARY SCENTED SALMON STEAKS

This recipe works for: Cancer Protection, Women's Health, Hair, Skin and Nails
Makes 6 servings:

Sizzle 2 TBS Olive Oil and 2 minced Cloves Garlic in a large skillet for 1 minute.
—Add 4 large Salmon Steaks and cook for 3-4 minutes on each side until browned. Pour 3 TBS Lemon Juice over and sprinkle with 2 TBS Fresh Rosemary Leaves or $^1/_2$ tsp. dried Rosemary Season to taste with Lemon-Pepper. Cover and simmer for 5-8 minutes, or until flesh flakes when tested with a fork.

PERFECT SHRIMP JAMBALAYA

This recipe works for: Boosting Sexuality, Men's Health, Heart Health
For 8 servings: Set oven to 375°F.

Combine in a large oven ready pot: 1 cup Brown Basmati Rice, 1/2 teasp. Sea Salt, 1 Clove Garlic minced, 1 large Onion diced, one Bay Leaf, 1/2 teasp. Chili Powder, 1/4 teasp. Nutmeg, 1/4 teasp. dry Thyme, 4 TBS snipped Fresh Parsley, 2 pinches Cayenne Pepper and 1 cup chopped Raw Oysters.

—Stir in one 16-oz. can Peeled Roma Tomatoes with juice, one 14-oz. can Organic Low Fat Chicken Broth, and one 8-oz. can Tomato Sauce. (Or use equivalent amounts of fresh ingredients.)

—Bake, stirring occasionally for 45 minutes, until rice is just tender. Top rice with 1 LB Raw Peeled Shrimp and bake covered until shrimp is pink, about 10 minutes. Serve hot in shallow soup bowls with sourdough bread and vegetable relishes.

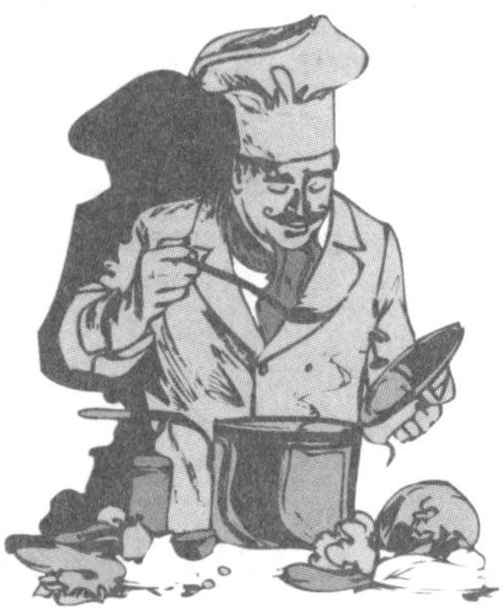

Nutrition: 139 calories; 17gm protein; 11gm carbohydrate; 1gm fiber; 3g total fat; 106mg choles.; 79mg calcium; 4mg iron; 51mg magnes.; 522mg potass.; 433mg sodium; Vit. A 137 IU; Vit. C 21mg; Vit. E 5 IU.

GINGER and SPICE SALMON with BRAISED BOK CHOY

This recipe works for: Srong Bones, Heart Health, Digestive Health
Makes 4 servings:

Have ready four 8-oz. Salmon Fillets.

—Rinse and trim 4 bunches Baby Bok Choy. Cut the leafy tops crosswise into 2-inch strips; cut the stems crosswise into 1-inch pieces.

—In a large frying pan over high heat, sizzle 2 teasp. minced Garlic in 2 teasp. Olive Oil for 2 minutes. Add bok choy and 3/4 cup Low Fat Organic Chicken Broth; cover and simmer 4 minutes; keep warm.

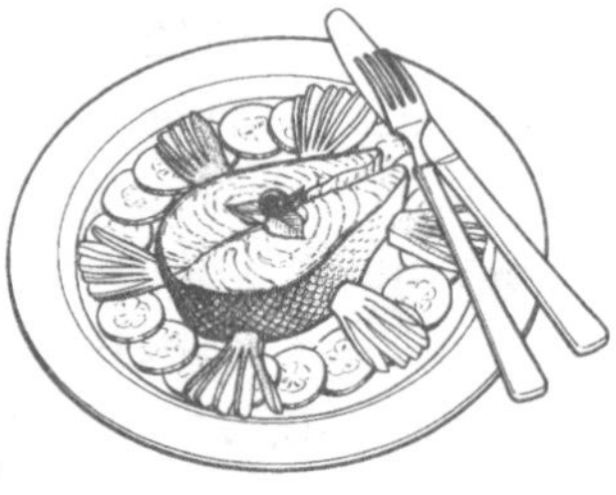

—Mix 2 TBS Chinese 5-Spice Powder, 2 TBS Tamari, 2 TBS minced Crystallized Ginger, 1 teasp. Lime Juice and 1/2 teasp. Black Pepper. Rub fish evenly with mixture.

—Add 2 more teasp. Olive Oil to skillet and heat 1 minute. Lay salmon skin down in pan; cook 3 minutes. With a wide spatula, turn fish and cook until it is opaque but still moist-looking in center of thickest part (cut to test), about 3 minutes more.

—Put salmon in wide soup bowls; spoon bok choy and broth equally around fish.

Nutrition: 441 calories; 49gm protein; 11gm carbohydrate; 2gm fiber; 19g total fat; 125mg choles.; 173mg calcium; 3mg iron; 95mg magnes.; 1491mg potass.; 321mg sodium; Vit. A 369 IU; Vit. C 53mg; Vit. E 5 IU.

BARBECUED SALMON with MUSTARD SAUCE

This recipe works for: Cancer Protection, Women's Health, Weight Control
Makes 18 to 20 servings:

Make the sauce: combine in a saucepan 1/2 cup diced Onion, 1 cup Vermouth, 6 TBS Dijon Mustard, 2 tsp. dry Tarragon, and 2 TBS Honey. Cook until reduced to 3/4 cup, stirring, 8 minutes.

—Spread onion mixture over top of salmon (6 to 7 lbs. total).

—Barbecue Salmon Fillets: Lay fish on a sheet of foil (about 12 by 17 inch). Trim foil to fit salmon. Have barbecue ready with indirect heat. Set foil with salmon on grill but not over heat. Cover barbecue as directed. Cook until fish is opaque but still moist in thickest part (cut to test), 30 to 40 minutes. Slide a rimless baking sheet under salmon and foil, then slide fish onto a large flat platter or board. Cut salmon and lift portions from skin with a wide spatula. Season to taste with Sesame Salt.

Nutrition: 233 calories; 29gm protein; 3gm carbohydrate; 1gm fiber; 9g total fat; 78mg choles.; 28mg calcium; 1mg iron; 43mg magnesium; 728mg potassium; 105mg sodium; Vit. A 18 IU, Vit. C 16mg; Vit. E 1 IU.

Low Fat Toppings, Dressings and Sauces

A topping dressing or sauce can send the fat calories in your meal soaring. The best solution is to use a lot less oil and more vinegar to escape the fat. You get the same gratifying taste - but in a more delicate way. Or, use no oil at all. Instead puree tomato or lemon juice with plain low fat yogurt. Use low-fat yogurt, low fat cheeses and light mayonnaise in place of full fat ingredients. To lower fat in a bottled dressing: mix it with equal parts of plain low-fat yogurt, lemon juice or your favorite vinegar.

VERY LOW FAT DRESSING or VEGGIE DIP

This recipe works for: Fatigue Syndromes, Women's Health, Weight Control
For about 2 cups:

Blender blend until smooth: 1/2 cup Low Fat Cottage Cheese, 1/2 cup Plain Low Fat Yogurt or Kefir Cheese, 1 teasp. Dijon Mustard, 2 Scallions minced, 1 TB Olive Oil, 1 teasp. Lemon Juice, 1/2 teasp. Lemon Pepper, dashes Hot Pepper Sauce.

Add if desired: 1 small diced Tomato, 1 teasp. dry Basil, 2 TBS Sweet Pickle Relish.

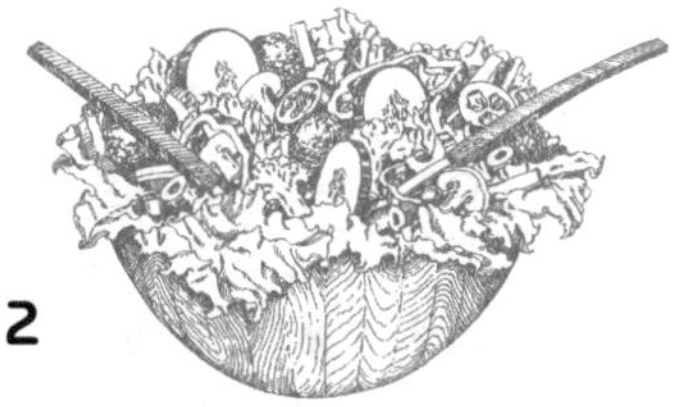

Nutrition: 76calories; 5gm protein; 4gm carbohydrate; 1gm fiber; 4g total fat; trace choles.; 86mg calcium; trace iron; 10mg magnesium; 140mg potassium; 149mg sodium; Vit. A 13 IU, Vit. C 4mg; Vit. E trace.

LOW FAT MEDITERRANEAN VINAIGRETTE

This recipe works for: Digestive Health, Women's Health, Weight Control
Makes about $^3/_4$ cup:

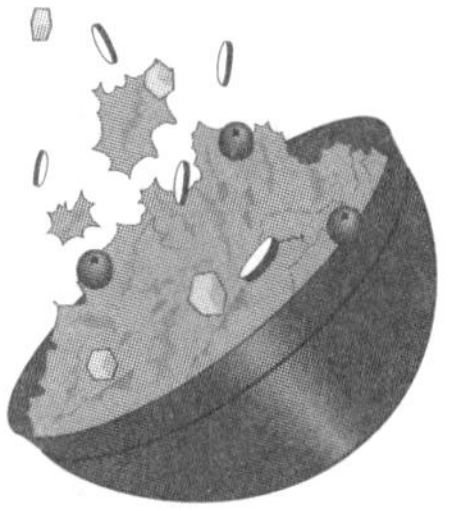

Mix with a fork and serve: 2 TBS Olive Oil, 2 TBS Balsamic Vinegar, 1 TB Dijon Mustard, 2 TBS minced Green Onion, 2 TBS Lemon Juice, 2 TBS Sparkling Water, 1 TB snipped Fresh Chives, $^1/_2$ teasp. Lemon-Pepper.

SIX HERB VINAIGRETTE

This recipe works for: Infections, Liver and Organ Health, Weight Control
Makes about 1 cup: Mix with 8-oz. Kefir Cheese for a great raw veggie dip.

Mix by hand in a bowl: $^2/_3$ cup White Wine Vinegar or Raspberry Vinegar, 3 TBS Olive Oil, $^1/_2$ TB EACH: fresh snipped Rosemary, fresh snipped Oregano, fresh snipped Basil, fresh snipped Thyme, fresh snipped Chives and fresh snipped Lemon Mint, $^1/_2$ teasp. dry Mustard, $^1/_2$ teasp. Sea Salt, dashes Paprika.

HOT and SOUR SALAD DRESSING

This recipe works for: Liver and Organ Health, Digestive Health, Weight Control
For about $1^1/_2$ cups:

Sauté 3 TBS Soy Bacon Bits in 3 TBS Olive Oil until fragrant. Sprinkle on 1 TB Whole Wheat Flour; stir until oil and flour combine and bubble. In a measuring cup, combine $^1/_3$ cup Brown Rice Vinegar and enough water to make 1 cup. Add and stir til dissolved: 2 teasp. Honey, 1 teasp. Sesame Salt, 1 teasp. Dry Mustard.

—Beat 1 Egg in a bowl and gradually add vinegar mix. Pour over mixture in the hot skillet, and cook over low heat, stirring for several minutes until thickened.

ROASTED VEGETABLE SPREAD

This recipe works for: Liver and Organ Health, Digestive Health, Weight Control
Makes 1 $^1/_2$ cups: Preheat oven to 450°F.

Rub a 12 x 15" pan with $^1/_2$ tsp. Olive Oil. Place 2 large Red Onions diced, 2 small firm-ripe Tomatoes diced, and 4 Cloves Garlic minced in it. Bake in an oven until liquid has largely evaporated and vegetable edges are brown, about 45 minutes; turn vegetables with a wide spatula every 15 minutes. Let cool.

—Blender blend: roasted vegetables, 1 cup jarred Roasted Red Peppers drained and chopped, and 2 TBS minced Parsley; add Salt and Pepper to taste. Mound roasted vegetable spread in a small bowl and serve.

Nutrition: 68 calories; 6gm protein; 6gm carbohydrate; 3gm fiber; 3g total fat; 0mg choles.; 85mg calcium; 1mg iron; 15mg magnesium; 216mg potassium; 160mg sodium; Vit. A 169 IU; Vit. C 56mg; Vit. E 1 IU.

KIWI NO OIL DRESSING

This recipe works for: Liver and Organ Health, Detoxification, Weight Control
For 1 cup: Perfect for greens with feta cheese crumbles and toasted walnuts.

Blender blend: 2 Kiwis, 2 TBS Raspberry Vinegar, 2 teasp. Lime Juice, 1 teasp. Fructose, Sea Salt and Pepper to taste.

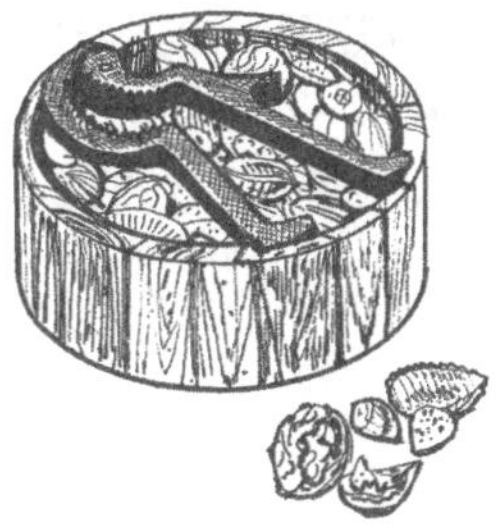

LOW FAT MINTY CUCUMBER RAITA

This recipe works for: Liver and Organ Health, Detoxification
Makes 8 servings:

Combine in a bowl: 2 cups Plain Low Fat Yogurt, 1 cup diced Cucumber, 2 TBS Fresh snipped Mint, 2 teasp. Lemon Juice, pinches ground Cumin and Lemon Pepper. Use as a topping for Beans and Rice, or Black Bean Chili.

Nutrition: 43 calories; 3gm protein; 5gm carbohydrate; trace fiber; 1g total fat; trace choles.; 117mg calcium; trace iron; 13mg magnesium; 138mg potassium; 44mg sodium; Vit. A 18 IU; Vit. C 3mg; Vit. E trace

VERY LOW FAT TOMATO BASIL SAUCE

This recipe works for: Prostate Cancer Control, Immune Breakdown Diseases
For 2 cups: Especially good for cold cucumber or yellow squash sticks.

Heat in a pan: 2 cups jarred Tomato Sauce with Mushrooms, 2 TBS snipped Fresh Basil Leaves, 1 Bay Leaf (Remove when ready to serve). Put into serving dish. Snip on Fresh Mint Leaves; then swirl a dollop of Low Fat Plain Yogurt on top.

LOW FAT DESERT DIP A good 'scoop' for toasted pita pieces.

This recipe works for: Sugar Imbalances, Liver and Organ Health, Men's Health
For 12 servings: Preheat oven to 400°.

Pierce and oven roast 2 LBS Eggplant until crinkly and soft; or parboil 2 LBS sliced Zucchini in vegetable broth until just tender. Scoop out eggplant meat into blender (no need to peel zucchini).

—Blender blend eggplant meat or zucchini until smooth. Add: 1/3 cup Lemon Juice, 4 TBS Sesame Tahini, 2 TBS snipped Fresh Parsley, 2 TBS chopped Green Onion, 1/2 teasp. Lemon-Pepper, 1/4 teasp. Cumin Powder.

Turn into a shallow serving dish and cover with finely diced Red and Yellow Tomatoes. Serve wth toasted Pita or Chapati Pieces, or Lavosh Cracker Bread.

Nutrition: 70 calories; 3gm protein; 10gm carbohydrate; 3g fiber; 3g total fat; 0 choles.; 17mg calcium; 1mg iron; 37mg magnesium; 257mg potassium; 26mg sodium; Vit. A 20 IU; Vit. C 8mg; Vit. E trace.

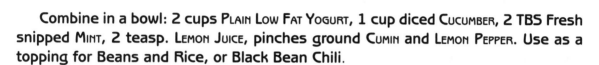

GOOD FAT GREEN and RED GUACAMOLE

This recipe works for: Hair, Skin and Nails, Arthritis, Sugar Imbalances
For about 2 cups:

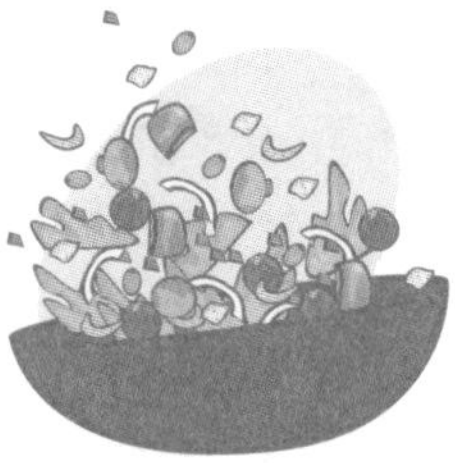

Mash together: 2 to 3 Avocados, 1 diced Tomato, 1/2 diced small Red Onion, 1 TB Lime Juice, 2 diced Green Chilies, 1/2 teasp. Lemon-Pepper.

YOGURT CHEESE SAUCE AND DIP

This recipe works for: Digestive Problems, Women's Health, Allergies - Asthma
For 3 cups: For veggies, baked potatoes, broiled fish, rice crackers, and chips.

Mix all in the blender until green; chill to intensify flavors: 1/2 cup Yogurt Cheese (See page 261 for how to make), 2 TBS Low Fat Soy Mayonnaise, 2 TBS snipped Fresh Cilantro or Parsley, 1 teasp. Lemon Zest, 1/2 teasp. Garlic-Lemon Seasoning.

Nutrition: 85 calories; 3gm protein; 16gm carbohydrate; trace fiber; 2g total fat; 3mg choles.; 119mg calcium; trace iron; 13mg magnesium; 173mg potassium; 73mg sodium; Vit. A 29 IU; Vit. C 7mg; Vit. E 1 IU.

Sweet and Low Desserts

Desserts can be fudgy, chewy, creamy, crusty, sweet and gooey - and still be low in fat and calories, and nutritious.

LIGHT ORANGE SOUFFLÉ with RASPBERRY SAUCE

This recipe works for: Digestive Problems, Women's Health, Allergies - Asthma
For 6 servings: Preheat oven to 375°.

Make the soufflé in the top of a double boiler over hot water. Blend 4 Egg Yolks and 1/2 cup Fructose until thick and creamy. Stir in 1/4 cup Unbleached Flour, 1 cup Plain Low Fat Yogurt, 1/2 cup Water, grated Zest from 1 Orange. Cook over low heat stirring, until mixture boils. Let cool, stirring gently every few minutes. Add 1/2 cup Orange Juice.

—Whip 6 Egg Whites to stiff peaks and fold into Orange Sauce with a pinch of Cream of Tartar. Turn into a lecithin-sprayed 2-qt. straight-sided soufflé dish. Bake for 30 minutes until light and puffy.

—While soufflé is baking, make the RASPBERRY SAUCE in a sauce pan: stir and heat 2 cups Raspberries, 3 TBS Sugar-Free Raspberry Jelly, 2 TBS Orange Juice until blended. Chill and pour over cold soufflé.

Nutrition: 211 calories; 9gm protein; 34gm carbohydrate; 2gm fiber; 4g total fat; 144mg choles.; 108mg calcium; 1mg iron; 24mg magnes.; 276mg potassium; 89mg sodium; Vit. A 82 IU; Vit. C 26mg; Vit. E 1 IU.

No-Guilt Cheesecakes are the essence of indulgence.

VERY LOW-FAT CHERRY CHEESECAKE Only one gram of fat.

This recipe works for: Arthritis, Women's Health, Digestive Health

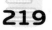

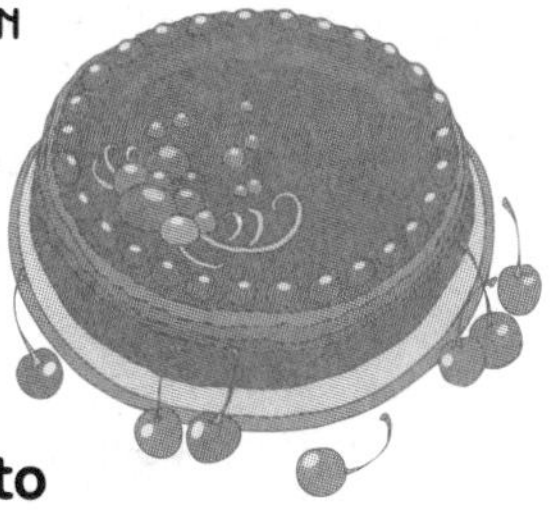

Make the filling in a double boiler: dissolve 2 TBS Plain Gelatin in $^1/_2$ cup Water. Add and stir until well blended: 2 cups Low Fat Lemon Yogurt, 4 TBS Cherry Juice from a package of thawed frozen Cherries, 4 cups Low Fat Cottage Cheese, 1 teasp. Almond Extract. Beat well until mixture is smooth. Then chill in the fridge.

—When mixture begins to thicken, add 8-oz. Kefir Cheese or Low Fat Cream Cheese, and 2 TBS Lemon Juice. Beat very well again to the consistency of thick whipped cream. Spoon into a spring form pan and chill until firm.

—Make the topping: stir 2 TBS more Cherry Juice from the thawed cherries with 2 TBS Arrowroot Powder or Kuzu Chunks until dissolved.

—Make the CHERRY GLAZE: Put the frozen Cherries from the package in a sauce pan on low heat with 1 cup Apple Juice. Gradually stir in arrowroot mixture until smooth, thickened and glossy. Remove from heat and cool.

—To serve, release the springform sides of the cheesecake pan. Leave the bottom on the cake, and put the cake on a plate. Spoon over sauce and cut.

Nutrition: 277 calories; 23gm protein; 30gm carbohydrate; 1gm fiber; 4gm total fat; 23mg choles.; 204mg calcium; trace iron; 23mg magnes.; 378mg potassium; 503mg sodium; Vit. A 90 IU; Vit. C 3mg; Vit. E trace.

LOW-FAT FUDGE

This recipe works for: Waste Management Problems, Sports Nutrition

Makes 16 pieces: Preheat oven to 350°F. Lightly oil an 8-inch square baking pan.

Have ready $^1/_2$ cup Pureed Prunes. Chop 1 $^1/_3$ cups Pitted Prunes in a blender. With motor running, add $^1/_3$ cup water and 3 TBS Orange Juice. Purée, stopping to scrape sides, until mixture resembles smooth paste, about 5 minutes.

—Place in heat-proof bowl: 4-oz. Unsweetened Low Fat Chocolate, cut into 1-inch pieces. Set bowl over low heat in small skillet containing $^1/_2$-inch simmering Water. Stir occasionally, just until chocolate is melted. Remove from heat; set aside.

—In a mixer bowl, combine: $^1/_2$ cup Pureed Prunes, 3 large Egg Whites, $^1/_2$ cup Honey, $^1/_4$ cup Fructose, 1 tsp. Sea Salt, 1 tsp. Vanilla. Beat to blend thoroughly. Add in $^1/_2$ cup Unbleached Flour. Spread batter in prepared pan; sprinkle with $^1/_3$ cup chopped Walnuts.

—Bake until center top of brownies springs back to the touch, about 30 minutes. Cool on a rack. Cut into 2-inch squares. Grate on fresh Orange Zest .

Nutrition: 162 calories; 3gm protein; 29gm carbohydrate; 3gm fiber; 5g total fat; 0mg choles.; 21mg calcium; 1mg iron; 39mg magnesium; 216mg potassium; 141mg sodium; Vit. A 39 IU; Vit. C 3mg; Vit. E 1 IU.

INSTANT CRANBERRY MOUSSE

This recipe works for: Bladder-Kidney Problems, Women's Health, Allergies - Asthma
For 4 people:

Briefly heat 1/2 cup MAPLE SYRUP. Blender blend 2 cups FROZEN UNSWEETENED CRANBERRIES with half the syrup. Add 2 TBS FRUCTOSE and rest of syrup; blend until smooth.

—Beat 2 EGG WHITES in a bowl with a pinch of CREAM OF TARTAR until stiff. Pour cold CRANBERRY purée over the whites and fold in. Mound into mousse cups and garnish with toasted slivered ALMONDS.

Nutrition: 161 calories; 2gm protein; 39gm carbohydrate; 2gm fiber; trace fat; 0mg choles.; 31mg calcium; trace iron; 10mg magnesium; 139mg potassium; 31mg sodium; Vit. A 2 IU, Vit. C 6mg; Vit. E 1mg.

EASY WALNUT STRAWBERRY COOKIES Delicious.

This recipe works for: Sugar Balance Problems, Kid's Health, Allergies and Asthma
Makes 15 to 18 cookies:

Blender blend WALNUTS to make 1/2 cup. Blender blend ROLLED OATS to make 1 cup. Pour each into a mixing bowl. Add 1 cup WHOLE WHEAT PASTRY FLOUR and a pinch SALT.

—In a separate bowl, mix: 2/3 cup BROWN RICE SYRUP, 2 TBS CANOLA OIL, 5-oz. SUGAR-FREE or HONEY SWEETENED STRAWBERRY JAM, 1/2 tsp. ALMOND EXTRACT, 1 tsp. VANILLA EXTRACT.

—Pour the liquid ingredients into the dry ingredients and mix until moistened. Let sit for 30 minutes. Then on an oiled cookie sheet, drop 1 TB of batter per cookie and bake in a 350°F oven for 20 minutes.

HIGH OCTANE GINGER COOKIES

This recipe works for: Heart and Circulatory Problems, Men's and Women's Health
Makes 4 dozen cookies: Preheat oven to 350°F.

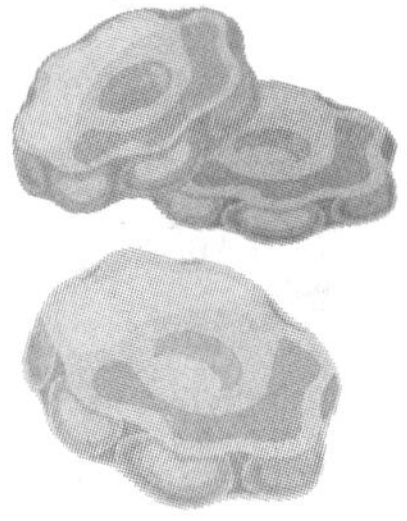

Whirl 3/4 cup chopped CRYSTALLIZED GINGER and 2 TBS FRUCTOSE in a blender until finely ground. Pour into a mixing bowl. Add 1 EGG, 3 TBS BUTTER, 3 TBS CANOLA OIL, 1/4 cup MOLASSES, 3 TBS FRUCTOSE; beat til fluffy. Blend in 2 cups UNBLEACHED FLOUR, 2 teasp. BAKING SODA, 3/4 tsp. ground CINNAMON and 1/2 tsp. ground NUTMEG. Cover dough and chill about 1 hour. Shape dough into 1-inch balls. Sprinkle with a mix of 3 TBS LEMON ZEST and 2 TBS FRUCTOSE. Place balls 2 to 3 inches apart on nonstick or oiled baking sheets.

—Bake in a 350°F oven until slightly dark brown, 11 to 12 minutes total (if using 1 oven, switch pan positions after about 6 minutes). Transfer cookies to racks to cool. Serve, or store airtight up to 1 week; freeze to store longer.

Nutrition: 55 calories; 1gm protein; 9gm carbohydrate; trace fiber; 2g total fat; 6mg choles.; 18mg calcium; 1mg iron; 6mg magnesium; 57mg potassium; 55mg sodium; Vit. A 9 IU; Vit. C trace; Vit. E trace; trace zinc.

FROZEN YOGURT BARS

This recipe works for: Digestive Problems, Women's Health, Weight Control
For 9 pieces:

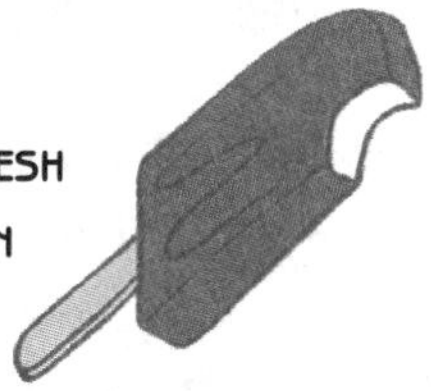

Freeze 2 cups Fruit Yogurt (any flavor). Freeze 1 cup chopped Fresh Fruits. Put the frozen ingredients in a blender and add 1 cup Frozen Rice Dream. Blend until smooth. Pour into an 8" square pan. Add 1 cup Grapenuts; gently mix them in.

—Top with one more cup Grapenuts; press into top. FREEZE SOLID. Cut in bars. Wrap in foil to keep, and freeze until just before you want to eat them.

Nutrition: 161 calories; 6gm protein; 34gm carbohydrate; 3gm fiber; 1g total fat; trace choles.; 130mg calcium; 7mg iron; 37mg magnes.; 206mg potass.; 142mg sodium; Vit. A 197 IU; Vit. C 11mg; Vit. E 1 IU.

LUSCIOUS PEACH CHEESECAKE Delicious with a crust or no crust.

This recipe works for: Hair and Skin, Women's Health, Digestive Health

To make a perfect cookie crust: just crumble your favorite cookies (I like macaroons), over the bottom of a cheesecake pan and toast for 10 minutes.

Make the cake: mix together 2$^1/_2$ cups thinly sliced Fresh Peaches, $^1/_2$ cup shredded Coconut, $^1/_4$ cup Fructose, 2 TBS Unbleached Flour, $^1/_2$ teasp. Cinnamon, $^1/_2$ teasp. Nutmeg, and $^1/_4$ teasp. each Ginger Powder, Lemon Peel Powder, Cardamom Powder and Ground Cloves. Turn into a lecithin-sprayed spring form pan.

—Make the topping; blender blend very smooth: 2 Eggs, 16-oz. Low Fat Cream Cheese or Soy Cream Cheese, or 8-oz. Kefir Cheese and 8-oz. Peach Yogurt. Add and blend until very smooth: $^3/_4$ cup Orange Honey, $^1/_2$ teasp. Cinnamon, 2 teasp. Vanilla. Pour over peach mixture. Do not stir, so that the integrity of the separate layers is maintained. Bake at 350°F 50 to 60 minutes until just set, and slightly wobbly in the center. Remove, cool and chill.

Nutrition: 220 calories; 6gm protein; 29gm carbohydrate; 1gm fiber; 6g total fat; 56mg choles.; 57mg calcium; 1mg iron; 11mg magnesium; 186mg potassium; 14mg sodium; Vit. A 119 IU; Vit. C 3mg; Vit. E 1 IU.

Try this delicious, low fat VANILLA CUSTARD SAUCE for a perfect PEACH CHEESECAKE, or spoon it over fresh fruit. *For 4 to 6 servings:*

Whirl 2 Eggs and 1 teasp. Vanilla in the blender to frothy.

—Heat 1 cup Vanilla Almond Milk or Vanilla Kefir and 3 TBS Fructose in a saucepan to just below a boil. Remove from heat and add to the eggs in the blender in a thin stream.... just to warm, but not cook them. Mixture should coat the back of a spoon. If it doesn't, return briefly to saucepan and simmer a little longer until thickened.

Nutrition: 74 calories; 4gm protein; 9gm carbohydrate; 0 fiber; 2g total fat; 80mg choles.; 95mg calcium; 1mg iron; 4mg magnesium; 47mg potassium; 32mg sodium; Vit. A 38 IU; Vit. C 0mg; Vit. E 1 IU.

GINGER-SPICED PEACHES and CHERRIES

This recipe works for: Digestive Problems, Women's Health, Hair and Skin
Makes 8 servings:

Slice 4 ripe, peeled Fresh Peaches in 1-inch sections. Pit 3 cups Fresh Cherries.

—In a 4 quart saucepan, heat 1 cup Orange Juice, $^{1}/_{2}$ cup Sparkling Water, 2 TBS Fructose, 2 TBS minced Crystallized Ginger and 2 TBS Lemon Juice.

—Add peaches and cherries, reduce heat and simmer, uncovered, 20 to 40 minutes, until tender when pierced with a fork. Transfer to a serving bowl, cover and chill hour before serving. Spoon on some of the poaching liquid; then crumble some Ginger Snaps or Macaroons on top.

Nutrition: 121 calories; 2gm protein; 28gm carbohydrate; 2gm fiber; 1g total fat; 0mg choles.; 21mg calcium; 1mg iron; 17mg magnesium; 306mg potassium; 47mg sodium; Vit. A 42 IU; Vit. C 24mg; Vit. E 1 IU.

LOW FAT HIGH FIBER COOKIES An easy 20 minutes, start to finish.

This recipe works for: Heart Health, Men's Health, Waste Management
For 24 cookies: Preheat oven to 350°.

Mix: 4 TBS Canola Oil, $^{1}/_{2}$ cup Honey, $^{1}/_{2}$ cup Apple Juice, 2 TBS Molasses, 1 Egg.

—Mix: 1 cup Rye Flour, $^{1}/_{2}$ cup Oat Flour, $^{1}/_{2}$ cup Oat Bran, 2 teasp. Cinnamon, 2 TBS minced Crystallized Ginger, 1 teasp. Sea Salt, 1 teasp. no-aluminum Baking Powder.

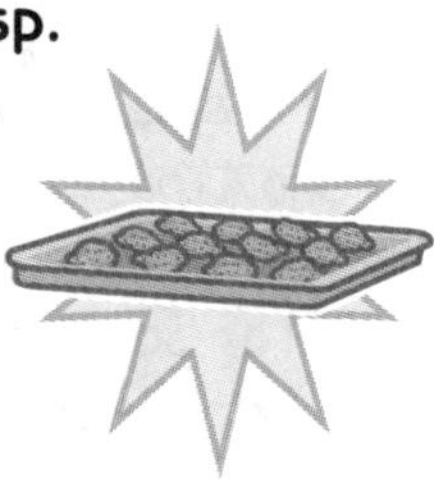

—Mix wet and dry ingredients together just to moisten. Drop by spoonfuls onto lecithin-sprayed sheets. Bake for 10 minutes until edges start to brown.

Nutrition: 88 calories; 1gm protein; 16gm carbohydrate; 1gm fiber; 3gm total fat; 8mg choles.; 35mg calcium; 1mg iron; 16mg magnesium; 92mg potassium; 108mg sodium; Vit. A 40 IU; Vit. C 2mg; Vit. E 1 IU.

BLUEBERRY CRUNCH

This recipe works for: Circulation Health, Kid's - Men's Health, Hair and Skin
Makes 4 servings: Preheat oven to 350°F.

In medium saucepan, combine 3 cups Fresh Blueberries or Unsweetened Frozen Blueberries with reserved juice, and $^{1}/_{2}$ cup Apple Juice Concentrate or Maple Syrup.

—In a small dish mix 1 TB Arrowroot Powder and $^{1}/_{4}$ tsp. Cinnamon with 2 TBS fruit liquid. Heat blueberries and juice until simmering; remove from heat and stir in arrowroot mixture. Stir over low heat until slightly thickened, about 5 minutes. Divide mixture among 4 individual ovenproof baking cups or custard cups.

—Crush $1^{1}/_{2}$ cups Macaroons and divide over cups. Bake until topping is lightly browned, about 15 minutes.

NO-FAT DESSERT DIP for FRUIT

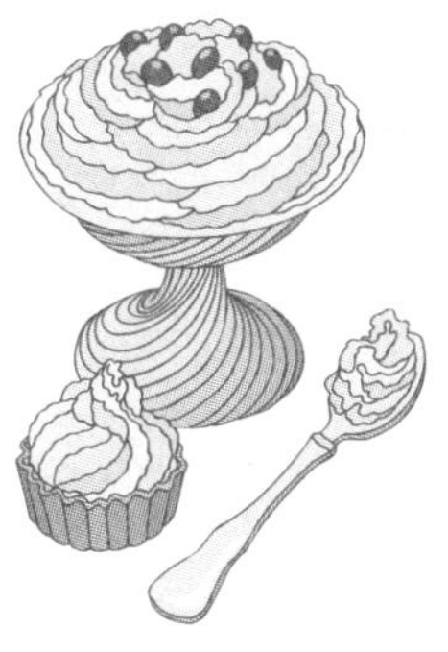

This recipe works for: Heart Health, Women's Health, Weight Loss
Makes 8 servings:

In a bowl, mix $^1/_2$ cup NON-FAT VANILLA YOGURT, $^1/_2$ cup NON-FAT CREAM CHEESE, 1 TB FRUCTOSE, and $^1/_4$ teasp. ground CINNAMON.

CHEESE STUFFED PEARS

This recipe works for: Stress Reactions, Illness Recovery, Overcoming Addictions
Makes 8 servings:

Slice 4 PEARS lengthwise. Core to form a pocket; brush surface with LEMON JUICE.
—Mix the filling: 1 cup LOW FAT COTTAGE CHEESE, $^1/_2$ cup LOW FAT YOGURT CHEESE, 2 TBS minced FRESH MINT, 2 TBS HONEY, $^1/_2$ cup diced WALNUTS. Mound filling on top of pears and smooth with a knife. Decorate with slivers of DRIED APRICOTS.

Nutrition: 179 calories; 7gm protein; 26gm carbohydrate; 3gm fiber; 5g total fat; 5mg choles.; 56mg calcium; 1mg iron; 27mg magnesium; 276mg potassium; 120mg sodium; Vit. A 53 IU; Vit. C 5mg; Vit. E 1 IU.

FRESH FRUIT SUNDAE

This recipe works for: Heart Health, Kid's - Men's Health, Sugar Imbalances
Makes 4 servings

Peel and section 2 ORANGES into a bowl. Add $^1/_2$ pint FRESH BERRIES, and $^1/_2$ pint HONEY and ORANGE SORBET. Set aside until ready to serve. Just before serving, evenly divide scoops of LOW-FAT or NON-FAT VANILLA FROZEN YOGURT among four serving bowls. Top with fruit mixture, sprinkle with 4 TBS TOASTED SLICED ALMONDS. Serve Immediately.

EASY LOW FAT CHEESECAKE with FRESH BERRIES

This recipe works for: Heart Health, Kid's - Men's Health, Sugar Imbalances
For 10 to 12 pieces: Preheat oven to 350°.

Make the crust: mix $1^1/_2$ cups GRAHAM CRACKER CRUMBS, 2 TBS BUTTER, 2 TBS CANOLA OIL. Press into bottom and sides of a springform pan. Bake 7 minutes. Remove and cool. Reduce oven heat to 300°.
—Blender blend filling until very smooth: 1 cup LOW FAT COTTAGE CHEESE, 1 EGG, 2 cups LOW FAT VANILLA YOGURT, 2 EGG WHITES, $^1/_3$ cup FRUCTOSE, 1 teasp. VANILLA. Pour into crust; bake until top feels dry when touched, and center jiggles when shaken slightly, about 55 minutes. Let cool; then chill for 8 hours.
—Just before serving, top with 2 cups WHOLE FRESH BERRIES.

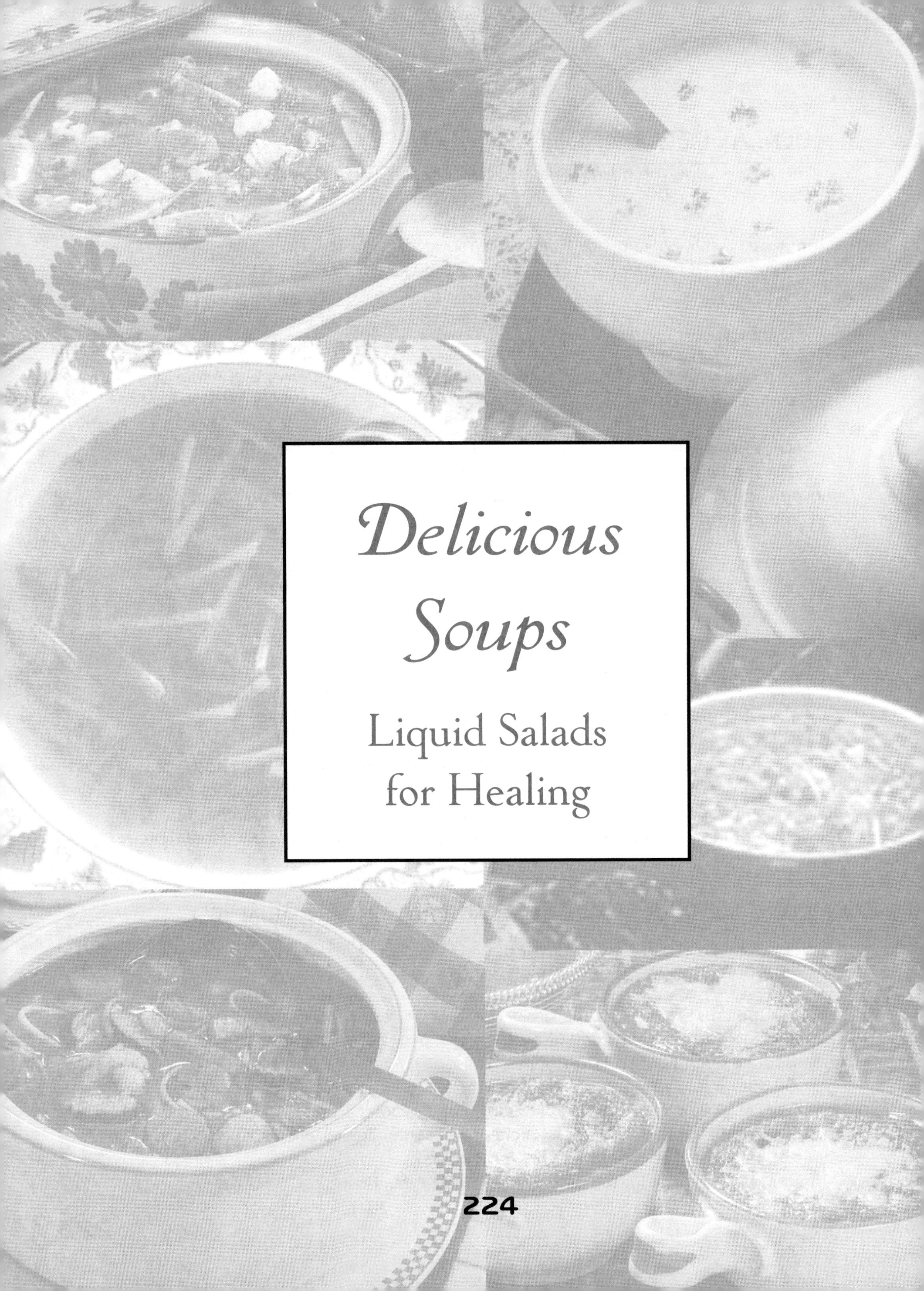

Delicious Soups

Liquid Salads for Healing

Soups - Liquid Salads

Soups are super foods for a healing diet, delicious therapy foods that work like liquid salads. Soups are vitamin-filled, easy-to-take nutrition that can allay hunger during a cleansing diet. They may be packed with high protein for faster healing, fiber and complex carbohydrates for rebuilding; yet they don't have the density of solid food that can slow things down.

I think of an herb-scented soup as a robust, healing tea. A hot broth is the perfect conductor for healing herbs. In fact, soups are the best medium for taking in the healing benefits of pungent herbs like garlic, (every healing tradition has a garlic soup), or sea vegetables for iodine therapy, or hot chilies or cayenne peppers.

Use soups hot or cold, as low-fat, low calorie meals or snacks for losing weight without feeling hungry, or toning muscle, and for keeping your circulation free of clogging fats.

A fragrant, simmered foundation is essential to delicious homemade soup taste. Today it's easy to buy good preservative-free soup mixes in health food stores and gourmet groceries. But to control the *nutrition* of a healing diet, it is best to make your soups from scratch with your own vegetables and seasonings, (see page 494 for stock recipes). Canned or commercially prepared stocks, broths and bouillons may be too high in salt or fat as well.

Make soups in a large open pot if possible. It gives the stock and ingredients room to "work," and allows the aroma to develop.

Soup Recipe Sections

Healing Broths

Broths are the world's most ancient way to heal. The basis of a cleansing, yet nourishing diet, purifying broths are used by every culture and every age to normalize human body functions and balance.

HEALING SHIITAKE BROTH

This recipe works for: Detoxification, Circulation, Cancer Control, Recovery
Makes 4 servings:

Have ready 4-oz. Fresh Shiitake Mushrooms stemmed and sliced, and 4-oz. thin wheat noodles (Somen), cooked and cooled.

—In a soup pot heat 1 teasp. Canola Oil. Add 1 piece Ginger Root, peeled and slivered, $^1/_4$ tsp. ground Tumeric and $^1/_2$ tsp. Chinese Five Spice Powder. Cook and stir until fragrant, 3 minutes. Add 6 cups Organic Low Fat Chicken Broth, 1 TB Tamari, 1 small Carrot and 1 small Daikon Radish cut in matchsticks, and the mushrooms. Simmer until mushrooms are very tender, about 15 minutes.

—Add noodles and $^1/_4$ cup Cilantro Leaves, and warm through, 2 minutes more. Season with 1 teasp. Toasted Sesame Oil, and Garlic-Lemon Seasoning to taste. Serve immediately in warmed soup bowls.

Nutrition: 141 calories; 6gm protein; 18gm carbohydrate; 3gm fiber; 4g total fat; 0mg choles.; 28mg calcium; 1mg iron; 19mg magnes.; 251mg potassium; 968mg sodium; Vit. A 509 IU; Vit. C 15mg; Vit. E 1 IU.

ORIENTAL DOUBLE PEA and MUSHROOM BROTH

This recipe works for: Detoxification, Recovery from Illness, Cancer Control
For 8 servings:

Soak 6 to 8 dry Shiitake Mushrooms until soft. Sliver, discard woody stems, and reserve soaking water. Sort and rinse 1 cup dry Split Peas.

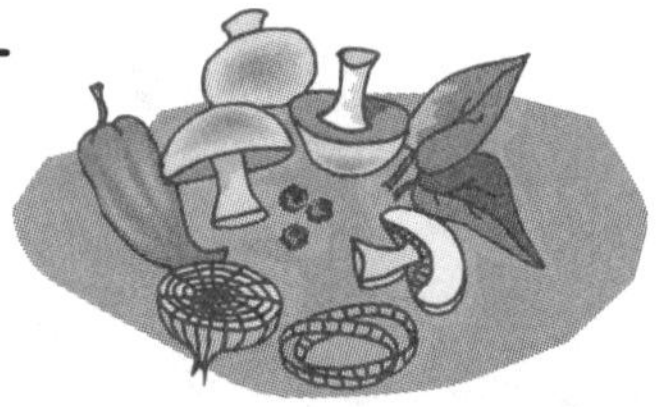

—Sauté in a large soup pot in 1 TB Canola Oil until aromatic, about 5 minutes: 1 small Onion chopped, 2 cups thin sliced Celery, 1 Carrot thin sliced, 2 TBS fresh minced Ginger.

—Add 6 cups Miso Soup or Low Fat Chicken Broth, the slivered mushrooms, the reserved soaking water and the split peas. Bring to a boil, partially cover and simmer until peas are tender - about $1^1/_2$ hours.

Remove from heat, remove cover and add a 10-oz. package Frozen Peas. Let peas heat until color changes to bright green. Season with 1 teasp. Hot Pepper Sauce and 1 teasp. Toasted Sesame Oil. Serve immediately.

Nutrition: 194 calories; 11gm protein; 31gm carbohydrate; 8gm fiber; 4g total fat; 0mg choles.; 56mg calcium; 2mg iron; 59mg magnesium; 531mg potassium; 709mg sodium; Vit. A 35 IU; Vit. C 12mg; Vit. E 3 IU.

DOUBLE MUSHROOM BROTH immune booster - blood cleanser

This recipe works for: Immune Breakdown Diseases, Recovery, Cancer Control
For 6 servings:

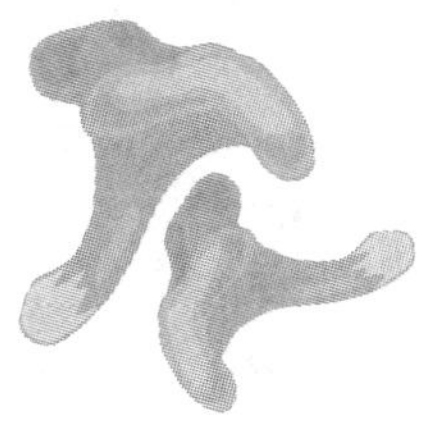

Heat 6 cups RICH BROWN BROTH (page 494) in a large soup pot. Soak 2 to 3 large dry SHIITAKE MUSHROOMS in water to cover until soft. Sliver, discard woody stems, and add soaking water to the soup pot. Slice 8-oz. BROWN CREMINI MUSHROOMS and 3 GREEN ONIONS. Add to soup pot and simmer for 45 minutes.

—Add 2 TBS LEMON JUICE, 2 TBS WHITE WINE, 1 teasp. snipped dry WAKAME SEA GREENS, 1 teasp. TAMARI, 1 teasp. HERB SEASONING, $^1/_2$ teasp. WHITE PEPPER.

Nutrition: 35 calories; 2gm protein; 7gm carbohydrate; 2gm fiber; trace fat; 0mg choles.; 23mg calcium; 1mg iron; 17mg magnesium; 243mg potassium; 256mg sodium; Vit. A 4 IU; Vit. C 7mg; Vit. E trace.

AYURVEDIC DETOX BROTH

This recipe works for: Respiratory Detoxification, Liver - Organ Health, Circulation
Makes 6 cups:

In a large pot, bring to a boil 6 cups ORGANIC LOW FAT CHICKEN BROTH to a simmer. Add $^1/_2$ cup thinly sliced GREEN ONIONS, 6 quarter size slices FRESH GINGER, 2 dried HOT RED CHILIES, 1 strip dry WAKAME SEA VEGETABLE, and 2 CLOVES GARLIC, peeled but left whole. Reduce heat, cover, and simmer 15 minutes. With a slotted spoon, lift out and discard ginger, wakame and chilies. Serve hot in small cups.

Nutrition: 57 calories; 3gm protein; 5gm carbohydrate; 2gm fiber; 2g total fat; 0mg choles.; 21mg calcium; 1mg iron; 5mg magnesium; 37mg potassium; 502mg sodium; Vit. A 4 IU; Vit. C 2mg; Vit. E trace.

CHINESE IMMUNE PROTECTION SOUP

This recipe works for: Immune Health, Immune Breakdown, Cancer Control
Drink 1 cup of the broth in the morning, afternoon, and evening.
Makes 6 cups:

Simmer 1-oz. dried REISHI or MAITAKE MUSHROOM, $1^1/_2$-oz. dried SHIITAKE MUSHROOMS (about 6), and 1-oz. ASTRAGALUS BARK in 6 quarts WATER for 30 minutes.

—Add $^1/_4$ cup ORGANIC PEARLED BARLEY, half a BEET slivered, 1 small CARROT sliced, 1 RIB CELERY diced. Simmer for another 30 minutes, adding $^1/_4$ cup crumbled dry NORI and WAKAME SEA VEGETABLES. Discard mushrooms and astragalus before serving.

Nutrition: 54 calories; 2gm protein; 13gm carbohydrate; 3gm fiber; trace fat; 0mg choles.; 27mg calcium; 1mg iron; 22mg magnesium; 164mg potassium; 56mg sodium; Vit. A 172 IU; Vit. C 2mg; Vit. E trace.

GREENS and HERBS SOUP

This recipe works for: Arthritis, Bone Building, Cancer Protection, Respiratory Health
For 6 people:

In a large soup pot, sauté 2 minced Cloves Garlic and 1 chopped Onion in 3 TBS Olive Oil until translucent. Add 1 diced Stalk Celery and sauté for 5 minutes.

—Add 1 cup V-8 VEGETABLE STOCK (pg. 495) and heat to a simmer. Add 1 Head Romaine Lettuce sliced, and 1 16-oz. Package Frozen Peas; braise for 2 minutes only. Remove from heat. Let cool slightly and pureé in the blender until smooth.

—Return to soup pot. Add 5 more cups Vegetable Stock, $^1/_2$ teasp. Lemon Pepper, $^1/_2$ teasp. dry Basil (or 1 TB snipped Fresh Basil), $^1/_4$ teasp. dry Thyme, $^1/_4$ teasp. dry Sage, and $^1/_4$ teasp. Savory. Top with dry snipped Sea Greens (any kind) to serve.

Nutrition: 125 calories; 5gm protein; 16gm carbohydrate; 5gm fiber; 5g total fat; 0mg choles.; 49mg calcium; 2mg iron; 29mg magnesium; 269mg potass.; 210mg sodium; Vit. A 124 IU; Vit. C 22mg; Vit. E 2 IU.

TRADITIONAL CHINESE FLUSHING GREEN SOUP

This recipe works for: Lymph Detoxification, Liver - Organ Health, Immune Health
For 6 servings:

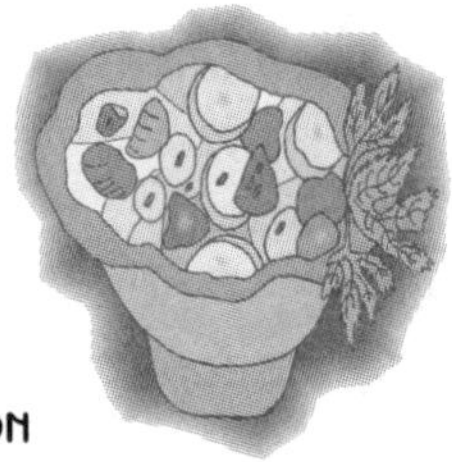

Sauté in 1 TB. Olive Oil for 5 minutes: 2 minced Cloves Garlic, 2 TBS minced Shallots, $^1/_2$ cup minced Scallions, $^1/_4$ cup minced white parts Leek. Add and toss just to wilt 1 minute, 1 cup finely sliced Spinach Leaves, $^1/_4$ cup Watercress Leaves, $^1/_4$ cup Cilantro Leaves, 1 minced Rib Celery with Leaves.

—Bring 4 cups Miso Soup to a boil. Add vegetables, 1 TB Lemon Juice, 1 teasp. Sesame Salt or Herb Seasoning Salt, and $^1/_4$ teasp. Chili Pepper.

—Heat just through, and garnish with slivers Daikon White Radish.

TRADITIONAL HEALING CHICKEN SOUP

This recipe works for: Respiratory Healing, Liver Health, Childhood Diseases
For 6 to 8 servings:

Rinse about 4 LBS Organic Chicken Pieces and put in a large soup pot with 5 Carrots, quartered, 3 Parsnips, quartered, 4 Leeks, quartered, 4 Celery Ribs in 2" lengths, 2 Whole Bay Leaves, 1 teasp. Sea Salt, $^3/_4$ teasp. Pepper, 2-Qts. Organic Chicken Stock, and 4 cups Water. Bring to a boil slowly. Reduce heat and simmer, uncovered, skimming off fat and foam until chicken is tender - about 1 hour.

—Strain; transfer chicken and veggies with a slotted spoon to a platter. Cover.

—Return broth to soup pot and boil until liquid is reduced to 6 cups, about 30 minutes. Season again. Remove bones from chicken, tear into bite size pieces; divide chicken and vegetables between soup bowls. Pour broth over and serve.

DETOX MORNING MELON SOUP loaded with EFA's

This recipe works for: Digestive Health, Hair and Skin, Bladder-Kidney Health
Makes 4 servings:

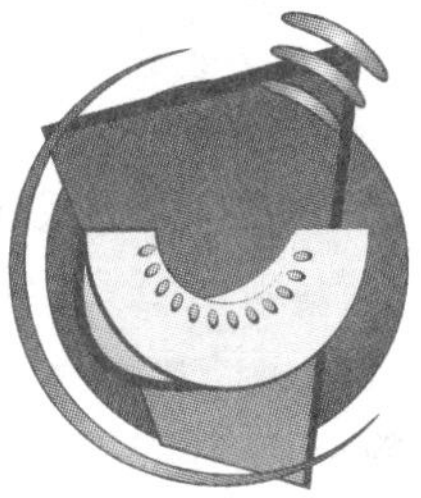

Quarter 1 ripe Cantaloupe, discard seeds, cut fruit from rind. Dice fruit into a food processor. Add 1 cup Orange Juice, 2 tsp. Fresh Lemon Juice and 1 cup Low-Fat Vanilla Yogurt; process until smooth. Top with 1 teasp. snipped Fresh Mint per serving.

OVERNIGHT REGULARITY SOUP

This recipe works for: Waste Management, Liver - Organ Health, Kid's Health
Makes 5 cups: Stores in the fridge easily for a week's worth of soup.

Bring 1 cup Raisins, 1 cup Prunes, and 8 cups Water to a boil and add $^1/_3$ cup Tapioca. Cook over low flame for 2 hours. Then add Juice of 1 Lemon, Honey to taste, and $^1/_4$ cup Apple Juice.

MEDITERRANEAN LEMON HEALING SOUP

This recipe works for: Stress Reactions, Addiction Recovery, Sugar Imbalances
For 4 servings:

Cut off green tops from 2 large Leeks; slice white parts in thin matchsticks. Slice half a head Romaine Lettuce. Braise lettuce and leeks in 2 TBS Olive Oil and 1 cup Miso Soup for 10 minutes. Add a 10-oz. Package Frozen Pea Pods, and steam 2 minutes until color is bright green. Remove from heat. Add 1 teasp. Lemon-Pepper, 4 Fresh Mint Leaves and 2 teasp. Lemon Juice. Add 2 scoops Plain Low Fat Yogurt and blend smooth.

HEALING GAZPACHO

This recipe works for: Liver-Organ Detox, Bladder-Kidney Health, Men's Health
Makes 8 servings:

Blender blend in batches: 3-lbs coarsely chopped Vine-ripened Tomatoes, 1 large Bell Pepper, 1 European Cucumber, 1 small Onion and 1 Clove Garlic. Transfer to large bowl with a pouring spout and stir in 1 cup Tomato Juice, $^1/_4$ cup Balsamic Vinegar and 2 TBS Olive Oil. Pour through a strainer set over a bowl; discard solids. Cover and chill several hours. Divide among small chilled bowls. Sprinkle with plenty of Lemon-Garlic Seasoning. and snip on Fresh Cilantro Leaves.

Nutrition: 96 calories; 3gm protein; 15gm carbohydrate; 3gm fiber; 4gm total fat; 0mg choles.; 27mg calcium; 1mg iron; 32mg magnes.; 579mg potassium; 22mg sodium; Vit. A 141 IU; Vit. C 51mg; Vit. E 3 IU.

WATERCRESS SOUP

This recipe works for: Bone Building, Liver - Organ Health, Illness Recovery
Makes 4 servings:

Cook 2 Potatoes, peeled and chopped in boiling water to cover until softened, about 10 to 15 minutes. Drain; season with Sea Salt and Pepper and set aside.

—Heat 2 TBS Canola Oil in a saucepan; sizzle 3 minced Shallots and 1/2 teasp. Lemon-Pepper until fragrant, 2 minutes. Remove from heat and add 1 large bunch Watercress, and 2 TBS Fresh Cilantro Leaves minced. Stir to blend flavors 2 minutes

—Place potatotes, watercress mixture, 2 cups Vegetable Broth, 2 TBS Lemon Juice, salt and pepper in a food processor or blender; blend til smooth. Chill. Divide between 4 soup bowls; top with a dollop of Plain Low-Fat Yogurt and grated Lemon Zest.

Low Fat, Low Calorie Soups

These soups are a good way to keep your middle little.

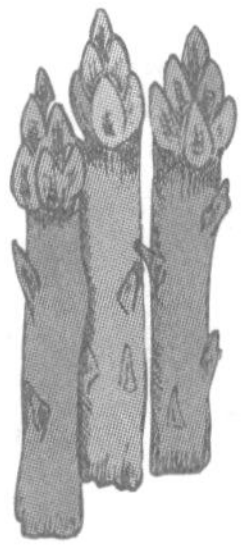

ASPARAGUS SOUP

This recipe works for: Arthritis, Liver - Organ Health, Weight Loss
Makes 4 servings:

In a pan, sizzle 1 TB Olive Oil, 1 finely chopped Onion, and 1 minced Clove Garlic for 5 minutes. Add 2 cups Water, 1 LB. Fresh Asparagus cut in 1" pieces, 1 stalk Lemon Grass, 1 tsp. Chervil, and 1 handful Fresh Parsley, stems trimmed off. Simmer 5 minutes ONLY. Remove lemon grass stalk and pour into blender or food processor and blend smooth. Add 1/4 cup White Wine. Season with Lemon-Pepper and serve hot.

FRESH TOMATO BASIL SOUP

This recipe works for: Arthritis, Men's Health, Weight Loss, Hair and Skin
Makes 6 servings:

Sauté in 2 TBS Olive Oil, 1 finely chopped Onion, and 1 minced Clove Garlic for 5 minutes. Add 1 diced Zucchini and 1 diced Bell Pepper. Sauté for 3 minutes.

—Add 4 cups Organic Vegetable Stock, and bring to a boil. Reduce heat; add 3/4 cup White Wine and 3 Fresh Tomatoes, diced. Simmer for 20 minutes. Add 4 minced Scallions, 1/2 cup snipped Fresh Basil and 1/2 teasp. White Pepper and heat for 5 minutes.

—Sprinkle with a little Parmesan-Reggiano Cheese if desired.

Nutrition: 104 calories; 2gm protein; 10gm carbohydrate; 3gm fiber; 4g total fat; 0mg choles.; 41mg calcium; 1mg iron; 28mg magnesium; 376mg potassium; 106mg sodium; Vit. A 86 IU; Vit. C 34mg; Vit. E 2 IU.

SWEET PEA and FRESH MINT SOUP

This recipe works for: Illness Recovery, Men's Health, Hair, Skin and Nails
For 8 servings:

Sizzle 2 cups diced Yellow Onions in 3 TBS Olive Oil until fragrant. Add 3 cups Organic Vegetable Broth; bring to a boil, reduce heat; simmer 10 minutes. Remove from heat. Finely chop 1 small bag Baby Spinach Leaves. Add half to the soup. Finely chop 2 cups Fresh Mint Leaves. Add half to the soup.

—Blender blend soup with 1 cup Plain Low Fat Yogurt until smooth. Return to soup pot. Add a 10-oz. package Frozen Peas. Heat soup until peas turn a bright green. Add rest of Spinach and Mint. Season with Herbal Seasoning and White Pepper.

Nutrition: 99 calories; 5gm protein; 12gm carbohydrate; 3gm fiber; 4g total fat; trace choles.; 98mg calcium; 2mg iron; 35mg magnes.; 319mg potassium; 136mg sodium; Vit. A 193 IU; Vit. C 24mg; Vit. E 2 IU.

WHITE GAZPACHO

This recipe works for: Arthritis, Heart Health, Bladder-Kidney Health, Hair and Skin
For 6 servings:

Peel and dice 1 long European Cucumber. Blender blend with 1/4 teasp. Garlic-Lemon Seasoning, 2 cups Plain Low-Fat Yogurt, 1/2 cup Onion Broth and 2 TBS Lemon Juice.

—Pour into a large soup pot with: 1 1/2 more cups Onion Broth, 1/2 cup White Wine, and 1/2 cup Water. Stir and heat gently til smooth. Remove from heat.

—Top with 2 TBS snipped Fresh Cilantro Leaves, 2 TBS snipped Green Onions, 1 TB snipped Fresh Basil. Chill in the fridge for 1 to 2 hours and serve.

Nutrition: 74 calories; 5gm protein; 9gm carbohydrate; 1gm fiber; 1g total fat; 4mg choles.; 158mg calcium; trace iron; 26mg magnesium; 332mg potassium; 81mg sodium; Vit. A 18 IU, Vit. C 8mg; Vit. E 1trace.

ORIENT EXPRESS HOT and SOUR SOUP

This recipe works for: Heart Health, Digestive Problems, Immune Health
Makes 4 servings:

Have ready 1/2 lb. Firm Tofu, frozen and thawed with excess water pressed out.

—Heat 1 TB Sesame Oil in a wok and sizzle 2 minced Shallots, 1/2 cup diced Scallions, 2 Carrots cut in match sticks and 1/2 cup sliced Fresh Shiitake Mushrooms for 5 minutes. Crumble tofu and stir into vegetable mixture.

—Mix in a bowl: 3 TBS Miso Paste, 4 cups Water, 1/4 cup Brown Rice Vinegar, 1 TB Honey, 1/2 tsp. Cracked Pepper, 2 TBS finely grated Ginger. Stir mixture into vegetables. Let simmer for 5 minutes.

Divide among soup bowls. Snip on 1 TB dried Arame or Sea Palm. Sprinkle on Sesame Seeds and serve hot with brown rice.

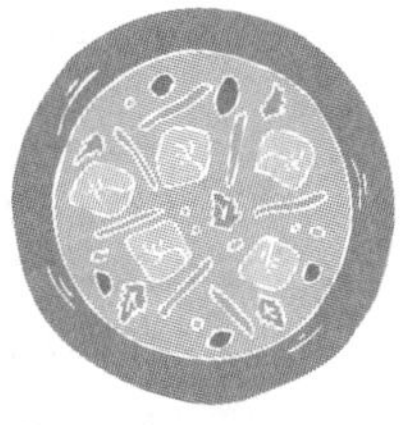

VERY LOW CALORIE VEGETABLE SOUP

This recipe works for: Heart Health, Bone Building, Allergies and Asthma
Makes 10 servings:

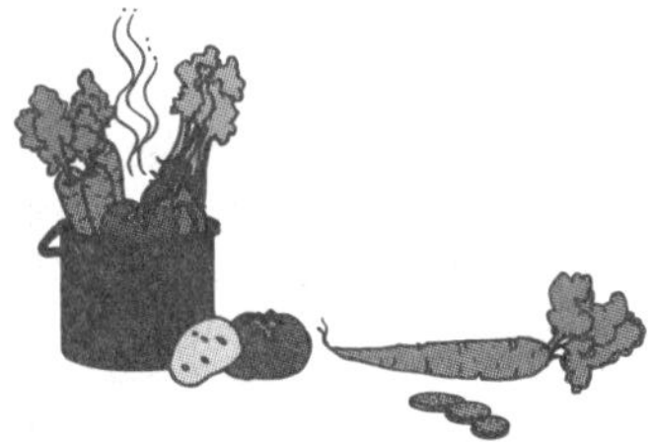

Heat 2 TBS Olive Oil in a pot. Add 4 Garlic Cloves minced, and 2 Yellow Onions diced; cook stirring, 3 to 4 minutes. Add 2 quarts Organic Vegetable Broth, 3 Ribs Celery diced, 2 Carrots diced, 4 peeled, diced Ripe Tomatoes, 1 cup chopped Broccoli, 1 cup French Cut Green Beans, $^1/_4$ cup snipped Fresh Basil, $^1/_4$ cup snipped Fresh Parsley, 1 TB snipped Fresh Summer Savory, 1 tsp. dry Herbs de Provence, and $^1/_4$ cup snipped Fresh Green Onions. Simmer, covered, for about 10 minutes.

—Add 4-oz. thin Egg Noodles (Capellini); cook, stirring occasionally until al dente, about 7 minutes. Add 1 cup sliced Zucchini or Yellow Crookneck Squash and cook about 2 minutes. Season with Lemon-Pepper to taste. Serve in heavy pottery bowls.

NO-FAT TOMATO GAZPACHO

This recipe works for: Heart Health, Detoxification, Allergies, Weight Loss
Makes 6 servings:

Heat $^1/_4$ cup Organic Vegetable Broth. Sizzle 4 chopped Cloves Garlic and $^1/_2$ cup chopped Red Onion for 7 minutes until fragrant. Scrape into a bowl and toss with: 2 cups chopped Tomatoes, 1 cup chopped Red or Yellow Bell Pepper, 1 cup peeled, chopped Cucumber, 2 chopped Scallions, $^1/_3$ cup Fresh Cilantro Leaves, $^1/_4$ cup Fresh Basil Leaves, 1 TB Honey, $^1/_4$ cup Fresh Lime Juice, 2 TBS Balsamic Vinegar, 1 tsp. snipped Fresh Tarragon or $^1/_4$ tsp. dried and 1 tsp. snipped Fresh Basil or $^1/_4$ tsp. dried. Add $^1/_2$ cup White Wine, 2 cups Tomato Juice or Water. Pour half into a food processor bowl or blender and blend to smooth.

—Pour into a large serving bowl. Blend remaining half, leaving some texture. Pour into serving bowl. Add Herbal Seasoning Salt and White Pepper to taste. Cover with plastic wrap and chill 15 minutes.

Nutrition: 73 calories; 2gm protein; 14gm carbohydrate; 2gm fiber; 1mg fat; 0mg choles.; 37mg calcium; 1mg iron; 24mg magnesium; 394mg potassium; 195mg sodium; Vit. A 93 IU; Vit. C 43mg; Vit. E 2 IU.

QUINOA CORN CHOWDER one of the few complete protein grains.

This recipe works for: Men's Health, Wheat Allergies, Sports Nutrition
Makes 4 servings: Mild, buttery flavor.

Simmer $^1/_2$ cup Quinoa, 1 cubed Potato, 1 diced Carrot and 1 chopped Yellow Onion in 2 cups Onion Broth until tender, about 15 minutes. Add one 16-oz. can Corn and $1^1/_2$ cups Plain Rice Milk. Simmer another 5 minutes. Season with Sea Salt and Cracked Pepper to taste. Sprinkle dried Parsley and dried Green Onions over top.

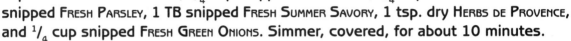

VELVET PUMPKIN SOUP with HONEY and CLOVES

This recipe works for: Men's Health, Sugar Imbalances, Stress Reactions
Makes 8 servings:

Sizzle in a soup pot for 10 minutes: 2 TBS Butter, 1 large Onion, chopped, 2 large Carrots, chopped, and 2 Celery Stalks, chopped. Add 6 cups cubed Pumpkin Flesh, 6 cups Organic Low-Fat Chicken Broth, 2 Sticks Cinnamon and 6 Whole Cloves. Cover and simmer until pumpkin is tender, 25 minutes. Discard cloves and cinnamon sticks.

—Blender blend soup in batches. Return to the soup pot. Stir in 1/2 cup Low Fat Plain Rice Milk, 2 TBS minced Crystallized Ginger and 2 TBS Honey. Bring to simmer. Season with Sea Salt and White Pepper. Thin with more stock if needed. Serve hot.

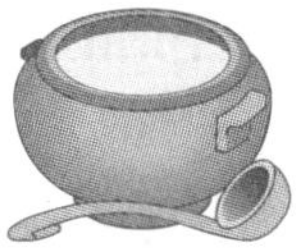

High Protein Soups

Soups can be strengthening and building as well as cleansing and purifying. The recipes in this section are a good way to get more protein for healing.

QUICK POTATO TOFU STEW

This recipe works for: Women's and Men's Health, Fatigue and Stress Syndromes
For 6 people:

Sauté 1 chopped Onion and 2 minced Cloves Garlic in 2 TBS Olive Oil for 3 minutes. Add 3 diced Red Potatoes, 1/2 teasp. Sea Salt, 1/4 teasp. Pepper; sauté 5 minutes.

—Add and bring to a bubble: 1 16-oz. jar Tomato Sauce, 1 cup Red Wine, 3 cups Water, 16-oz. Tofu, diced, and 1 TB Miso Paste. Reduce heat and simmer for 20 minutes til potatoes are tender but not crumbly. Remove from heat and stir in 1 1/4 cups grated Cheddar. Swirl briefly until cheese is just melted.

EASY CHICKEN SOUP with BROWN RICE

This recipe works for: Kid's-Men's Health, Respiratory Healing, Sports Nutrition
For 4 servings:

Have ready 1 1/2 cups cooked Brown Rice.

—Combine in a pot: 3 1/2 cups Organic Chicken Broth, 1 small Onion, chopped, 1/2 cup diced Celery, 1/2 teasp. Garlic Lemon Seasoning and 2 TBS snipped Fresh Parsley. Bring to a boil; simmer 30 minutes. Divide vegetables between soup bowls. Add rice to broth and simmer until rice is hot. Spoon soup and rice over veggies.

Nutrition: 105 calories; 4gm protein; 18gm carbohydrate; 2gm fiber; 1g total fat; 0mg choles.; 23mg calcium; trace iron; 31mg magnesium; 141mg potassium; 149mg sodium; Vit. A 12 IU; Vit. C 7mg; Vit. E trace.

SPICY CHICKEN TORTILLA SOUP

This recipe works for: Kid's-Men's Health, Liver - Organ Health, Sports Nutrition
Makes 6 servings:

In a pot, stir for 1 minute on high heat: $^1/_3$ cup chopped Onion, 3 minced Cloves Garlic, $^3/_4$ tsp. ground Cumin, $^3/_4$ tsp. dried Oregano, $^1/_4$ tsp. Chili Powder, and $^1/_4$ tsp. Pepper. Add 6 cups Organic Low Fat Chicken Broth, 1 can (14-oz.) Diced Tomatoes (with juice), and 1 can (4-oz.) Diced Green Chilies. Cover, reduce heat, simmer 15 minutes.

—Cut $1^1/_2$ lbs. boned skinned Chicken Breasts into strips. Add chicken to broth, cover, and simmer until chicken is done (about 5 minutes). Stir in 2 TBS snipped Fresh Cilantro and Garlic Salt to taste. Thinly slice one Avocado. Swirl slices into the soup.

—Divide 1 package Baked Tortilla Corn Strips between 6 soup bowls. Ladle soup over strips, swirl in avocado slices and sprinkle with $^1/_2$ cup shredded Cheddar Cheese.

VEGETABLE JAMBALAYA

This recipe works for: Men's Health, Sports Nutrition, Immune Breakdown
Makes 6 servings:

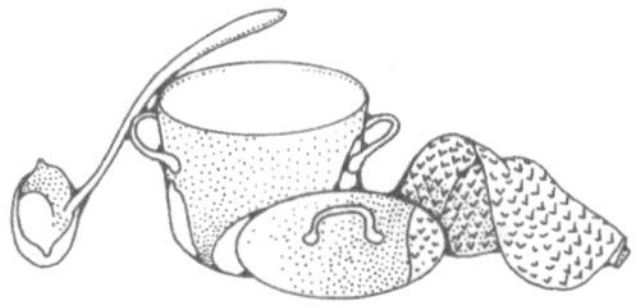

Freeze 12-oz. Fresh Firm Tofu. Thaw tofu and crumble in a bowl. Set aside. Marinate 2 cups chopped Italian Plum Tomatoes in 1 cup dry Red Wine for 1 hour.

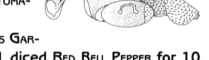

—Heat 2 TBS Olive Oil in a large pot. Sizzle 3 Cloves Garlic, minced, 1 diced Yellow Onion, 1 diced Rib Celery, 1 diced Red Bell Pepper for 10 minutes. Add $1^1/_2$ cups Organic Vegetable Broth and bring to a boil.

—Add 1 cup Raw Brown Basmati Rice, a 12-oz. package Baked Tempeh, cut in bite-size chunks, the crumbled thawed tofu, the marinated tomatoes and wine marinade. Add enough Water to cover ingredients. Return to a boil, reduce heat and simmer 50 minutes, stirring occasionally, until rice absorbs the liquid. Season with $^1/_2$ tsp. dry Thyme, $^1/_2$ tsp. dry Sage, $^1/_2$ tsp. Marjoram, $1^1/_2$ teasp. Lemon-Pepper. Fluff with a fork. Top with $^1/_2$ cup snipped Arugula Leaves and dashes Hot Pepper Sauce.

ASIAN TURKEY EGG DROP SOUP

This recipe works for: Cancer Protection, Immune Breakdown, Recovery
Makes 8 servings:

Bring 4 cups Water to a boil. Add 2 cups Brown Rice. Reduce heat and cook 40 minutes. Remove from heat and divide among 6 soup bowls. In a saucepan bring about 4 cups Fat-Free Organic Chicken Broth to a boil. Add $^1/_3$ cup Tamari and 2 TBS Brown Sugar. Add 8-oz. slivered Fresh Shiitake Mushrooms. Stir in $1^1/_2$ cups shredded, cooked Turkey, 6 Scallions thin-sliced and $1^1/_2$ TB Crystallized Ginger, minced.

—In a bowl beat 4 Eggs. Gently pour into hot soup. Let eggs spread naturally; do not stir. Cook until eggs ripple around the edges, 1 minute. Ladle soup over rice.

TAOS TURKEY and BLACK BEAN SOUP

This recipe works for: Kid's-Men's Health, Liver - Organ Health, Illness Recovery
Makes 6 servings:

Purée 2 cups Black Beans (16-oz. can) and 1 cup Turkey Stock or Organic Chicken Broth in a food processor. Set aside.

—Heat 1 TB Olive Oil in a soup pot. Add 2 minced Garlic Cloves, 2 cups chopped Onions, and 1 cup diced Red Bell Pepper; sauté about 10 minutes. Add 2 tsp. ground Cumin and stir 1 minute. Add 1 large Tomato diced, the bean mixture and 1 more 16-oz. can Whole Black Beans, rinsed and drained. Add 2 more cups Turkey Stock or Organic Chicken Broth. Simmer until vegetables are tender and soup is slightly thickened, about 20 minutes. Thin soup with more stock if needed.

—Add 1 cup diced cooked Turkey and 1 can diced Green Chilies and simmer just to heat through. Season with drops Hot Pepper Sauce and top with Cilantro Leaves.

Nutrition: 234 calories; 18gm protein; 30gm carbohydrate; 12gm fiber; 4gm total fat; 20mg choles.; 115mg calcium; 5mg iron; 16mg magnes.; 196mg potass.; 537mg sodium; Vit. A 100 IU; Vit. C 41mg; Vit. E 1 IU.

CHICKEN DUMPLING SOUP

This recipe works for: Kid's-Men's Health, Sugar Imbalance, Respiratory Infections
For 6 people:

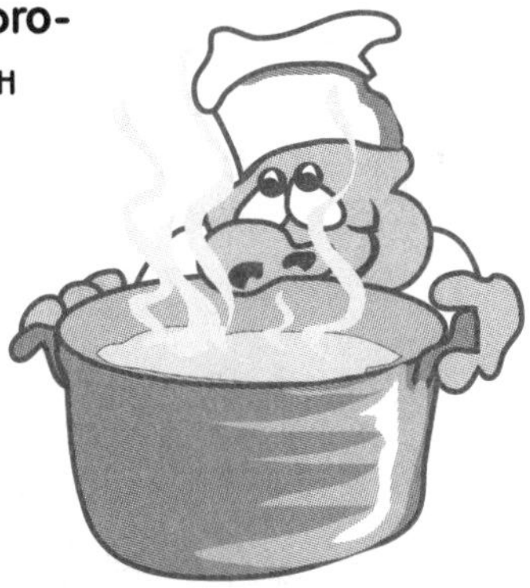

Make the chicken dumplings. Grind in a blender or food processor: 1 1/2 cups cooked diced Chicken, 2 TBS minced Fresh Parsley, 1/2 cup Whole Grain Bread or Cracker Crumbs, 1 Egg, 1 TB grated Parmesan Cheese, 1/4 teasp. Lemon-Pepper. Form into 6 balls. Chill for 1 hour. (If you don't have time for dumplings, use 1 1/2 cups cooked diced Chicken instead.)

—Bring 6 cups Organic Low Fat Chicken Broth to a simmer. Add the chicken balls, 1/4 teasp. Oregano, and 1/4 teasp. Garlic-Lemon Seasoning. Simmer for 10 minutes. Remove balls with a slotted spoon and set aside. Keep the soup stock hot.

—Sizzle 1 TB Olive Oil for 5 minutes in a skillet. Add 1/2 cup sliced Mushrooms, 1 teasp. Lemon Juice, 1/4 cup minced Green Onions, 1/2 teasp. Italian Herbs and dashes Paprika. Add to hot stock and stir in 4-oz. Orzo Rice Pasta. Simmer 5 minutes. Add chicken balls to heat.

—Beat together in a bowl: 3 Eggs, 1 cup Plain Yogurt, 1/3 cup grated Parmesan Cheese. dd 1/2 cup soup to warm the eggs and return mixture to the soup pot. Heat just briefly to warm. Do not boil. Serve hot sprinkled with more Parmesan, dashes Paprika and Italian Herbs.

Nutrition: 351 calories; 32gm protein; 25gm carbohydrate; 3gm fiber; 12g total fat; 197mg choles.; 236mg calcium; 3mg iron; 63mg magnes.; 407mg potassium; 546mg sodium; Vit. A 107 IU; Vit. C 4mg; Vit. E 2 IU.

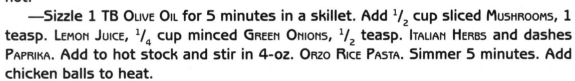

HEARTY LENTIL SOUP

This recipe works for: Fatigue Syndromes, Sports Nutrition, Controlling Addictions
For 8 people:

Cover 1 1/2 cups Lentils with water in a bowl; let soak while making soup base.
—In a soup pot, sauté 3 minced Cloves Garlic, 2 diced Onions in 3 TBS Olive Oil for 5 minutes. Add 2 sliced Carrots and 1 minced Rib Celery with Leaves. Add 1/3 cup Brown Rice and sauté until coated and shiny, about 2 minutes. Add drained lentils.
—Add 1 1/2 qts. Water, 3 TBS Nutritional Yeast, 1 teasp. Sea Salt, 1/2 teasp. Cracked Pepper, 1/2 teasp. dry Basil and 1/4 teasp. Cumin Powder.
—Mix about half a cup of soup with 2 TBS Miso Paste. Add back to soup. Simmer for 20 minutes until fragrant. Remove from heat, cool slightly and purée in the blender til smooth. Return to soup pot. Add 1 teasp. Herbal Seasoning Salt, and 1 TB. Soy Bacon Bits. Heat through and serve with thin Lemon slices on top.

Nutrition: 259 calories; 14gm protein; 35gm carbohydrate; 7gm fiber; 7g total fat; 0mg choles.; 61mg calcium; 5mg iron; 7mg magnesium; 571mg potassium; 453mg sodium; Vit. A 510 IU; Vit. C 11mg; Vit. E 5 IU.

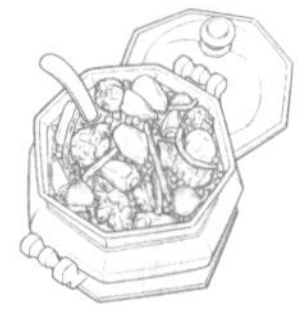

Homestead Stews

Hearty, whole meal stews have been a mainstay of human nourishment since the discovery of fire. They're as important now as they were then.... hot nutrition that reaches throughout our bodies to fuel and energize us quickly.

HOMESTEAD MINESTRONE

This recipe works for: Kid's-Men's Health, Fatigue Syndromes, Bone Building
For 12 people:

Soak 1 1/2 cups dry Kidney Beans overnight in enough water to keep covered, then drain and put them in a 2 gallon kettle or larger, with 3 quarts water. Add 4 chopped Cloves Garlic, 1 large chopped Onion, 1/4 tsp. Celery Seeds and 5 TBS Olive Oil. Simmer for about 1 1/2 hours.
—Cut 3 scrubbed Potatoes into large pieces; add to the pot. Slice and add 2 Carrots, white parts of 4 Leeks, and 6 Zucchini. Season with Lemon-Pepper, snipped Fresh Parsley, 2 TBS snipped Fresh Basil, 1 tsp. dry Oregano, 1/4 tsp. dry Marjoram. Simmer 30 minutes. Add 1/2 cup Brown Basmati Rice. Add 1 10-oz. package frozen French-Cut Green Beans. Simmer 20 more minutes.
—Five minutes before soup is ready to serve, add 6 firm Beefsteak Tomatoes, cut into wedges, 1 cup grated Parmesan Cheese, and more snipped Fresh Parsley.

Nutrition: 287 calories; 12gm protein; 42gm carbohydrate; 9gm fiber; 8gm total fat; 6mg choles.; 181mg calcium; 3mg iron; 93mg magnes.; 962mg potassium; 60mg sodium; Vit. A 443 IU; Vit. C 35mg; Vit. E 3 IU.

FRENCH ONION STEW

This recipe works for: Hair, Skin and Nails, Allergies and Asthma, Recovery
For 6 people:

Sizzle 4 large sliced Onions in 2 TBS Olive Oil until translucent. Add 4 cups Onion Broth, $1\frac{1}{2}$ cups sliced Red Potatoes, 1 teasp. Herbal Seasoning and $\frac{1}{2}$ teasp. Pepper. Cover and cook until tender. Remove from heat. Cool slightly, and purée in the blender, in batches with 1 cup Plain Yogurt. Return to the soup pot, and re-season.

Trim 6 slices Whole Wheat Sourdough Bread and lay on a baking sheet. Sprinkle with grated Swiss Cheese and toast until cheese melts. Put one slice of toast in the bottom of each soup bowl and pour soup over. Serve at once.

MIXED MUSHROOM RAGOÛT

This recipe works for: Cancer Protection, Immune Breakdown, Brain Boosting
For 6 people: Preheat oven to 425°F.

Have ready 6 cups cooked Brown Basmati Rice.

—In a large bowl mix: 1 cup each Button, Porcini, Brown Cremini and Shiitake Mushrooms, or a 16-oz. package frozen Mixed Mushrooms, 6 minced Cloves Garlic, 6 sliced Shallots, 2 TBS snipped Fresh Rosemary. Toss to coat with 3 TBS Olive Oil, 2 TBS White Wine Vinegar, Sea Salt and Pepper to taste. Arrange mushrooms in one layer in a heavy roasting pan. Roast in oven about 15 minutes. Remove mushrooms to a soup pot.

—Put the roasting pan on a stovetop burner over medium heat. Add 1 cup White Wine and stir to deglaze until wine is reduced by half, then add 2 cups Organic Low Fat Chicken Broth. Cook five minutes to blend. Add mushrooms and $\frac{1}{4}$ cup snipped Fresh Parsley; simmer for 5 minutes longer. Serve over rice.

Nutrition: 372calories; 8gm protein; 57gm carbohydrate; 7gm fiber; 10g total fat; 0mg choles.; 107mg calcium; 4mg iron; 102mg magnes.; 490mg potassium; 298mg sodium; Vit. A 13 IU; Vit. C 9mg; Vit. E 2 IU.

TURKEY STEW with POLENTA BALLS

This recipe works for: Kid's-Men's Health, Sugar Imbalance, Fatigue Syndromes
For 6 people:

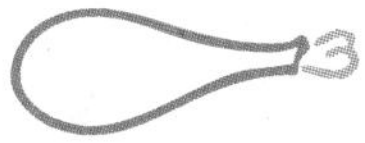

Bring 5 cups Low-Fat Organic Chicken Broth to a boil in a soup pot. Add $1\frac{1}{2}$ cups Yellow Cornmeal and whisk to smooth. Bring to boil again, cover and cook 45 minutes stirring occasionally. Season to taste. Remove from heat. Spoon up polenta into balls and divide between 6 pasta bowls.

—Heat 1 TB Olive Oil in a large skillet. Sizzle $\frac{1}{2}$ diced Red Onion and 6-oz. slivered Portobello Mushrooms 10 minutes. Stir in 3 cups canned crushed Roma Tomatoes, 4 TBS Sun dried Tomatoes in Oil and $\frac{1}{2}$ teasp. Lemon Garlic Seasoning. Stir in $1\frac{1}{2}$ cups shredded cooked Turkey; season to taste and sprinkle with Parmesano-Reggiano Cheese.

OLD SOUTH STEW

This recipe works for: Men's Health, Stress Reactions, Sports Nutrition
For 6 people:

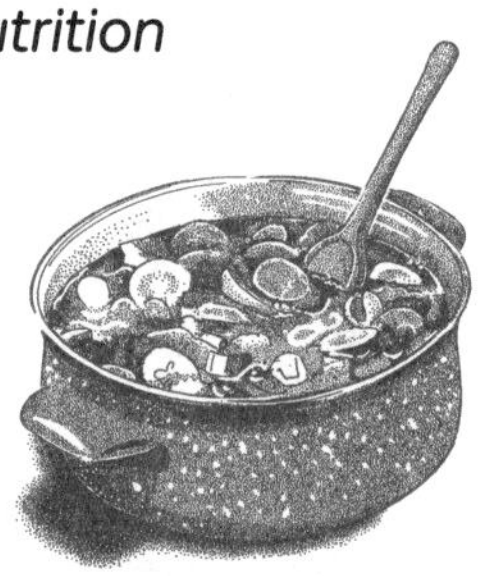

Have ready 6 cups cooked Brown Rice.

—Drain 1 large can Black-eyed Peas, reserving liquid. Rinse, drain and set aside. In a large pot, sizzle 1$^1/_2$ TBS Olive Oil, 2 large chopped Onions, and 2 minced Cloves Garlic for 10 minutes.

—Stir in 3 large chopped Tomatoes, $^1/_4$ cup snipped Fresh Basil (or 2 tsp. dried), 1 tsp. Fresh Thyme Leaves (or $^1/_2$ tsp. dried) and $^1/_4$ cup Water; bring to a boil. Reduce heat to low and simmer until tomatoes soften slightly, 5 minutes.

—Stir in the cooked rice, the black-eyed peas, 1 teasp. Lemon-Pepper and $^1/_2$ tsp. Sea Salt. Simmer until flavors have blended, 5 minutes. Add a little reserved liquid from peas as needed to keep mixture moist. Spoon into serving bowls and garnish with Fresh Basil Leaves.

Nutrition: 336 calories; 9gm protein; 66gm carbohydrate; 9gm fiber; 6g total fat; 0mg choles.; 120mg calcium; 1mg iron; 127mg magnesium; 550mg potass.; 197mg sodium; Vit. A 89 IU; Vit. C 17mg; Vit. E 3 IU.

SPICY TOFU GOULASH

This recipe works for: Liver and Organ Health, Arthritis
For 4 to 6 people:

In a soup pot, sauté 2 TBS Olive Oil and 1 large chopped Onion for 5 minutes. Add 1 chopped Red Bell Pepper, 2 sliced Carrots and 3 cubed Red Potatoes. Stir for 5 minutes more. Add 8-oz. Tomato Sauce, $^1/_2$ cup Water, and $^1/_2$ cup White Wine; simmer for 10 minutes to blend flavors. Add 2 cubed Cakes Tofu, 1 TB Paprika, 1 teasp. Herbal Seasoning, $^1/_2$ teasp. Nutmeg and 1 teasp. Pepper. Simmer for 10 minutes more. Remove from heat. Add 1 cup soup to a blender with 1 cup Plain Yogurt. Whirl until smooth and add back to the pot. Sprinkle with more paprika, nutmeg and pepper.

EASY LENTIL-BARLEY STEW

This recipe works for: Addiction Recovery, Women's and Men's Health
For 4 to 6 people:

In a stew pot, sizzle 1 chopped Yellow Onion and 2 minced Cloves Garlic for 5 minutes. Add 1 cup rinsed Lentils and 1 cup Barley, stir for 5 more minutes. Add 2 $^1/_2$ quarts Organic Vegetable Broth, 2 cups sliced Celery, 2 large sliced Carrots, $^1/_2$ teasp. dry Sage and 2 tsp. dried Rosemary. Bring to a boil over high heat, stirring frequently. Reduce heat, cover and simmer, stirring occasionally, 15 minutes.

—Add 5 to 6 chopped Tomatoes, cover and stir occasionally until lentils are tender to bite, about 15 minutes more. Season to taste with Sea Salt and Lemon-Pepper.

BEDOUIN STEW

This recipe works for: Liver and Organ Health, Arthritis, Respiratory Infections
Makes 6 servings

Grind the CARAVAN SPICE in a blender or with mortar and pestle: 2 TBS. Cumin Seeds, 1 teasp. Cardamom Pods, $^1/_2$ tsp. Fennel Seeds, 2 teasp. Coriander Seeds, 1 TB Mixed Peppercorns, 1 TB Whole Allspice Berries, 3 Whole Cloves, 1 TB fresh grated Ginger, 2 TBS Paprika, $^1/_2$ tsp. Cinnamon, $^1/_2$ tsp. Tumeric and a pinch Saffron. Set aside.

—Make the stew: heat 2 TBS Olive Oil in a large soup pot. Add 3 Cloves Garlic, minced, 1 large chopped Yellow Onion, 1 chopped Red Bell Pepper, 1 chopped Yellow Bell Pepper, 2 large chopped Tomatoes, 2 chopped Carrots, 3 cups peeled, chopped Red Potatoes, 1 small Butternut Squash, peeled, seeded and cubed. Add $1^1/_2$ TBS Caravan Spice and simmer, stirring for 5 minutes.

—Add 4 cups Water or Onion Broth and simmer 20 to 25 minutes, until vegetables are tender. Add more spices if needed. Stir in $^1/_4$ cup minced Cilantro Leaves.

Nutrition: 168 calories; 4gm protein; 29gm carbohydrate; 5gm fiber; 5g total fat; 0mg choles.; 65mg calcium; 3mg iron; 52mg magnesium; 837mg potassium; 27mg sodium; Vit. A 42 IU; Vit. C 57mg; Vit. E 2 IU.

SAVORY CHICKEN POT-AU-FEU

This recipe works for: Immune Recovery, Bone Building, Respiratory Infections
For 4 people:

Sizzle and brown in 1 teasp. Olive Oil for 5 minutes: 4 boned, skinned Organic Chicken Breast Halves, each half sliced in 4 or 5 slices. Remove and set aside.

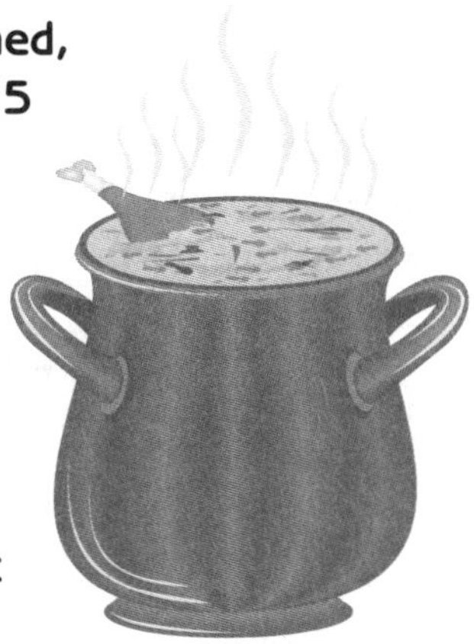

—Add to pot 3 cups Organic Low Fat Chicken Broth, 1 cup White Wine and 2 teasp. Fresh Tarragon Leaves. Peel 12 Baby Red Potatoes. Bring broth to a boil and add potatoes. Cover, and simmer for 5 minutes. Add 8 peeled Baby Carrots. Arrange chicken in a single layer on vegetables. Cover and cook for 10 minutes. Slice 4 Baby Bok Choy in half. Lay bok choy on chicken; cover and simmer until chicken is white in center of thickest part (cut to test), about 5 minutes longer.

—In a small bowl, mix a MUSTARD-CHEESE sauce: $^1/_3$ cup Low Fat Cream Cheese, 1 TB Dijon Mustard, 2 TBS chopped Shallots, 1 TB drained Capers, pinches Sea Salt and Pepper.

—With a slotted spoon, divide chicken and vegetables between wide soup bowls. Ladle hot broth equally into bowls and swirl in MUSTARD-CHEESE sauce. Snip 1 teasp. Fresh Parsley on each bowl.

Nutrition: 294 calories; 23gm protein; 26gm carbohydrate; 6gm fiber; 8g total fat; 47mg choles.; 38mg calcium; 3mg iron; 49mg magnes.; 843mg potass.; 781mg sodium; Vit. A 1119 IU, Vit. C 138mg; Vit. E 1 IU.

Soup Toppers

Dumplings can make any soup into dinner. Dumpling tidbits make an ordinary soup into a speciality. They are tender and light, very easy to make, and may be used in all kinds of soups.

Here's how: Mix ingredients. Roll into balls. Chill to set. Drop into simmering soup. Do not open pot lid while cooking so dumplings will steam properly. They are ready when they rise to the surface.

LEMON HERB DUMPLINGS

For 25 dumplings: mix $^1/_2$ cup Vegetable Broth, 1 TB. Lemon Juice, 2 TBS Butter, 1 Egg, $^1/_2$ teasp. Herb Seasoning, 6 TBS Unbleached Flour, $^1/_4$ teasp. ground Celery Seed, 1 TB snipped Fresh Parsley, 1 TB snipped Fresh Chives, $^1/_4$ teasp. Lemon-Pepper.

TENDER TOFU DUMPLINGS

For 18 dumplings: 2 mashed Cakes Tofu, $^1/_2$ cup Whole Wheat Pastry Flour, 1 Egg, 2 TBS chopped Fresh Parsley, 2 teasp. Baking Powder, 1 teasp. Herbal Seasoning Salt.

CHICKEN SOUP WITH RICOTTA DUMPLINGS

Sift the dry ingredients together: 2 cups Unbleached Flour, 3 tsp. Non-Aluminum Baking Powder, 1 tsp. Sea Salt. In a small bowl, combine 2 Eggs, $^1/_2$ cup Ricotta Cheese, $^1/_4$ cup Low-Fat Rice Milk, 1 TB snipped Fresh Thyme and 1 TB snipped Fresh Parsley. Combine with flour mixture. Stir just until dough holds together. Using a tablespoon, form dumplings and drop into boiling chicken soup broth. Simmer 15 minutes.

TOASTED ALMOND DUMPLINGS

Mix for 30 dumplings: Sizzle 3 TBS Butter to very dark in a saucepan. Add and mix in: 1 cup crushed Whole Grain Cracker Crumbs, $^1/_2$ cup Plain Yogurt, $^1/_2$ cup chopped Almonds, 1 Egg, 1 teasp. Sea Salt, 2 pinches Pepper.

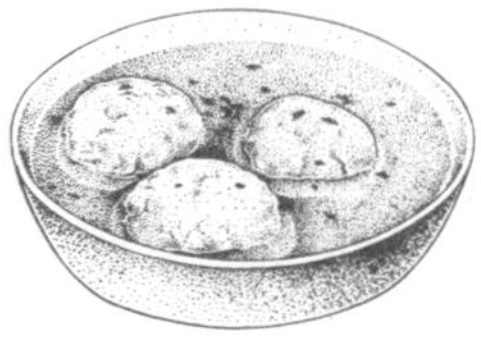

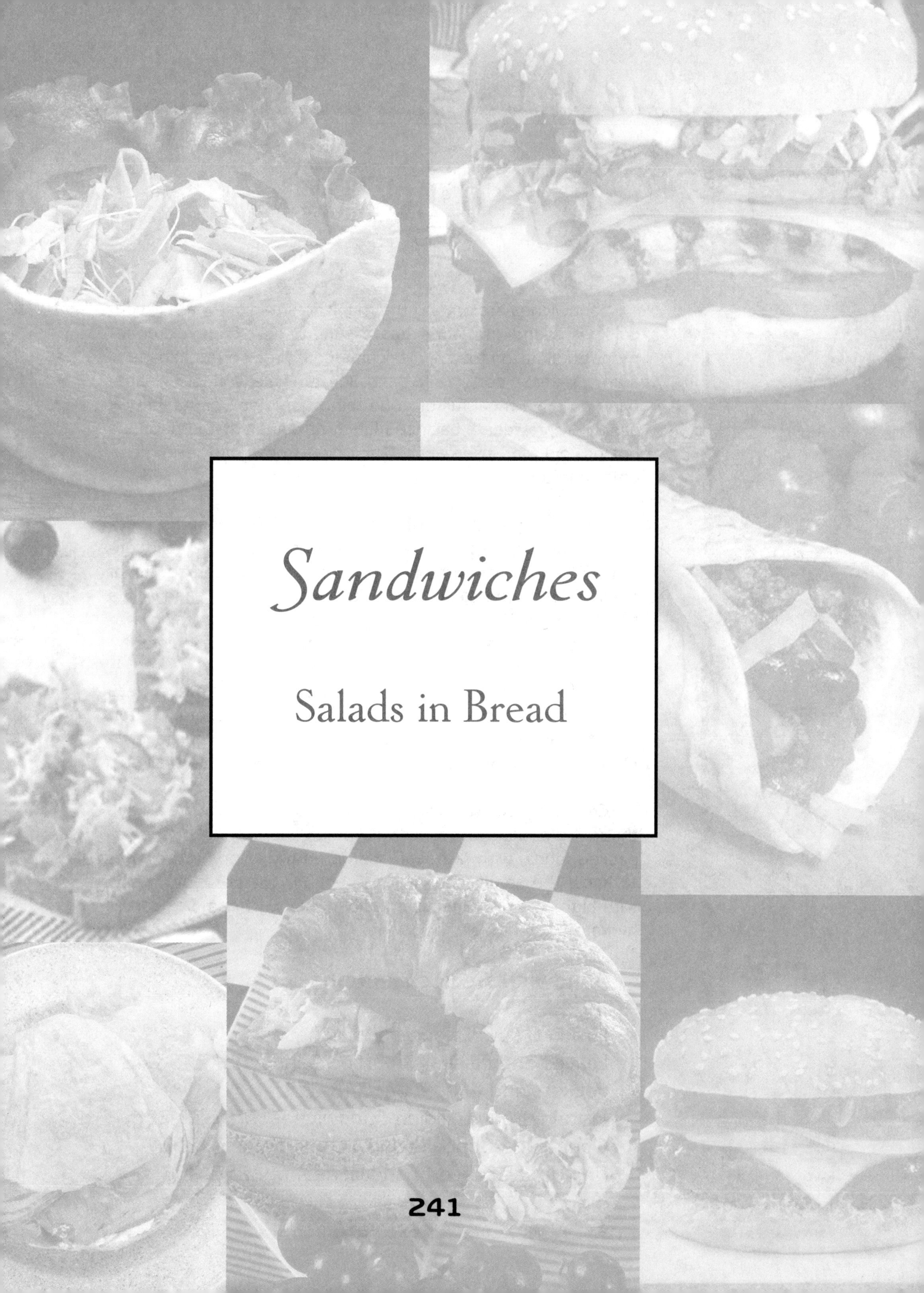

Sandwiches

Salads in Bread

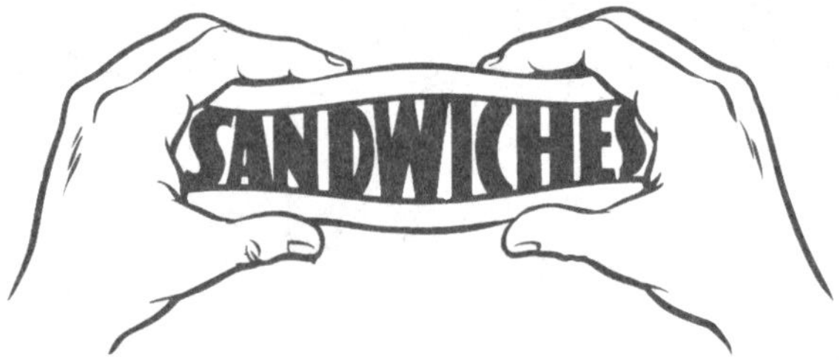

Sandwiches are among the mankind's earliest foods. Every cuisine around the world has a sandwich.... French croque-monsieurs, Italian tostas, Mexican tacos, Greek pitas, Lebanese arams, Chinese egg rolls. A sandwich can be a wonderful, satisfying portable meal full of good things to keep you healthy. A sandwich provides a balanced lunch or dinner that is delicious hot or cold, and uses almost anything from gourmet ingredients to leftovers.

Pack your sandwich with protein. Seafoods, poultry, vegetables, beans, tofu and seasoned grains offer high quality energy. Put your sandwich on whole grain sandwich bread, full of body building complex carbohydrates. Make your sandwich a salad in bread. Load it with fresh greens and vegetables, low-fat or non-dairy dressings and cheeses, and herbal seasonings.

An open-face sandwich is a salad on toast, with even less density. Pita breads are a good choice for weight control..... fun to eat, low in calories, fat and cholesterol. Stuff your favorite fillings in a neat pita pocket so that everything doesn't fall out.

Create a great sandwich. It's good for you! If you've always thought that sandwiches just fill you up and out, (heavy, meat-packed foods, with fatty spreads on empty calorie bread), get to know the sandwiches in this section. They're tasty meals with high protein, minerals and fiber, plenty of complex carbohydrates, low fats and no sugars.

Sandwich Recipe Sections

Low Fat Low Calorie Sandwiches

Sandwiches are satisfying and healthy, convenient, all-in-one meals. They're really salads in whole grain bread. It's a shame that they have a reputation as junk food.

MEAL SIZE ROASTED VEGGIE SUB

This recipe works for: Kid's and Men's Health, Liver - Organ Health, Heart Health
For 4 servings: Preheat oven broiler.

Slice 4 large Portobello Mushrooms in thin slices. Lay on a lecithin-sprayed baking sheet and drizzle 2 TBS Olive Oil over mushrooms. Sprinkle with Granulated Garlic and broil 4 to 5 minutes until mushrooms begin to sweat. Remove, but leave oven on.

—Peel and slice 1 Eggplant in thin slices. Brush with 1 TB Balsamic Vinegar and 2 TBS Red Wine and broil until slices brown and soften, about 5 to 7 minutes. Remove.

—Sliver 2 large Roasted Red Bell Peppers from a jar.

—Split and broil to brown, 4 Individual Submarine Rolls. Divide mushrooms, red peppers and eggplants on the bottom half of each roll. Top with Fresh Tomato Slices overlapped. Sprinkle liberally with shredded Low-Fat Provolone Cheese and minced Black Olives. Broil briefly to melt cheese and blend flavors.

Nutrition: 347 calories; 13gm protein; 57gm carbohydrate; 7gm fiber; 11g total fat; 4mg choles.; 160mg calcium; 4mg iron; 34mg magnes.; 430mg potass.; 434mg sodium; Vit. A 212 IU; Vit. C 45mg; Vit. E 3 IU.

SEA VEGGIE D.L.T Enjoy courtesy of Maine Coast Sea Vegetables

This recipe works for: Overcoming Addictions, Liver - Organ Health, Hair and Skin

Toast Whole Grain Bread Slices. Snip dried Dulse with kitchen shears in bacon-size strips. Sprinkle strips with Teriyaki Sauce before making sandwiches.

—Sprinkle toast with drops of Olive Oil, or spread Low Fat Mayonnaise. Cover each slice toast with Boston Lettuce Leaves, top each slice with Tomato Slices, cover tomatoes with Dulse Strips. Let sit 5 minutes to remoisturize dulse; put sandwiches together.

BREAKFAST FRUIT 'N' FIBER TORTILLA SANDWICHES

This recipe works for: Waste Management, Men's Health, Stress Reactions
For 2 sandwiches: Preheat a heavy skillet.

Soften 2 Whole Wheat Flour Tortillas on the skillet. Top each with a slice of Low Fat Cheddar Cheese or Rice Cheddar Cheese. Spread cheese with 1 tsp. Jam or Fruit Butter, and top with 1 more slice Cheese. Fold up bottom, fold in sides, and roll snugly to secure top flap. Arrange seam side down; skillet toast until tortillas cheese melts, 4 minutes per side.

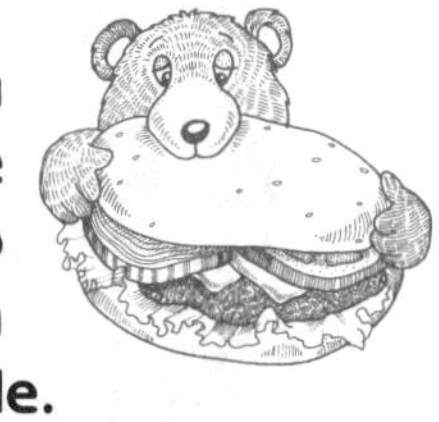

MAKE YOUR OWN GOURMET VEGGIE BURGER

This recipe works for: Allergies and Asthma, Weight Control, Candida Infection
For 6 Burgers:

Heat 2 teasp. Toasted Asian Sesame Oil in a skillet. Add an 8-oz package Tempeh and brown on each side. Add 1 cup Water and 1 TB Tamari. Simmer turning occasionally until liquid is absorbed, then remove tempeh and crumble into a mixing bowl.

—Toast 4 TBS chopped Walnuts in the skillet until aromatic. Add to tempeh. Toast $^1/_2$ cup cooked Brown Rice or Soy Nuts, and 2 Cakes Tofu in the skillet for 3 minutes. Add $^2/_3$ cup Organic Chicken Broth and simmer until liquid is absorbed. Add to tempeh. Add 2 TBS snipped Fresh Cilantro or Parsley.

—Sizzle 2 minced Garlic Cloves, $^1/_2$ cup minced Scallions, 3 TBS minced Oil-Packed Sun-dried Tomatoes in the skillet for 2 minutes. Add 1 cup fine-chopped <u>each</u>: Portobello Mushrooms, Cremini Mushrooms and Button Mushrooms. Stir in 1 TB Miso, 1 TB minced Ginger and 1 tsp. Thai Chili Paste. Sizzle 5 minutes. Then blender blend to a paste and add to tempeh. Form into 6 patties. Chill while you make the ASIAN SLAW TOPPING.

ASIAN SLAW Great burger topping or pita pocket stuffing.

This recipe works for: Digestive Health, Liver - Organ Health, Cancer Control
Makes enough for 8 tofu burgers or 6 pockets: Also a black bean wrap sauce.

Slice off leafy top of a 2-lb. Nappa Cabbage. Reserve leafy top for another use. (I mix it with wet and dry dog food for extra pet food nutrition.) Thinly slice rest of cabbage and place in a large bowl. Sliver 2 large Olive Oil-packed Roasted Red Bell Peppers from a jar. Toss peppers with cabbage. Thinly slice 2 large Broccoli Stems and toss with cabbage mix. Cut 1 Jicama into thin matsticks and toss with cabbage mix.

—Blend 2 TBS Olive Oil, $^1/_2$ teasp. Toasted Sesame Oil, 4 TBS Brown Rice Vinegar, 12 teasp. Fructose, 1 TB minced Crystallized Ginger and 2 pinches Sea Salt. Pour over slaw and chill 1 hour to blend flavors.

Nutrition filling: 117 calories; 3gm protein; 18gm carbohydrate; 6gm fiber; 4gm total fat; 0mg choles.; 57mg calcium; 2mg iron; 43mg magnes.; 399mg potass.; 140mg sodium; Vit. A 234 IU; Vit. C 83mg; Vit. E 6 IU.

LOW FAT PARTY SANDWICHES

This recipe works for: Anti-Aging, Weight Control, Women's Health
For 24 cocktail sandwiches:

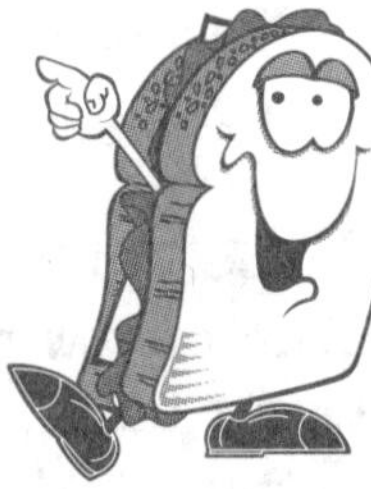

Mix together: 16-oz. Low Fat Cottage Cheese, half a carton (about 4-oz.) Kefir Cheese or Soy Cream Cheese, 1 peeled minced Cucumber, $^1/_2$ cup snipped Watercress or Parsley; chill. Pile on Toasted Rye Rounds and serve.

Nutrition: 55 calories; 5gm protein; 9gm carbohydrate; 1gm fiber; trace fat; 1mg choles.; 37mg calcium; 1mg iron; 4mg magnesium; 53mg potassium; 216mg sodium; Vit. A 10 IU; Vit. C 2mg; Vit. E trace.

MEDITERRANEAN FETA CHEESE SANDWICHES

This recipe works for: Women's and Men's Health, Sports Nutrition, Weight Loss
Makes 6 sandwiches: Preheat broiler.

Combine 1 teasp. Garlic Granules and 3 TBS Olive Oil in a bowl. Set aside.

—Split a 12-inch Italian Bread Baguette lengthwise, then cut each half into 3 pieces. Brush cut sides with Garlic-Olive Oil mix and toast pieces under a broiler for 3 minutes. Transfer baguettes to sandwich plates.

—Peel 1 small Eggplant and cut into 6 lengthwise slices. Lay on a baking sheet and brush with Garlic-Olive Oil mix. Broil about 6 minutes on each side until soft.

—Top each bread slice with a thin slice of Feta Cheese. Overlap eggplant slices, then put Fresh Tomato slices on top to cover. Sprinkle with snipped Fresh Basil Leaves. Broil briefly to brown top and serve immediately.

Nutrition: 306 calories; 10gm protein; 35gm carbohydrate; 3gm fiber; 14g total fat; 25mg choles.; 221mg calcium; 3mg iron; 21mg magnes.; 253mg potassium; 640mg sodium; Vit. A 93 IU; Vit. C 12mg; Vit. E 1 IU.

ROLLED SHRIMP SANDWICHES

This recipe works for: Heart Health, Hair and Skin, Weight Loss
For 8 rolls: 2 per person

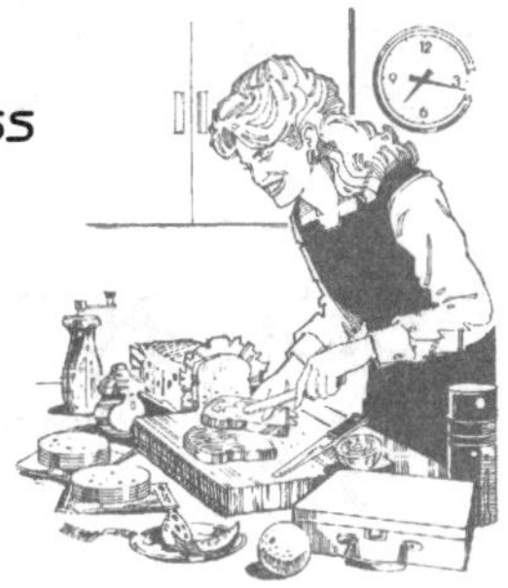

Cook $^1/_2$ cup Short Grain Brown Rice in $1^1/_4$ cups Water with 1 strip of Kombu Seaweed added for flavor, covered, for 20 minutes. Uncover, fluff, and set aside.

—Make the VINEGAR SHRIMP FILLING. Mix together: 3-oz. cooked Salad Shrimp, 2 TBS Sweet Pickle Relish, drained, 1 teasp. Brown Sugar, 2 TBS Brown Rice Vinegar and 2 teasp. grated Lemon Zest; add to the rice.

—Dip 8 Large Romaine Lettuce Leaves in boiling water until limp, then immediately put into ice water until cold. Lay on paper towels to dry. Divide filling between leaves. Fold sides over, and roll from stem end, tucking in edges as you go to make a packet. Chill before serving.

Nutrition: 62 calories; 3gm protein; 11gm carbohydrate; 1gm fiber; 1g total fat; 0mg choles.; 14mg calcium; 1mg iron; 22mg magnes.; 96mg potass.; 196mg sodium; Vit. A 45 IU; Vit. C 5mg; Vit. E trace

LOW FAT TURKEY HERO Use Pita Pocket Bread for lowest fat.

This recipe works for: Women's and Men's Health, Sports Nutrition, Heart Health

<u>For each sandwich</u>: Lay 1 slice peeled Eggplant and 1 Red Onion Ring on a baking sheet; drizzle with Olive Oil. Preheat broiler and broil for 6 minutes <u>each side</u>. Slice one end off a pita to make a pocket, spread with Dijon-Honey Mustard. Stuff with eggplant slice, onion slice, several thin slices Roast Turkey, 1 slice Beefsteak Tomato and 1 slice Avocado. Top with 1 big spoonful Sweet Pickle Relish or Sunflower Sprouts.

Loaves and Fishes: Seafood Sandwiches

Ocean foods are widely acknowledged as some of the Earth's healthiest harvest. Americans enhance their love affair with sandwich meals by enthusiastically embracing seafood sandwiches of all kinds.

SALMON-ARTICHOKE SANDWICHES

This recipe works for: Hair and Skin, Arthritis, Brain Enhancement
For 8 open-face sandwiches: Preheat broiler.

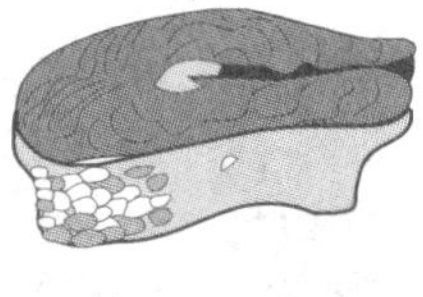

Mix in a bowl: $^1/_2$ cup LOW FAT CREAM CHEESE or KEFIR CHEESE, 1 TB minced FRESH ROSEMARY LEAVES, $^1/_4$ teasp. LEMON-PEPPER and 2 TBS LEMON JUICE. Shred about 4 ounces thin-sliced SMOKED SALMON and mix in.

—Split a 12-inch ITALIAN BREAD BAGUETTE lengthwise, then cut each half into 4 pieces. Spread cream cheese mix over each cut side. Drain an 11-oz jar of WATER-PACKED ARTICHOKES; chop coarsely and place on baguette pieces. Cover artichokes with LOW FAT HAVARTI CHEESE slices. Broil about 6" from heat for 3 minutes until golden.

Nutrition: 172 calories; 12gm protein; 20gm carbohydrate; 3gm fiber; 5g total fat; 16mg choles.; 193mg calcium; 2mg iron; 31mg magnes.; 205mg potassium; 546mg sodium; Vit. A 52 IU; Vit. C 5mg; Vit. E trace.

DELICIOUS SALMON BURGERS Loaded with healthy EFA's.

This recipe works for: Arthritis, Cardiac Health, Hair, Skin and Nails
For 2 servings: Preheat broiler.

Run 2 halves of a large WHOLE WHEAT SOURDOUGH ROLL under the broiler to brown.

—Make the patties easily in a food processor: mix about 6-oz. leftover SALMON FILET, 2 SCALLIONS, $^1/_3$ cup TOASTED WHEAT GERM, 1 EGG and 3 TBS KETCHUP. Scrape into a bowl and season with SEA SALT and LEMON-PEPPER. Form into 2 patties. Brown patties in a hot, LECITHIN-sprayed skillet about 3 minutes on each side. Remove and keep warm.

—Make the topping: Mix $^1/_3$ cup LOW FAT MAYONNAISE, 2 minced SCALLIONS and 2 TBS minced FRESH DILL WEED (or 2 teasp. dried). Spread a dollop on the roll halves, top with salmon patties, spoon on a sauce dollop, top with a TOMATO slice and serve.

TENDER GRILLED CRAB CAKES

This recipe works for: Arthritis, Cardiac Health, Hair, Skin and Nails
For 2 servings: Preheat BBQ grill. Grill French Bread slices first and have ready.

Mix: a 6-oz. can CRABMEAT, 1 cup WHOLE GRAIN CRACKER CRUMBS, $^1/_2$ cup snipped SCALLIONS, 2 TBS LOW FAT MAYONNAISE, 1 teasp. SEAFOOD COCKTAIL SAUCE and 1 EGG. Form into 2 cakes. Coat with $^1/_2$ cup more CRACKER CRUMBS and grill 4 minutes each side. Remove; spread toast with more MAYONNAISE and DIJON MUSTARD. Top with crab cakes and serve.

LOW FAT CRAB ROLLS

This recipe works for: Brain Boosting, Women's Health, Hair, Skin and Nails
For 4 to 6 people as appetizers: Preheat oven broiler when ready to serve.

Whisk together: $^1/_4$ cup Low Fat Mayonnaise, $^1/_2$ cup Plain Low Fat Yogurt, 2 teasp. Lime Juice, 2 teasp. Lemon Juice. Stir in: 1 to 2 minced Celery Ribs, 1 minced Green Onion, $^1/_4$ teasp. Tarragon, $^1/_2$ teasp. Dry Parsley, $^1/_4$ teasp. Lemon-Pepper. Fold in: 1-LB Dungeness Crabmeat picked over for shells, or 16-oz. canned Crabmeat. Cover and chill.
—Broil 24 Rye Cocktail Rounds until brown on top. Top with spoonfuls of crab mix. Broil briefly again just to brown. Sprinkle with snipped Watercress or Fresh Parsley.

Nutrition: 250 calories; 26gm protein; 33gm carbohydrate; 4gm fiber; 3g total fat; 58mg choles.; 143mg calcium; 3mg iron; 50mg magnes.; 400mg potass.; 900mg sodium; Vit. A 31 IU; Vit. C 6mg; Vit. E 1 IU.

SALMON CLUB

This recipe works for: Stress Relief, Liver - Organ Health, Hair, Skin and Nails
For 4 sandwiches: Preheat broiler.

Toast 8 slices Whole Grain Bread under broiler until golden. Remove; set aside.
—Season 1 LB Smoked Salmon slices with Lemon-Pepper. Spread all toast slices with Lemon Mayonnaise or Low Fat Mayonnaise seasoned with 1 TB Lemon Juice and pinches Lemon-Pepper. Top 4 toast pieces with Salmon slices, Boston Lettuce Leaves, and thin overlapping Tomato slices. Top with remaining 4 bread slices. Cut in half and serve.

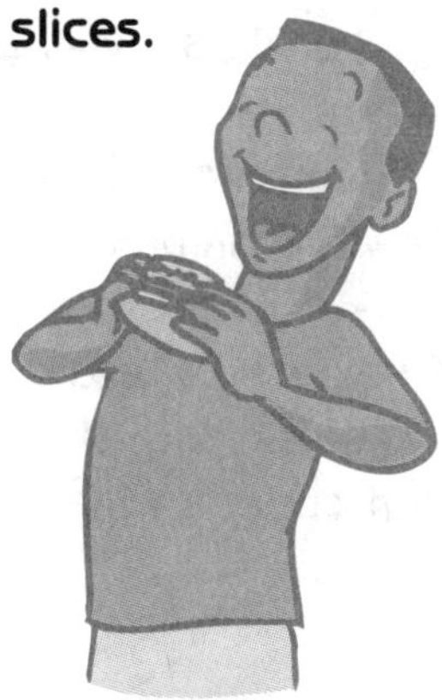

Terrific Tuna Sandwiches. Americans are only now realizing how healthy this oldy but goody really is.... a tasty, low fat source of protein loaded with heart-wise Omega-3 oils. Pile any of these on whole grain toast or stuff in pita pockets

TUNA ITALIAN

This recipe works for: Stress and Energy, Men's Health, Liver and Organ Health
For 4 sandwiches:

Mix: a 6-oz. can Water Packed White Tuna, 4 TBS Red Bell Pepper, 3 minced Scallions, $^1/_4$ cup snipped Fresh Cilantro Leaves, $^2/_3$ cup diced Mozzarella Cheese, 16 Black Olives, sliced, 3 TBS Low Fat Italian Vinaigrette Dressing. Pile onto Whole Grain Toast, and top with another slice of toast.

Nutrition: 415 calories; 31gm protein; 34gm carbohydrate; 5gm fiber; 18g total fat; 45mg choles.; 389mg calcium; 4mg iron; 84mg magnes.; 391mg potass.; 798mg sodium; Vit. A 162 IU; Vit. C 17mg; Vit. E 6 IU.

TUNA MEXICANO

This recipe works for: Weight Control, Kid's and Men's Health, Allergies and Asthma
For 4 sandwiches:

Mix: a 6-oz. can Water Packed White Tuna, $^{1}/_{2}$ cup shredded Jalapeño Jack Cheese, 4 minced Green Onions, 1 large diced Tomato, 2 cups Shaved Lettuce and 3 TBS Hot Salsa or Barbecue Sauce. Pile on Whole Grain Toast, top with another slice, or stuff into Pitas.

Nutrition: 203 calories; 20gm protein; 17gm carbohydrate; 3gm fiber; 6g total fat; 38mg choles.; 152mg calcium; 2mg iron; 56mg magnes.; 419mg potass.; 373mg sodium; Vit. A 209 IU; Vit. C 36mg; Vit. E 1 IU.

HOT DOG TUNA

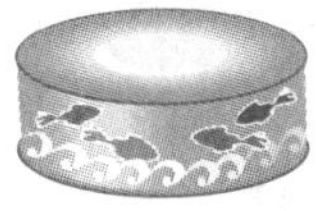

This recipe works for: Sports Nutrition, Kid's and Men's Health
For 4 sandwiches:

Mix: a 6-oz. can Water Packed White Tuna, 4 TBS Low Fat Mayonnaise, 4 teasp. Sweet Pickle Relish, 2 Hard Boiled Egg, crumbled, 2 teasp. Tamari and 2 teasp. Yellow Mustard. Pile on half a Toasted Bun. Top with Alfalfa Sprouts; cover with the other half.

SALSA TUNA MELT Loaded with valuable Omega oils.

This recipe works for: Sports Nutrition, Men's Health, Overcoming Addictions
For 4 sandwiches: Preheat broiler. Toast whole grain buns first.

Combine filling in a bowl: $^{3}/_{4}$ cup minced Celery, 2 TBS minced Red Onion, 4 TBS Low Fat Mayonnaise, and $^{1}/_{2}$ teasp. Dill Weed. Spread on toasted whole grain buns.
—Cut a thick 16-oz Ahi Tuna Steak into 12 thin slices. Season with Lemon-Pepper. Drizzle with Lemon Juice. Broil for 5 minutes. Place 3 slices on each of 4 bun halves.
—Top with shredded Low Fat Mozzarella Cheese and broil again until cheese bubbles. Top cheese with dollops of Hot Salsa and cover with the top bun.

Pockets and Wraps

Middle Eastern cuisine pioneered the use of pita pockets by stuffing them with falafel, a spicy garbanzo bean mix. Today, almost every type of cuisine has a pocket or a wrap in its repertoire.... Italian calzones, Mexican tacos and burritos, Japanese sushi, Chinese eggrolls, Vietnamese rice wraps, Thai spring rolls.... for every kind of filling imaginable. They are fun to eat, and low in fat and calories. They come in all sizes from minis for appetizers to large ones the size of tortillas. They can be split at the top, cut in half for filling, or sliced lengthwise for open-face rounds or pizzas. They are delicious broiled, toasted or cold. Use whole wheat pitas for better health.

HOT SALSA PIZZARITO A fresh salad in a pocket

This recipe works for: Arthritis, Kid's and Men's Health, Overcoming Addictions
For 4 sandwiches:

Mix in a bowl: $^1/_4$ cup diced Zucchini, $^1/_4$ cup chopped Tomato, 2 TBS Green Onion, 2 TBS chopped Red Bell Pepper, 2 TBS sliced Black Olives, 2 teasp. Parmesan Cheese, 4 TBS Low Fat Mozarrella Cheese, 2 TBS slivered Oil-Packed Sun-Dried Tomatoes, and 2 TBS Roasted Sunflower Seeds. Stuff filling into split, halved pita pockets.

—Blender blend the fresh HOT TOMATO SALSA: (Makes $1^1/_2$ cups sauce. I like to keep some in the fridge for all kinds of uses.) $1^1/_4$ cups chopped Tomatoes, $^1/_4$ cup grated Low Fat Cheddar Cheese, 1 TB Soy Bacon Bits, 2 TBS chopped Green Chilies, $^1/_2$ teasp. Oregano and $^1/_2$ teasp. Hot Chili Sauce. Top pita pockets with dollops of sauce.

—Oven-toast to melt cheese; top with 2 TBS Mixed Spicy Sprouts per sandwich.

Nutrition: 129 calories; 6gm protein; 16gm carbohydrate; 33gm fiber; 5g total fat; 5mg choles.; 89mg calcium; 1mg iron; 31mg magnes.; 174mg potass.; 212mg sodium; Vit. A 43 IU; Vit. C 11mg; Vit. E 3 IU.

CHICKEN and ASPARAGUS CALZONE

This recipe works for: Arthritis, Kid's and Men's Health, Sugar Imbalances
Makes 4 servings - 1 large calzone: Preheat oven to 400°F.

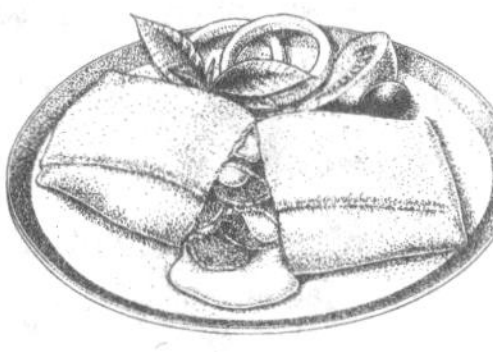

Prepare Basic Pizza Dough pg. 205 as directed. Set aside.

—Sprinkle 1 large Zucchini, sliced with Sea Salt; drain in a sieve for 20 minutes. Rinse and pat dry with paper towels. Blanch 8-oz. trimmed Fresh Asparagus spears in boiling water until bright green, and cut into 2-inch pieces.

—Mix filling: $1^1/_2$ cups cooked cubed Organic Chicken, 2 TBS Soy Bacon Bits, $^1/_3$ cup Low Fat Ricotta Cheese drained, 1 minced Scallion and 1 TB grated Parmesan Cheese. Season with $^1/_3$ tsp. Cracked Pepper, 1 teasp. Balsamic Vinegar and 1 teasp. Olive Oil.

—Roll dough to $^1/_4$-inch thick circle, about 12-inches in diameter. Pile filling onto one half. Fold uncovered side over filling; fold edges up and in to seal, then crimp. Transfer to a greased cookie sheet, brush top with Olive Oil and bake for 20-25 minutes, or until golden brown. Stand for 5 minutes before serving.

POCKET GYROS

This recipe works for: Digestive Health, Liver and Organ Health, Arthritis
Makes 2 Pitas:

Mix: $^1/_2$ cup shredded Arugula Leaves, $^1/_4$ cup crumbled Feta Cheese, $^1/_4$ cup chopped Black Olives, 2 TBS Jarred Roasted Red Peppers, and 1 small Tomato diced. Mix with 1 TB Balsamic Dressing. Stuff Small Pitas and serve.

LOW-FAT POCKET FALAFELS

This recipe works for: Sports Nutrition, Kid's and Men's Health, Heart Health
For 4 large pitas split; enough for 8 pita pockets: Preheat oven to 350°.

Blender blend FALAFEL BALLS. (Makes 48 balls): 4 cups canned GARBANZO BEANS, 3 CLOVES GARLIC, 1/3 cup diced CELERY, 1/2 cup diced ONION, 3 TBS TOASTED WHEAT GERM, 2 TBS SESAME TAHINI, 1/2 teasp. CUMIN SEED, 1/4 teasp. TURMERIC, 1/4 teasp. CAYENNE, 1/4 teasp. SEA SALT, 1/4 teasp. PEPPER. Chill in the fridge to blend flavors. Form mixture into 1-inch balls. Place on a LECITHIN-sprayed baking sheet; bake until golden brown.

—Divide 1 thin sliced CUCUMBER, 4 thin sliced TOMATOES, a 4-oz. tub ALFALFA SPROUTS, and FALAFEL BALLS among pita pocket halves. Top with spoons of PLAIN LOW-FAT YOGURT.

Nutrition: 260 calories; 13gm protein; 43gm carbohydrate; 10gm fiber; 5g total fat; 0mg choles.; 89mg calcium; 4mg iron; 95mg magnes.; 580mg potass.; 208mg sodium; Vit. A 49 IU, Vit. C 17mg; Vit. E 3 IU.

THAI LETTUCE WRAP

This recipe works for: Weight Loss, Women's Health, Bone Building
Makes 15 servings:

Soak 6 large dried SHIITAKE MUSHROOMS until soft; sliver and save soaking water.

—Make the sauce in a bowl: 2 TBS HOISIN SAUCE, 2 TBS TAMARI, 1 TB SAKE or SHERRY, 1 teasp. ARROWROOT POWDER, 1/4 teasp. WHITE PEPPER, 1/4 teasp. WASABI PASTE; set aside.

—Make the filling: Heat 2 TBS CANOLA OIL in a large wok. Add shiitakes and 1 TB minced CRYSTALLIZED GINGER; stir until fragrant, about 30 seconds. Add 2 STALKS CELERY diced, 1 large CARROT diced, 1 DAIKON WHITE RADISH or JICAMA diced; stir 1 minute. Add 1/2 cup chopped BAMBOO SHOOTS, 1/2 cup chopped WATER CHESTNUTS; stir 1 minute more. Add 2 sliced GREEN ONIONS, 1/2 cup chopped DRY ROASTED PEANUTS and sauce; cook until sauce boils and thickens a bit, about 1 minute.

—Wilt in hot water for 1 minute <u>only</u>, 15 big outer leaves from 1 large HEAD ICEBERG LETTUCE. To serve, divide filling on each leaf; roll and eat with your hands.

HAWAIIAN CHICKEN PITAS

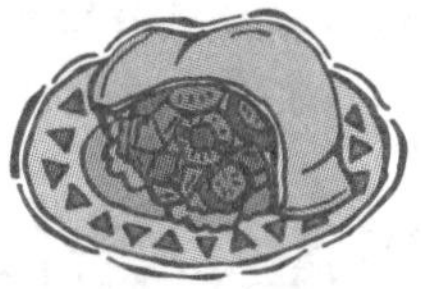
Pita

This recipe works for: Allergies and Asthma, Arthritis
For 6 pita pockets:

Sauté in a wok until opaque, 3/4 LB boneless, skinless ORGANIC CHICKEN BREASTS in bite-size chunks. Remove from heat and set aside.

—Mix in a bowl: 1/2 cup PLAIN LOW-FAT YOGURT, 1/4 cup diced CELERY, 1 cup diced PINEAPPLE, 1 TB LIME JUICE, 1/2 cup halved RED SEEDLESS GRAPES, 1/4 cup toasted slivered ALMONDS. Chill to let flavors blend. Add chicken to yogurt mix and fill pita pockets.

Nutrition: 193 calories; 21gm protein; 19gm carbohydrate; 2gm fiber; 3g total fat; 49mg choles.; 52mg calcium; 1mg iron; 39mg magnes.; 294mg potass.; 175mg sodium; Vit. A 11 IU; Vit. C 7mg; Vit. E 1 IU.

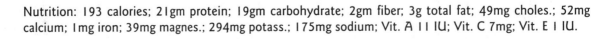

VIETNAMESE RICE PAPER WRAPS

This recipe works for: Liver and Organ Health, Allergies and Asthma, Arthritis
Makes 12 servings:

Make the DIPPING SAUCE: Bring to a boil over high heat, stirring until smooth: $^1/_4$ cup Hoisin Sauce, 1 TB Peanut Oil, and $^1/_3$ cup White Wine. Remove from heat; stir in 3 TBS chopped Dry Roasted Peanuts. Pour into serving bowl and set aside.

—In a pan, cover a Sweet Potato with Cold Water. Simmer until fork-tender, about 15 minutes. Cut in half lengthwise; peel and cut into 12 fat french fry size sticks.

—In a wok, heat 1 TB Peanut Oil. Add 1 LB Firm Tofu cut into 12 fat french fry size sticks; cook until golden turning on all sides, 5 to 7 minutes. Drain on paper towels.

–Peel 1 Cucumber, cut in 24 thin slices. Chop $^1/_4$ cup each: Chives, Cilantro Leaves and Mint. Rinse $1^1/_2$ cups Bean Sprouts, and 1 head Boston Lettuce Leaves.

—Place all filling ingredients on a platter. Place dipping bowl in center. Brush 12 Rice Paper Wrapper Triangles (find in an Oriental Food market) well with Water and arrange overlapping, on a large plate; they soften after standing for a few minutes.

—To make Vietnamese rolls, place a softened rice triangle on a flat surface, pointed end toward you. Lay 1 piece each tofu and sweet potato vertically in center. Top with 2 slices cucumber and a sprinkling of herbs. Roll up from one side into a cone. Distribute some bean sprouts on a lettuce leaf. Place rice cone on top and roll lettuce around it. Repeat with remaining ingredients. Serve with DIPPING SAUCE.

Nutrition: 143 calories; 8gm protein; 18gm carbohydrate; 1gm fiber; 5g total fat; 0mg choles.; 94mg calcium; 4mg iron; 48mg magnes.; 222mg potass.; 93mg sodium; Vit. A 351 IU; Vit. C 7mg; Vit. E 1 IU.

RED SALAD SANDWICH PITA

This recipe works for: Liver and Organ Health, Allergies, Digestive Health
Serves 4: Rinse and drain all beans.

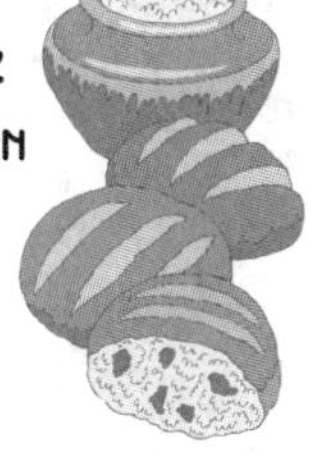

Combine: 3 TBS Balsamic Vinegar Dresssing, 2 TBS Lime Juice, 1 16-oz can Red Kidney or Pinto Beans, 1 diced Red Bell Pepper, 1 cup cooked Brown Rice, $^1/_2$ cup diced Red Onion, and 1 Red Tomato. Stuff in Pitas.

BARBECUED TURKEY WRAPS

This recipe works for: Stress Reduction, Respiratory Problems, Weight Control
For 6 wraps:

Sizzle 1 TB Canola Oil, 2 TBS Chipotle Chili Sauce and 2 large diced Onions for 5 minutes. Reduce heat and simmer over low until onions carmelize, 20 minutes. Stir in 2 cups shredded cooked Turkey, $^2/_3$ cup Smoky Barbecue Sauce, 2 TBS Dijon Mustard.

—Warm large Flour Tortillas one at a time in a dry skillet until soft. Spoon turkey mix down tortilla center. Cover with Baby Spinach Leaves. Roll up and eat.

High Protein Sandwiches

Want more protein for healing? A sandwich is an easy way to get usable protein without high fats or calories.

PEANUT BUTTER TOMATO CLUB

This recipe works for: Kid's Health, Illness Recovery, Sports Nutrition
For 2 sandwiches:

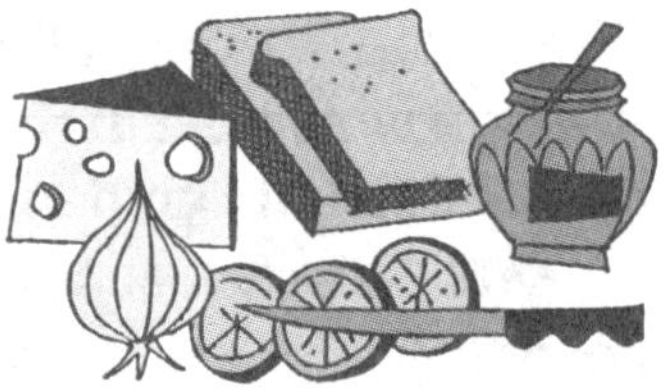

Spread 2 slices Whole Grain Toast with Peanut Butter. Top each with a Boston Lettuce Leaf. Sprinkle with 1 teasp. Soy Bacon Bits, 2 pinches Granulated Dulse and top with a Tomato slice. Spread 2 more slices of toast with Peanut Butter; place face up on top of the tomatoes. Cover each with a lettuce leaf and a slice of Low Fat Cheddar Cheese. Top with 1 more Tomato slice; spread Low Fat Mayonnaise on the last 2 pieces of toast. Cover, press down to set the sandwich and cut diagonally into quarters.

CLASSIC AVO JACK

This recipe works for: Recovery, Hair, Skin and Nails, Sugar Imbalances, Arthritis
For 1 sandwich:

Mix $^{1}/_{4}$ teasp. Herbal Seasoning Salt with 2 TBS Low Fat Mayonnaise. Spread on 2 slices Whole Grain Toast. Thin-slice several leaves Romaine Lettuce; cover toast slices.
—Fill sandwich with: 2 or 3 thin slices Avocado, 1 slice Jack Cheese or Rice Cheddar Cheese, Alfalfa Sprouts, and thin slices Cucumber. Sprinkle with Toasted Sunflower Seeds and Soy Bacon Bits. Cover with 2 slices Whole Grain Toast.

Nutrition: 420 calories; 17gm protein; 34gm carbohydrate; 8gm fiber; 25g total fat; 31mg choles.; 278mg calcium; 3mg iron; 110mg magnes.; 434mg potass.; 657mg sodium; Vit. A 108 IU; Vit. C 6mg; Vit. E 8 IU.

TURKEY PITAS

This recipe works for: Stress and Energy, Illness Recovery, Women's Health
Makes enough for 6 Pitas:

Mash together: 1 rinsed, drained 15-oz can Chickpeas, $^{1}/_{2}$ cup Plain Low Fat Yogurt, 2 TBS Olive Oil, $^{1}/_{2}$ cup Mixed Spicy Sprouts, 1 TB Tamari, 1 teasp. Garlic-Lemon Seasoning and 1 teasp. Ground Cumin.
—Combine in a bowl with: $1^{1}/_{2}$ cups shredded cooked Turkey, 2 cups diced European Cucumber, 2 cups diced Tomatoes, 4 TBS minced Red Onion, 2 TBS Lemon Juice, 2 TBS toasted Pine Nuts. Let stand 5 minutes to blend and stuff into Pitas.

SHIITAKE and FRESH TUNA HEAVENLY SANDWICH

This recipe works for: Brain Health, Hair, Skin and Nails, Fatigue Syndromes
For 4 sandwiches:

Mix 1 teasp. Honey, 1 TB Dijon Mustard and 1 TB Lemon Juice with 6 TBS Low Fat Mayonnaise. Let sit to blend. Soak 4 to 6 large dry Shiitake Mushrooms until soft. Sliver and discard woody stems.

—Slice a 16-oz. Fresh Ahi Tuna Filet into 4 slices. Brush tuna and mushrooms with Olive Oil, and let sit while you heat a griddle (or heavy skillet) to hot. Place tuna and mushrooms on griddle and grill one minute on each side.

—Spread spiced mayonnaise on 4 Whole Grain Toast slices. Top each slice with 2 Butter Lettuce Leaves, tuna and mushrooms. Sprinkle with Lemon Juice and Lemon-Pepper.

Nutrition: 292 calories; 38gm protein; 24gm carbohydrate; 3gm fiber; 4g total fat; 60mg choles.; 58mg calcium; 2mg iron; 109mg magnes.; 825mg potass.; 490mg sodium; Vit. A 27 IU; Vit. C 4mg; Vit. E trace

BLACK BEAN TORTILLA WRAP Protein and chlorophyll-rich

This recipe works for: Men's Health, Overcoming Addictions, Sports Nutrition
For 4 sandwiches:

Have ready 2 cups cooked, Short Grain Brown Rice; and 4 large Wheat Tortillas.

—Combine in a bowl: a 15-oz. can Black Breans, rinsed and drained, 1 diced Red Bell Pepper, 1 diced Tomato, 2 TBS minced Fresh Cilantro Leaves, 1 TB Olive Oil and 1 teasp. Garlic-Lemon Seasoning.

—Warm each Tortilla in a dry skillet until pliable. Lay flat and spread $^1/_2$ cup Brown Rice down center. Cover rice with bean filling. Roll up, tucking sides toward the center to form a bundle. Slice each in half and serve with Plain Yogurt dollops.

Nutrition: 321 calories; 12gm protein; 61gm carbohydrate; 10gm fiber; 6g total fat; 0mg choles.; 87mg calcium; 5mg iron; 75mg magnes.; 269mg potass.; 616mg sodium; Vit. A 23 IU; Vit. C 24mg; Vit. E 1 IU.

VEGETARIAN TUNA SALAD SANDWICH

This recipe works for: Recovery, Allergies and Asthma, Women's Health
Enough for 4 servings:

Mash spread in a bowl: 1 rinsed, drained 16-oz. can Chickpeas, $^1/_3$ cup diced Celery, $^1/_4$ cup diced Red Onion, $1^1/_2$ TBS Lemon Juice, 2 TBS Soy Mayonnaise, 1 cake Silken Tofu, $^1/_2$ tsp. Garlic-Lemon Seasoning, 2 teasp. Granulated Dulse and $^1/_4$ tsp. Cracked Pepper. Serve on crusty Whole Grain Bread.

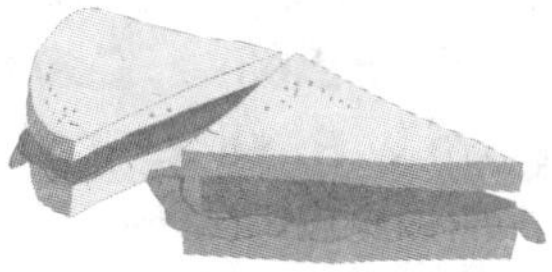

Open Face Topper Sandwiches

Want less density in your sandwich? Want to reduce your carb intake? Try these open face delights. Great for brunches, light lunches, weight control diets.

TOMATO HERB BRUSCHETTA

This recipe works for: Cancer Protection, Respiratory Problems, Men's Health
Makes enough for 8:

Cut a 12-oz. Loaf Italian Bread, diagonally into 8 slices; toasted under a broiler for 2 minutes. Cut 2 Cloves Garlic in half and let sit in 2 TBS Olive Oil in a small bowl.

—Combine TOMATO TOPPNG: mix $^1/_2$ teasp. Garlic Granules with 1 TB Olive Oil, 4 or 5 large, thin-sliced Roma Tomatoes, 1 thin sliced Yellow Bell Pepper, 1 TB Balsamic Vinegar, 2 TBS snipped Fresh Basil, 2 teasp. Fresh Oregano and $^1/_2$ teasp. Cracked Pepper. Toss to coat and set aside for 15 minutes to blend flavors.

—Brush Garlic-Olive Oil mix over toasted bread slices. Spoon on topping. Sprinkle with Parmesano-Reggiano Cheese. Run under broiler for 2 minutes only to heat.

Nutrition: 191 calories; 8gm protein; 24gm carbohydrate; 2gm fiber; 7g total fat; 5mg choles.; 138mg calcium; 2mg iron; 22mg magnes.; 166mg potass.; 257mg sodium; Vit. A 93 IU; Vit. C 26mg; Vit. E 1 IU.

CHICKEN MELT CROISSANTS

This recipe works for: Allergies and Respiratory Problems, Men's and Kid's Health
For 8 sandwich halves: Preheat broiler.

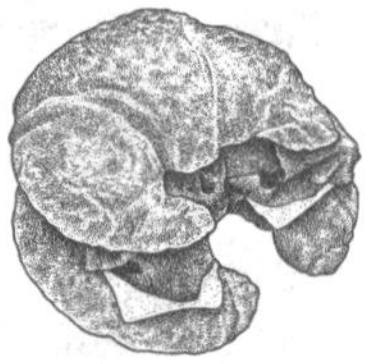

Split and toast 4 Whole Wheat Croissants to golden on a baking sheet, 2 minutes.

—Shred 2 cups cooked Chicken Breast into a bowl. Mix with Low Fat Mayonnaise. Add 3 minced Green Onions, 1 TB Lemon Juice, 1 TB Sweet Pickle Relish, 1 tsp. dry Tarragon, Dijon Mustard and Hot Pepper Sauce to taste.

—Spread each croissant half with chicken mix. Form the filling to the shape of the croissant half and let chill on the baking sheet before broiling. Top with grated Low Fat Swiss or Rice Swiss Cheese. Broil until cheese melts, about 30-45 seconds.

TERIYAKI TOFU SANDWICH

This recipe works for: Immune Breakdown Infection, Women's Health
For 4 sandwiches: Slice into 4 diagonal sandwiches.

Slice 12-oz. Extra Firm Tofu into slabs and marinate in 4 TBS bottled Teriyaki Sauce. Split a Whole Grain Italian Bread Loaf lengthwise. Cover cut halves with Low Fat Mayonnaise and Sweet-Hot Asian Mustard. Top with slices of Low Fat Swiss or Rice Swiss Cheese. Top with tofu slices. Pour over any remaining teriyaki sauce and broil until brown.

HOT BROWN

This recipe works for: Heart Health, Stress Reactions, Men's Health
For 4 sandwiches: Preheat broiler.

Make the sauce: Melt together 3 TBS Butter, 3 TBS Whole Wheat Flour and 2 TBS Soy Bacon Bits. Stir until bubbly; stir in 1 teasp. Sweet-Hot Mustard. Add 1 cup diced Low Fat Cheddar Cheese and 1/2 cup Low Fat Jack Cheese. Mix in 2 TBS Sherry and 2 TBS Plain Low Fat Yogurt.

—Toast 4 Whole Grain Bread slices. Cover each with a tablespoon of sauce, and slices of cooked Turkey Breast. Spoon rest of cheese sauce over. Top with Fresh Beefsteak Tomato slices and broil until sauce browns. Serve hot.

Nutrition: 327 calories; 25gm protein; 23gm carbohydrate; 5gm fiber; 14g total fat; 48mg choles.; 380mg calcium; 2mg iron; 81mg magnes.; 398mg potass.; 465mg sodium; Vit. A 144 IU; Vit. C 3mg; Vit. E 1 IU.

GRILLED BRIE with MUSHROOMS

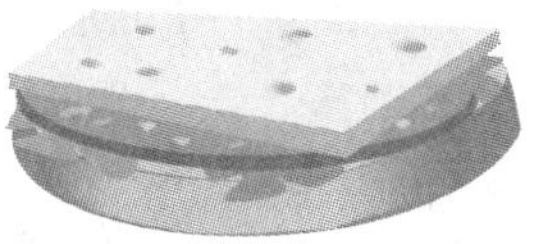

This recipe works for: Immune Health, Stress
For 4 sandwiches: Preheat griddle or broiler.

Sauté in 2 TBS Olive Oil: 6 Button Mushrooms or Chanterelles until soft, about 2 minutes. Add 2 snipped Green Onions and sauté until bright green. Remove from heat and season with Lemon-Pepper. Slice 4-oz. cold Brie Cheese into 4 slices. Put each slice of cheese on a slice of Whole Grain Bread. Soak 2 teasp. dry Tarragon in 2 TBS White Wine for 10 minutes. Drain and divide over each cheese slice. Divide mushroom mix on cheese and broil on an oiled sheet until cheese melts.

FOCACCIA with SWEET CARMELIZED ONIONS

This recipe works for: Heart Health, Stress Reactions, Hair, Skin and Nails
Makes 48 squares: Preheat oven to 375°F.

Sizzle 2 TBS Olive Oil in a skillet. Add 3 large diced Sweet Onions, 1 teasp. Sea Salt and Cracked Pepper to taste. Cook stirring occasionally about 15 minutes.

—Mix in a bowl: 4 TBS Frozen Orange Juice Concentrate, 2 TBS Tarragon Vinegar, 2 TBS Lemon Juice, 1 1/2 TBS grated Lemon Zest, 1 TB Lime Juice and 2 teasp. dry Tarragon. Add to onions and cook stirring until onions are very soft and sweetly aromatic.

—Cream topping together in a bowl: 4 TBS Parmesan-Reggiano Cheese, 4 TBS grated Provolone Cheese, 4 TBS Low Fat Cream Cheese, 2 TBS snipped Parsley.

—Break off tips of 48 Asparagus. (Save stems for another use.) Blanch tips in hot Water 1 minute only. Drizzle with 1 TB Olive Oil and season with Italian Herbs.

—Cut 1 large Focaccia with Olive Oil and cut into 48 squares; place them on a baking sheet. Divide cheese mix, onion mix and asparagus tips among squares. Bake 3 to 5 minutes until bubbly. Serve hot.

CALIFORNIA SUNSHINE MELT

This recipe works for: Weight Control, Arthritis, Allergies
For 2 sandwiches: Preheat broiler.

Toast 2 slices Whole Grain Bread. Spread with 2 TBS Low Fat Cream Cheese.
—Top each with thin-sliced Radishes, thin-sliced Tomatoes, thin-sliced Mushrooms, shredded Carrot, and a slice of Low Fat Swiss Cheese or Rice Swiss Cheese. Run under the broiler just to melt cheese. Top with Sunflower Sprouts or Spicy Mixed Sprouts.

Nutrition: 267 calories; 19gm protein; 24gm carbohydrate; 5gm fiber; 12g total fat; 30mg choles.; 365mg calcium; 2mg iron; 59mg magnes.; 446mg potass.; 493mg sodium; Vit. A 813 IU; Vit. C 13mg; Vit. E 1 IU.

SPICY NEW ORLEANS EGG SALAD

This recipe works for: Heart Health, Arthritis, Women's Health
For 4 sandwiches:

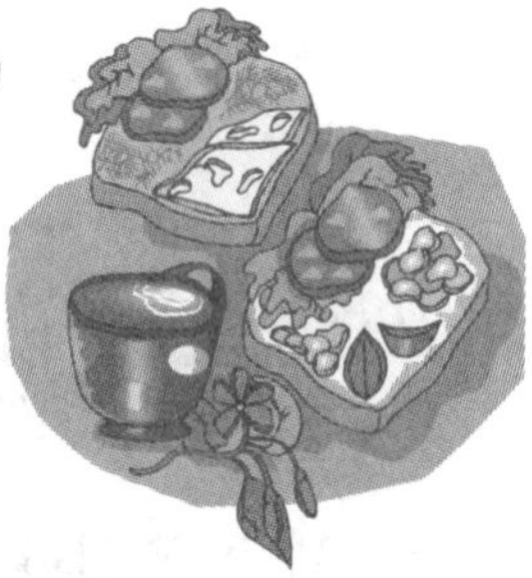

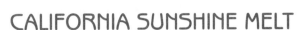

Hard boil 4 Eggs. Chop into a bowl.
—Sauté 1 slice Red Onion, diced, 1 slice Red Bell Pepper, diced, and 1 minced Clove Garlic in 1 TB Olive Oil until soft. Remove from heat and moisten with 2 TBS Low Fat Mayonnaise.
—Add 4 TBS diced Celery, 3 TBS Sweet Pickle Relish, 2 teasp. Sherry, 2 teasp. Sweet Paprika, 1 teasp. Lemon Juice, 1/2 teasp. Dill Weed, 1/2 teasp. Hot Pepper Sauce and, 1/2 teasp. Lemon-Pepper. Combine gently with eggs. Spread on Whole Grain Toast slices covered with Watercress or Arugula Leaves. Top with snipped Cilantro Leaves.

Nutrition: 230 calories; 10gm protein; 21gm carbohydrate; 3gm fiber; 12g total fat; 214mg choles.; 79mg calcium; 2mg iron; 42mg magnes.; 269mg potass.; 346mg sodium; Vit. A 222 IU; Vit. C 18mg; Vit. E 3 IU.

OPEN FACE LENTIL-WALNUT BRUSCHETTAS

This recipe works for: Liver and Organ Health, Sexuality Boost, Men's Health
For 1 long French Bread Loaf, about 8 servings:

Bring to a boil 3/4 cup rinsed Lentils and 1 1/2 cups salted Water; reduce heat, cover and simmer until lentils water is absorbed, about 40 minutes. Drain and set aside.
—In a small food processor, blend 3/4 cup chopped Walnuts to a paste. Scrape into lentils and combine the two with a fork. Mash in 1 TB Lemon Juice and 1/2 teasp. Lemon-Pepper, 1 cup minced Watercress or Arugula Leaves, 3 TBS Sherry, 1/4 teasp. ground Cumin, 1/4 teasp. dry Tarragon, and 1/4 teasp. ground Coriander. Spread on toasted French Bread slices, sprinkle with Soy Bacon Bits and broil until brown.

Nutrition: 253 calories; 11gm protein; 634m carbohydrate; 4gm fiber; 8 total fat; 0mg choles.; 79mg calcium; 4mg iron; 40mg magnes.; 245mg potass.; 510mg sodium; Vit. A 23 IU; Vit. C 5mg; Vit. E trace

Roll Up Party Sandwiches

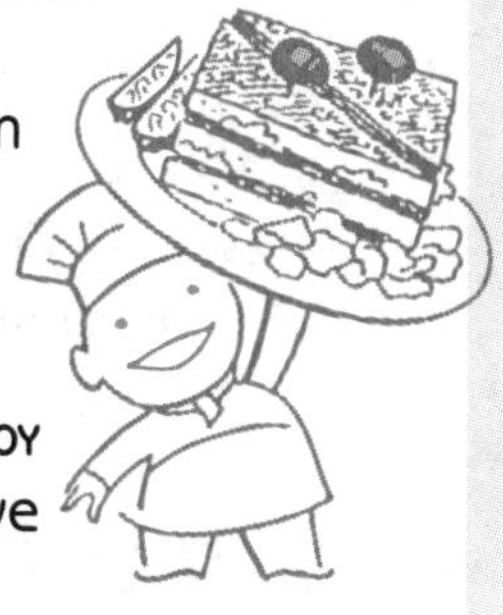

Roll up sandwiches are great party food.... light, neat, inexpensive, satisfying and easy-to-make for a crowd.

Buy the crackerbread dough circles for roll-ups from any deli section in a supermarket. They're big, soft, flat circles all ready to fill, available in plain, spinach or tomato flavors. The result is delicious either way.

Whatever filling you choose, basic roll up directions are the same:

1: Cover entire round with **Low Fat Cream Cheese, Kefir Cheese or Soy Cream Cheese**. Layer all filling ingredients pizza fashion on the circle. Leave 4 inches at one end covered only with the cream cheese.

2: Beginning at the end covered with filling, roll the bread tightly jelly-roll fashion toward the end covered with only the cream cheese. Ingredients will move down as you roll. Just tuck them under and keep rolling. The last roll acts as a seal.

3: Wrap in plastic to chill several hours. To serve, slice like a jelly roll into rounds. Each roll makes about 16 one-inch slices - about 30 calories per slice, and 3gm. fat.

ROAST TURKEY ROLL UP

This recipe works for: Weight Control, Hair and Skin, Anti-Aging

Mix 3-oz. Low Fat Cream Cheese with 2 TBS Plain Yogurt, 2 TBS Sweet Pickle Relish and 2 teasp. Dijon Mustard. Spread on entire round. Sprinkle with Lemon-Pepper. Layer on about 8-oz. thin Roast Turkey slices. Cover with slices Low Fat Swiss Cheese. Cover everything with plenty of Baby Spinach Leaves. Roll and chill as in directions above.

FRESH VEGETABLE and HERB ROLL UP

This recipe works for: Liver and Organ Health, Women's and Men's Health

Mix 3-oz. Low Fat Cream Cheese with 2 TBS Low Fat Mayonnaise, 1 TB Lemon Juice and 1 TB snipped Fresh Basil. Spread on entire round. Sprinkle with Sesame Salt and Cracked Pepper. Layer on thinly sliced Beefsteak Tomatoes, thin-sliced Black Olives and Cucumber. Sprinkle with grated Carrot and 2 TBS Roasted, Salted Sunflower Seeds. Cover everything with plenty of Baby Spinach Leaves. Roll and chill as in directions above.

HOT SALSA ROLL UP

This recipe works for: Sports Nutrition, Sexuality Boost, Men's Health

Mix 3-oz. Low Fat Cream Cheese with 2 TBS Plain Yogurt and 2 teasp. Hot Salsa. Spread on entire round. Sprinkle with pinches ground Cumin and Onion Salt. Cover with a layer of Refried Beans (no lard), thinly sliced Tomatoes, and a layer of thinly sliced Monterey Jack Cheese Slices. Roll and chill as in directions above.

WASABI CUCUMBER ROLL UPS

This recipe works for: Liver and Organ Health, Kidney- Bladder Health, Arthritis

Mix 3-oz. Low Fat Cream Cheese with 2 TBS Plain Yogurt, $^1/_2$ teasp. Granulated Dulse (or thin dry Dulse slices) and $^1/_4$ to $^1/_2$ teasp. Wasabi Paste. Spread on entire round. Top with 1 English Cucumber sliced paper thin, and $^1/_2$ cup Watercress or Arugula Leaves. Roll and chill as in directions on previous page.

SALMON and CREAM CHEESE ROLL UPS

This recipe works for: Hair, Skin and Nails, Sexuality Boost, Brain Enhancing

Mix 3-oz. Low Fat Cream Cheese with 2 TBS Low Fat Mayonnaise, and 2 teasp. Dijon Mustard. Spread on entire round. Sprinkle with Lemon-Pepper. Layer on about 8-oz. thin Smoked Salmon slices. Cover with slices Low Fat Swiss Cheese. Cover everything with plenty of Baby Spinach Leaves. Roll and chill as in directions on previous page.

GUACAMOLE ROLL UP

This recipe works for: Arthritis, Men's Health, Hair and Skin

Mash 3-oz. Low Fat Cream Cheese with 1 Avocado, 2 TBS Lemon Juice, 2 teasp. Hot Salsa, and 1 TB Tamari. Spread on entire round. Sprinkle with 2 teasp. Lemon-Garlic Seasoning. and 3 TBS snipped Fresh Cilantro. Layer on thinly sliced Tomatoes, and thin-sliced Green Olives. Roll and chill as in directions on previous page.

VERY LOW FAT PARTY ROLL UPS

This recipe works for: Weight Loss, Waste Management, Brain Enhancing

Mix 3-oz. Low Fat Cream Cheese with 2 TBS Plain Yogurt, 2 TBS Sweet Pickle Relish and 2 teasp. Dijon Mustard. Spread on entire round. Sprinkle with Lemon-Pepper. Layer on thinly sliced Beefsteak Tomatoes and Cucumber. Cover with slices Low Fat Swiss Cheese. Cover everything with plenty of Watercress or Arugula Leaves. Roll and chill.

TOMATO ROLL-UPS with BASIL MAYONNAISE

This recipe works for: Women's Health, Men's Health, Hair and Skin

Mix 3-oz. Low Fat Cream Cheese with 3 TBS Low Fat Mayonnaise, 2 TBS minced Red Onion, 3 TBS minced Fresh Basil Leaves and 1 teasp. Dijon Mustard. Spread on entire round. Layer on thinly sliced Beefsteak Tomatoes and slices Low Fat Cheddar Cheese. Roll and chill.

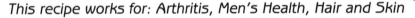

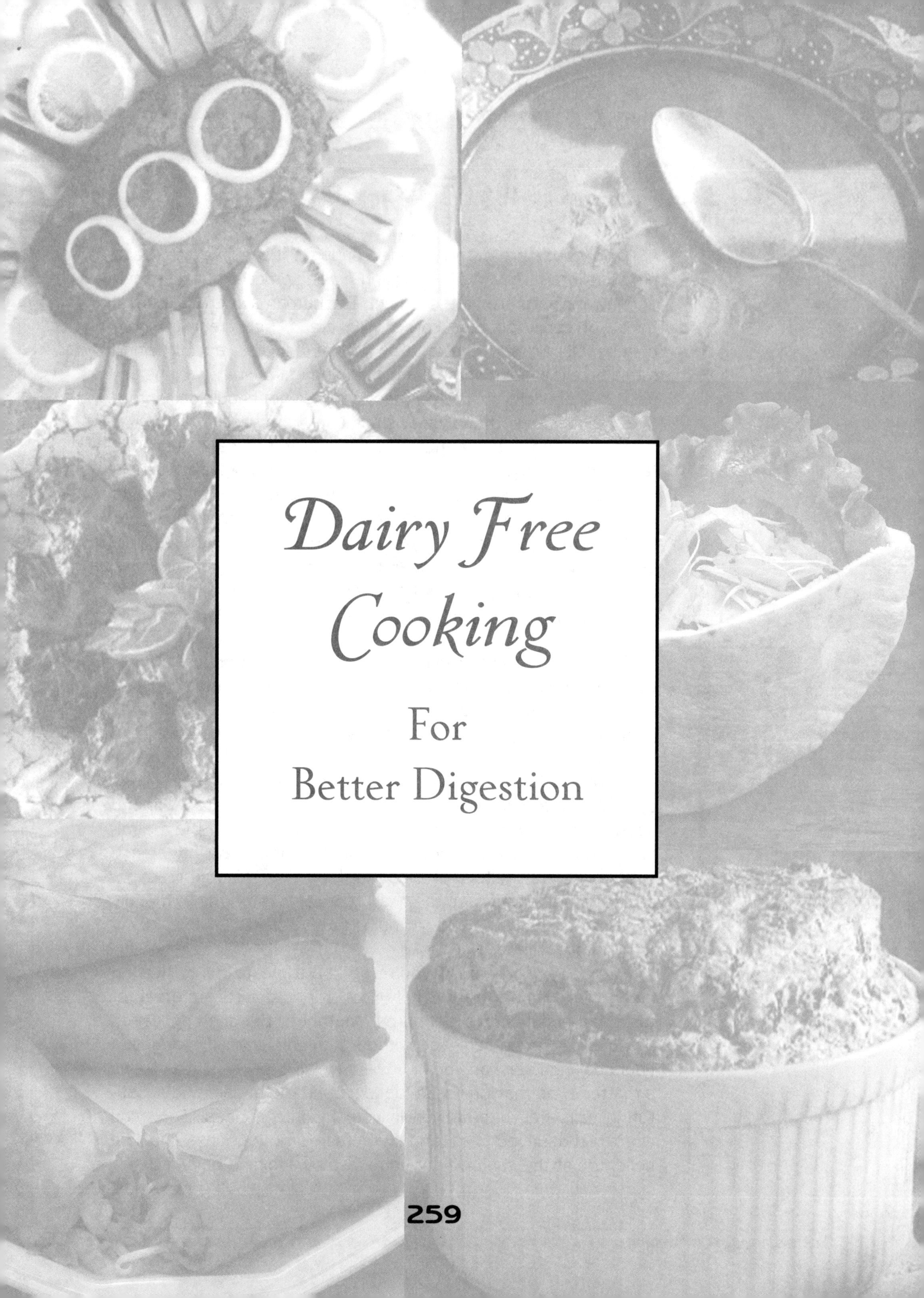

Dairy Free Cooking

For Better Digestion

Dairy Free Cooking

Dairy foods are better avoided during a cleansing diet. Dairy products interfere with the cleansing-healing process because their density and saturated fats are high. The human system in general does not easily process cow's milk, cream, ice cream or hard cheese. Our bodies tend to throw off dairy excess, accumulating strain on eliminative organs, and clogging our systems as the unused matter backs up. Women especially, do not handle dairy products well because their systems back up more easily.

For over 25% of Americans, dairy intolerance causes allergic reactions, poor digestion, and heavy mucous build-up. Even people with no noticeable sensitivity to dairy products report a rise in energy when they stop using them as a main part of their diet. Reducing high dairy fats usually means effective weight loss, reduced blood pressure and lower cholesterol levels. Female problems, such as fibrous growths, bladder and kidney ailments are improved by avoiding dairy foods.

Do you need dairy foods for calcium? Dairy products are not our best source of calcium. Heavy processing, high fat content, and an unbalanced ratio with phosphorus mean absorbability is poor. Vegetables, nuts, seeds, fish and sea greens have calcium that is much easier to assimilate. Soy cheese and milk, rice cheese and milk (delicious), almond cheese and milk, and tofu among other foods, are all good substitutes for dairy products. Kefir and yogurt, although made from milk, are normally free of the assimilation problems of dairy products. Unless your lactose intolerance is quite severe, neither of these foods causes allergic reaction, and they are beneficial to the healing process through the friendly bacteria cultures they add to your digestive tract.

Are dairy foods OK if you're <u>not</u> on a cleansing or healing diet? A little is fine - a lot is not. Most dairy products are great for taste, but questionable for optimum nutrition. But don't despair.... rich quality can be achieved without rich dairy. Small changes in your cooking habits and point of view are all it takes..... it's mostly a matter of not having these foods around the house, and substituting dairy-free alternatives in your favorite recipes. Soon you won't feel deprived at all; and if you're like most people, you'll be delighted at the easy weight you'll lose by avoiding dairy fats.

Your Dairy Food Options

See the Diet Book page 86 and 476 for more on dairy foods.

—**Rice Milk:** Made of brown rice, brown rice syrup, canola oil, seasonings and sea greens, rice milk is my personal favorite as a dairy substitute. The taste is delicious, it's full of nutrition and it works beautifully in recipes (Use the plain in savory recipes, vanilla in sweet dishes.)

—**Amazake Rice Drink**: a macrobiotic favorite widely available in health food stores, amazake may also be used cup for cup as a milk substitute in recipes. Simply blend 1/2 cup amazake with 2 cups water in a blender.

—**Rice Cheese:** Made from rice milk, rice cheese is a mild, delicious cheese replacement. With a small amount of casein, it is meltable for cooked dishes.

—**Rice Dream Frozen Dessert:** now available in several flavors, it is sweeter and has a better texture than frozen soy desserts.

—**Yogurt**: smooth and creamy, yogurt is a good intestinal cleanser, beneficial for health. To use cup for cup as a replacement for milk in recipes: mix 1/2 cup plain yogurt with 1/2 cup broth, white wine, water or sparkling water for lightness. For baking, where richness is needed (like a cheesecake), or for whipped cream consistency, whip one-third the amount of heavy cream called for in the recipe, then fold in the remaining two-thirds with non-fat plain yogurt.

—**Yogurt Cheese, cream cheese style**: much lighter in fat and calories than sour cream or cream cheese, but with the same richness and consistency.

How to make it: Use a piece of cheesecloth or a sieve-like plastic funnel, (available from kitchen catalogs or hardware stores). Spoon in as much plain yogurt as you want, usually use about 16-oz. Hang the cheesecloth over the sink faucet (put the funnel over a large glass). It takes about 14 to 16 hours for the whey to drain out. Voila! you have yogurt cheese. (Use the whey as a delicious part of the liquid in soups and stews). Stored in a covered container in the refrigerator, it will keep for 2 to 3 weeks.

—**Yogurt Cheese, block cheese style**: available in health food and gourmet food stores. A dairy food with yogurt, acidophilus cultures and enzymes added, yogurt cheese is a block cheese made in the semi-soft Farmer cheese style.

—**Yogurt Sour Cream**: for 1 cup: mix 1/2 cup low-fat soy mayonnaise and 1/2 cup low-fat plain yogurt for a healthy non-dairy food.

—**Kefir**: a cultured food made by adding kefir grains (naturally formed milk proteins), to milk and letting it incubate to milkshake consistency. Kefir has 350mg of calcium per cup. Use plain kefir cup for cup as a replacement for whole milk, buttermilk or half-and-half; use fruit flavored kefir in sweet baked recipes.

—**Kefir Cheese**: an excellent replacement for sour cream or cream cheese in recipes, kefir cheese is low in fat and calories, and has a slight tangy-rich flavor that enhances snack foods. Use it cup for cup in place of sour cream, cottage cheese, cream cheese or ricotta.

—**Soy Milk**: nutritious, versatile, smooth and delicious, soy milk is vegetable-based, lactose/cholesterol free. With unsaturated or poly-unsaturated fats, soy milk in your diet can help reduce serum cholesterol. Soy milk contains less calcium and calories than milk, and more protein and iron. It adds a slight rise to baked goods. Use it cup for cup as a milk replacement in cooking; plain flavor for savory dishes, vanilla for sweet dishes or on cereal.

—**Soy Cheese**: made from soy milk, the small amount of calcium caseinate (a milk protein) added allows it to melt. Mozarrella, cheddar, jack and cream cheese types are available. Use it cup for cup in place of any low-fat or regular cheese.

—**Soy Ice Cream**: frozen desserts and soy yogurt are available in many flavors.

—**Soy Yogurt Cheese**: use the recipe for yogurt cheese on the preceeding page

—**Soy Mayonnaise**: has the taste and consistency of regular mayonnaise.

—**Soy Lecithin**: low in fat and cholesterol, lecithin helps thicken and emulsify ingredients. It can make many recipes extra rich and smooth. Add a tablespoon of lecithin granules to a sauce, custard dessert or homemade ice-y dessert.

—**Tofu:** a white, digestible curd made from soybeans, tofu is a good replacement for dairy foods, in texture, taste and nutritional content. It is high in protein, low in fat and contains no cholesterol. Available in a wealth of varieties, tofu is extremely versatile, and may be used in place of eggs, sour cream, cheese and cottage cheese. See the *Cultured Foods* section, page 400 in this book for more information and recipes.

—**Miso**: a fermented paste made from cooked aged soybeans and certain whole grains, miso is a good dairy substitute in macrobiotic and cleansing-alkalizing diets. Light miso mixed with vegetable or onion stock is a tasty replacement for milk.

—**Coconut Milk:** a bittersweet liquid made by simmering equal parts of shredded fresh coconut and water. May be used in place of oil, fat and butter, but it's high in calories and fat, so use in moderation. A good complete protein source for children.

—**Frozen Fruit:** use in smoothies, shakes and dessert sauces and toppings. Simply peel, chunk and freeze fresh fruit. Then blend it in the blender. It may be used cooked or as is, or combined with other ingredients, and 1 to 2 TBS lecithin granules.

—**Fruit Juice:** may be used to replace milk in baked recipes. Apple and pear juices on cereals (either hot or cold) instead of milk are delicious.

—**Tapioca:** a sweet sun-dried starch made by crushing cassava roots with water, tapioca is natural thickener in cooking, a dessert favorite with children and easily digested by the elderly and small children.

—**Low Fat Cottage Cheese**: a low-fat, cultured dairy product, cottage cheese is well tolerated by those with only slight lactose intolerance, and is a good substitute for ricotta, commercial cream cheese, and processed cottage cheese foods that are full of chemicals. Mix with non-fat or low-fat plain yogurt to add the richness of cream or sour cream to recipes without the fat.

—**Almond Milk**: rich and nutty tasting; use one to one in place of milk in baked recipes, sauces or gravies. To make 1 cup almond milk: blender blend 1 teasp. almond butter, 1 teasp. honey and 1 cup water until very smooth.

—**Almond Cheese**: made from almond milk, a nutty, non-melting cheese, good in salads, spreads, dips, dressings or sandwiches.

—**Sesame Tahini**: sesame butter made from ground sesame seeds. Use tahini in place of cream or sour cream in dips, sauces and gravies. Mix with water to milk consistency as a high protein milk substitute for baking. Tahini complements greens and vegetables. Mix tahini with oil and other dressing ingredients for salads. Use tahini on toast or bread instead of peanut butter, on pancakes instead of butter. May be used almost anywhere you would use sesame seeds.

—**Tahini Milk**: use as a cup for cup dairy substitute in recipes: add 1 TB sesame tahini and 1 teasp. honey to 8-oz. water in a blender and blend smooth.

—**Butter:** Although butter is a saturated fat, it is relatively stable and the body can use it in small amounts for energy. Its make-up, like that of raw cream, is a whole and balanced food, used by the body better than its separate components might indicate. if you use butter, use raw unsalted butter, never margarine, pasteurized butter or shortening. Don't let butter get hot enough to sizzle or smoke.

For less fat saturation, simply clarify the butter by melting it and skimming off the top foam. Remove from heat. Let rest a few minutes, and spoon off the clear butter for use. Discard whey solids that settle to the bottom of the pan.

High quality vegetable oil (or a blend of butter and oil) may be substituted for butter without loss of taste.

The new trans fat free soy spreads are acceptable vegetarian alternatives in baking recipes and on breads and pancakes.

Organic vegetable, chicken and onion broths are good substitutes for butter in stir fried recipes and sautés

—**Eggs:** although they contain cholesterol, eggs are also high in balancing lecithins and phosphatides, and do not increase the risk of atherosclerosis. The difference in nutrition-rich, fertile eggs from free "scratch and run" chickens and the products from commercial egg factories is remarkable; the yolk color is brighter, the flavor clearly fresher, and the workability in recipes better. The distinction is particularly noticeable in poached and baked eggs, where the yolks firm up and rise higher. Eggs should be lightly cooked for the best nutrition, preferably poached, soft-boiled, or baked, never fried.

—Egg Replacer Mix, a product made from potato starch and tapioca flour is a viable substitute for baking needs.

—Tofu may be used in place of eggs in quick breads, cakes, custards and quiches.

—Flax seeds and water mixed can replace eggs in quick breads, pancakes and muffins. Use $^1/_4$ cup flax seeds to $^3/_4$ cup water. Whirl in the blender until thoroughly crushed, and add to batter in place of 3 eggs.

—Dry yeast or sourdough starter may be used as a leavener in place of eggs.

—Starchy vegetables may be used as thickeners in place of eggs in savory recipes. Apple sauce may be used as a thickener in sweet recipes.

When you do opt for dairy foods, purchase low-fat or non-fat products; buy goat's milk, or raw milk and cheeses that provide immediately usable protein, with a proper calcium/phosphorus/sodium ratio. There is a world of difference in taste. Raw, fresh cream cheese is light years ahead of commercial brands with gums, fillers and thickeners. Raw mozzarella, farmer's cheese, ricotta and cheddar are notably superior in taste to pasteurized cheeses or cheese foods with high salt and additives.

Dairy Free Recipe Sections

The dairy free recipes here emphasize traditional areas of diet where dairy's richness and creaminess are hard to omit.

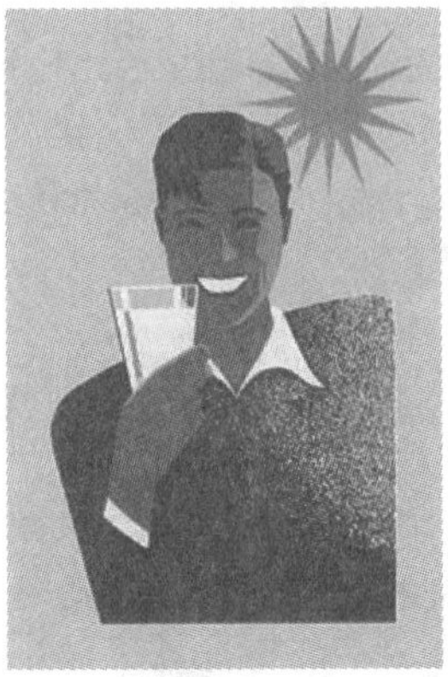

Dairy Free Appetizers and Starters

Appetizers and snacks without cheese or dairy-rich fillings seem almost like a contradiction in terms. A small sampling is offered in this section to give you inspiration in the right direction. I have served these recipes many times to compliments, even at gatherings where no one had a problem with dairy foods.

ITALIAN TOMATO TOAST

This recipe works for: Kid's and Men's Health, Liver - Organ Health, Heart Health
For 6 servings: Preheat oven to 350°.

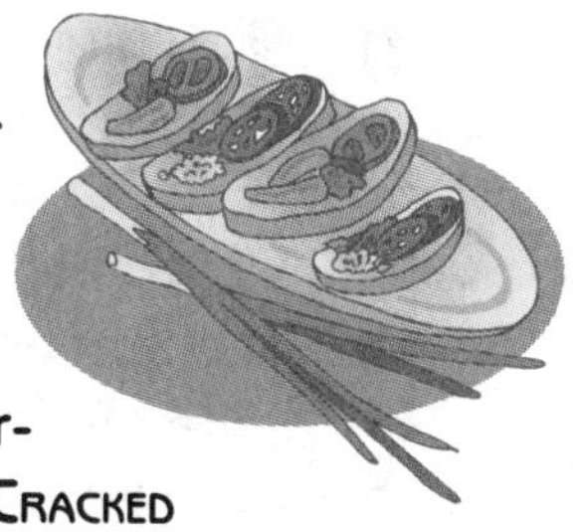

Slice 1 long Italian Bread Loaf in 1/4" slices. Lay on a lecithin-sprayed baking sheet and drizzle 4 TBS Olive Oil over the slices. Toast in the oven for 10 minutes. Remove, but leave oven on.

—Line a shallow baking dish with half the slices. Patch empty spaces with bits of toast. Slice 4 large Tomatoes and arrange overlapped on top. Drizzle with 2 TBS Olive Oil. Season with Sea Salt, Cracked Pepper and pinches Fructose. Top with 2 TBS minced Green Onion. Cover with the rest of the toast. Drizzle with 2 TBS Olive Oil more.

—Toast 2 Whole Wheat Sourdough Bread slices in the oven (or use equivalent Seasoned Bread Crumbs). Crumb in the blender with 6 TBS Soy Parmesan or Rice Parmesan Cheese, and scatter over dish. Bake uncovered for 45 minutes until light brown. Then cover with foil and bake for 15 minutes until soft.

Nutrition: 249 calories; 6gm protein; 22gm carbohydrate; 2gm fiber; 15g total fat; trace choles.; 106mg calcium; 2mg iron; 26mg magnesium; 329mg potass.; 271mg sodium; Vit. A 56 IU; Vit. C 15mg; Vit. E 5 IU.

FRESH HERB EGGPLANT ROLLS

This recipe works for: Overcoming Addictions, Liver - Organ Health, Men's Health
For 8 to 10 appetizer servings: Preheat oven to 375°.

Peel 1 large Eggplant. Cut into quarters, then into 8ths for 32 slices 1/8" thick.

—Mix 3 TBS Olive Oil with 2 teasp. Garlic-Lemon Seasoning. Brush on 3 baking pans. Lay eggplant slices in a single layer. Brush with rest of oil and bake until soft and brown, about 12 minutes. Do not let scorch. Loosen with a spatula and let cool.

Mix topping in a small bowl: 1 TB Olive Oil, 2 teasp. Fresh or Dry Rosemary Leaves, 3 TBS snipped Fresh Basil Leaves (or 1 teasp. dry), 2 teasp. Fresh Oregano Leaves (1/2 teasp. dry) and 8-oz. Soy or Rice Mozzarella. Cut into 32 two-inch long pieces.

—Place a piece of cheese on the narrow end of the eggplant slice. Roll to enclose. Place seam side down on an ovenproof platter. Season lightly and heat just before serving. Even people who haven't liked eggplant (like my husband), like this.

Nutrition: 116 calories; 2gm protein; 3gm carbohydrate; 1gm fiber; 11g total fat; 0 choles.; 40mg calcium; 2mg iron; 26mg magnesium; 104mg potass.; 352mg sodium; Vit. A 13 IU; Vit. C 2mg; Vit. E 5 IU.

QUICK DAIRY-FREE SAVORIES

This recipe works for: Allergies and Asthma, Digestive Health, Candida Infection

Spread 1 package Thin Savory Rice Crackers on a baking sheet. Cut slices of Rice Cheddar Cheese into 4 squares. Lay on top of crackers and top with minced Red Bell Pepper and Green Onion. Sprinkle with Hot Pepper Sauce and broil til bubbly.

SULTAN'S PURSES

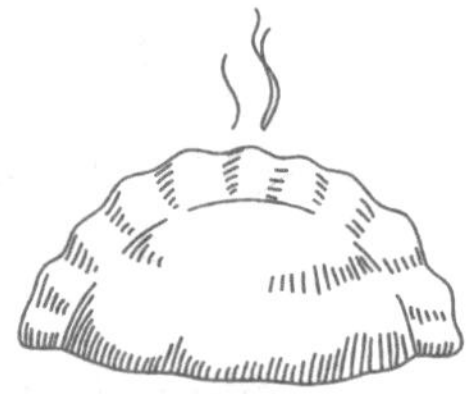

This recipe works for: Arthritis, Liver - Organ Health, Cancer Control
For 60 steamed pouches:

Soak 6 dried Shiitake Mushrooms to soften. Sliver and set aside. Reserve soaking water. Separate white and green parts from a large bunch of Scallions. Sliver $^1/_4$ cup green slices for topping and set aside. Separate the white and yolk of 1 Egg.

—Bring 2 cups Water to a rapid boil. Add $^1/_4$ teasp. Baking Soda and the Scallions and blanch until bright green, 2 minutes. Rinse under cold water and sliver.

—Blender blend the SAVORY FILLING: 8-oz. tiny cooked Salad Shrimp, 1 teasp. Tamari, 2 TBS Arrowroot Powder, $1^1/_2$ teasp. Fructose, 1 teasp. Sesame Salt (gomashio), 1 Egg White, $1^1/_2$ teasp. Toasted Sesame Oil, $1^1/_2$ teasp. grated Ginger, $1^1/_2$ teasp. Canola Oil, 1 TB Sake and $^1/_4$ teasp. Black Pepper. Turn into a bowl, add $^1/_4$ cup diced Water Chestnuts and $^1/_4$ cup Green Peas. Mix lightly, and chill.

—Separate 60 skins from a package of won ton wrappers. Put about 1 teaspoon of filling in the center of each. Draw the four points of the sides together, seal edges with Egg Yolk, and twist the top to form a drawstring "purse." Chill.

—Use a large steamer or wok with a steaming rack, and bring an inch of water to a boil. Cover with Spinach Leaves, and put purses in a single layer on the leaves. Steam for 10 minutes. Transfer purses to a serving plate lined with Boston Lettuce Leaves. Sprinkle with reserved scallions.

—Make the DIPPING SAUCE: Mix 3 TBS Dry Mustard or Chinese Hot Mustard Powder in a bowl with $1^1/_2$ teasp. Hot Pepper Sauce and enough water to make a dip.

Nutrition per: 20 calories; 1gm protein; 2gm carbohydrate; trace fiber; 1g total fat; 10mg choles.; 6mg calcium; 1mg iron; 14mg magnesium; 42mg potass.; 30mg sodium; Vit. A 10 IU; Vit. C 1mg; Vit. E trace

SHERRY MUSHROOMS on RYE

This recipe works for: Anti-Aging, Liver - Organ Health, Immune Health
For 8 to 10 servings:

Heat 6 TBS Olive Oil and 1 teasp. Garlic-Lemon Seasoning in a skillet until hot. Add 1 small Red Onion chopped and sizzle for 10 minutes. Add $1^1/_2$ LBS Button or Cremini Mushrooms; sizzle and toss for 20 minutes. Add $^3/_4$ cup Sherry, dashes Sesame Salt and Pepper, and simmer for about 10 minutes. Serve hot on toasted Rye Cocktail Rounds.

WHITE BEAN PATÉ STEEPED in HERBS

This recipe works for: Brain Boosting, Sports Nutrition, Fatigue Syndromes
For 8 servings:

Blender blend: 2 cups cooked White Beans, 1 teasp. Garlic-Lemon Seasoning or 2 Cloves Garlic minced, $^1/_2$ cup peeled diced Shallots, and $^1/_2$ teasp. each dry Basil, snipped Fresh or dry Rosemary, dry Sage, dry Lemon Peel, dry Thyme, Dill Weed and dry Tarragon. Add 1 teasp. Dijon Mustard, 1 TB Sesame Tahini, 1 TB Capers, $^1/_2$ teasp. Sea Salt, $^1/_2$ teasp. White Pepper and $^1/_4$ teasp. Nutmeg.

—Transfer to a serving dish. Snip on top 2 TBS Fresh Parsley, add dashes Hot Pepper Sauce. Snip on more fresh herbs to taste. Chill briefly; serve on crackers.

Nutrition: 87 calories; 5gm protein; 14gm carbohydrate; 4gm fiber; 1g total fat; 0 choles.; 52mg calcium; 2mg iron; 44mg magnesium; 275mg potass.; 70mg sodium; Vit. A 12 IU; Vit. C 3mg; Vit. E 1 IU.

DAIRY FREE MUSHROOM PATÉ

This recipe works for: Allergies and Asthma, Cancer Protection, Immune Health
For 1 cup - 4 servings:

Soak 1-oz. Shiitake Mushrooms in water until soft. Sliver and discard woody stems. Save soaking water. Mix shiitakes with 5-oz. chopped Button Mushrooms and $^1/_3$ cup minced Onion. Sauté the mixture in 2 TBS Olive Oil for 15 minutes until softened. Remove from heat and stir in 1 TB Sherry, $^1/_2$ carton Kefir Cheese or Soy Cream Cheese, or 2 crumbled Cubes Tofu, and $^1/_4$ cup chopped Parsley.

—Whirl in the blender if a smooth paté is desired, or pack into a thick crock. Chill overnight or longer (it just gets better if covered well, up to a week). Use cocktail knives to spread on Toasted Rye Rounds.

Nutrition: 242 calories; 15gm protein; 19gm carbohydrate; 4gm fiber; 14g total fat; 0 choles.; 176mg calcium; 9mg iron; 86mg magnesium; 460mg potass.; 151mg sodium; Vit. A 32 IU; Vit. C 6mg; Vit. E 1 IU.

JALAPEÑO POTATO Mibbles

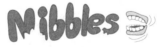

This recipe works for: Liver and Organ Health, Men's Health, Sports Nutrition

Cut 12 small Red Potatoes in half and steam until tender. Scoop out some of the meat from the cut side to leave a shell for filling.

—Mix potato meat with Soy Bacon Bits and grated Soy or Rice Jalapeño Cheese to taste. Add 1 teasp. Worcestershire Sauce and $^1/_4$ teasp. Black Pepper.

—Stuff potato shells. Arrange on a baking sheet and broil until brown and crispy on top. Sprinkle with drops Hot Pepper Sauce and serve with toothpicks.

Nutrition: 55 calories; 2gm protein; 9gm carbohydrate; 1gm fiber; 1g total fat; 0 choles.; 10mg calcium; 1mg iron; 16mg magnesium; 165mg potass.; 9mg sodium; Vit. A 5 IU; Vit. C 5mg; Vit. E 1 IU.

Creamy Dairy Free Dips and Spreads

Today's dairy free foods are great in your favorite dip and spread recipes, without depriving you of any creamy richness. Try soy and rice cheeses or tofu in place of cheese. Lactobacillus cultured dairy foods like yogurt, yogurt cheese or kefir cheese are healthful for all but those with the most severe dairy allergies; use them in place of sour cream, cream cheese or cottage cheese. If you choose a total vegan diet, use sesame tahini, tofu, avocados and ground nuts or nut milk to replace dairy foods.

TRIPLE HOT TOFU GUACAMOLE

This recipe works for: Sugar Imbalances, Fatigue Syndromes, Respiratory Healing
For about 8 servings:

Mash together in a bowl: 1 large Avocado, peeled and seeded, 1 teasp. Onion Powder, 1 teasp. Chili Powder, $^1/_4$ teasp. Hot Pepper Sauce, 2 TBS Lemon Juice, 1 Tomato, seeded and diced, and 2 Cakes Tofu mashed. Sprinkle $^1/_4$ teasp. Sweet Paprika on top. Serve with rice chips, tamari chips or vegetable crackers.

Nutrition per: 87 calories; 4gm protein; 6gm carbohydrate; 3gm fiber; 6gm total fat; 0mg choles.; 45mg calcium; 2mg iron; 48mg magnesium; 249mg potass.; 36mg sodium; Vit. A 47 IU; Vit. C 8mg; Vit. E 3 IU.

DANNY'S HOT ASPARAGUS DIP People wax poetic over this dip.

This recipe works for: Arthritis, Women's Health, Hair, Skin and Nails
For 2 to 3 servings:

Sauté 2 teasp. Canola Oil and 1 small chopped Red Onion until soft and fragrant.
—Lightly steam 1 bunch Fresh Asparagus. Chop asparagus and blender blend until smooth with an 8-oz. carton Soy Cream Cheese, $^1/_2$ teasp. Sesame Salt and the onions. Serve warm.

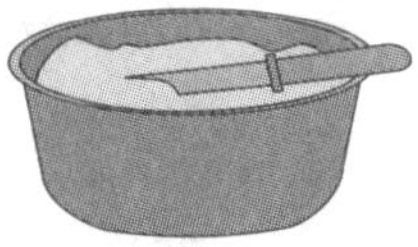

ALWAYS SURPRISING DIP and SPREAD

The base of this dip is pureed vegetables - excellent for those with dairy sensitivities. Every combination is surprisingly different, and almost every combination works. If you liked it yesterday as a soup or salad or casserole, you will like it as a dip today. Leftover lentil, black bean or pea soup are especially good.

Take any left-over salad and dressing, or leftover steamed veggies and sauce, or the last serving of a vegetable casserole, or the remains of yesterday's vegetable soup, and puree it in the blender. Sometimes that's all there is to it; a delicious raw veggie or cracker spread just as it is.

If it needs more spice, add something for richness.... your favorite Spices and Herbs, a Tofu Cube, an Avocado, Sesame Tahini, or Kefir Cheese.

AUTUMN SWEET POTATO SPREAD for PITA CHIPS

This recipe works for: Arthritis, Women's Health, Hair, Skin and Nails
Makes about 12 servings:

Have ready a big bowl of baked Pita Chips.

—Bake 2 Sweet Potatoes at 350° until soft, 40-60 minutes. Let cool. Then peel potatoes and drop into a blender.

—Heat 2 tsp. Canola Oil in a saucepan: sizzle 1 minced Yellow Onion until dark gold, about 20 minutes. Add onions to the blender. Add 1 TB Maple Syrup, 2 TBS Sesame Tahini and 1/2 teasp. Lemon-Pepper. Blend smooth. Spread warm or chilled on pita chips.

Nutrition per: 98 calories; 3gm protein; 17gm carbohydrate; 3gm fiber; 2g total fat; 0mg choles.; 17mg calcium; 1mg iron; 30mg magnesium; 138mg potass.; 78mg sodium; Vit. A 443 IU; Vit. C 5mg; Vit. E 1 IU.

GINGER DIP with TOFU Serve with sliced, chunked raw vegetables.

This recipe works for: Candida Recovery, Liver - Organ Health, Heart Health
Makes about 2 cups:

Blender blend: 16-oz. Silken Soft Tofu, 1/4 cup chopped Green Onion, 3 TBS minced Crystallized Ginger, 2 TBS Tamari, 1 teasp. Toasted Sesame Oil, 1/2 teasp. Garlic-Lemon Seasoning and a pinch Cayenne Pepper; chill to let flavors bloom.

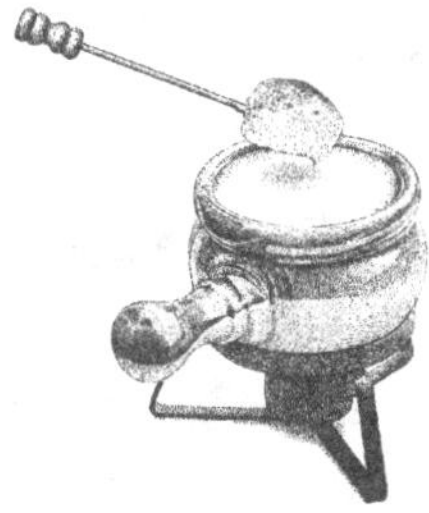

THREE STAR DIP for RAW VEGETABLES

This recipe works for: Arthritis, Liver - Organ Health, Hair, Skin
Makes about 8 servings:

Blender blend 1 large Avocado, seeded and peeled, 1 Grapefruit, seeded and sectioned, 1 large Tomato, seeded and chopped, 1 teasp. Sesame Salt, 1/2 teasp. Chili Powder, 1/4 teasp. Cracked Pepper, 1 TB minced Fresh Herbs of your choice.

Nutrition per: 53 calories; 1gm protein; 5gm carbohydrate; 3gm fiber; 4g total fat; 0mg choles.; 10mg calcium; trace iron; 15mg magnesium; 223mg potass.; 93mg sodium; Vit. A 31 IU; Vit. C 15mg; Vit. E 1 IU.

NUTTY DELIGHT delicious chilled on celery sticks or apple crescents.

This recipe works for: Men's and Kid's Health, Sports Nutrition, Heart Health
For 2 cups:

Toast in the oven until golden and fragrant: 3 TBS Sunflower Seeds, 3 TBS Sesame Seeds, 4 TBS Cashews. Then blender blend until buttery with 1 cup Peanut Butter, 1/2 cup Sesame Tahini. Add Sea Salt to taste.

TOFU TAHINI DIP

This recipe works for: Women's Health, Hair, Skin and Nails, Fatigue Syndromes
For 1 cup:

Blender blend everything: 2 TBS Raspberry Vinegar, 1 minced Green Onion, $^1/_2$ cup snipped Fresh Parsley, 1 Cube Tofu, 1 teasp. Toasted Sesame Oil, $^1/_4$ cup Sesame Tahini, 2 TBS White Wine, 1 TB Lemon Juice, 1 TB Tamari, $^1/_2$ teasp. Sesame Salt, $^1/_4$ teasp. Black Pepper, $^1/_4$ teasp. Paprika.

HOT GREEN BEAN and POTATO PUREE

This recipe works for: Arthritis, Liver - Organ Health, Weight Loss
For 6 servings: Preheat oven to 450°.

Cook 1 LB small, thin skinned White Potatoes in boiling salted water for 10 minutes. Add 1 LB frozen French-Cut Green Beans, partially cover pot, and cook for 5 minutes more. Drain. Puree in the blender with 5 TBS Canola Oil and dashes of Nutmeg, Sea Salt and Pepper. Scrape into a lecithin-sprayed baking dish. Bake for 15 minutes until a skin forms on the top. Serve immediately with Crackers or Rye Rounds.

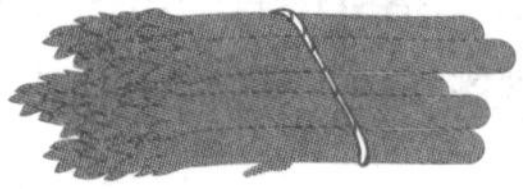

Creamy Soups without the Cream

Hearty cream soups often get their richness from the fats in dairy foods. These soups are creamy and satisfying without the dairy. You'll never miss it.

"CREAM" of ASPARAGUS SOUP

This recipe works for: Arthritis, Liver - Organ Health, Weight Loss
Makes 4 servings:

Cut off woody bottoms and slice 1 bunch Fresh Asparagus. Blanch in hot water until color is bright green, about 3 minutes. Drain and rinse in cold water. Place asparagus pieces <u>except tops</u> in the blender and whirl briefly with $^1/_3$ cup White Wine.

—Heat 4 TBS Canola Oil and add 4 TBS Unbleached Flour in a soup pot. Stir until well blended. Add 1 cup Organic Chicken Broth and blend well. Add asparagus to the soup pot. Add 2 more cups Chicken Broth and heat until blended. Add in 1 TB mixed herbs of your choice, like Thyme, Rosemary or Basil. Season with Herbal Seasoning Salt and Pepper. Top with reserved asparagus tops and serve.

Nutrition per: 188 calories; 4gm protein; 10gm carbohydrate; 2gm fiber; 14g total fat; 0mg choles.; 50mg calcium; 1mg iron; 34mg magnesium; 386mg potass.; 197mg sodium; Vit. A 88 IU; Vit. C 31mg; Vit. E 5 IU.

CREAMY SPINACH SOUP

This recipe works for: Allergies and Asthma, Men's Health, Bone Building
Makes 6 servings:

Place 1 large chopped ONION in a soup pot with 1 cup simmering WATER. Simmer about 3 minutes. Add 4 more cups WATER, 1 cup WHITE WINE, 3 POTATOES, peeled and chopped, 3 ZUCCHINI, thickly sliced and 1 TB BRAGG'S LIQUID AMINOS. Bring to a boil, reduce heat, cover and simmer for 30 minutes. Add 1 small bag BABY SPINACH LEAVES and CRACKED PEPPER to taste. Immediately remove from heat. Puree soup in batches in blender. Return to pan; heat gently for 2 minutes. Spoon hot into soup bowls and sprinkle on plenty of toasted, salted PINE NUTS or PUMPKIN SEEDS.

Nutrition per: 161 calories; 6gm protein; 21gm carbohydrate; 5gm fiber; 4g total fat; 0mg choles.; 59mg calcium; 3mg iron; 103mg magnes.; 682mg potass.; 167mg sodium; Vit. A 213 IU; Vit. C 21mg; Vit. E 1 IU.

DAIRY FREE CREAMY BROCCOLI SOUP Intense flavor

This recipe works for: Arthritis, Women's Health, Bone Building, Weight Loss
Serves 6:

In a soup pot, heat 1/4 cup CANOLA OIL and 2 pinches ground CORIANDER. Add 6 cups diced BROCCOLI, stems and florets. Add 2 diced RIBS CELERY and 1 diced YELLOW BELL PEPPER. Season with HERBAL SEASONING SALT and WHITE PEPPER. Cook 30 minutes.

—Make the soup: Puree broccoli mix in batches with 1 cup ORGANIC VEGETABLE BROTH or LOW FAT CHICKEN BROTH in a blender. Strain through a sieve into a large bowl and discard any fibrous material that sticks to the sieve. When all broccoli mix is pureed, pour soup back into the pot and reheat, thinning with more broth if needed. Ladle into bowls and top with snipped FRESH PARSLEY, CILANTRO or MINT. Each topping gives a different taste to the soup.

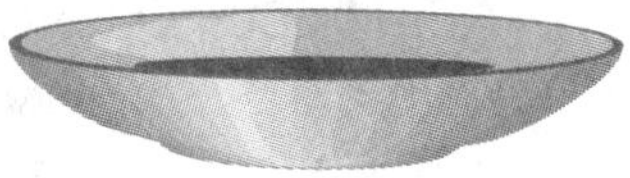

NO DAIRY CREAM of LEMON GRASS

This recipe works for: Immune Breakdown, Women's Health, Candida Infection
Makes 4 servings:

Combine 3 cups ORGANIC LOW FAT CHICKEN BROTH, 2 small POTATOES, peeled and quartered and 1/2 small YELLOW ONION, diced in a soup pan. Cook about 15 minutes. Add 1 medium bunch of FRESH LEMON GRASS washed and chopped; cook 2 minutes.

—Blender blend a 10 1/2-oz. package SILKEN TOFU and 1/2 cup RICE MILK until creamy. Transfer to a bowl. Puree potato-lemon grass-mixture until smooth. Add 2 TBS snipped PARSLEY. Pour mixture into saucepan; stir in tofu purée. Heat gently, but do not allow to boil or soup will curdle. Season to taste. Garnish with 1 teasp. LEMON ZEST.

Nutrition: 199 calories; 14gm protein; 29gm carbohydrate; 7gm fiber; 4g total fat; 0mg choles.; 326mg calcium; 31mg iron; 99mg magnes.; 372mg potass.; 520mg sodium; Vit. A 17 IU; Vit. C 10mg; Vit. E 2 IU.

NON-DAIRY CREAM of MUSHROOM SOUP

This recipe works for: Stress Reduction, Allergies, Heart Health
Makes 6 servings:

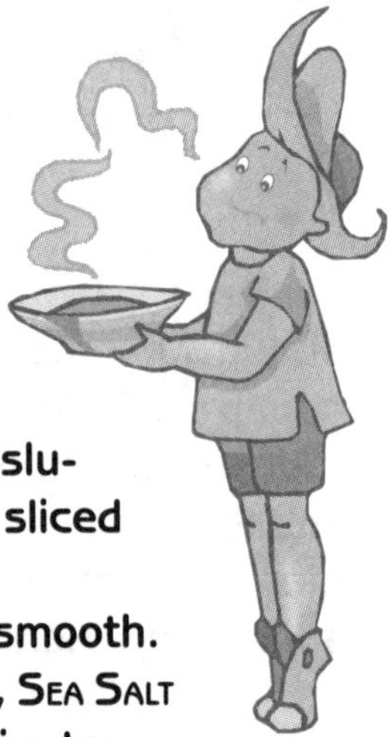

Blender blend smooth: 10 1/2-oz. Silken Tofu, 1/2 cup Rice Cream Cheese and 1/2 cup Water.

—In a large skillet, sizzle 1 chopped Yellow Onion and 5 minced Cloves Garlic in 2 TBS Canola Oil and 2 TBS Sherry until onion is translucent, 5 minutes. Add 8-oz. Button or Brown Cremini Mushrooms, thickly sliced and 1 tsp. Thyme; add 1/2 cup more Sherry; simmer 5 minutes.

—Add a ladleful of cooking liquid to tofu-water mixture; blend smooth. Pour tofu mixture into skillet with mushrooms and add 1 tsp. Tamari, Sea Salt to taste and a pinch Cayenne. Simmer to blend flavors, about 10 minutes.

Nutrition per: 171 calories; 10gm protein; 11gm carbohydrate; 3gm fiber; 9g total fat; 1mg choles.; 153mg calcium; 6mg iron; 66mg magnes.; 402mg potass.; 159mg sodium; Vit. A 25 IU; Vit. C 6mg; Vit. E 1 IU.

FRESH CORN CHOWDER with CHICKEN and POPCORN

This recipe works for: Stress Reduction, Allergies, Heart Health
Makes 6 servings: This soup is a complete meal.

Use a serrated knife to strip 6 cups Fresh Corn Kernels from their cobs. Set aside.

—In a soup pot, sizzle 1 chopped Yellow Onion and 2 TBS Soy Bacon Bits in 2 TBS Canola Oil for 5 minutes. Add 1 large peeled, cubed Russet Potato and half a Red Bell Pepper, diced; sizzle 5 minutes more. Add the fresh corn and sizzle 5 minutes more.

—Dump a whole 15-oz. can Corn Kernels and 1 cup Plain Yogurt into a blender and puree. Pour into the soup pot and add fresh corn-onion-potato mix. Cover pan; simmer 5 minutes.

—Add 4 cups Organic Low Fat Chicken Broth, 2 cups cooked diced Organic Chicken, 1 TB snipped Fresh Tarragon and 1 TB snipped Fresh Thyme. Partially cover pan; simmer until potatoes are tender, about 15 minutes. Season chowder to taste with Sea Salt and Pepper. Ladle into bowls. Sprinkle with plenty of Popcorn and serve.

VELVETY VEGETABLE SOUP

This recipe works for: Sports Nutrition, Liver Health, Overcoming Addictions
For 4 servings:

In a soup pot, sauté 2 sliced Yellow Onions and 2 sliced Ribs Celery in 2 TBS Olive Oil for 5 minutes. Add 4 cups Organic Low Fat Chicken Broth, 2 peeled, cubed Russet Potatoes, 2 sliced Carrots and cook on low heat until vegetables are soft. Pour soup into blender in batches and blend until smooth. Divide among soup bowls. Season with Sea Salt and Pepper. Sprinkle with snipped Fresh Parsley.

SWEET CARROT CREAM

This recipe works for: Kid's and Women's Health, Liver Health, Bone Building
For 6 people: Use a large soup pot.

Bring 2 TBS Canola Oil, $^1/_2$ teasp. Lemon-Garlic Seasoning and 1 cup Organic Vegetable Broth to a simmer. Add $1^1/_2$ lbs. Carrots sliced, 2 Ribs Celery sliced, and 3 cups Leeks, sliced (mostly white parts); simmer 5 minutes. Pureé in the blender with 1 cup Plain Yogurt until smooth. Return to soup pot. Add 5 more cups Vegetable Broth, $^1/_3$ cup snipped Fresh Parsley, $^1/_4$ tsp. Nutmeg and $^1/_4$ tsp. White Pepper. Heat just gently.

—Cook 1 teasp. Brown Sugar for 3 minutes in a saucepan until caramelized. Add $^1/_2$ cup minced Carrots, $^1/_4$ cup Plain Yogurt, $^1/_2$ teasp. Sea Salt, $^1/_4$ teasp. White Pepper. Cook for 10 minutes until carrots are tender crisp. Swirl into hot soup. Spoon into soup bowls. Sprinkle with 1 TB snipped Fresh Mint.

SESAME MUSHROOM SOUP Rich, non-dairy high protein.

This recipe works for: Kid's and Women's Health, Liver Health, Bone Building
For 6 people:

Sauté in 2 TBS Canola Oil until fragrant: 1 large Onion diced, 1 teasp. grated Ginger, $^1/_2$ teasp. Dry Basil (or 1 TB Fresh Basil snipped) and a pinch Cayenne Pepper.

—Add: 2 cups sliced Mushrooms, 3 Stalks Celery thin sliced, $^1/_2$ teasp. Sesame Salt, $^1/_4$ teasp. Black Pepper; sauté for 7 to 10 minutes.

—Add 4 cups chopped Tomatoes, $^1/_2$ cup Organic Vegetable Broth, $^1/_2$ cup White Wine, 3 TBS Sesame Tahini, 2 TBS Peanut Butter; simmer 15 to 20 minutes. Add 1 Cake Very Firm Tofu cubed; heat through. Serve hot sprinkled with snipped Fresh Cilantro.

Dairy Free Sauces, Dressings, Toppings

It may be hard to imagine creamy sauces without the dairy products that give them richness. But nut rice and soy milks are easy to substitute for great taste.

ALMOND or CASHEW NUT MILK

Almond milk is a rich, non-dairy liquid that may be used as a base for soups, sauces, gravies and protein drinks. Use it in baking for cakes and desserts, including cheesecakes. It makes any recipe rich.

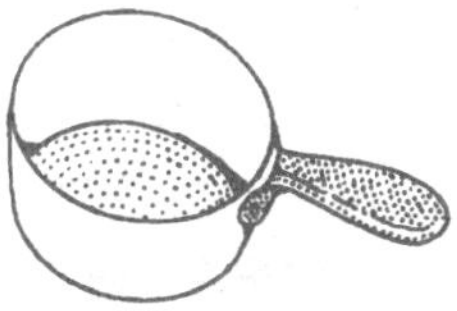

Whirl 1 cup Almonds or Cashews (toasted or raw) in a blender with 1 tsp. Honey and about 3 cups Water, depending on consistency you want, (milk, half and half, cream).

Nutrition per cup: 215 calories; 8gm protein; 8gm carbohydrate; 4gm fiber; 18g total fat; 0mg choles.; 98mg calcium; 1mg iron; 107mg magnes.; 260mg potass.; 9mg sodium; Vit. A 0 IU; Vit. C 0mg; Vit. E 12 IU.

ALMOND MILK GRAVY

This recipe works for: Allergies and Asthma, Respiratory Infections, Digestive Health
For four 5-oz. servings:

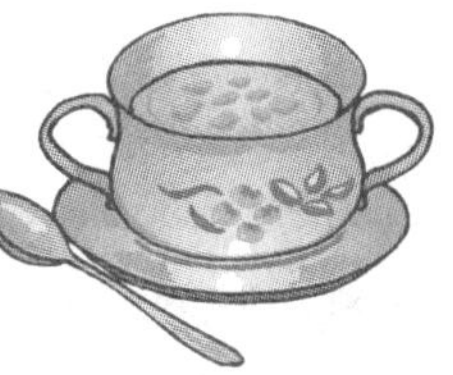

Blender blend until smooth: 2 cups Water, 2 TBS Toasted Wheat Germ, 1 cup chopped Almonds, 1 teasp. chopped Dry Onion, 2 TBS diced Celery, 2 TBS snipped Fresh Parsley, 2 TBS Canola Oil, 1/2 teasp. Tamari. Pour into a pan and cook, stirring over medium heat until thick and creamy.

CREAMY TOMATO DRESSING Tastes like gourmet Thousand Island.

This recipe works for: Men's and Women's Health, Digestive Health, Bone Building
For 3 cups:

Blender blend until smooth: 1/3 cup toasted, salted Sunflower Seeds or toasted, salted, diced Almonds, 3 1/3 cup Balsamic Vinegar, 1/4 cup White Wine, 3 TBS Honey, 2 cups chopped Fresh Tomatoes, 2 chopped Green Onions, 1/4 cup snipped Fresh Basil Leaves, 2 TBS Tamari, 2 TBS Lemon Juice, 1 teasp. Herbal Seasoning Salt, 1 teasp. dry Tarragon Leaves, 1/4 teasp. Granulated Dulse and 4 TBS snipped Fresh Parsley.

—Slowly add 1 cup Virgin Olive Oil in a thin stream to get a mayonnaise-like consistency. Pour into a serving container, and stir in 2 TB. Sweet Pickle Relish.

Nutrition: 164 calories; 1gm protein; 7gm carbohydrate; 1gm fiber; 14g total fat; 0mg choles.; 15mg calcium; 1mg iron; 11mg magnes.; 113mg potass.; 170mg sodium; Vit. A 28 IU; Vit. C 8mg; Vit. E 5 IU.

DEFINITELY GOURMET MUSHROOM SAUCE

This recipe works for: Immune Power, Cancer Protection, Sugar Imbalances
For eight (4 teasp. servings):

Soak 6 large dry Shiitake Mushrooms in a mixture of half Water and half White Wine until soft. Slice into thin strips; discard woody stems and reserve soaking liquid.

—Mix with half a package or half a bunch Fresh Enoki Mushrooms, stems removed. Add 4 to 6 thin-sliced Fresh Chanterelles or Cremini Mushrooms.

—Bring 1/2 cup Mushroom Soaking Liquid to a boil in a saucepan. Add 1 minced Onion, 1/2 diced Red Bell Pepper, 1 teasp. Tamari, 1/4 teasp. Rosemary and 1/2 teasp. Garlic-Lemon Seasoning. Cover, reduce heat and cook 15 minutes. Uncover and cook to evaporate liquid. Continue cooking until onions are brown and aromatic.

—Add 2 TBS Balsamic Vinegar to the pan. Stir, scraping up brown bits. Puree in the blender using more soaking water if needed for consistency. Return to saucepan; add mushrooms and rest of soaking water. Simmer 30 minutes to intensify flavor.

Nutrition: 24 calories; 1gm protein; 6gm carbohydrate; 2gm fiber; trace total fat; 0mg choles.; 7mg calcium; trace iron; 9mg magnes.; 170mg potass.; 10mg sodium; Vit. A 27 IU; Vit. C 11mg; Vit. E trace.

CREAMY "CHEESE-Y" SAUCE for STEAMED VEGGIES

This recipe works for: Immune Health, Sugar Imbalances, Digestive Health
Makes 8 servings:

Blender blend until creamy: $^1/_2$ cup Lemon Juice, 4 TBS Sesame Seeds, 1 carton Kefir Cheese or Rice Cream Cheese, 6 TBS Honey, 4 TBS Bragg's Liquid Aminos, 2 teasp. Sesame Seeds, $^1/_2$ teasp. Lemon-Pepper.

Nutrition: 104 calories; 4gm protein; 18gm carbohydrate; 1gm fiber; 3g total fat; 1mg choles.; 68mg calcium; 1mg iron; 27mg magnes.; 131mg potass.; 431mg sodium; Vit. A 6 IU; Vit. C 4mg; Vit. E trace.

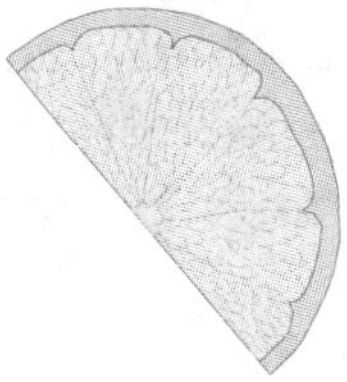

LEMON SESAME SAUCE

This recipe works for: Candida Control, Allergies, Liver Health
For 6 servings:

Whisk together: $^1/_2$ cup Sesame Tahini, $^1/_4$ cup White Wine or Organic Chicken Broth, 1 teasp. Sesame Seeds, $^1/_4$ cup Lemon Juice, 1 TB Honey, $^1/_2$ tsp. Sea Salt, $^1/_2$ tsp. Lemon Zest.

Nutrition: 144 calories; 4gm protein; 8gm carbohydrate; 2gm fiber; 11g total fat; 0mg choles.; 36mg calcium; 1mg iron; 75mg magnes.; 115mg potass.; 185mg sodium; Vit. A 2 IU; Vit. C 6mg; Vit. E trace.

SPINACH TOFU TOPPING with FRESH BASIL chlorophyll-rich

This recipe works for: Brain Health, Hair, Skin and Nails, Fatigue Syndromes
For 8 servings:

Steam 1 bunch washed, stemmed Spinach Leaves and 2 cups loosely packed washed, stemmed Fresh Basil Leaves <u>briefly</u> until just wilted and color changes to bright green. Add 1 teasp. Garlic-Lemon Seasoning, and 1 teasp. Tamari. Toss to coat.

—Blender blend 1 LB cubed Firm Tofu and $^1/_2$ cup Sesame Tahini until smooth. Add spinach mixture and blend until creamy. Reheat briefly. Serve hot sprinkled with 2 TBS Toasted Sesame Seeds.

PARSLEY ALMOND PESTO a delicate pesto for pasta, rice or potatoes.

This recipe works for: Heart Health, Hair, Skin and Nails, Women's Health
Enough for 6 servings:

Blender blend: 1 cup packed Fresh Parsley, $^1/_2$ cup Olive Oil, $^1/_2$ cup chopped Toasted Almonds, 2 TBS Lemon Juice, $^1/_4$ tsp. Garlic-Lemon Seasoning and $^1/_4$ tsp. Pepper.

Nutrition: 232 calories; 2gm protein; 4gm carbohydrate; 2gm fiber; 24g total fat; 0mg choles.; 47mg calcium; 1mg iron; 40mg magnes.; 150mg potass.; 10mg sodium; Vit. A 52 IU; Vit. C 12mg; Vit. E 5 IU.

TOFU or TEMPEH PASTA SAUCE A meaty-textured sauce.

This recipe works for: Men's Health, Sports Nutrition, Bone Building
For 8 servings: Serve hot over spaghetti or rotelli.

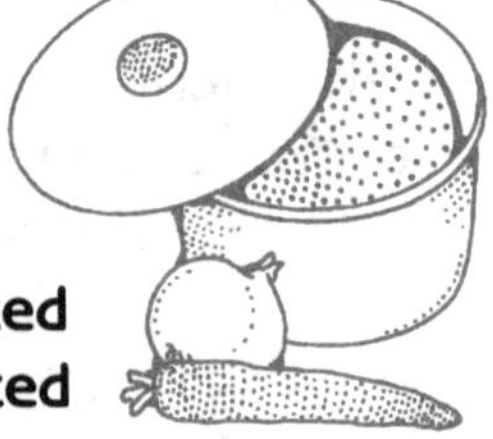

Shake 8-oz. cubed Firm Tofu or Tempeh in a bag with $^1/_2$ cup Unbleached Flour, Sea Salt and Pepper. Brown in 2 TBS hot Olive Oil in a skillet. Remove and set aside.

—Keep skillet hot; sauté 2 minced Cloves Garlic and 2 diced Yellow Onions until fragrant. Add 1 diced Orange Bell Pepper, 1 diced Red Bell Pepper, 4-oz. thin-sliced Cremini Mushrooms and 1 teasp. dry Basil; sauté for 5 minutes. Add tofu or tempeh cubes back to skillet. Then add one 28-oz. can Roma Tomatoes with juice, 1 TB Honey, $^1/_2$ teasp. Tarragon and $^1/_2$ teasp. Oregano. Bring to a boil. Reduce heat. Cover and simmer 10 minutes; uncover and simmer 10 minutes.

Nutrition: 108 calories; 5gm protein; 16gm carbohydrate; 3g fiber; 4g total fat; 0mg choles.; 77mg calcium; 3mg iron; 58mg magnesium; 455mg potass.; 71mg sodium; Vit. A 124 IU; Vit. C 44mg; Vit. E 3 IU.

COLD CUCUMBER SAUCE for SALMON or PRAWNS

This recipe works for: Bladder-Kidney Health, Hair, Skin and Nails, Women's Health
For 6 servings:

Blender blend until smooth: 2 Cucumbers, peeled and chunked, 4 to 6 Green Onions sliced, $^1/_3$ cup Plain Yogurt, 2 TBS snipped Fresh Parsley, 1 TB snipped Fresh Dill Weed, 1 TB snipped Fresh Mint, 2 teasp. Tarragon Vinegar, $^1/_4$ teasp. Celery Seed, $^1/_4$ teasp. Lemon-Pepper, $^1/_4$ teasp. Herbal Seasoning Salt. Chill and serve.

Nutrition: 25 calories; 1gm protein; 5gm carbohydrate; 2g fiber; trace total fat; trace choles.; 54mg calcium; 1mg iron; 18mg magnesium; 233mg potassium; 14mg sodium; Vit. A 21 IU; Vit. C 8mg; Vit. E trace.

CREAMY GREENS DRESSING

This recipe works for: Bone and Brain Health, Fatigue Syndromes, Recovery
For 6 servings:

Blender blend briefly: $^1/_2$ cup Olive Oil, $^1/_4$ teasp. dry Basil (or 1 teasp. snipped Fresh Basil), $^1/_2$ cup packed Baby Spinach Leaves, 2 sliced Green Onions, 2 TBS snipped Fresh Parsley, 2 TBS Tarragon Vinegar (or Lemon Juice), 1 teasp. Honey, $^1/_2$ teasp. Sesame Salt, $^1/_4$ teasp. Marjoram, and $^1/_4$ teasp. Cracked Pepper. (Add 1 teasp. Dijon Mustard and, $^1/_4$ teasp. Dill Weed if desired.) Add slowly while blending, $^1/_2$ cup Plain Yogurt and $^1/_4$ cup Water until dressing thickens. Chill to blend flavors before serving.

Nutrition: 180 calories; 1gm protein; 3gm carbohydrate; trace fiber; 18g total fat; 1mg choles.; 53mg calcium; 1mg iron; 14mg magnesium; 127mg potassium; 74mg sodium; Vit. A 88 IU; Vit. C 5mg; Vit. E 4 IU.

CREAMY CAESAR DRESSING

This recipe works for: Weight Control, Immune Health, Waste Management
Makes 5 servings:

Blender blend: 1 Clove Garlic, 4-oz. Low-Fat Soft Silken Tofu, $^1/_4$ cup Fresh Lemon Juice, 2 TBS Soy Parmesan Cheese, 1 TB White Miso Paste, 2 tsp. Dijon Mustard, $1^1/_2$ tsp. Garlic-Lemon Seasoning and $^1/_2$ tsp. White Worcestershire Sauce. Add enough Water or White Wine to give good dressing consistency. Store in a glass jar in the refrigerator.

Nutrition per: 44 calories; 3gm protein; 3gm carbohydrate; 1mg fiber; 2g total fat; 0mg choles.; 40mg calcium; 2mg iron; 32mg magnesium; 74mg potassium; 398mg sodium; Vit. A 3 IU; Vit. C 6mg; Vit. E trace

TAHINI POPPY SEED DRESSING

This recipe works for: Men's and Women's Health, Fatigue Syndromes, Hair, Skin
For 6 servings:

Add to a blender: 4 TBS Sesame Tahini, 2 TBS Honey, 2 TBS Poppy Seeds, 1 TB Lemon Juice, 1 teasp. Tamari, $^1/_2$ teasp. Black Pepper, $^1/_2$ teasp. grated Orange Zest, $^1/_4$ teasp. Nutmeg. Fill to blender 1 cup line with Canola Oil and blend until combined and creamy.

Nutrition: 203 calories; 3gm protein; 10gm carbohydrate; 2g fiber; 17g total fat; 0mg choles.; 41mg calcium; 1mg iron; 41mg magnesium; 106mg potassium; 15mg sodium; Vit. A 1 IU; Vit. C 3mg; Vit. E 8 IU.

CALIFORNIA GUACAMOLE DRESSING

This recipe works for: Overcoming Addictions, Liver Health, Hair, Skin and Nails
For $1^1/_2$ cups:

Blender blend smooth: 1 sliced Avocado, 3 TBS Olive Oil, half a Red Onion, sliced, $^1/_4$ cup Light Bottled Salsa, 2 TBS Lemon Juice, 2 TBS Wine Vinegar, $^1/_2$ teasp. Lemon-Pepper. Pour into a bowl and add in 1 large Tomato diced.

SWEET TAHINI CREAM for FRUIT SALAD

This recipe works for: Digestive Health, Hair and Skin, Anti-Aging
Makes 1 pint:

Blender blend until creamy: $^2/_3$ cup Plain Yogurt, 1 teasp. Vanilla, 3 TBS Honey, 1 TB Lime Juice. Fill to the 2 cup mark with Sesame Tahini. Add more honey if desired.

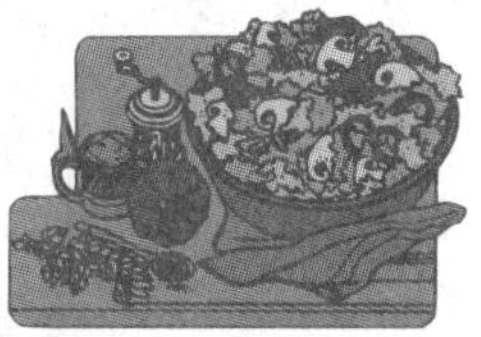

Dairy Free Desserts

These desserts are guaranteed creamy and delicious without dairy products; rich and satisfying without the saturated fat. The recipes here are for inspiration, to give you an idea of how to substitute in your own favorites.

NO-DAIRY CHERRY DELIGHT

This recipe works for: Heart Health, Kid's - Men's Health, Sugar Imbalances
For 4 servings: Chill dishes for ice cream.

Blender blend $^{1}/_{2}$ cup Ground Almonds and 1 cup Boiling Water for 1 minute. Add $^{1}/_{2}$ cup Rice Syrup and 2 TBS Lecithin Granules and blend for 1 minute. Add 4 cups pitted Cherries and $^{1}/_{4}$ tsp. Almond Extract; process until smooth. Pour the mixture into ice cube trays and freeze until solid. When frozen, place cubes in the food processor and process until creamy. Serve in chilled dishes.

NO-DAIRY PAPAYA ICE CREAM

This recipe works for: Allergies and Asthma, Digestive Health, Sugar Imbalances
For 6 servings: Chill dishes for ice cream.

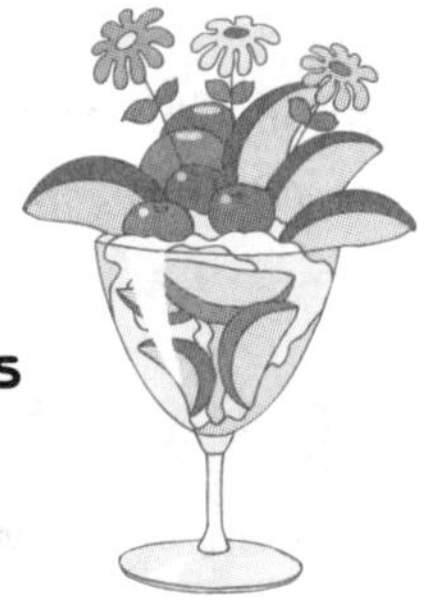

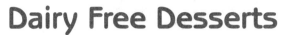

Blender blend to smooth: 2 $^{1}/_{2}$ cups Vanilla Rice Dream Dessert, (if you use Vanilla Rice Dream Milk, add 2 TBS Lecithin Granules), 2 large mashed Papayas. Pour the mixture into ice cube trays and freeze until solid. When frozen, place cubes in the food processor and process until creamy. Serve in chilled dishes.

CHEESECAKE without the CHEESE Rich in absorbable calcium

This recipe works for: Heart Health, Kid's - Men's Health, Sugar Imbalances
For 8 servings: Preheat oven to 350°.

Crush about 15 Whole Grain Graham Crackers and mix with 3 TBS Almond Butter or Sesame Tahini for the crust. Press into a Lecithin-sprayed, spring form-pan and sprinkle with Cinnamon. Chill crust while you mix the filling ingredients.

—Crumble into a blender and blend until absolutely smooth: 3 $^{1}/_{2}$ LBS Very Fresh Tofu into a bowl. Add $^{2}/_{3}$ cup Vanilla Rice Milk, $^{1}/_{4}$ cup Sesame Tahini, $^{3}/_{4}$ cup Maple Syrup, 2 TBS Lemon Juice and 2 teasp. Vanilla. (Add 2 Eggs if your diet and system can tolerate them. They can be easily omitted. Taste will not suffer, only lightness.)

—Pour into the chilled springform crust, smooth the top and bake until filling sets and begins to turn golden. Remove and cool on a rack. Cover and chill. Arrange drained, sliced Fresh Fruits on top in an artistic pattern and serve.

Nutrition: 370 calories; 19gm protein; 36gm carbohydrate; 4g fiber; 19g total fat; 0mg choles.; 273mg calcium; 12mg iron; 264mg magnes.; 314mg potass.; 104mg sodium; Vit. A 18 IU; Vit. C 2mg; Vit. E 12 IU.

LOW CALORIE LEMON TOFU CHEESECAKE

This recipe works for: Overcoming Addictions, Liver - Organ Health
For 8 servings: Preheat oven to 350°.

Blender blend until very smooth: $1^1/_2$ LBS Very Fresh Tofu, one 8-oz. carton Lemon Yogurt, 2 TBS Lemon Juice, $^1/_2$ cup Honey, $^1/_4$ cup Canola Oil, $1^1/_2$ teasp. Vanilla, 1 teasp. grated Lemon Zest. Pour into oven-ready custard cups or a straight-sided casserole dish, and bake for 40 minutes until set.

—Top with $1^1/_2$ cups sliced, drained Fresh Fruits and fresh snipped Mint Leaves.

—Or top with this all-natural, showy FRUIT GLAZE: Blender blend well: 1 cup Fresh Fruits, (like Raspberries, Peaches or Apricots), in the blender. Add 2 to 3 teasp. Honey, 2 TBS Kuzu Chunks or Powdered Arrowroot dissolved in 3 TBS Water and 1 TB Lemon Juice. Pour into a saucepan and bring to a boil. Simmer until glaze thickens and clears, about 1 minute. Spoon over cheesecake immediately; chill and serve.

Nutrition per: 235 calories; 9gm protein; 28gm carbohydrate; 2g fiber; 11g total fat; trace choles.; 151mg calcium; 5mg iron; 94mg magnesium; 223mg potass.; 28mg sodium; Vit. A 10 IU; Vit. C 7mg; Vit. E 3 IU.

FRESH PEACH COBBLER with GRAPENUTS TOPPING

This recipe works for: Stress Reactions, Kid's Health, Healthy Pregnancy
For 8 servings: Preheat oven to 350°. Use a 8 x 11 x $2^1/_2$" Lecithin-sprayed pan

Mix in a bowl: 8 sliced Fresh Peaches, $^1/_4$ cup Orange Juice, $^1/_4$ cup Honey, 2 $^1/_2$ TBS Tapioca Pearls. Pour into prepared baking pan.

—Mix topping and sprinkle over to cover, $^3/_4$ cup Grapenuts Cereal, $^1/_2$ cup chopped Pecans, 1 TB minced Crystallized Ginger, 2 TBS Maple Syrup, 1 teasp Cinnamon, 1 teasp. Nutmeg. Bake for 40 minutes til browned, bubbly and fragrant.

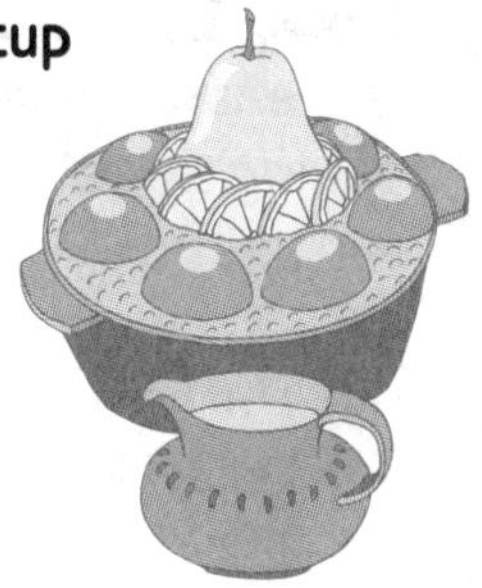

ORANGE PUDDING

This recipe works for: Digestive Allergy Control, Kid's Health, Healthy Pregnancy
Makes 12 servings: Preheat oven to 350°F.

In a bowl combine 4 TBS Canola Oil and 6 TBS Brown Sugar. Add $^1/_2$ cup Frozen Apple-Juice Concentrate, thawed and $^1/_2$ cup Egg Replacer; mix well (mix may look curdled).

—In a separate bowl, combine 1 cup Whole Wheat Pastry Flour and $^1/_2$ cup Unbleached Flour, 1 tsp. Ground Allspice, 1 tsp. non-aluminum Baking Powder, and 1 teasp. Baking Soda. Add to liquid ingredients; mix well. Add 2 TBS Orange Juice, 2 tsp. Orange Zest and 8 oz. grated Carrots; mix gently. Pour batter into 9-inch round cake pan; bake 25 to 30 minutes, or until a tester inserted in center comes out clean.

Nutrition per: 146 calories; 3gm protein; 24gm carbohydrate; 3g fiber; 5g total fat; 0mg choles.; 50mg calcium; 1mg iron; 31mg magnesium; 221mg potass.; 148mg sodium; Vit. A 533 IU; Vit. C 5mg; Vit. E 1 IU.

CLASSIC HASTY PUDDING CAKE

This recipe works for: Hair, Skin and Nails, Allergies, Sports Nutrition
For 6 old fashioned servings: Preheat oven to 350°.

Make the HOT MOLASSES SAUCE. Bring $\frac{1}{3}$ cup Molasses, $\frac{1}{3}$ cup Honey, and $\frac{1}{3}$ cup Water to a boil in a saucepan; then set aside.

—Mix together until smooth: 1 cup Unbleached Flour, $\frac{1}{3}$ cup Vanilla Rice Milk, Soy Milk or Almond Milk, $\frac{1}{4}$ cup Honey, $\frac{1}{4}$ cup Canola Oil, $1\frac{1}{2}$ teasp. Vanilla, $\frac{1}{2}$ teasp. non-aluminum Baking Powder, and $\frac{1}{2}$ teasp. Baking Soda.

—Stir in $\frac{1}{3}$ cup Raisins. Pour into an oiled casserole. Sprinkle on more raisins. Pour hot molasses syrup over top and bake about 40 minutes. Serve warm.

Nutrition per: 341 calories; 3gm protein; 63gm carbohydrate; 1g fiber; 10g total fat; 0mg choles.; 193mg calcium; 5mg iron; 53mg magnesium; 572mg potass.; 149mg sodium; Vit. A 1 IU; Vit. C 1mg; Vit. E 3 IU.

KATE'S OATMEAL COOKIES

This recipe works for: Kid's Health, Stress Reactions, Bone Building
For about 4 dozen: Preheat oven to 350°.

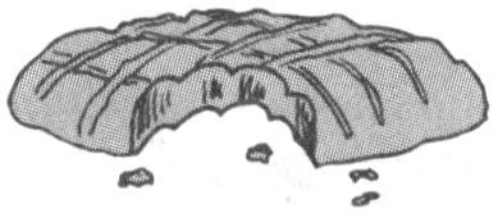

Mix $\frac{1}{2}$ cup Canola Oil, $\frac{1}{2}$ cup Honey, and 3 TBS Sesame Tahini (or 3 TBS Vanilla Yogurt) in a large bowl til well blended.

—Add and mix just to moisten: $1\frac{1}{2}$ cups Whole Wheat Pastry Flour, $1\frac{1}{4}$ cups Oats, 1 teasp. non-aluminum Baking Powder, $\frac{1}{4}$ teasp. Baking Soda, $\frac{1}{2}$ teasp. Nutmeg, 1 teasp. Cinnamon and $\frac{1}{2}$ cup Raisins. Drop onto Lecithin-sprayed baking sheets. Sprinkle each with Sesame Seeds and flatten with a fork dipped in cold water so it won't stick. Bake for 8 minutes until golden brown.

Nutrition per 2 cookies: 132 calories; 3gm protein; 16gm carbohydrate; 2g fiber; 7g total fat; 0mg choles.; 23mg calcium; 1mg iron; 29mg magnesium; 153mg potass.; 7mg sodium; Vit. A 1 IU; Vit. C 1mg; Vit. E 5 IU.

SWEET SAVORY SCONES

This recipe works for: Overcoming Addictions, Sugar Imbalances, Candida
For 8 scones: Preheat oven to 425°.

Mix until just moistened: $1\frac{1}{2}$ cups Unbleached Flour, $\frac{1}{2}$ cup Oat Flour, $\frac{1}{4}$ cup Canola Oil, $\frac{1}{2}$ cup Plain Yogurt mixed with $\frac{1}{4}$ cup Water, or $\frac{3}{4}$ cup Plain Kefir or $\frac{3}{4}$ cup Plain Soy Milk, 2 TBS Honey, 2 teasp. Baking Powder, $\frac{1}{2}$ teasp. Baking Soda, 1 teasp. dry Savory, $\frac{1}{2}$ teasp. Sea Salt and $\frac{1}{2}$ cup Currants (better than raisins here). Turn dough onto floured board and knead just 12 turns. Pat into a round on a greased baking sheet. Score into 8 wedges with a knife. Bake until browned, about 30 minutes.

Nutrition per: 205 calories; 6gm protein; 30gm carbohydrate; 3g fiber; 8g total fat; trace choles.; 104mg calcium; 1mg iron; 45mg magnesium; 543mg potass.; 67mg sodium; Vit. A 4 IU; Vit. C 1mg; Vit. E 6 IU.

MIDGET PEANUT BUTTER COOKIES

This recipe works for: Men's and Kid's Health, Sports Nutrition
For 36 cookies: Preheat oven to 350°.

Mix together: 1 1/4 cup Whole Wheat Pastry Flour, 1/4 cup Canola Oil, 1/2 cup Peanut Butter, 1/4 cup Whole Grain Granola, 1/2 cup Honey, 2 TBS Maple Syrup, and 1 teasp. Vanilla; drop onto greased baking sheets. Flatten each cookie with a fork dipped in cold water and bake for about 10 minutes.

Nutrition per: 68 calories; 2gm protein; 8gm carbohydrate; 1mg fiber; 4g total fat; 0mg choles.; 6mg calcium; trace iron; 12mg magnesium; 66mg potass.; 2mg sodium; Vit. A trace; Vit. C trace; Vit. E trace

SESAME OATMEAL COOKIES

This recipe works for: Kid's Health, Skin and Hair, Women's Health
For 12 cookies: Preheat oven to 350°.

Stir together until well blended: 1/2 cup Honey, 1 1/2 cups Oatmeal, 1/2 cup diced Walnuts, 1/3 cup Sesame Tahini, 1/2 teasp. Cinnamon, 1/4 teasp. Nutmeg. Drop teaspoonfuls on Lecithin-sprayed baking sheets. Bake for 10 minutes til edges are brown. Cool.

OATMEAL RAISIN WHEELS

This recipe works for: Sports Nutrition, Illness Recovery, Overcoming Addictions
For 18 cookies: Preheat oven to 375°.

Mix to make a stiff dough: 1/2 cup dry-roasted, chopped Peanuts or Almonds, 1/2 cup Peanut Butter or Almond Butter, 1/2 cup Whole Wheat Pastry Flour, 1/2 cup Toasted Wheat Germ, 2 cups diced Dates, 2 cups Raisins, 1 cup Rolled Oats, 1/4 cup Canola Oil, 2 TBS Apple Juice, 1 teasp. Vanilla, 1 teasp. Cinnamon, 1/2 teasp. Nutmeg, and 1/2 teasp. Ginger Powder.

—Process about 1/3 of the dough in a food processor or blender; then mix back in so cookies will hold together, but still have nice chewy chunks. Bake about 15 minutes until brown, and crusty around the edges.

Nutrition per: 245 calories; 5gm protein; 38gm carbohydrate; 5g fiber; 10g total fat; 0mg choles.; 52mg calcium; 2mg iron; 68mg magnesium; 411mg potassium; 4mg sodium; Vit. A 2 IU; Vit. C 1mg; Vit. E 8 IU.

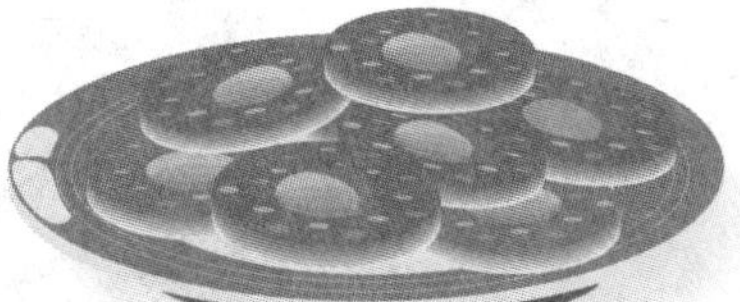

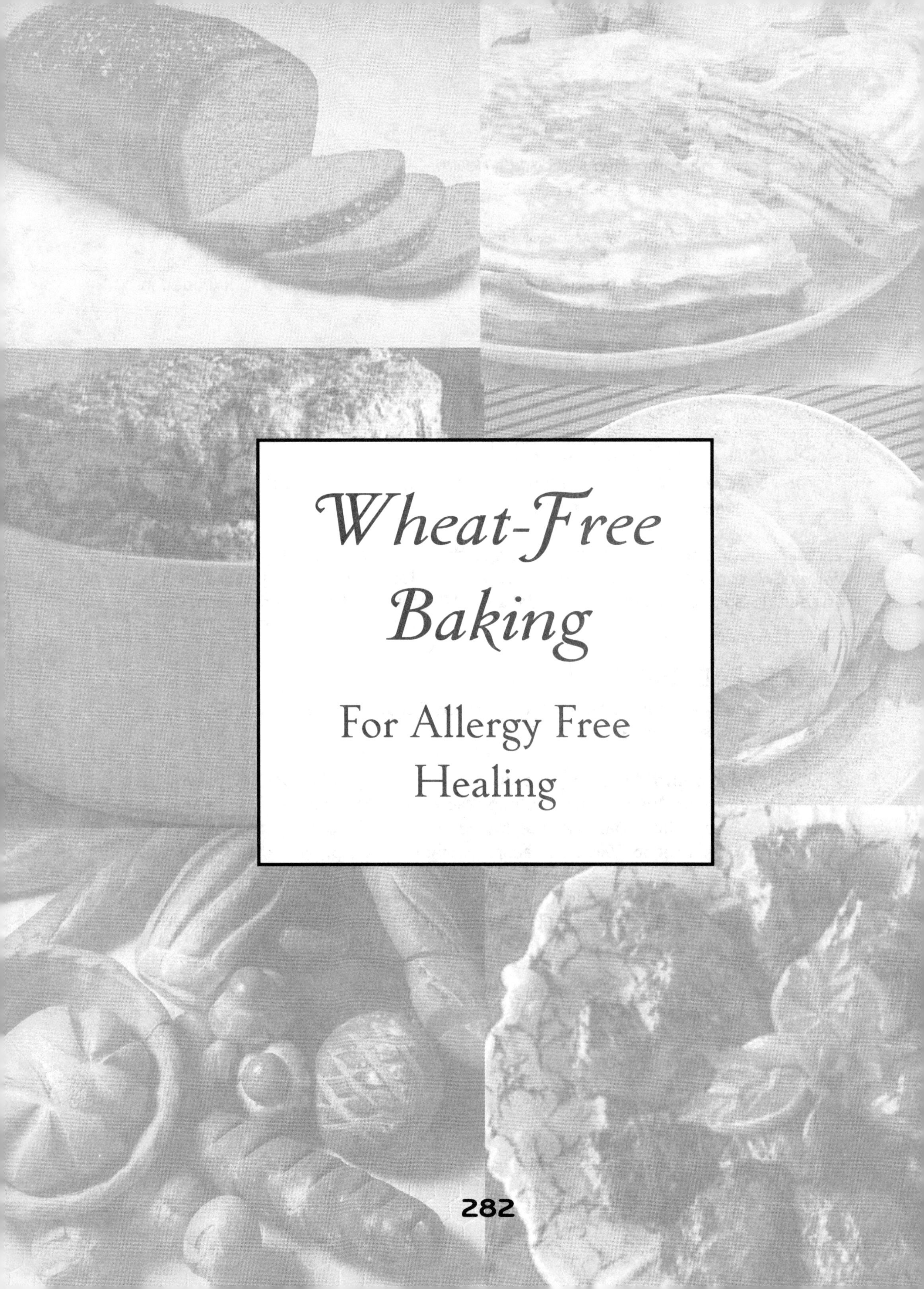

Wheat-Free Baking

For Allergy Free Healing

Wheat Free Living

Over 38 million Americans suffer from food allergies.... the fastest growing type of allergic reactions in the U.S. today. Wheat products and high gluten foods are clearly major offenders. They're really protein intolerances, largely caused by diet and environmental chemical sensitivities. Over time, left untreated, wheat or gluten allergies can lead to serious disorders like Irritable Bowel Syndrome (I.B.S.), Crohn's disease and Celiac disease.

Do you have a wheat or gluten allergy?

Here are some symptoms to watch for: Chronic headaches, moodiness, fatigue and depression are usually the first stages of sensitivity, followed by itchy, watery eyes or blurred vision, and mental fuzziness. Most people get an excessively swollen stomach and feel nauseous after eating, closely followed by gas and constipation, or diarrhea. **Children** become overly irritable, hyperactive, flushed in the face and get chronic ear infections. **Women** with wheat or gluten allergies regularly suffer from hypothyroidism, heart palpitations and osteoarthritis. **Men** regularly experience hypoglycemia, muscle weakness or poor coordination and excessive sweating. **The elderly** often get hives and ringing in the ears. Chronic congestion and unexplained obesity are universal symptoms of wheat allergies and gluten reactions.

Sensitivity to wheat and gluten was once rare. Ancient civilizations in every climate zone enjoyed whole wheat grains as a regular part of their daily diet. Yet today, commercial wheat is one of our most problematic allergen foods.

What's causing today's wheat allergy problem?

1: Agriculture chemicals and fertilizers: Research on the chemicals used in agriculture pesticides and fertilizers shows that they affect the way our bodies use and absorb wheat and gluten. When sugar and wheat are combined, as they are in almost 50% of commercially prepared foods, the problems are aggravated, because the carbohydrates in the wheat cannot be fully digested. The poorly digested carbohydrates are then attacked by bacteria in the intestines, and contribute to gas and loose bowels. (This is true even with whole wheat products; refined wheat flour foods cause even more problems.)

2: **Heavily treated, overly refined grains:** Wheat crops are heavily sprayed with the types of pesticides that are major suspects in food allergies (see previous page). Even "whole grain" products are made today with refined, bleached wheat flour, a process which strips it of 80% of its vitamins and minerals. (Four nutrients, iron, thiamin, riboflavin and niacin, are added back as "enrichments," but in synthetic forms that are less usable by the body.)

Most commercial wheat products are what I call non-food foods, nutrient stripped and loaded with chemicals. Additives, preservatives, colorings and sugars are also added, contributing to the chemical overload, difficult for even the strongest digestive system to process over a long period of time.

3: **Enzyme deficiency:** Scientists suspect that most of us are enzyme deficient today... largely from a lack of enzymes from fresh foods. Over time, the effects of undigested or partially digested food in the intestinal system can be devastating. The gut wall becomes more permeable and undigested proteins leak out into the bloodstream. The immune system sees the proteins as invaders, so it brings in inflammation... and we get a food allergy response. Gluten proteins (found in wheat) are especially difficult to process and are a main factor in the development of Celiac disease, and Candida yeast overgrowth. Poor food combining hampers enzyme activity, too. High gluten grains are often combined with heavy meat proteins or high fruit sugars, further impairing digestion.

TIP: Get wheat sensitivities and poor digestion under control by adding more enzymes from raw foods or supplements to your diet. A 1995 Italian study shows supplementing with pancreatic enzymes enhances the benefits of a gluten-free diet for Celiac patients. See "Enzyme Rich Foods and Recipes," on pg. 142 of this book.

If you suspect a wheat or gluten sensitivity, begin by eliminating dubious foods from your diet. During the initial stages of healing, stick closely to the wheat and gluten free recipes in this section. Eat at home as much as possible, preparing your food from scratch during healing, so you can control its contents. You can't effectively know or control everything you are eating away from home. Gluten-containing grains - wheat, barley, bulgur and rye - appear in a wide variety of restaurant and deli food products, including ice cream, candies, salad dressings, meats, soups, sauces and condiments, foods you might not suspect. Even small amounts of gluten may initiate an allergic reaction.

TIP: In spite of pesticide and pollutant problems, real whole grains still offer important health benefits. They're a good source a complex carbohydrates, for slow calorie burning and increased energy. Their protective fiber, antioxidants and plant chemicals like phytic acid deter cancer and heart disease. A study from Harvard Medical School reveals that eating just two servings of whole grains a day cuts risk for heart disease by 30%! Whole grains also reduce depression because they naturally stimulate your brain's production of mood stabilizing serotonin. I recommend organic, real whole grains from the health food store to help correct a wheat sensitivity.

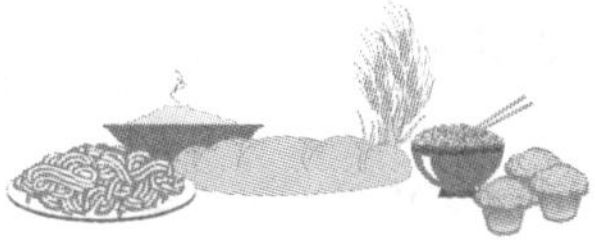

Your Non-Wheat Options

See my "Food Pharmacy Digest," page 476 in the Diet Book for more.

What's left after you've eliminated wheat? Healthy options available at health food stores ease the transition. Pasta, cereals (hot and cold), whole grain flours, breads and snack foods are all available in wheat and gluten-free forms. Ancient grains like spelt and kamut can be enjoyed by 70% of people allergic to commercial wheat. Look for spelt and kamut breads in the refrigerated section. Rice breads are a tasty option for a wheat free sandwich. (They're a little crumbly, but are often sweetened with fruit juice to enhance flavor, and are well tolerated by the gluten intolerant.)

Try vegetable pastas made with quinoa or rice. Soba noodles made from buckwheat are a good wheat-free choice, but are not for people with gluten intolerance. For a wheat-free hot breakfast, cream of rice, buckwheat and oat bran are tasty. Amaranth, muesli, brown rice crisps and corn flakes are wheat-free cereals.

Here's a short list of wheat-free, low gluten grains:

- **KAMUT**: wheat-free. An ancient grain around since 4000 B.C., kamut, is related to durum. It's available in the U.S. as a powdered drink mix, in cereals, pastas, and bread. It has a rich, buttery flavor that enhances recipes where you would normally use wheat, including yeasted breads. It's not a good choice for gluten sensitivity because it contains gluten. Green Kamut drink mixes are a good choice for cleansing.

- **RICE**: ok for gluten sensitivity, wheat-free. Rice is the staple grain for over half of the world's population. Available as a grain, flour, bread, pasta, cereal, and in dairy-free milk and cheese, it is one of the most versatile grains known and one of the most easily digested. Choose organic rice; commercial rice is often loaded with pesticides. For people who are also lactose intolerant, I recommend delicious rice cheeses.

- **CHICKPEA**: ok for gluten sensitivity, wheat-free. Chickpeas are not a true grain, but a legume cultivated in Mesopotamia since 5000 B.C. A nice addition to pudding and casseroles, they are best enjoyed in hummus and falafel dishes. Chickpea flour (from ground chickpeas) is gluten-free and a good thickener in soups and sauces.

• **AMARANTH**: ok for gluten sensitivity, wheat-free. There are over 500 species of amaranth. Amaranth is available today as a flour for wheat-free baking. Mixing a little amaranth with grains like rice, millet or oats adds a peppery flavor. Popped amaranth makes a good snack. After toasting, popcorn-like amaranth seeds are added to soups or vegetables or eaten alone. Amaranth cereals are popular in a wheat-free breakfast.

• **SPELT**: ok for gluten sensitivity, wheat-free. An ancient European grain, spelt is available in the U.S. as a bread, flour and in berries. Although spelt isn't gluten-free, most people with gluten sensitivity can tolerate it. *Note: Italian spelt pastas are sometimes made with whole wheat flour. If you're unsure, choose domestic products.*

• **CORN**: ok for gluten sensitivity, wheat-free. A staple food for Native Americans, corn still feeds much of the Americas, human and animal. It's extremely versatile, excellent in baking, in cereals, and with quinoa in pasta. Sweet corn is the favorite American vegetable (next to the potato), great on the grill, roasted, gently steamed and in casseroles. You really can't go wrong with corn. It's inexpensive and easy to prepare.

• **MILLET**: ok for gluten sensitivity, wheat-free. An ancient grain, the Chinese used it as their staple grain before rice came along. The ancient Egyptians used millet to make bread. Millet is available today as a grain, flour, meal and in cereals.It's excellent in flatbreads, puffed in snack foods, and to add heartiness to stuffed veggies and casseroles.

• **BUCKWHEAT**: wheat-free. Buckwheat became popular in Europe during the Middle Ages for its ability to withstand poor growing conditions. Buckwheat is available today as a flour, cereal and pasta (Soba noodles). Nutty, roasted buckwheat (kasha) is good with vegetables like onions, mushrooms and winter squash. Buckwheat is a great choice for chemical sensitivities because it's rarely treated with pesticides.

• **OATS**: wheat-free. Popular since 2500 B.C., oats are known today for their fiber providing ability. Oats are available as a grain, cereal, bran and flour. Old fashioned hot oatmeal cereal is still an American favorite. Because they are high in gluten, oats are also often used as a thickener in soups, and in meat loaf, baked goods and granola. *Note: A 1997 study in the New England Journal of Medicine says celiac patients in remission can tolerate oats in moderate amounts. Ask your physician.*

• **BARLEY**: ok for gluten sensitivity, wheat-free. Most frequently used in the West in hearty soups, barley is also good as a breakfast cereal, and in bread and casseroles. Unrefined whole barley is the best choice. Barley is also a healing green grass. See the Cooking for Healthy Healing Diet Book section on "Nature's Superfoods," pg.44.

• **RYE**: may be ok for gluten sensitivity, wheat-free. Most of Medieval Europe ate rye as a staple grain. Rye is available as a flour, berry, cereal, grits and meal. I like rye bread in a healthy Reuben sandwich with raw sauerkraut and hormone-free turkey. It's lower in gluten than wheat and may be tolerated by some people with mild gluten sensitivity.

• **QUINOA**: ok for gluten sensitivity, wheat-free. Considered by many a nearly perfect protein, quinoa has been cultivated in the Andes mountains for 5,000 years. It has a rich, nutty flavor and works well as a wheat free grain and pasta. Prepare quinoa just like rice; it only takes about 5 to 10 minutes before it's ready. *Note: If you're allergic to wheat, make sure the quinoa pasta you buy isn't made with semolina flour.*

• **SOY FLOUR**: ok for gluten sensitivity, wheat-free. Soy flour is available for baking, but because it contains no gluten, it doesn't work well by itself in raised breads. It's usually mixed with an all purpose flour (not gluten-free) in baking. Soy flour can also be used to add a creamy texture to fruit smoothies.

• People with gluten sensitivity can also usually tolerate potato starch and tapioca, but they are not as nutritious as the grains listed above.

If you're affected by wheat or gluten allergies, read product labels to make sure there is no wheat or gluten on the ingredient list. Gluten can also be found in some vitamin supplements. Always inquire if you are unsure.

Wheat Free Baking

Healthy Crusts, Toppings, and Coatings: Crusts, toppings, sprinkles and coatings are an important part of a recipe. The foundation of a dish should be as healthy as the filling. (See index for individual crust and topping recipes.)

Low-fat, thin crusts for pizzas, quiches, and vegetable tarts:

—Use crushed, wheat-free whole grain cracker crumbs, plain, or sprinkled with a little low oil dressing or tamari. Bake until crispy - about 10 minutes at 375° - then fill.

—Use any cooked wheat-free whole grain or vegetable leftovers, and whirl in the blender to a paste. Press into a lecithin-sprayed baking dish, crisp in a 400° oven for 10 minutes.

—Thin slice tofu blocks horizontally. Bake with a little oil for 10 minutes to firm.

—Cover bottom of a baking dish with crisp wheat-free Chinese noodles. Oven toast; then fill.

—Sprinkle toasted nuts and seeds to cover bottom of the baking dish. Season with herbal seasoning salt and fill.

—Spread cooked brown rice to cover the bottom and sides of a lecithin-sprayed baking dish. Toast at 375° to crisp and dry slightly, then fill.

Low-fat crusts for dessert pies, tarts and custards: A blend of all or some of the whole non-wheat grains like amaranth, buckwheat, oats and barley, make a lovely, nutty, lighter pastry crust for desserts. Buy them already ground into flour from your health food store. Barley flakes and rolled oats are easy to toast in the oven until fragrant, then mix with a sweetener, toast again and use as a crust

—Toast cooked rice and cooked quinoa in the oven. Mix with a little date sugar or honey to sweeten, and spread on bottom and sides of baking dish. Toast again briefly and fill.

—Use toasted nuts and seeds, ground and sweetened with date sugar or honey. Spread on bottom and sides of baking dish. Toast again briefly for crunch, and fill.

—Use juice-sweetened, sugar-free, wheat-free cookie crumbs. Press onto bottom and sides of baking dish. Toast briefly and fill.

—Sprinkle date sugar, maple syrup granules, or maple sugar on bottom of a custard dish. Broil briefly to caramelize; then fill and bake as usual. Yum.

Casserole foundations -a unique cooking art: Cover the bottom of the baking dish with: hard boiled eggs; Left over cooked brown rice or other wheat-free whole grain; spaghetti squash, cooked and briefly toasted; zucchini or tomato rounds.

For both bottoms and toppings: Chinese-noodles, toasted; Wheat-free whole grain granola, toasted; Wheat-free whole grain chips, crushed slightly and toasted.

Healthy low-fat, low salt coatings for seafood, poultry and veggies: Mix with yogurt, or egg and water; coat food and chill briefly before baking. Wheat-free crushed whole grain chips, falafal or tofu burger mix.

Wheat Free Recipe Sections

Wheat free baking isn't very difficult. There are many other good grains to choose from. Recipe categories include:

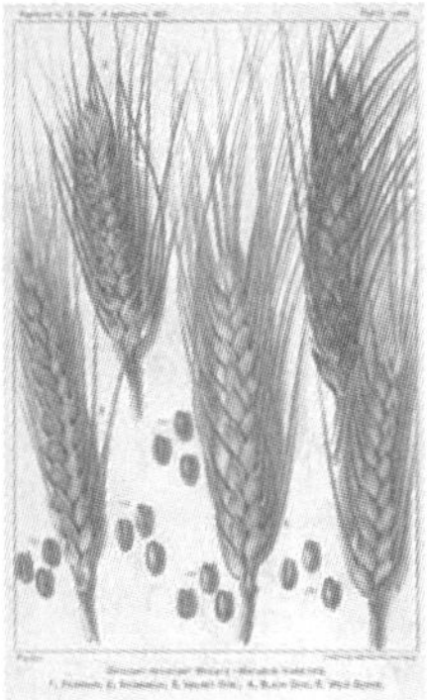

Wheat Free Crusts

If you have to deny yourself delicious fresh dessert and vegetable pies, tarts or quiches because of the wheat flour in the crust, try the recipes in this chapter. It offers several choices for both sweet and savory fillings - all wheat free.

SESAME OAT CRUST Good for creamy pies like BANANA SOUR CREAM

For one 10" pie: Preheat oven to 350°. Makes 8 servings.

Mix: 1 1/2 cups OATS, 1 TB VANILLA, 1/4 cup TOASTED SESAME SEEDS, 1/2 teasp. SESAME SALT, 1/4 cup chopped ALMONDS, 2 TBS melted BUTTER, 2 TBS CANOLA OIL, 1/2 cup RICE FLOUR, 3 TBS HONEY, 1/2 teasp. CINNAMON, 1/4 teasp. NUTMEG and 1/4 teasp. ALLSPICE. Press into a pie pan. Bake for 10 minutes; cool before filling.

Nutrition per: 256 calories; 6gm protein; 26gm carbohydrate; 3gm fiber; 13gm total fat; 7mg choles.; 40mg calcium; 2mg iron; 46mg magnesium; 118mg potass.; 4mg sodium; Vit. A 28 IU; Vit. C 1mg; Vit. E 3 IU.

COCONUT CAROB CHIP CRUST

For one 8" pie: Makes 8 servings.

Sauté 3 TBS MELTED BUTTER and 2 cups shredded COCONUT until golden and toasty. Add 1/2 cup CHOCOLATE or CAROB CHIPS. Press mixture into a pie plate. Cool and fill.

Nutrition per: 205 calories; 2gm protein; 11gm carbohydrate; 4gm fiber; 18gm total fat; 8mg choles.; 9mg calcium; 1mg iron; 30mg magnesium; 146mg potass.; 9mg sodium; Vit. A 27 IU; Vit. C 1mg; Vit. E 1 IU.

MACAROON COOKIE CRUST

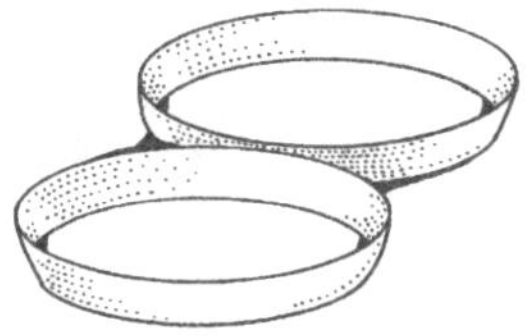

This crust is very rich, but absolutely delicious with any fruit or cream filling.... heavenly with a frozen yogurt filling.

Crumble chewy WHEAT-FREE MACAROONS (made of non-fat dry milk, sweetener, coconut, egg whites) into a pie plate. Add 3 TBS melted BUTTER over and press onto top and sides.

MIXED NUT CRUST Good for both savory and dessert fillings.

Mix: 1/2 cup finely chopped NUTS (WALNUTS and PECANS are good for sweet fillings, CASHEWS and PEANUTS for savory fillings), 1/2 cup ROLLED OATS, 1/2 cup RICE FLOUR, 1/4 cup BUCKWHEAT FLOUR, 2 TBS melted BUTTER, 2 TBS CANOLA OIL, and 4 TBS COLD WATER. Pat into a pie pan and chill.

SPINACH-CHARD CRUST Good for quiches, vegetable or chicken pies.

For one 10" pie: Preheat oven to 375°. Makes 8 servings.

Sauté 1 TB Olive Oil, 1 small bag Baby Spinach Leaves, 1 TB Sesame Seeds and 1/2 bunch chopped Chard Leaves in a hot skillet for 2 minutes. —Add and mix in: 1/2 cup Oat Flour, 1/2 cup Rice Flour, 2 TBS Olive Oil, 1/2 teasp. Sea Salt, and 1/2 teasp. Nutmeg. Pat into the bottom of an oiled pie pan. Bake for 10 minutes to set. Cool and fill.

Nutrition per: 104 calories; 2gm protein; 12gm carbohydrate; 2g fiber; 5g total fat; 0mg choles.; 37mg calcium; 1mg iron; 41mg magnesium; 179mg potassium; 156mg sodium; Vit. A 151 IU; Vit. C 7mg; Vit. E 2 IU

BROWN RICE CRACKER CRUST Very low-fat...for weight loss diets

For one 8" pie:

Crush 15 to 20 savory Brown Rice Crackers, (3/4 cup). Combine with 3 TBS Canola Oil, and 1 small minced Zucchini. Press into bottom and sides of pie plate and fill.

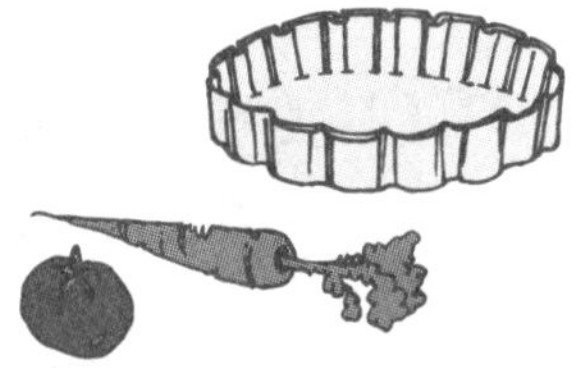

POPPY SEED CRUST

Freeze for 15 minutes before filling for best texture.

Mix together to make a dough ball: 1/2 cup Oat Flour, 1/2 cup Cornmeal, 1/4 cup Buckwheat Flour, 2 TBS Poppy Seeds, 2 TBS melted Butter, 2 1/2 to 3 TBS Ice Water, 1/2 teasp. Sea Salt. Chill, roll out and pat into a pie plate.

Wheat Free Fillings for Quiches, Tarts and Pies

The quiche, pie and tart fillings in this section are healthy, and have already been tested with the crusts in the previous section Just mix and match. They're delicious.

SOUR CREAM APPLE PIE FILLING Try it with a SESAME OAT CRUST.

This recipe works for: Sugar Imbalances, Immune Recovery, Allergies-Asthma
For about 8 slices: A rich, but no-sugar apple pie. Preheat oven to 375°.

Mix: 5 cups tart thin sliced Apples, 1/4 cup Honey or Maple Syrup, 2 TBS Rolled Oats, Juice and grated Zest of 1 Lemon, 1/2 teasp. Cinnamon, 1/4 teasp. Nutmeg, 1 Egg and 1/2 cup Low Fat Sour Cream. Pour into crust and bake for 40 minutes until bubbly.

Nutrition per: 108 calories; 2gm protein; 21gm carbohydrate; 2gm fiber; 3gm total fat; 32mg choles.; 29mg calcium; 0mg iron; 8mg magnesium; 120mg potass.; 15mg sodium; Vit. A 33 IU; Vit. C 6mg; Vit. E 1 IU.

SWEET, SAVORY CARROT FILLING

This recipe works for: Bone Building, Candida Recovery, Respiratory Healing
For 8 servings: Preheat oven to 375°.

Sauté 1 cup sliced Red Onions and $^1/_2$ teasp. Sea Salt in 2 TBS Butter and 1 TB Canola Oil until fragrant. Add 1 LB thin sliced Carrots, and simmer, covered 5 minutes. Add 1 TB Sherry and 1 TB Honey.

—Beat together in a bowl: 1$^1/_2$ cups Low Fat Cottage Cheese, $^1/_4$ teasp. White Pepper, 1 Egg and $^1/_2$ cup grated Low Fat Cheddar Cheese, Rice Cheddar or Almond Cheese.

—Combine with carrot mixture. Pour into pie shell and sprinkle with Nutmeg. Bake for 15 minutes, then reduce heat and bake at 350° for 30 minutes more.

Nutrition per: 123 calories; 7gm protein; 11gm carbohydrate; 2g fiber; 6g total fat; 36mg choles.; 50mg calcium; 1mg iron; 14mg magnesium; 263mg potass.; 332mg sodium; Vit. A 1638 IU; Vit. C 7mg; Vit. E 1 IU

SUN-DRIED TOMATO-BASIL FILLING

This recipe works for: Sugar Imbalances, Fatigue Syndromes, Men's Health
For 8 servings: Preheat oven to 350°.

Cover a pre-baked 9" crust with $^3/_4$ cup grated Low Fat Mozzarella Cheese, 1 grated Zucchini, 3 minced Scallions and $^1/_2$ cup slivered, oil-packed Tomatoes.

—Mix together: 3 Eggs, $^1/_2$ cup Plain Low Fat Yogurt, 2 TBS Red Wine, 2 TBS Balsamic Vinegar, $^1/_4$ cup Water, $^1/_4$ teasp. Italian Seasoning, and $^1/_4$ teasp. Sea Salt.

—Pour over cheese and vegetables; snip on 2 TBS Fresh Basil and bake for 25 minutes til set. Let stand for 5 minutes before cutting.

CREAMY ONION-MUSTARD FILLING

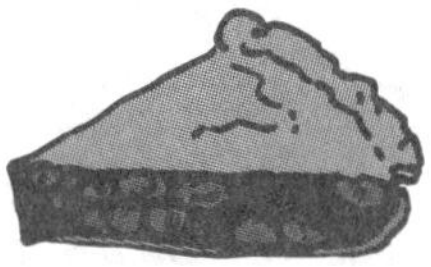

This recipe works for: Hair, Skin, Fatigue Syndromes, Arthritis
For 8 pieces: Preheat oven to 375°.

Sizzle 4 cups thin-sliced Yellow Onions in 3 TBS Olive Oil til onions are translucent. Stir in 1 teasp. Dijon Mustard, 1 teasp. Sesame Salt and 3 TBS White Wine Vinegar.

—Sprinkle on 3 TBS Oat or Rice Flour. Stir to blend well, and add 3 TBS White Wine.

—Beat together until smooth: $^1/_2$ cup Low Fat Cream Cheese or Kefir Cheese, 1 Egg, 1 cup Plain Low Fat Yogurt, $^1/_3$ cup grated Parmesan Cheese, 3 TBS Low Fat Mayonnaise, 2 TBS Lemon Juice, 2 TBS snipped Fresh Parsley, $^1/_4$ teasp. Black Pepper, $^1/_2$ teasp. Wasabi Paste or $^1/_2$ teasp. Hot Pepper Sauce.

—Pour into shell, and bake for 45 minutes. Sprinkle with Sweet Paprika and Sesame Seeds to serve.

Nutrition per: 190 calories; 9gm protein; 15gm carbohydrate; 2gm fiber; 7gm total fat; 43mg choles.; 218mg calcium; 1mg iron; 29mg magnesium; 278mg potass.; 213mg sodium; Vit. A 73 IU, Vit. C 8mg; Vit. E 1 IU.

HONEY CHEESECAKE Very low calorie.... perfect with a nutty crust.

This recipe works for: Recovery, Fatigue Syndromes, Weight Control
For 8 servings: Preheat oven to 350°.

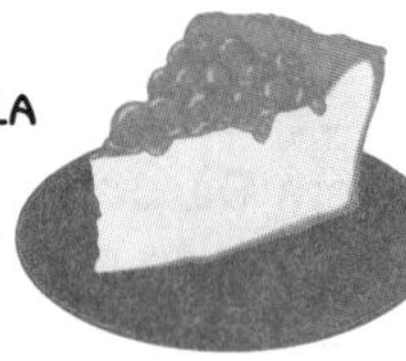

Blender blend: 1 cup Low Fat Cottage Cheese, 1 cup Low Fat Vanilla Yogurt, 3 Eggs, 1/2 cup Honey, 1/2 cup Low Fat Cream Cheese, 1 TB Lemon Juice, 3/4 teasp Cinnamon, 1 teasp. Vanilla. Pour into a prepared NUT CRUST and bake for 40 minutes. Cool and chill for 2 hours.

Nutrition per: 170 calories; 9gm protein; 21gm carbohydrate; trace fiber; 4gm total fat; 90mg choles.; 103mg calcium; 1mg iron; 11mg magnesium; 158mg potass.; 161mg sodium; Vit. A 77 IU; Vit. C 2mg; Vit. E trace

QUICK ITALIAN CHEESE PIE

This recipe works for: Men's Health, Fatigue Syndromes, Recovery
For 6-8 servings: Preheat oven to 350°.

Combine in a bowl: 1/2 cup shredded Low Fat Mozzarella Cheese, 1/4 teasp. dry Basil, 1 Egg, 1/4 cup Low Fat Plain Yogurt, and 1/4 teasp. Sea Salt. Lay on 1 sliced Tomato. Lightly sprinkle with grated Parmesan-Reggiano Cheese and 1/4 teasp. Nutmeg. Pour into a prepared SPINACH-CHARD CRUST. Bake for 30 minutes until set.

CRANBERRY JAM FILLING Try this with an almond nut crust.

This recipe works for: Sugar Imbalances, Women's Health, Bladder-Kidney Health
For 10 small slices: Preheat oven to 350°.

Cook 4 cups Fresh Cranberries and 1 cup Orange Honey until berries pop, about 30 minutes. Set a strainer over a bowl. Pour in berries, and let cool.

—Return strained juice to the pan; blend in 2 teasp. Arrowroot Powder or Kuzu Chunks for a high gloss. Bring to a rolling boil, stirring. Add 1/2 cup Sugar-Free Raspberry Jam and stir until melted. Mix in berries and pour into crust.

—Mix your nut crust choice. Bake until crust is browned, about 25 to 30 minutes. Remove and cool. Loosen crust with a long spatula from sides. Chill.

—Remove the sides when chilled and set. I have made this with the HONEY CUSTARD top layer, and also plain with just the glossy fruit top. Both ways are very rich and very good.

—Make the <u>CUSTARD TOPPING</u>: Whisk together 2 Egg Yolks, 3 TBS Honey and a pinch Sea Salt in the top pan of a double boiler over hot water. Gently heat 1 cup Vanilla Rice Milk. Pour slowly into egg yolk mix and whisk. Place pan over hot water and stir with a wooden spoon til custard coats the back of the spoon. Remove from heat, and add 2 TBS Sherry and 1 teasp. Almond Extract. Smooth over cranberries. Chill again to set. Remove sides of spring form pan and serve.

Wheat-Free Breads and Muffins

Breads are the most difficult foods to buy or make without wheat or gluten grains. The recipes here show you how easy it can be without loss of taste or function.

OAT BRAN MUFFINS

A delicious way to get oat bran's benefits.

This recipe works for: Allergies, Fatigue Syndromes, Waste Management
For 9 small or 6 large muffins: Preheat oven to 400°.

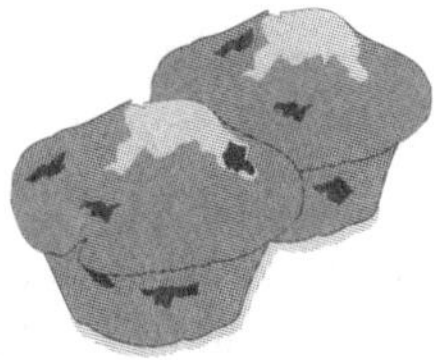

Mix in a bowl: 1 cup Oat Bran, 1 TB Lecithin Granules, 1 teasp. non-aluminum Baking Powder, 1 teasp. Cinnamon, 1/2 teasp. Stevia Leaves. —Blender blend: 1 Egg Yolk, 1/4 cup Apple Juice, 1/4 cup Raisins, 1 teasp. Vanilla, 1 chunked Apple, and 1/4 cup chopped Pecans. Mix wet and dry ingredients in a bowl. Beat 1 Egg White to stiff peaks and fold into batter.

—Fill muffin tins lined with paper muffin cups, and bake for 15 to 20 minutes, until a toothpick inserted in the center of a muffin comes out clean.

Nutrition per: 89 calories; 3gm protein; 15gm carbohydrate; 2gm fiber; 4gm total fat; 23mg choles.; 57mg calcium; 1mg iron; 37mg magnesium; 171mg potass.; 49mg sodium; Vit. A 13 IU; Vit. C 1mg; Vit. E trace.

SWEET CORN LOAF

Toast and top with sweet toppers for a great snack.

This recipe works for: Sugar Imbalances, Men's Health, Allergies and Asthma
For 8 servings: Preheat oven to 350°. Place loaf pan in the oven to preheat.

Stir together: 2 cups Yellow Cornmeal, 1/3 cup Honey, 1/4 cup Oat Flour, 1/4 cup Rice Flour, 2 teasp. Baking Powder, 1 teasp. Baking Soda and 1 teasp. Sea Salt.

—Add and mix just to moisten: 2 Eggs, 1 cup Plain Yogurt, 1 cup Water, 1 TB Canola Oil. Oil bottom and sides of a loaf pan with 1 TB Canola Oil. Return loaf pan to oven to heat to smoky. Bake for 1 hour until browned and crusty. Turn out on a rack to cool before slicing.

Nutrition per: 234 calories; 6gm protein; 43gm carbohydrate; 3gm fiber; 4gm total fat; 54mg choles.; 152mg calcium; 2mg iron; 56mg magnesium; 205mg potass.; 540mg sodium; Vit. A 44 IU; Vit. C 1mg; Vit. E 1 IU.

EASY WHEAT-FREE APPLE MUFFINS

This recipe works for: Sugar Imbalances, Fatigue Syndromes, Kid's Health
For 12 to 18 muffins: Preheat oven to 375°.

In a food processor, mix: 7 Tart Apples, 3 cups rolled Oats, and 1 TB Sherry, leaving apples chunky. Let stand 5 minutes. Mix in 1/2 cup Raisins and 1/2 cup Walnut Pieces. Spoon into paper-lined muffin tins, and bake for 25 minutes until firm.

BROWN BATTER BREAD

This recipe works for: Sugar Imbalances, Overcoming Addictions, Candida Albicans
For 2 loaves: Preheat oven to 350°. Makes 16 servings.

Cream together until smooth: $^1/_2$ cup HONEY, 3 TBS CANOLA OIL, 3 TBS UNSULPHURED MOLASSES, 1 cup PLAIN YOGURT, 1 cup WATER, 1 cup chopped WALNUTS and 1 cup RAISINS.

—Add and mix well: 1 cup CORNMEAL, 1 cup BUCKWHEAT FLOUR, 1 cup AMARANTH FLOUR, 2 teasp. BAKING SODA and 1 teasp. SEA SALT.

—Divide batter into 2 greased loaf pans; bake for 40 minutes until centers test done with a toothpick.

Nutrition per: 246 calories; 6gm protein; 38gm carbohydrate; 4gm fiber; 8gm total fat; 1mg choles.; 1mg calcium; 3mg iron; 88mg magnesium; 357mg potass.; 311mg sodium; Vit. A 8 IU; Vit. C 2mg; Vit. E 1 IU.

YAM BREAD

This recipe works for: Anti-Aging, Fatigue Syndromes, Women's Health
For 2 loaves: Preheat oven to 350°. Makes 24 servings.

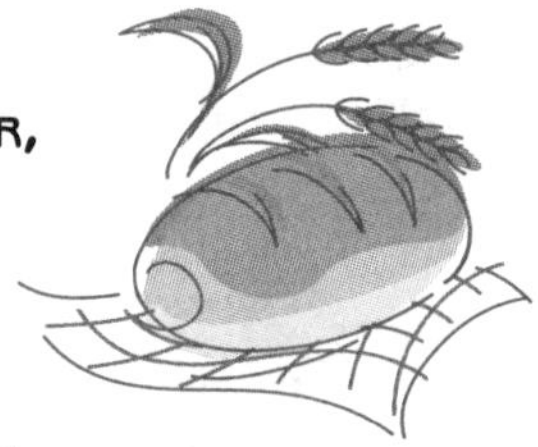

Mix dry ingredients: 1 cup BUCKWHEAT FLOUR, 1 cup AMARANTH FLOUR, $^1/_2$ cup RICE FLOUR, $^1/_2$ cup OAT FLOUR, 1 TB CHINESE FIVE-SPICE POWDER, $1^1/_2$ tsp. BAKING SODA, 1 tsp. ground GINGER, $^1/_2$ tsp. SEA SALT.

—Blend wet ingredients: 3 EGGS, $^1/_2$ cup soft BUTTER, 1 cup DATE SUGAR, $^1/_4$ cup CANOLA OIL, $^1/_2$ cup PLAIN YOGURT, $^1/_2$ cup MAPLE SYRUP, $^1/_2$ cup HONEY, 2 TBS WATER and 2 tsp. VANILLA. Pour wet into dry ingredients and mix.

—Mash in 2 small cooked YAMS. Blend in 1 cup each: chopped DATES and chopped WALNUTS. Pour into 2 lecithin-sprayed loaf pans and bake for 60 to 70 minutes, until bread pulls away from sides, and a center inserted toothpick comes out clean.

Nutrition per: 257 calories; 5gm protein; 38gm carbohydrate; 9gm fiber; 9gm total fat; 37mg choles.; 48mg calcium; 1mg iron; 58mg magnesium; 254mg potass.; 141mg sodium; Vit. A 294 IU; Vit. C 3mg; Vit. E 1 IU.

WHEAT FREE HERB BREAD

This recipe works for: Heart Health, Brain Boosting, Respiratory Healing
For 1 skillet: Makes 12 servings.

Put 2 TBS OLIVE OIL in a 12" iron skillet and heat in a 425° oven while you make the bread. Mix all ingredients: 2 cups YELLOW CORNMEAL, 2 EGGS, 3 teasp. BAKING POWDER, $^1/_4$ cup OAT FLOUR, $^1/_4$ cup RICE FLOUR, $^1/_2$ cup PLAIN YOGURT, $^1/_2$ cup WATER, $^1/_2$ teasp. dry OREGANO, 1 TB CHIVES, $^1/_2$ teasp. SEA SALT, $^1/_2$ teasp. SAGE and $^1/_2$ teasp. ROSEMARY.

—Pour into sizzling hot skillet. Bake for 20 minutes until center springs back when touched. Cut in squares, and top with a pat of butter.

Nutrition per: 132 calories; 4gm protein; 20gm carbohydrate; 2gm fiber; 4gm total fat; 36mg choles.; 112mg calcium; 1mg iron; 36mg magnesium; 110mg potass.; 205mg sodium; Vit. A 28 IU; Vit. C 1mg; Vit. E 1 IU.

DARK CHEWY CRANBERRY BREAD

This recipe works for: Kidney Problems, Fatigue Syndromes, Women's Health
For 1 loaf: Preheat oven to 350°. Makes 12 servings.

Sauté 1/2 cup chopped Walnuts, 1 1/2 cups Fresh Cranberries, 1/2 teasp. Cinnamon and 1/4 teasp. Nutmeg in 4 TBS Butter and 4 TBS Canola Oil for 10 minutes until fragrant. Remove from heat and set aside.

—Mix together: 1 cup Buckwheat Flour, 3/4 cup Amaranth Flour, 1/4 cup Oat Flour, 1/2 teasp. Sea Salt and 1/2 teasp. Baking Soda.

—Mix together: 2 Eggs, 1/4 cup Unsulphured Molasses, 2 TBS Maple Syrup, 4 TBS Date Sugar and 1/2 teasp. Vanilla.

—Combine all mixtures. Spread in a lecithin-sprayed loaf pan and bake 45 minutes. Cool 10 minutes in the pan. Rap bottom of pan sharply to loosen and remove.

Nutrition per: 239 calories; 6gm protein; 25gm carbohydrate; 4gm fiber; 13gm total fat; 44mg choles.; 97mg calcium; 3mg iron; 84mg magnesium; 347mg potass.; 160mg sodium; Vit. A 54 IU; Vit. C 2mg; Vit. E 1 IU.

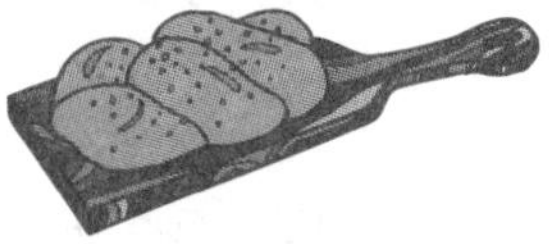

Breakfast without Wheat or Gluten

It may seem impossible considering the commercial choices available on grocery shelves today, but you can have a great, satisfying breakfast without wheat or gluten. Try the delicious pancakes and spoonbreads in this section.

REAL COUNTRY SKILLET CORN BREAD

This recipe works for: Stress Reactions, Allergies and Asthma, Men's Health
For 8 servings: Preheat oven to 375°. Make this in a cast iron skillet for best results.

Heat 2 TBS Olive Oil in an iron skillet; sauté 2 minced Cloves Garlic and 1/2 cup diced Onion til translucent. Add 1 cup Salsa or Tomato Sauce, 1/2 cup diced Red Bell Pepper and 1/2 cup Corn Kernels. Sizzle briefly, remove from heat and add 3 TBS snipped Fresh Cilantro.

—Mix lightly in a separate bowl: 2 cups Polenta, 2 Eggs, 1/2 cup Sparkling Water (for lightness), 1/2 cup Plain Yogurt, 1/4 cup Honey and 2 TBS Olive Oil.

—Pour over the vegetables in the skillet and sprinkle with Jalapeño Cheese or Soy Jalapeño Cheese. Turn oven down to 325° and bake for 20 minutes until set, and cheese bubbles and browns.

Nutrition per: 169 calories; 5gm protein; 23gm carbohydrate; 2gm fiber; 7gm total fat; 53mg choles.; 18mg calcium; 1mg iron; 18mg magnesium; 241mg potass.; 36mg sodium; Vit. A 99 IU; Vit. C 18mg; Vit. E 1 IU.

WHEAT FREE BREAKFAST MUFFINS

This recipe works for: Sugar Imbalances, Fatigue Syndromes, Allergies
For 12 muffins: Preheat oven to 375°.

Stir everything together just to moisten: 1 cup any Wheat Free Dry Breakfast Cereal, 1 Egg, 1 cup Buttermilk (or $^{1}/_{2}$ cup Plain Yogurt mixed with $^{1}/_{2}$ cup Water), $^{1}/_{2}$ cup Oat Bran, $^{1}/_{4}$ cup Peanut Butter, $^{1}/_{4}$ cup any Fruit Yogurt, $^{1}/_{2}$ cup Raisins, $^{1}/_{4}$ cup chopped Walnuts, 1 TB Fructose, $^{1}/_{2}$ teasp. Baking Soda, $^{1}/_{2}$ teasp. Baking Powder, 3 TBS Maple Syrup and 1 TB Canola Oil. Spoon into paper-lined muffin cups, and bake for 20 to 25 minutes til a toothpick comes out clean.

OLD VIRGINIA SPOONBREAD

This recipe works for: Digestive Health, Fatigue Syndromes, Candida Healing
For 8 servings: Preheat oven to 400°.

Butter a 1-qt. soufflé or 8" square pan and heat it in the oven until sizzling.

—Bring 2 cups Cold Water, 1 cup Yellow Cornmeal and $^{3}/_{4}$ teasp. Sea Salt to a boil in a pan over high heat. Reduce heat to low and simmer for 5 minutes, stirring til stiff. Remove from heat and stir in 1 cup Cold Buttermilk, 2 Eggs, and 2 TBS Butter.

—Pour batter into hot baking dish and bake 40 minutes until firm in the center and well-browned on top. Serve hot.

CINNAMON OATCAKES with MANGO TOPPING

This recipe works for: Kid's and Men's Health, Digestive Health, Heart Health
Makes 4 servings (3 pancakes per serving):

Make the topping: Put 1 package (12-oz.) frozen Mango Chunks in a saucepan with 3 TBS Brown Sugar and $^{1}/_{2}$ tsp. Cinnamon; set aside to thaw.

—Make the pancake batter: In a bowl, mix 2 cups Low-Fat Buttermilk, 1 cup Quick-Cook Oatmeal, grated Zest of 1 Orange and 1 tsp. Anise Seed. Set aside for about 15 minutes to soften oatmeal. Beat in 1 Egg, 2 TBS Brown Sugar, and 1 teasp. Canola Oil.

—In a separate bowl, sift together $^{1}/_{2}$ cup Oat Flour, $^{1}/_{2}$ cup Buck-wheat Flour, 1 tsp. non-aluminum Baking Powder, $^{1}/_{4}$ tsp. Baking Soda, 2 pinches Sea Salt; stir into the batter.

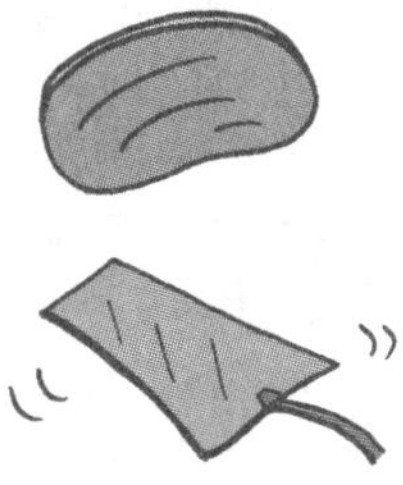

—Heat 1 teasp. Canola Oil in a nonstick skillet over medium and spoon portions of the batter into the pan. Cook, flipping once when top becomes bubbly. While the pancakes cook, add $^{1}/_{2}$ cup of water to the mango mix and simmer just until the mango chunks and syrup are hot. Serve the pancakes sauced with the berries.

Nutrition per: 340 calories; 13gm protein; 61gm carbohydrate; 7gm fiber; 6gm total fat; 57mg choles.; 289mg calcium; 3mg iron; 104mg magnes.; 571mg potass.; 376mg sodium; Vit. A 370 IU; Vit. C 33mg; Vit. E 3 IU.

HERB PANCAKES Wheat-Free and Dairy-Free

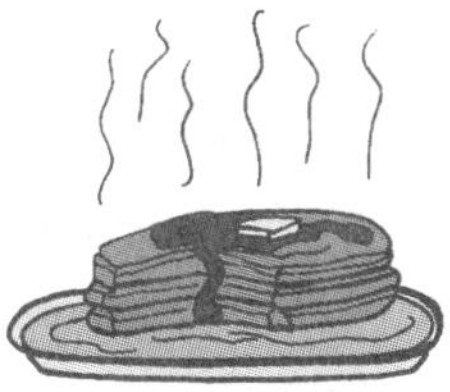

This recipe works for: Candida Infections, Fatigue Syndromes
For 16 small pancakes:

Combine in a large bowl: 3 Eggs, 1/2 cup snipped Scallions, 1/4 cup snipped Fresh Cilantro, 1/2 cup snipped Fresh Parsley, 1 teasp. Herbal Seasoning Salt, 1/2 cup snipped Fresh Basil Leaves, 1/4 teasp. White Pepper.

—Heat a griddle or skillet brushed with oil to sizzling. Drop on 2 TBS pancake mix for each pancake. Make four at a time, and cook 3 minutes until golden and crispy on the edges. Serve alone or with a mushroom sauce (page 274).

BROCCOLI PANCAKES

This recipe works for: Cancer Protection, Arthritis, Candida, Fatigue Healing
For 6 dinner pancakes: Preheat griddle to medium hot.

Finely chop 1 1/2 cups Broccoli. Blanch in boiling water until color changes to bright green. Drain.

—Mix together: 1 Egg, 1/2 cup Buckwheat Flour, 2 TBS Plain Low Fat Yogurt, 2 TBS Water, 1 teasp. Baking Powder, and 1/4 teasp. Sea Salt. Mix in broccoli.

—When water beads on the hot griddle, ladle 4 pancakes and cook until bubbles appear. Turn, cook 1 minute and remove. Serve plain or with a mushroom sauce.

Nutrition per: 49 calories; 3gm protein; 7gm carbohydrate; 1gm fiber; 9gm total fat; 34mg choles.; 84mg calcium; 1mg iron; 28mg magnesium; 141mg potass.; 8mg sodium; Vit. A 51 IU; Vit. C 21mg; Vit. E trace.

POTATO PANCAKES with HERB SPRINKLES

This recipe works for: Stress Reactions, Fatigue Syndromes, Sports Nutrition
Makes about 18: Preheat oven to 250°F.

Peel and grate 2 1/2 lbs. White Potatoes and 1 large White Onion into cold water to cover. Let stand 15 minutes. Then drain in a large colander. With your hands, squeeze the mixture to extract most of liquid. Put the mixture into a bowl and stir in 1/2 cup snipped Scallions, 1/2 cup snipped Fresh Cilantro, 1/2 cup Chickpea Flour, 2 Eggs, 2 teasp. Chipotle Chili Sauce, 2 tsp. ground Coriander, 1 1/2 tsp. Sea Salt and 1/2 tsp. Cracked Black Pepper.

—Heat 2 TBS Olive Oil in large nonstick skillet over medium heat. Add 1 1/2 tsp. Cumin Seeds and 1/2 tsp. Ground Tumeric. Let stand 30 minutes for flavors to blend.

—Heat 1 TB Olive Oil in the same skillet over medium heat. Spoon on 3 TBS potato mixture for each pancake; flatten to 4-inch rounds with a spatula. Cook until golden, 5 minutes per side. Keep pancakes in an ovenproof dish. Repeat with remaining potato mixture, adding more oil to skillet as necessary. Serve warm.

WILD RICE and PECAN PANCAKES

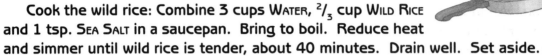

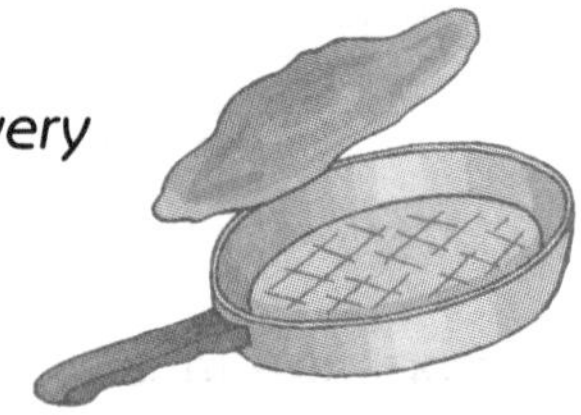

This recipe works for: Overcoming Addictions, Illness Recovery
Makes about 12:

Cook the wild rice: Combine 3 cups Water, $^2/_3$ cup Wild Rice and 1 tsp. Sea Salt in a saucepan. Bring to boil. Reduce heat and simmer until wild rice is tender, about 40 minutes. Drain well. Set aside.

—Mix $^1/_2$ cup Buckwheat Flour, $^1/_2$ tsp. Baking Powder, $^1/_2$ tsp. Baking Soda, $^1/_4$ tsp. Black Pepper and $^1/_2$ tsp. Sea Salt in a bowl. Whisk in 5 TBS Plain Yogurt, 4 TBS Water, and 1 Egg. Add wild rice, $^1/_4$ cup toasted chopped Pecans and 1 minced Shallot.

—Heat 1 TB Olive Oil in large nonstick skillet over medium-high heat. Drop batter by spoonfuls to form 3-inch-diameter panckes. Cook about 2 minutes per side. Repeat, adding more olive oil as necessary. Transfer pancakes to plates and serve.

ALMOND BUTTER PANCAKES So rich they melt in your mouth.

This recipe works for: Men's Health, Candida Recovery, Allergies and Asthma
For 9 to 10 pancakes: Preheat griddle to medium hot.

Combine just to moisten: 1 cup Buckwheat Flour, $^1/_4$ cup Oat Flour, 1 Egg, $^1/_2$ cup Plain Yogurt, $^1/_2$ cup Water, 1 TB Honey, 3 TBS Canola Oil, 2 TBS Almond Butter, $^1/_2$ teasp. Sea Salt, $^1/_2$ teasp. Vanilla and 2 drops Almond Extract.

—Brush Canola Oil on a hot griddle. Use 3 TBS batter per pancake to make 4" circles. Cook until bubbles appear; turn and brown on the bottom.

—Make the ALMOND BUTTER TOPPING: Melt and mix: $^1/_2$ cup Almond Butter, $^1/_2$ cup Peanut Butter, 3 teasp. Honey and 2 drops Almond Extract. Stir until fragrant.

Nutrition per: 270 calories; 8gm protein; 18gm carbohydrate; 3gm fiber; 19gm total fat; 22mg choles.; 74mg calcium; 1mg iron; 94mg magnesium; 303mg potass.; 127mg sodium; Vit. A 12 IU; Vit. C 1mg; Vit. E 7 IU.

PUFFY VEGETABLE PANCAKES

This recipe works for: Fatigue Syndromes, Candida Recovery, Sports Nutrition
For 16 pancakes: Preheat griddle to medium hot.

Separate 3 Eggs. Combine: 1 cup Buckwheat Flour, $^1/_3$ cup Amaranth Flour, 1 TB Baking Powder and $^1/_2$ teasp. Sea Salt. Whisk in: the Egg Yolks, 1 cup Plain Yogurt, 1 cup Water, 4 TBS Canola Oil, 2 teasp. Honey. Set aside.

—Sizzle in a small skillet for 3 minutes in 1 TB Olive Oil: 1 minced Onion, 2 minced Ribs Celery, $^1/_2$ minced Green Bell Pepper, and 2 small diced Carrots. Remove from heat. Stir into batter mix. Beat 3 Egg Whites to stiff peaks, and fold into batter.

—When water beads on skillet or griddle, ladle on 3 to 4 pancakes. Turn when bubbles appear on the surface, and cook 1 minute more (no longer, or they will be tough). Serve with a LIGHT CHEESE SAUCE (page 218, 275).

SWEET POTATO PANCAKES

This recipe works for: Allergies and Asthma, Candida Infections, Women's Health
Makes 8 cakes: Preheat oven to 400°.

Bake 4 large Sweet Potatoes until soft. Peel and mash in a bowl. Beat in 1 cup Soy Flour, 3 Eggs, 1 tsp. Sea Salt, 2 tsp. Canola Oil, $^1/_2$ teasp. Ginger Powder and $^1/_2$ tsp. Cardamom Powder. Heat a griddle or heavy skillet to hot. Drop on spoonfuls batter and cook until crispy on the edges, about 5 minutes per side. Serve with Maple Syrup.

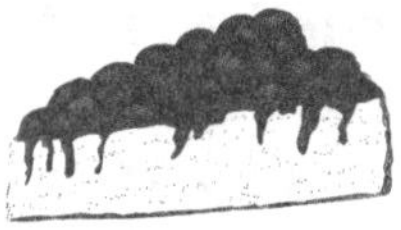

Wheat Free Cakes and Cookies

Think you can't satisfy a craving for sweet baked treats if you have a wheat or gluten allergy? Check out these wheat free cookies and cakes.

NO WHEAT, NO BAKE FRUITCAKE

This recipe works for: Allergies - Asthma, Sugar Problems, Women's Health
For 10 pieces:

Have ready 1 MACAROON COOKIE CRUST (page 289) in a spring form pan.

—Combine in a large bowl: 3 cups crumbled Sweet Rice Cakes (Honey-Nut, Caramel and Apple-Lemon flavors are all good), 1 LB mixed, diced Dried Fruits, 1 cup Raisins, 4-oz. shredded Unsweetened Coconut, $^1/_2$ cup Sherry, $^1/_4$ cup Orange Honey, grated Zest from 1 Orange, grated Zest from 1 Lemon, 3 TBS Lemon Juice, 2 TBS Crystallized Ginger, $^1/_2$ teasp. each Cinnamon, Allspice and Nutmeg.

—Pack mixture firmly into macaroon lined pan. Cover with foil; chill for 3 days. To serve, remove from pan, peel off foil and slice thin with a very sharp knife.

Nutrition per: 290 calories; 3gm protein; 56gm carbohydrate; 6gm fiber; 7gm total fat; 0mg choles.; 36mg calcium; 2mg iron; 43mg magnesium; 656mg potass.; 12mg sodium; Vit. A 166 IU; Vit. C 8mg; Vit. E 1 IU.

WHEAT FREE CARROT NUT CAKE

This recipe works for: Allergies - Asthma, Bone Building, Women's Health
For 12 slices: Preheat oven to 350°.

Beat til fluffy: 5 Egg Yolks, $^1/_3$ cup Honey, 3 TBS Fructose, 1 teasp. Almond Extract, $^1/_4$ teasp. Sea Salt. Whirl 2 Carrots, 8-oz. Whole Almonds and $^1/_3$ cup Rolled Oats in a food processor; stir into egg mixture. Beat 5 Egg Whites to stiff peaks; fold into cake.

—Bake in an oiled spring form pan for about 1 hour until cake springs back when touched. Cool in pan and then remove sides.

FRESH FRUIT WHEEL on a GIANT WHEAT-FREE COOKIE

Arrange the fruits in expressive patterns. Kids love to build this dessert.
This recipe works for: Heart Health, Waste Management, Kid's Health
Serves 10-12: Preheat oven to 325°.

Combine dry cookie ingredients: $^1/_2$ cup chopped Nuts, $^1/_3$ cup Oat Flour, $^1/_3$ cup Amaranth Flour, $^1/_3$ cup Rice Flour, 1 TB Baking Powder, 1 cup diced Dates.

—Heat $^1/_3$ cup Honey, $^1/_3$ cup Orange Juice and 4 TBS Butter. Add to a blender and blend with 2 Eggs, 2 TBS Frozen Orange Juice Concentrate and 2 teasp. Vanilla.

—Mix wet and dry ingredients together, and pour the whole thing onto a Lecithin-sprayed round pizza pan with a lip. Spread batter to the edges. Bake for 5 minutes, then turn down oven to 300° and bake for 10 more minutes. Watch closely to avoid burning. Remove when center is springy. Cool completely before topping.

—Blender the topping: 2 cups Low Fat Cottage Cheese, 3 TBS Low Fat Cream Cheese, 2 TBS Maple Syrup, 2 TBS Honey, 2 tsp. grated Lemon Peel, 1 tsp. grated Orange Peel and 1 tsp. Lemon Extract. Spread over cool crust. Top with seasonal fresh, sliced drained Fruits..... raspberries, peaches, kiwi, blueberries, nectarines in artful patterns.

Nutrition per: 270calories; 10gm protein; 38gm carbohydrate; 3gm fiber; 9gm total fat; 49mg choles.; 141mg calcium; 1mg iron; 47mg magnesium; 300mg potass.; 257mg sodium; Vit. A 79 IU; Vit. C 10mg; Vit. E 1 IU.

WHEAT FREE RAISIN SPICE COOKIES

This recipe works for: Allergies and Asthma, Digestive Health, Kid's Health
For 24 to 30 pieces: Preheat oven to 400°.

Combine dry ingredients: $^1/_4$ cup Rice Flour, $^1/_4$ cup Amaranth Flour, $1^1/_2$ cups Rolled Oats, 1 TB minced Crystallized Ginger, 2 tsp. Cinnamon, $1^1/_2$ tsp. Nutmeg, $^1/_2$ tsp. Allspice, 1 tsp. Baking Powder and 1 tsp. Baking Soda.

—Combine wet ingredients: $^1/_2$ cup Apple Sauce, $^1/_2$ cup Frozen Apple Juice Concentrate, 1 teasp. Vanilla, $^1/_2$ cup Raisins, $^1/_4$ cup diced Dates and 2 Eggs.

—Mix all together. Drop by heaping tablespoons onto lecithin-sprayed baking sheets. Bake 12 to 15 minutes. Leave in the turned-off oven to cool and harden. Remove from baking sheets.

Nutrition per: 63 calories; 2gm protein; 12gm carbohydrate; 1gm fiber; 1gm total fat; 16mg choles.; 26mg calcium; 1mg iron; 16mg magnesium; 94mg potass.; 67mg sodium; Vit. A 8 IU; Vit. C 1mg; Vit. E trace

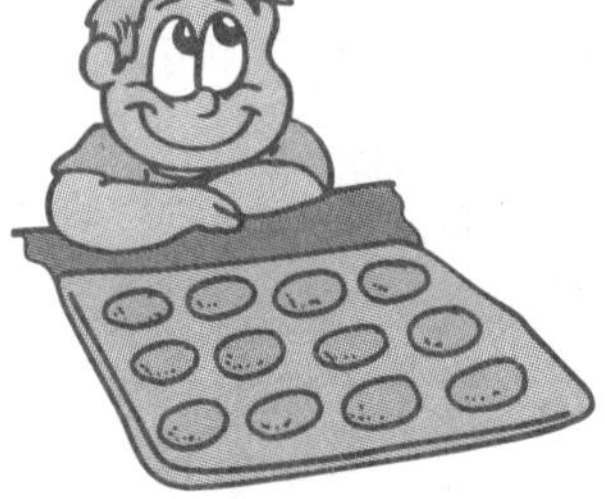

Main Dishes with Non-Wheat Grains

The living is easy (and so is dinner) with these wheat free entrees.

POLENTA SOUFFLÉ

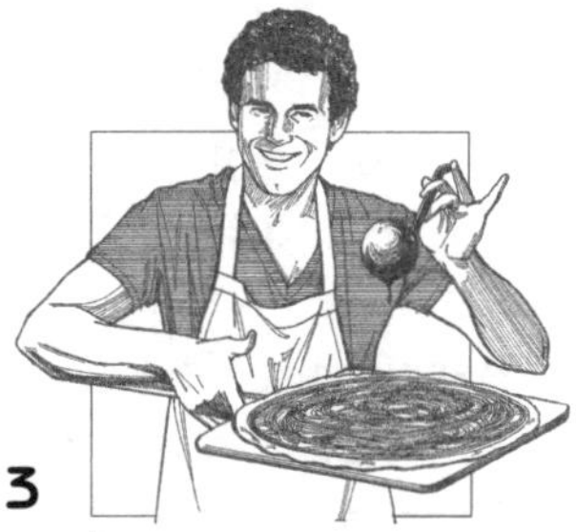

This recipe works for: Heart Health, Men's Health
Serves 4: Preheat oven to 350°F.

Separate 3 Eggs. Heat 2 cups Rice Milk to boiling. Stir in $^1/_3$ cup Yellow Cornmeal and 1 TB Butter. Reduce heat and stir in 3 TBS grated Jalapeño Jack Cheese and 1 tsp. Sea Salt. Cook to consistency of hot cereal. Season with $^1/_4$ tsp. Paprika, 3 shakes Cajun Seasoning or Hot Pepper Sauce. Whisk in egg yolks.

—Stir off heat 1 minute to let yolks thicken. Beat egg whites stiff and fold into corn meal mixture. Bake in ungreased baking dish for 25 minutes until crusty.

CORN BREAD PIZZA

This recipe works for: Arthritis, Sugar Imbalances, Kid's Health
For 8 servings: Preheat oven to 375°.

Cut about 2 lbs. Zucchini in chunks and steam until tender. Puree in a blender to make 2 cups. Add and mix in: 2 Eggs, 2 $^1/_2$ cups Yellow Cornmeal, 2 TBS Olive Oil, 2 teasp. Baking Powder, and 1 teasp. Sea Salt. Turn into a Lecithin-sprayed, large pizza pan. Bake for 12 to 15 minutes until crust begins to pull away from sides.

—While crust is baking, sauté filling ingredients briefly in Olive Oil until fragrant: 1 chopped Onion, 1 teasp. dry Oregano, 1 teasp. dry Basil, 1 teasp. Chili Powder, 1 teasp. Cumin Powder, $^1/_2$ teasp. ground Coriander. Scatter 3 chopped Tomatoes on top. Sprinkle with 1$^1/_2$ cups Low Fat Jalapeño Jack Cheese and bake for 10 more minutes.

Nutrition per: 298 calories; 16gm protein; 35gm carbohydrate; 5gm fiber; 6gm total fat; 52mg choles.; 379mg calcium; 3mg iron; 84mg magnes.; 555mg potass.; 620mg sodium; Vit. A 211 IU; Vit. C 20mg; Vit. E 2 IU.

2 CHEESE WHEAT FREE PIZZA

This recipe works for: Allergies, Kid's and Men's Health, Candida Healing
For 6 servings: Preheat oven to 350°.

Sizzle 1 diced Onion in 2 TBS Olive Oil for 5 minutes. Add 4 sliced Button Mushrooms and sizzle 5 minutes. Add $^1/_2$ cup White Wine, 1 TB snipped Fresh Basil and $^1/_4$ teasp. Black Pepper; stir until liquid evaporates. Remove from heat and set aside.

—Combine 3 Eggs, $^1/_4$ cup Buckwheat Flour, 2 TBS Oat Flour, 2 TBS Plain Yogurt and 2 TBS Water; pour into an oiled quiche pan. Spoon onion mix over top. Cover with grated Mozzarella Cheese. Bake about 25 minutes. Let cool 10 minutes; cut in wedges.

WHEAT FREE LENTIL NUT LOAF

This recipe works for: Heart Health, Cancer Protection, Men's Health

Soak $1^1/_2$ cups Dry Lentils overnight in water to cover (makes about 2 cups). Drain. Mince 1 Clove Garlic, shred $^1/_2$ cup Carrots, dice $^1/_2$ cup Tomato and $^1/_2$ cup Celery, chop $^1/_2$ cup Parsley, $^1/_2$ cup Red Onion and $^1/_2$ cup Avocado. Place lentils and other ingredients in a food processor. Add $^1/_4$ cup Oat Bran, $1^1/_2$ TB Tamari, $^1/_2$ tsp. Herbs de Provence, 2 teasp. Lemon Juice and blend well; leave in processor. Mix 2 TBS Arrowroot Powder with $^1/_3$ cup Water. Add to food processor; whirl to blend.

—Spoon lentil mixture onto a lightly oiled sheet of wax paper and roll into a log. Tuck in ends and place in a bread pan. Chill one hour. Unwrap loaf and roll in $^1/_2$ cup chopped ALMONDS until covered. Place loaf on a bed of Greens with halved Cherry Tomatoes dotted over top of loaf as garnish.

QUINOA PASTA SALAD

This recipe works for: Allergies and Asthma, Candida Healing, Arthritis
For 6 servings:

Rinse 2 cups Quinoa Grain in a colander under running water. Put in a pan with 2 cups Water. Bring to a boil, reduce heat and simmer for 20 to 25 minutes until water is absorbed. Drain and cool.

—Toss with: $^1/_2$ cup chopped Green Onion, 1 minced Shallot, 1 cup snipped Fresh Parsley, $^1/_4$ cup sliced Black Olives, 1 TB snipped Fresh Basil (1 teasp. dry), 1 TB snipped Fresh Mint Leaves and 24 Cherry Tomatoes, halved. Chill well.

—Whisk $^1/_2$ cup Fresh Lemon Juice and $^1/_4$ cup Olive Oil together. Pour over and toss with salad. Serve on Baby Spinach Leaves.

Nutrition per: 346 calories; 11gm protein; 49gm carbohydrate; 7gm fiber; 14gm total fat; 0mg choles.; 127mg calcium; 8mg iron; 181mg magnes.; 1021mg potass.; 153mg sodium; Vit. A 481 IU; Vit. C 54mg; Vit. E 9 IU.

PEPPER TACO CUPS

This recipe works for: Digestive Health, Candida Infections, Heart Health
Makes 12 cups: Preheat oven to 450°F.

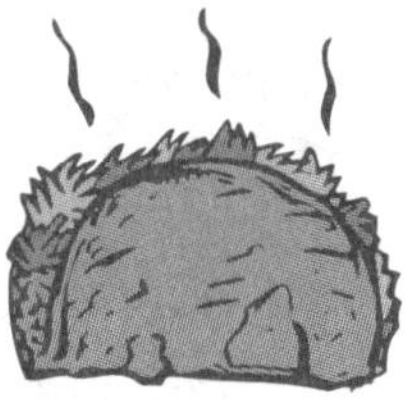

In a bowl, beat 2 Eggs to blend. Stir in 1 TB Chili Powder, $^1/_2$ tsp. dry Oregano, and $^1/_2$ tsp. Sea Salt. Add 2 cups diced mixed Red, Orange and Yellow Bell Peppers, 1 cup coarsely crushed Tortilla Chips, $^1/_2$ cup shredded Cheddar Cheese, and $^1/_3$ cup minced Green Onion.

—Spoon mixture into 12 nonstick muffin cups. Cover with more shredded Cheddar Cheese. Bake until taco cups are deep golden, 15 minutes. Loosen taco cups with a knife; lift to a platter. Top with Salsa. Serve warm.

GOURMET POT PIE, WHEAT FREE

This recipe works for: Candida Healing, Immune Health, Women's Health
Makes enough for 6: Preheat oven to 350°. Use a $1^1/_2$ qt. casserole dish.

Bake a Russet Potato in the oven until semi-soft. Peel and cut into cubes.

—Sizzle 1 small diced Onion and 1 diced Carrot in 2 TB Olive Oil for 5 minutes. Add 1 LB Extra-Firm Tofu in chunks and sizzle 5 more minutes. Turn into casserole and add $^1/_2$ cup frozen Peas, $^1/_3$ cup diced Walnuts, half the potato cubes and 1 TB snipped Fresh Basil.

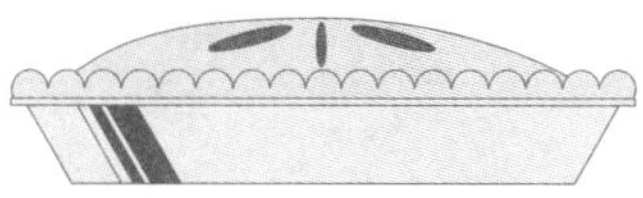

—Heat 2 cups Organic Chicken Broth in the skillet with 1 TB Tamari (wheat free), 1 tsp. dry Thyme, 1 tsp. dry Tarragon and $^1/_2$ tsp. dry Rosemary. Whisk in 2 TBS Arrowroot Powder dissolved in $^1/_4$ cup Red Wine. Stir until thickened. Season with Sea Salt and Pepper. Stir into vegetables in casserole.

—Make the pastry top in a food processor: 1 cup Rice Flour, $^1/_2$ cup Soy Flour, 1 tsp. Baking Powder, $^1/_2$ teasp. Sea Salt, 4 TBS Olive Oil and remaining Potato chunks. Slowly add Ice Water, 1 TB at a time, until dough forms a ball. Turn dough onto a lightly floured surface and roll out to fit casserole dish. Place crust on casserole and crimp edges. Bake about 45 minutes until light brown and fragrant. Serve warm.

Nutrition per: 460 calories; 23gm protein; 42gm carbohydrate; 4gm fiber; 23gmtotal fat; 0mg choles.; 236mg calcium; 11mg iron; 151mg magnes.; 861mg potass.; 269mg sodium; Vit. A 365 IU; Vit. C 9mg; Vit. E 3 IU.

SESAME GINGER CHICKEN with RICE NOODLES

This recipe works for: Allergies and Asthma, Candida Infections, Women's Health
Serves 6:

Have ready 1 cooked Organic Chicken Breast, shredded.

—Have ready a 6-oz. package Cellophane Rice Noodles, cooked briefly until soft and cooled.

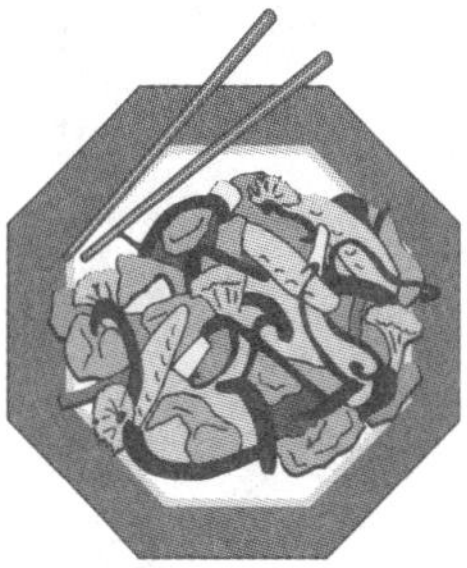

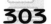

—Make the VINAIGRETTE SAUCE: whisk in a bowl, 4 TBS Olive Oil, 3 TBS Honey, 3 TBS Tamari (wheat free), 2 TBS minced Crystallized Ginger, 4 TBS Lime Juice, 1 teasp. Toasted Sesame Oil, 2 TBS Sesame Seeds, 2 shakes Hot Pepper Sauce and 2 shakes Granulated Garlic.

—Heat 2 TBS Olive Oil in a wok to hot; add 2 cups chopped Baby Bok Choy, and 1 cup shredded White Daikon Radish; sizzle with 2 to 3 pinches Garlic-Lemon Seasoning for 2 minutes.

—Mix the salad in a serving bowl: 1 cup Baby Spinach Leaves, 1 Carrot shredded, 1 Red Bell Pepper, diced, and the chicken and cooked vegetables. Pour on Vinaigrette and serve.

Nutrition per: 299 calories; 7gm protein; 42gm carbohydrate; 2gm fiber; 12gm total fat; 12mg choles.; 64mg calcium; 2mg iron; 37mg magnesium; 306mg potass.; 189mg sodium; Vit. A 565 IU; Vit. C 47mg; Vit. E 2 IU.

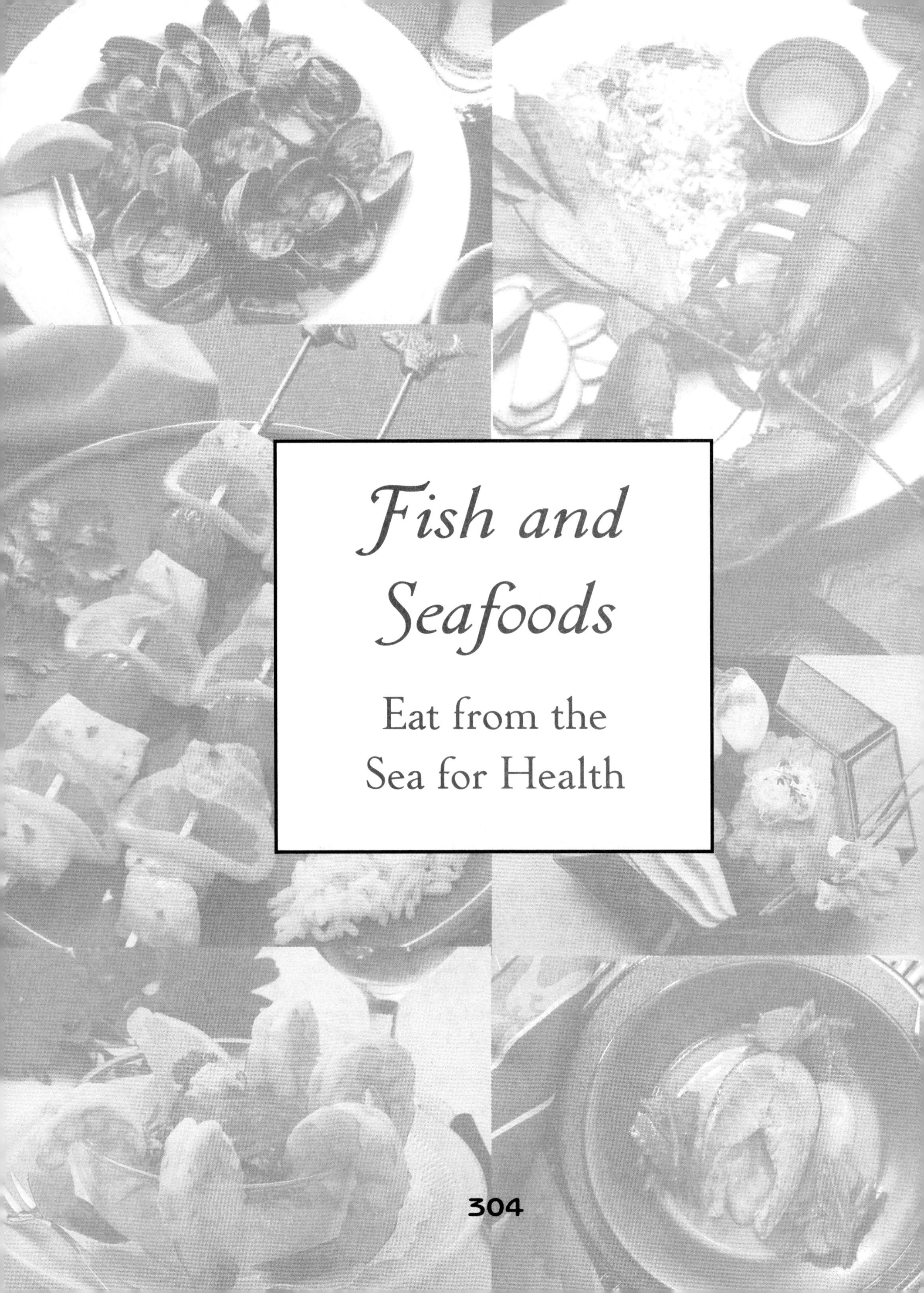

Fish and Seafoods

Eat from the Sea for Health

Healing from the Sea

Scientists have focused a great deal of research on complex Omega-3 fatty acids from sea foods for protection against heart and circulatory disease. They've been rewarded with test results showing that these oils not only deter blood clogs, clots, and platelet aggregation, but also help neutralize the bad effects of saturated fats already in the bloodstream.

Tests show that even with no other diet changes, both cholesterol and triglyceride levels drop substantially after the addition of Omega-3 oils and essential fatty acids from ocean foods. Further, the beneficial effects of these healthy oils have direct action on blood viscosity (thickness) and the blood's propensity to clot - factors that can help prevent heart attacks.

There's a lot to choose from for your healing diet. Salmon heads the list, but tuna (especially fresh tuna), mackerel, shad, cod, shark, bass, halibut, trout, red snapper and swordfish are all loaded with helpful fatty acids. Many of the Hawaiian and Alaskan fish from unpolluted waters are rich in EFA's, too.

Ocean foods are quick and easy to prepare, and low in saturated fat, cholesterol and calories. If you've heard that shellfish is high in cholesterol (initial studies had faulty measurements and incomplete information about cholesterol types), newer tests show that shellfish is heart healthy even with moderate cholesterol levels, because of its low saturated fats and high Omega-3 oils.

I was raised on the Chesapeake Bay, where fresh crab is a favorite food, and my mother had lots of delicious ways to fix it. As kids, we took chicken necks tied on a string, sat in an old abandoned row boat in an inlet behind our house, and caught fresh crabs for supper. The crabs always "knew" when we had chicken necks. They would even float close to the surface and watch us tie on the chicken necks. We'd just barely let the string down in the water before two or three of them grabbed it. We'd pull them up, pick them off the string, throw them in a bucket, and take them home to eat. I can still see my father sitting at our newspaper-covered kitchen table, cracking crab claws. The Chesapeake's coastal waters are too polluted now, (as are so many of America's waterways) but those were days of really fresh seafood at home.

Get the Best Healing Results from Ocean Foods

The secrets to moist, tender, delicious seafood are freshness and timing. Whether you broil, poach, bake, sauté or grill it, the moment your fish turns from its natural translucent white or pink, to opaque white (like egg whites), it is done. Remove it from the heat immediately. Even a *little* overcooking toughens and dries out the meat. Seafood is an investment. Pay attention to it; learn to gauge its thickness correctly; test it for doneness. When you're making a seafood meal, the rest of the meal should either already be together or done later. Once you put seafood on to cook, it needs your undivided attention for the few minutes it takes to come to perfection.

—Use the professional 10 minute rule for best results: cook 10 minutes for each inch of thickness.

—To bake or barbecue fish in foil or parchment, or simmer it in sauce, 15 minutes per inch of thickness is about right.

—Do not fry fish! Poach, bake, steam, broil or grill it for the best health benefits. For thick cuts, sear on a hot grill first to seal in juices, then barbecue. Cook it less and leave the meat firmer and fresher.

—To test for doneness: lightly poke the fish with your finger, if it springs back it is done; or cut into the thickest part of the fish, if it is just opaque, it is just right. If it flakes easily, it is probably overcooked. Older recipes recommend flaking as the proper doneness point, but years of eating seafoods tell me that the best flavor and texture have already gone by then.

Fish and Seafood Recipe Sections

I find myself eating largely from the sea for optimum health.

Seafood Appetizers

Meal starters are the perfect place for light, fresh seafood.

CRAB CAKES with WASABI CREAM

This recipe works for: Women's Health, Liver and Organ Health, Weight Control
Serves 4, 2 each: Preheat oven to 400°.

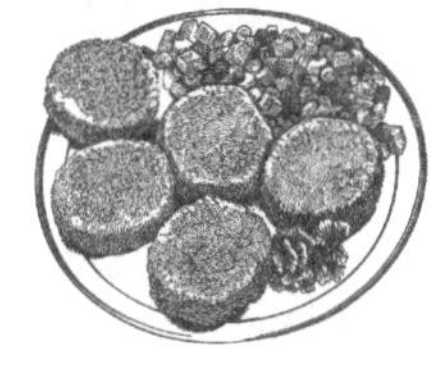

Mix: 16-oz. Crabmeat (or Surimi) with $^1/_4$ cup Plain Yogurt, 1 Egg, $^1/_4$ cup each, snipped Scallions, Red Bell Pepper and grated Parmesan, 1 TB each snipped Fresh Parsley and grated Lemon Zest, 1 teasp. Teriyaki Sauce, 1 cup Whole Wheat Bread Crumbs and $^1/_4$ cup Toasted Wheat Germ. Form into patties. Bake on Canola Oil-sprayed baking sheets until slightly browned and puffy, about 8 minutes on each side.

—Mix topping: 1 teasp. Wasabi Paste, 2 teasp. Lemon Juice and 4 TBS each Low Fat Cream Cheese and Low Fat Plain Yogurt. Spoon on top of warm crab cakes at serving.

Nutrition per: 280 calories; 34gm protein; 15gm carbohydrate; 2gm fiber; 7gm total fat; 169mg choles.; 304mg calcium; 3mg iron; 85mg magnesium; 673mg potass; 467mg sodium; Vit. A 118 IU; Vit. C 31mg; Vit. E 5 IU.

ENDIVE SURIMI SCOOPS Arrange in a design on a serving platter.

This recipe works for: Brain Health, Liver and Organ Health, Women's Health
For 32 scoops:

Have ready 32 rinsed Belgian Endive Leaves. Mix: 8-oz. Low Fat Cream Cheese, 2 TBS minced Scallions, 1 TB Lemon Juice, 1 TB White Worcestershire Sauce, and $^1/_2$ teasp. Lemon-Pepper. Stir in 6-oz. shredded Surimi (or canned Crab). Mound 2 teasp. filling onto root end of each endive leaf. Sprinkle with snipped Scallions or Cilantro.

SEA GREENS APPETIZERS

This recipe works for: Women's Health, Bone Building, Hair, Skin and Nails
For 8 people as an appetizer: Preheat oven to 350°.

Have ready 24 Button Mushrooms, wiped, with stems removed and minced.

—Soak $^1/_2$ cup crumbled, dried Arame Sea Greens and 6 dried Shiitake Mushrooms for 15 minutes in water to cover. Drain and rinse well. Remove woody mushroom stems. Cover mushrooms and arame again with water. Bring to a boil; simmer 15 minutes. Drain. Squeeze out liquid and mince both vegetables.

—Heat 1 teasp. Toasted Sesame Oil; sizzle 1 small diced Onion and the minced mushroom stems for 5 minutes. Add minced arame and shiitakes, 2 TBS Lemon Juiice, 2 TBS bottled Teriyaki Sauce, 1 TB minced Crystallized Ginger; simmer 5 minutes more.

—Stuff mushroom caps; cover and bake for 20 minutes. DON'T OVERCOOK, or mushrooms will not be juicy.

LEMON PRAWNS

This recipe works for: Digestive Health, Weight Control, Anti-Aging
For 8 people as an appetizer:

Simmer 1 lb. shelled Prawns in $^3/_4$ cup Brown Rice Vinegar and $^3/_4$ cup Lemon Juice with 1 teasp. Dijon Mustard until opaque. Remove with a slotted spoon to a bowl. Boil liquid over high heat until reduced to 1 cup - 5 minutes. Pour over prawns and chill overnight. Mix 4 thin sliced Green Onions, 2 diced Tomatoes, Sea Salt and Cracked Pepper to taste. Place drained prawns on Boston Lettuce leaves. Top with green onion mix; offer Lemon Wedges to squeeze over.

HOT CLAM BALLS

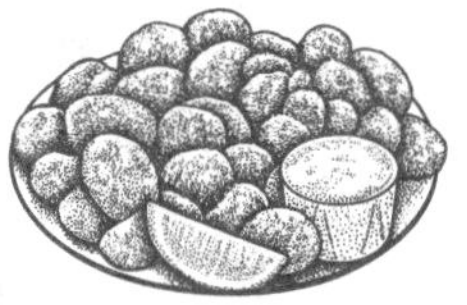

This recipe works for: Sexuality Boost, Bone Building
For about 12 servings: Preheat oven to 325°.

Drain juice from two 7-oz. cans chopped Clams into a bowl. (Save the clam juice for your pets if you don't have other uses for it. They love it.) Blend clams briefly in a blender to chewy chunks. Pour into a mixing bowl.

—Add to the blender and blend: $^1/_2$ cup crushed Whole Grain Crackers, 1 small chopped White Onion, $^1/_4$ cup chopped Red Bell Pepper, 1 TB White Worcestershire Sauce, 1 TB snipped Fresh Parsley, 1 teasp. Lemon-Garlic Seasoning, 1 teasp. Paprika, $^1/_2$ teasp. Hot Pepper Sauce, $^1/_2$ teasp. Sesame Salt, $^1/_4$ teasp. White Pepper. Mix with the clams. Form into balls. Add a little Toasted Wheat Germ if necessary to hold them together. Roll in Toasted Wheat Germ for crusty outside. Set on Lecithin-sprayed baking sheets and chill for 1 hour to set. Bake for 15 to 20 minutes. Serve hot with toothpicks.

Nutrition; 85 calories; 10gm protein; 8gm carbo.; 1gm. fiber; 1gm total fats; 22mg choles.; 38mg calcium; 10mg iron; 85mg magnesium; 272mg potassium; 126mg sodium; Vit. A 72 IU; Vit. C 13mg; Vit. E 2 IU.

CRAB STUFFED MUSHROOMS

This recipe works for: Women's Health, Immune Health, Hair and Skin
For 24 appetizers: Preheat oven to 400°.

Clean, stem, scoop out ribs from 24 large White Mushrooms to make a filling cavity. Mince stems and sizzle in 2 teasp. Olive Oil until soft. Scrape into a blender.

—Add to the blender for the filling: 8-oz. rinsed, picked over Lump Crabmeat, 2 teasp. Lemon Juice, $^1/_4$ cup Low Fat Cream Cheese or Soy Cream Cheese, $^1/_4$ teasp. dry Basil, $^1/_4$ teasp. Garlic Powder, $^1/_4$ teasp. Onion Powder. Turn into a bowl; mix in $^1/_3$ cup minced Black Olives and 2 TBS snipped Fresh Parsley. Fill mushroom caps.

—Rinse a baking sheet with water. Shake off excess and place filled caps on the sheet. Cover with foil and bake 12 to 15 minutes. Remove foil and bake for 5 more minutes until tops are golden. Serve hot.

CRAB PUFFS

This recipe works for: Digestive Health, Bone Building, Anti-Aging
For 12 puffs: Preheat oven to 350°.

Pick over 1 lb. rinsed, drained, LUMP CRAB MEAT.

—Melt 2 TBS BUTTER in a skillet. Stir in 2 TBS UNBLEACHED FLOUR and simmer until bubbly. Stir in 1/2 cup PLAIN YOGURT, 4 TBS WATER and 4 TBS WHITE WINE, 1/2 teasp. SEA SALT and 2 pinches WHITE PEPPER. Stir until a smooth sauce forms. Remove from heat.

—Separate 2 EGGS. Beat the EGG YOLKS to frothy. Add a little of the hot sauce to the yolks to warm them, then add them back to the sauce and stir in well. Add 1/4 teasp. PAPRIKA, 1 cup KEFIR CHEESE or LOW FAT CREAM CHEESE and the crab. Mix well.

—Beat the EGG WHITES to stiff peaks with 1 pinch CREAM OF TARTAR so they will hold up better, and fold into crab mixture. Place into 12 oiled ramekins. Place the ramekins in a pan of hot water, and bake for 40 to 45 minutes til puffs are high and firm.

—Offer an easy HOMEMADE TARTAR SAUCE: blend together in a bowl: 1/2 cup PLAIN LOW FAT YOGURT, 1/4 cup LIGHT MAYONNAISE, 2 TBS chopped GREEN ONIONS, 2 TBS SWEET PICKLE RELISH, 1 HARD BOILED EGG crumbled, 2 TBS WHITE WINE. Chill and serve.

Nutrition; 146 calories; 13gm protein; 5gm carbo.; 1gm fiber; 5gm total fats; 104mg choles.; 109mg calcium; 1mg iron; 23mg magnesium; 254mg potassium; 267mg sodium; Vit. A 93 IU, Vit. C 2mg; Vit. E 1 IU.

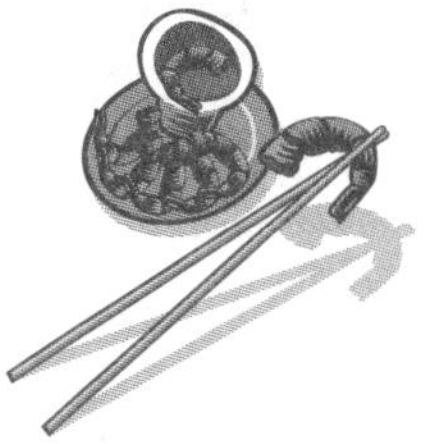

SALMON WRAPPED PRAWNS

This recipe works for: Brain Health, Heart and Artery Health
Makes 12: Preheat broiler or grill.

In a bowl marinate: 12 raw, peeled PRAWNS, 1/2 cup WHITE WINE, 1 teasp. GARLIC-LEMON SEASONING and 1/4 teasp, HOT PEPPER SAUCE. Set aside.

—Drain prawns; reserve marinade. Cut thin SMOKED SALMON into 12 inch-wide strips. Wrap prawns and secure with toothpicks. Broil or grill about 6" from heat until salmon is crispy on the edges. Watch closely. Serve with LEMON squeezes.

BABY POTATOES STUFFED with SMOKED SALMON

This recipe works for: Men's Health, Hair and Skin Health, Anti-Aging
Makes 24: Preheat oven to 400°.

Cut 12 BABY RED POTATOES in half crosswise. Drizzle with Olive Oil, place cut side down on a baking sheet; bake about 25 minutes until tender. Set aside.

—Make the filling: mix 4-oz. minced SMOKED SALMON with 2 TBS LOW FAT CREAM CHEESE, 2 teasp. SWEET PICKLE RELISH, 2 teasp. minced RED ONION and LEMON-PEPPER to taste.

—Cut a thin slice off the rounded end of each potato so it will stand upright. Scoop out a center pocket of each potato, spoon in filling. Run under a broiler for 1 minute to brown tops and serve hot.

Seafood Salads

Far from ho hum "shrimp and sauce" salads, these recipes have a load of health benefits, but none of the boredom. They're sea foods and sea greens with a healing difference. *Note: Lobsters are endangered or overfished on many coasts (and incredibly expensive). As good as this sea food is, Langoustinos, or some of the small Australian or Phillipine lobster cousins, are a good substitute.*

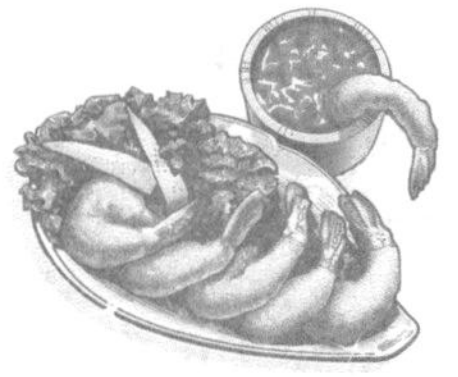

GRILLED SCALLOP - PRAWN SALAD

This recipe works for: Arthritis, Hair, Skin and Nails
Makes 4 servings: Have barbecue ready with heat at hot.

Skewer 8 large rinsed SCALLOPS onto a thin metal skewer. Push a second skewer through scallops, parallel to and 1/2 inch from the first to steady scallops on the grill. Thread 24 large PRAWNS onto metal skewers. Lay scallops and shrimp on hot grill. Turn until scallops are light brown and shrimp are pink, about 5 minutes. Remove.

—Rinse and drain 1 HEAD RADICCHIO, 1 head BELGIAN ENDIVE, and 1 package ARUGULA (4 to 6-oz.). Separate leaves from radicchio and endive heads. Discard tough arugula stems. Place in a big salad bowl. Toss with 6 TBS OLIVE OIL, 2 TBS LEMON JUICE, 2 TBS BALSAMIC VINEGAR and 1 TB snipped CHIVES.

—Divide salad onto individual plates. Divide scallops and shrimp from skewers onto salads. Sprinkle with LEMON-PEPPER to taste.

Nutrition; 313 calories; 23gm protein; 7gm carbo.; 1gm fiber; 21gm total fats; 82mg choles.; 105mg calcium; 2mg iron; 85mg magnesium; 608mg potass.; 232mg sodium; Vit. A 149 IU; Vit. C 16mg; Vit. E 5 IU.

FRESH AHI SALAD

This recipe works for: Bone Building, Brain-Bone Enhancement, Skin and Hair
Serves 6:

Mix a marinade in a bowl: 1/2 cup TAMARI, 1/4 cup SAKE, 3 sprigs snipped FRESH BASIL, 1 teasp. FRESH LEMON ZEST, 2 teasp. TOASTED SESAME OIL. Marinate 1 1/2 lbs. VERY FRESH AHI TUNA for 1 hour. —Sear Ahi in a very hot, heavy skillet about 10 seconds on each side. Remove and chill while you make the salad.

—Sizzle for 1 minute: 2 diced CARROTS, 2 TBS minced CRYSTALLIZED GINGER, 1/2 teasp. OLIVE OIL, 1/2 teasp. TOASTED SESAME OIL. Add 1/2 cup WATER, 1/2 cup WHITE WINE and 1/2 teasp. LEMON PEPPER; simmer 3 minutes. Remove from heat and blend in 1/4 cup LOW FAT CREAM CHEESE, and 4 snipped MINT LEAVES. Divide sauce onto 6 salad plates; divide tuna slices on top of sauce. Snip on FRESH CILANTRO LEAVES.

Nutrition; 255 calories; 30gm. protein; 8gm. carbo.; 1gm. fiber; 8gm total fats; 48mg choles.; 42mg calcium; 2mg iron; 76mg magnesium; 463mg potassium; 422mg sodium; Vit. A 1459 IU; Vit. C 4mg; Vit. E 4 IU.

TUNA and ASPARAGUS SALAD

This recipe works for: Arthritis, Brain Boosting, Women's Health
For 4 servings: Have ready a pot of boiling salted water or an asparagus cooker.

Cut off bottom inch from $1^1/_2$ lbs. Fresh Asparagus Spears. Blanch in boiling Salted Water for 4 minutes until bright green. Immediately plunge into ice water to stop cooking and set color. Remove from ice water and drain and dry on paper towels.

—Make the TUNA SAUCE: Grate 2 teasp. Fresh Lemon Zest. Blender blend the zest, $^1/_4$ cup Lemon Juice and 1 can water-packed White Tuna, 1 Green Onion and 2 teasp. Olive Oil til smooth. Arrange asparagus spears on 4 salad plates. Pour on Tuna Sauce, sprinkle with Lemon-Pepper and snip Fresh Parsley on top.

SEARED TUNA SALAD NICOISE

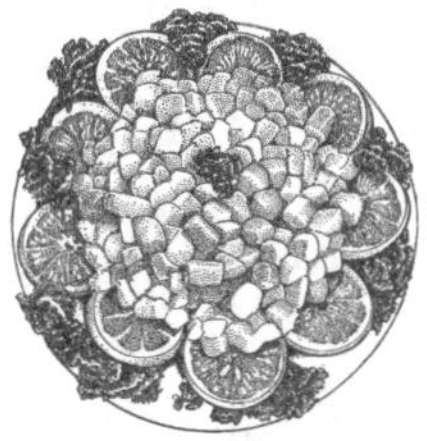

This recipe works for: Recovery, Brain, Weight Control
For 4 servings:

Have ready 1-lb. cooked small, yellow Dutch Potatoes, quartered. Have ready 8-oz. cooked French-cut Green Beans. Have ready 16 Cherry Tomatoes, halved.

—Sear an 8-oz. Fresh Ahi Steak in a very hot, heavy skillet about 1 minute on each side. Remove to a bowl and keep covered while you make the salad.

—Mix the tuna dressing: 2 TBS Olive Oil, 1 TB Sweet Hot Mustard, 3 TBS Balsamic Vinegar, 2 teasp. dry Tarragon, $^1/_2$ teasp. Lemon-Pepper. Brush on tuna.

—Divide 1 package Baby Asian Greens onto large salad plates. Divide tuna steak among plates. Surround with potatoes and green beans. Top with tomatoes and drizzle with remaining dressing from the tuna bowl. Sprinkle with Cracked Pepper.

Nutrition; 276 calories; 17gm protein; 29gm carbo.; 3gm fiber; 10gm total fats; 22mg choles.; 61mg calcium; 1mg iron; 68mg magnes.; 815mg potassium; 256mg sodium; Vit. A 475 IU; Vit. C 26mg; Vit. E 4 IU.

SPRING SALAD with SALMON and ASPARAGUS

This recipe works for: Hair and Skin, Fatigue Syndromes, Arthritis Recovery
For 4 servings:

Cut off bottom inch from 8-oz. Fresh Asparagus Spears. Blanch in boiling Salted Water for 4 minutes until bright green. Immediately plunge into ice water to stop cooking and set color. Remove from ice water, drain and dry on paper towels.

—Cover individual salad plates with a mixture of Watercress and Arugula. Arrange asparagus on top. Divide 1 thin-sliced Avocado on top.

—Separate 1 small head Belgian Endive. Wrap each asparagus spear with thin slices Smoked Salmon. Nestle into endive leaf and place on top of avocado.

—Whisk dressing: Zest of 1 Lime, Juice of 1 Lime, Zest of 1 Lemon, Juice of 1 Lemon, 1 TB Honey, 1 TB Olive Oil, 1 thin-sliced Kiwi Fruit. Pour on top.

DELUXE SHRIMP SALAD

This recipe works for: Liver - Organ Health, Respiratory Recovery, Hair and Skin
For 8 servings:

Make the vinaigrette in a bowl: 3 TBS Olive Oil, 2 TBS Fresh Lemon Juice, 2 thin sliced Green Onions, $^{1}/_{2}$ tsp. Honey, Lemon-Pepper to taste. Set aside.

—Combine in a bowl: 2 lbs. cooked medium Shrimp, 3 cups thin-sliced Kiwi, 3 cups ripe Papaya, scooped into small balls, 2 cups diced Plum Tomatoes, 2 cups peeled, diced Cucumber, $^{1}/_{4}$ cup snipped Fresh Basil, and 1 TB grated Lime Zest. To serve, toss with vinaigrette. Divide on salad plates and sprinkle with Cracked Pepper.

SEAFOOD RICE SALAD

This recipe works for: Brain Health, Arthritis and Candida, Hair and Skin
For 6 servings:

Have ready 3 cups cold cooked Brown Rice.

—Bring about 1 qt. Salted Water to a boil. Add $^{1}/_{2}$ lb. Bay Scallops and $^{1}/_{2}$ lb. peeled, deveined Shrimp, cover pan and remove from heat. Let stand until scallops and shrimp are opaque, 5 minutes. Drain and pour into a bowl; place bowl in ice water. Add 1 can (7-oz.) picked over, rinsed Crab Meat.

—In a blender or food processor, whirl 2 Tomatoes, 2 TBS Lime Juice and $^{1}/_{2}$ cup lightly packed Fresh Cilantro until puréed. Pour over shellfish. Add $^{1}/_{2}$ cup finely chopped Red Onion and 1 cup chopped Red Bell Pepper. Toss occasionally until salad cools, 30 minutes. Add rice; season to taste with Sea Salt.

—Cover large salad plates with seafood salad and sprinkle with Thai Hot Sauce.

Nutrition; 228 calories; 23gm protein; 28gm carbo.; 3gm fiber; 2gm total fats; 114mg choles.; 74mg calcium; 2mg iron; 96mg magnesium; 531mg potass.; 290mg sodium; Vit. A 155 IU; Vit. C 45mg; Vit. E 3 IU.

LOBSTER SALAD with GINGER DRESSING

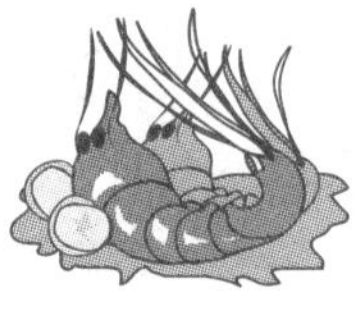

This recipe works for: Brain Health, Heart Health, Bone Health
For 4 servings:

Trim and blanch 8-oz. Fresh Pea Pods in boiling water until color changes to bright green. Remove pods and rinse in ice water to set color. Return water to a boil, and add 2 Lobster Tails (8-oz. each) or 16-oz. Langoustinos. Simmer covered until meat turns opaque in the center, about 7 minutes. Drain, clip fins and shell, and lift out meat. Slice meat into chunks and chill. Cover 4 salad plates with Baby Greens. Arrange 2 thin-sliced Kiwi in a ring over top. Fill the middle of the ring with fresh sliced Strawberries. Top with lobster and pea pods. Chill again while you make the dressing.

—Make the GINGER DRESSING: Mix 1 teasp. grated Orange Zest, $^{3}/_{4}$ cup Orange Juice, 2 TBS Brown Rice Vinegar and 2 TBS minced Crystallized Ginger. Pour over salad.

Seafood Loves Pasta

Sea foods compliment light vegetable or whole grain pastas beautifully, offering high protein and complex carbohydrates with low fat. Cook everything with a light hand for a healing diet.

FETTUCINI and FRESH AHI TUNA Melts in your mouth.

This recipe works for: Heart and Artery Health, Weight Control, Sexuality
For 8 servings: Use a heavy skillet.

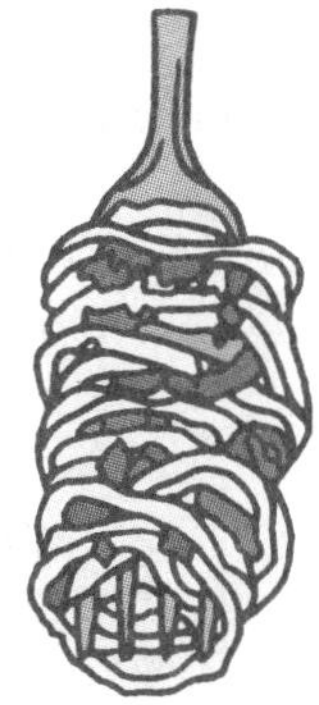

Bring a pot of Salted Water to boil with 3 Cloves Garlic for pasta.

—In a skillet, sauté 1 large Onion, diced in 2 TBS Olive Oil until soft, about 10 minutes. Add 2-lbs. Roma Tomatoes, diced and 1 TB snipped Fresh Basil. Season with $^3/_4$ teasp. Sea Salt and $^1/_2$ teasp. Cracked Pepper. Cook, partially covered until juices thicken to form a sauce, about 5 minutes. Remove vegetables from the skillet and set aside in a bowl.

—Heat 2 TBS Olive Oil in the skillet. Cube a 1-lb Fresh Tuna Steak and season with Lemon-Pepper. Sizzle in the hot skillet, tossing for 4 minutes only. Add the tomato sauce back to the skillet with $^1/_2$ cup snipped Fresh Mint, 1 teasp. Lemon Juice and 3 diced Scallions. Cook for 2 or 3 minutes only. Do not overcook. Remove from heat.

—Cook 1-lb. Fettucini in the boiling water to al dente, about 9 minutes. Drain, and transfer to a shallow serving bowl. Pour on the hot Tuna/Tomato Sauce; toss quickly to mix. Serve hot with more Basil snipped on top.

Nutrition; 367 calories; 22gm protein; 50gm carbo.; 8gm fiber; 8gm total fats; 21mg choles.; 61mg calcium; 3mg iron; 146mg magnes.; 693mg potass.; 190mg sodium; Vit. A 493 IU; Vit. C 30mg; Vit. E 1 IU.

STEAM-SMOKED SALMON and LINGUINI

This recipe works for: Heart and Artery Health, Hair, Skin, Nails, Arthritis
For 4 people:

Remove the skin from 1-LB Salmon Filet. Cut in $^1/_2$" wide strips. Pour about 3 TBS Liquid Smoke Flavoring into a wok. Set a steaming rack on top, put the salmon on the rack, cover tightly, and steam for 10-12 minutes. Remove and set aside.

—Make the sauce in a small pan: cook 2 TBS Balsamic Vinegar and $^1/_2$ cup chopped Red Onion until liquid evaporates. Add 1 cup Plain Low Fat Yogurt, $^3/_4$ cup White Wine, and 1 TB Dijon Mustard. Cook until liquid is reduced to about a cup.

—Bring 2-qts Salted Water to a boil. Cook 12-oz. Dry Linguini for 10 minutes to al dente. Drain and toss with the sauce. Divide pasta onto serving plates. Top each with smoked salmon slices, Fresh Parsley, Parmesan Reggiano Cheese and Cracked Pepper.

Nutrition; 480 calories; 35gm protein; 55gm carbo.; 3gm fiber; 10gm total fats; 66mg choles.; 174mg calcium; 4mg iron; 83mg magnes.; 826mg potassium; 198mg sodium; Vit. A 33 IU; Vit. C 4mg; Vit. E 2 IU.

EASY TUNA MAC

This recipe works for: Heart and Artery Health, Men's and Kid's Health, Brain
For 4 servings: Preheat oven to 350°.

In 1 TB Olive Oil, sizzle 1 chopped Green Onion, 1/4 cup diced Red Bell Pepper and 1 diced Rib Celery for 5 minutes. Add 2 TBS Whole Wheat Flour and stir until bubbly.

—Stir in 1 cup Low Fat Cottage Cheese and 1/3 cup Water; cook until thickened. Add a small can (7-oz.) Water Packed White Tuna with juice. Remove from heat.

—Bring 3-qts. Salted Water to a boil, and add about 1 1/2 cups Vegetable Elbow Macaroni. Cook for 7 minutes only. Drain immediately and mix with tuna. Pour into a Lecithin-sprayed casserole and bake covered for 15 minutes until hot through.

Nutrition; 311 calories; 25gm protein; 47gm carbo.; 2gm fiber; 2gm total fats; 14mg choles.; 60mg calcium; 3mg iron; 49mg magnesium; 307mg potassium; 375mg sodium; Vit. A 53 IU; Vit. C 13mg; Vit. E 1 IU.

TRADE WINDS TUNA CASSEROLE

This recipe works for: Arthritis, Men's and Kid's Health, Brain Booster
For 4 people: Preheat oven to 350°. Use a 1-qt. covered casserole dish.

Sauté 1/2 cup diced Onion in 1 TB Olive Oil for 10 minutes. Remove from heat; add an 8-oz. can sliced Water Chestnuts. Add 1 can (14-oz.) Cream of Celery Soup or Cream of Mushroom Soup. Add 1 can (7-oz.) Water-Packed White Tuna, 4 TBS Low Fat Cream Cheese, 1/2 tsp. Curry Powder, 2 cups Crispy Chinese Noodles (from 1 small package), 2 TBS snipped Fresh Parsley. Pour into a Lecithin-sprayed casserole. Top with remaining package of Chow Mein Noodles; cover and bake 35 minutes until light brown.

Nutrition; 274 calories; 19gm. protein; 26gm. carbo.; 3gm. fiber; 11gm total fats; 16mg choles.; 47mg calcium; 3mg iron; 34mg magnesium; 306mg potassium; 749mg sodium; Vit. A 22 IU; Vit. C 6mg; Vit. E 2 IU.

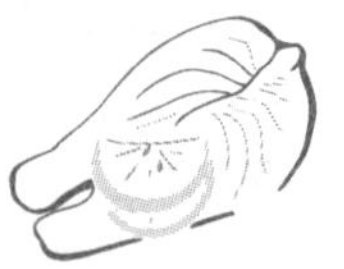

SEA BASS and RED PEPPER PASTA

This recipe works for: Hair and Skin, Men's Health, Sports Nutrition
Makes 4 servings: Preheat oven to 450°F. Use an 9-inch square baking dish.

Pour 3 TBS Lime Juice over 4 skinned Sea Bass Filets 2-inches thick (1 1/2 lb. total) and arrange in a single layer. Tightly cover dish with foil. Bake until fish is opaque but still moist-looking in thickest part (cut to test), 12 to 14 minutes. Set aside.

—In a blender or food processor, purée 1/2 cup jarred Roasted Red Bell Peppers, 1/2 cup grated Parmesan-Reggiano Cheese, 1 cup Organic Chicken Broth, 1 TB Arrowroot Powder, 2 tsp. minced Fresh Jalapeño Chili, 1/4 cup snipped Fresh Cilantro and 1 teasp. Garlic-Lemon Seasoning. Pour into a hot skillet. Stir in juices from the baked salmon.

—Cook 8-oz. dry Angel Hair Pasta (Cappellini) in 3 quarts boiling water until al dente, 7 minutes. Drain; return to pan. Mix 1 1/2 cups sauce with pasta. Spoon pasta onto plates. Top with fish and drizzle with remaining sauce. Serve hot.

SALMON with PASTA PRIMAVERA

This recipe works for: Sexuality, Women's Health, Bone Building
For 6 servings:

Sliver a 6-oz. package Smoked Salmon. Set aside.

—Bring 2-qts. Salted Water to a boil. Blanch 2 Carrots, in matchsticks, and 8-oz. French Cut Green Beans until color changes. Remove with a slotted spoon; set aside.

—Mix the PARMESAN SAUCE in a bowl: 6 TBS Olive Oil, 3 TBS Tarragon Vinegar, $^1/_2$ cup thin-sliced Green Onions, $^1/_2$ cup Frozen Green Peas, 2 TBS Parmesan-Reggiano Cheese, 1 teasp. Garlic-Lemon Seasoning and $^1/_2$ teasp. crushed Chilies; set aside.

—Bring salted water to boil again. Add 8-oz. small Ziti or Bow Tie Pasta and cook to al dente. Drain and toss with sauce.

—Set large Boston Lettuce cups on salad plates. Fill with pasta salad. Top with Smoked Salmon slivers; sprinkle with diced Tomatoes; season with Lemon-Pepper.

Nutrition; 341 calories; 13gm protein; 36gm carbo.; 6gm fiber; 16gm total fats; 8mg choles.; 86mg calcium; 2mg iron; 87mg magnesium; 422mg potass.; 390mg sodium; Vit. A 760 IU; Vit. C 85mg; Vit. E 4 IU.

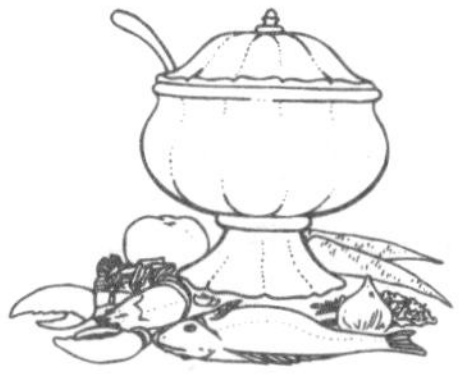

Seafood Stews

What's the Catch?

From cioppino to paella to bouillabaisse, you can use almost any fish or seafood in these wonderful stews. Every world class cuisine has discovered them - and they represent a delicious way to get healthy food from the sea. Serve them in big shallow soup bowls for best effect.

GINGER CRAB in WINE BROTH

This recipe works for: Weight Control, Women's Health, Brain Health
For 8 servings:

Melt 2 TBS Olive Oil and 2 TBS Butter in a large soup pot. Add 4 cups Organic Low Fat Chicken Broth, 2 cups White Wine, $^1/_4$ cup minced Scallions, 6 slices Fresh Ginger, peeled, 1 TB Tamari and 1 TB Lemon Juice.

—Simmer for 10 minutes until fragrant. Add the meat of 3 cooked, cleaned Dungeness Crabs. Heat and ladle into soup bowls.

Nutrition; 166 calories; 12gm protein; 2gm carbo.; 1gm fiber; 6gm total fats; 40mg choles.; 38mg calcium; 1mg iron; 34mg magnesium; 337mg potassium; 212mg sodium; Vit. A 40 IU; Vit. C 4mg; Vit. E 1 IU.

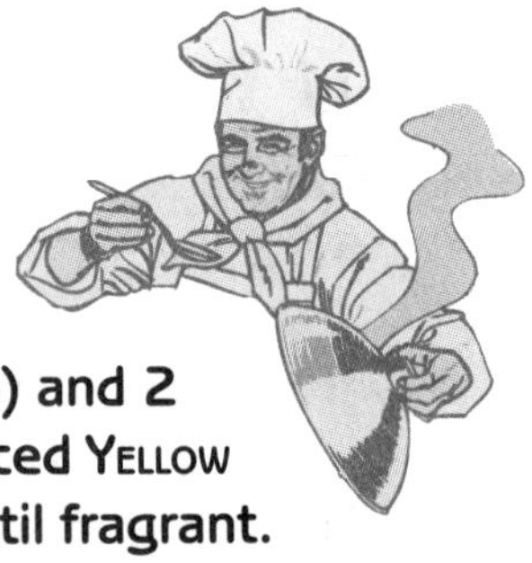

FRENCH BOUILLABAISSE

This recipe works for: *Stress Reactions, Heart Health*
For 8 servings: Preheat oven to 375°.

Sizzle 1½ cups sliced Leeks (white parts with a little green) and 2 minced Cloves Garlic in 2 TBS Olive Oil until aromatic. Add 1 diced Yellow Bell Pepper and 1 diced Red Bell Pepper; sizzle 6 to 7 minutes until fragrant.

—Stir in and cook 10 minutes: 2 tsp. ground Fennel, 2 tsp. dry Basil (or 2 TBS Fresh Basil), 1 tsp. Sea Salt, 1 tsp. Herbs de Provence and 3 diced Plum Tomatoes.

—Stir in and cook for 10 minutes more: 1 cup Vegetable or Fish Stock, 1 can (8-oz.) chopped Tomatoes with juice, 2 TBS Lemon Juice, 1 TB grated Lemon Zest, 1 teasp. Tarragon, 2 TBS snipped Fresh Parsley, 1 tsp. Saffron Threads, 1 tsp. Sweet Paprika.

—Place 3-lbs. White Fish Fillets about 1" thick, or 3-lbs mixed Shellfish (shrimp, scallops, clams, prawns, mussels, etc.) in a shallow oiled baking dish. Pour Bouillabaisse Sauce over, and bake covered for 20 minutes until fish or seafood is opaque. Snip on Fresh Parsley or Fresh Cilantro and serve in shallow soup bowls.

LIGHT ITALIAN CIOPPINO

This recipe works for: *Women's and Men's Sexual Health, Heart and Brain Health*
For 12 bowls: Serve in big shallow soup plates with crusty sourdough bread.

In a large heavy soup pot, heat ½ cup Olive Oil, and sauté 2 cups chopped Onions and 2 minced Cloves Garlic for 5 minutes. Add 1 diced Red Bell Pepper and 6 sliced Brown Cremini Mushrooms; sauté for 5 minutes until fragrant.

—Add 1½ cups chopped Plum Tomatoes, 1½ cups Rosé Wine, 3 TBS snipped Fresh Parsley, 2 teasp. Italian Seasoning Herbs, pinches Cayenne Pepper and Sweet Paprika to taste. Cover and cook over low heat for 1 hour.

—Add 3-lbs. Fresh Fish Fillet Chunks, 8-oz. Sea Scallops, 1 Lobster Tail in chunks and 8-oz. Prawns. Simmer 15 minutes until sea foods are just tender and opaque.

QUICK BASQUE FISH STEW

This recipe works for: *Skin and Hair Health, Heart Health, Brain Boosting*
For 8 servings: Serve in large shallow soup bowls.

Sauté 2 large diced Onions and 3 diced Cloves Garlic in 3 TBS Olive Oil until fragrant, 10 minutes. Add one can (28-oz.) Plum Tomatoes with their juice, 2 pinches Cayenne Pepper, 2 teasp. Saffron Threads, and 1 small (7-oz.) bottle Clam Juice.

—Add 2-lbs. mixed seafood: scrubbed Mussels and Oysters, Sea Scallops, thick chunks Sea Bass, Calamari Rings, etc.; heat through. Do not overcook!

Nutrition; 251 calories; 25gm protein; 11gm carbo.; 2gm fiber; 11gm total fats; 52mg choles.; 77mg calcium; 7mg iron; 73mg magnesium; 758mg potassium; 479mg sodium; Vit. A 135 IU; Vit. C 26mg; Vit. E 5 IU.

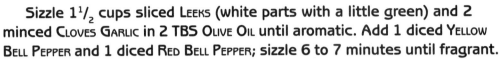

YOSENABE, JAPANESE FISH STEW

This recipe works for: Stress Reactions, Heart Health, Brain Boosting
Makes about 8 servings: Preheat oven to 250°F.

Heat a wok: Sizzle 2 TBS Canola Oil, 1 teasp. Toasted Sesame Oil, 3 minced Cloves Garlic, and 2 TBS minced Fresh Ginger until fragrant, about 5 minutes.

—Add 1 small (7-oz.) bottle Clam Juice, 2 large King Crab Legs in big chunks, 16-oz. Calamari in bite-size chunks, 12 Fresh Clams (or canned), 12 large shelled Prawns, 8-10 oz. thick White Fish Filet, and 2 TBS snipped Fresh Cilantro. Let bubble 1 minute.

—Stir in 1 more small (7-oz.) bottle Clam Juice, 2 TBS Sake, 2 TBS Oyster Sauce, 1 TB Arrowroot Powder or Kuzu Chunks dissolved in 2 TBS Water, 2 teasp. grated Lemon Zest and 1 teasp. Honey.

PAELLA

This recipe works for: Overcoming Addictions, Illness Recovery
Serves 9:

Heat 6 TBS Olive Oil in a paella pan or your widest heavy skillet. Sizzle 1-lb. large shelled Shrimp. Remove with a slotted spoon to a large bowl and set aside. Add 24 Mussels and cook 3 minutes until shells open (discard any that don't open). Remove to bowl with slotted spoon. Add 1-lb. Sea Bass or Monkfish Fillets in chunks. Sizzle 5 minutes and remove to bowl.

—Sprinkle fish with PAELLA SPICES and let flavors blend: 1 TB Sweet Paprika, 3 teasp. Saffron Threads, $^1/_2$ cup snipped Fresh Cilantro and 3 TBS Lemon Juice.

—Sizzle 2 cups diced Yellow Onions, 5 minced Cloves Garlic and 3 cups chopped Tomatoes in the pan for 10 minutes. Add $2^1/_2$ cups Arborio Rice, 4 cups Fish Stock or Vegetable Broth, 1 cup White Wine, 1 can Garbanzo Beans and 1 Jar Artichoke Hearts, quartered. Reduce heat, cover and simmer untouched for 15 minutes until rice is done but still chewy. You'll have a rich, crusty brown layer on the bottom of the pan.

—Turn off heat. Add entire contents of seafood bowl to paella. Cover and let stand to rewarm for 10 minutes. Serve with lots of Lemon Wedges and Cracked Pepper.

SEAFOOD CHOWDER

This recipe works for: Men's Health, Addictions Recovery, Allergies and Asthma
Serves 6: Preheat griddle to medium hot.

Heat 1 TB Olive Oil in a soup pot. Sizzle 1 diced Yellow Onion and 4 diced Yellow Dutch Potatoes for 10 minutes. Add 2 diced Carrots and 2 diced Ribs Celery and 16-oz. Corn Kernels; cook for 5 minutes. Add 4 cups Organic Chicken Broth, $1^1/_2$ cups Plain Low Fat Yogurt, 1 cup White Wine. Add 1 teasp. Herbs de Provence; simmer 5 minutes.

—Add 1-lb. shelled Shrimp and 1-lb. shelled Scallops. Cook 3 minutes. Top with snipped Fresh Chives, Fresh Parsley and Cracked Pepper.

Stars of the Sea

Seafoods are incredibly versatile, their healing powers amazing. There's something for everybody in this section - main dishes, with tastes ranging from delicate to hearty, from familiar to exotic.

CRUSTED SALMON with CITRUS-MINT SAUCE

This recipe works for: Weight Control, Heart / Artery Health, Hair and Skin
Serves 8: Preheat oven to 325°.

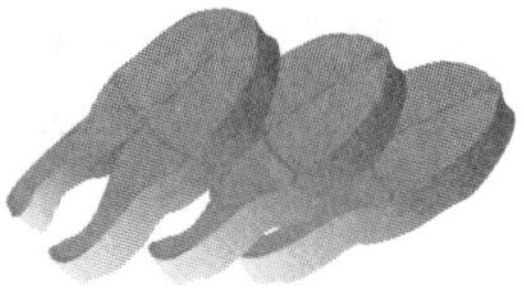

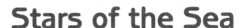

Blender blend the crust: whirl 3 slices Whole Grain Sourdough Bread, $^1/_3$ cup Pumpkin Seeds, $^1/_3$ cup chopped Almonds and $^1/_3$ cup Sunflower Seeds. Spread on a baking tray and bake in the oven until browned, 12 minutes. Turn into a shallow bowl.

—Peel and section 1 large Orange, 1 Red Grapefruit and 1 Lemon. Set aside.

—Beat 2 Egg Whites to frothy in a bowl. Dip 6 inch-thick Salmon Fillets in the whites. Then roll fillets in the crumb mixture to coat. Lay fillets on wax paper to rest.

—Heat a large skillet to hot with 1 TB Olive Oil. Sear salmon fillets about 2 minutes each side. Repeat til each piece is seared. Place fillets on the baking tray and bake for about 6 to 8 minutes.

—Make the sauce while salmon is baking: boil 1 cup Grapefruit Juice until reduced to $^1/_3$ cup. Remove from heat and stir in $^1/_2$ cup Low Fat Cream Cheese and $^1/_4$ cup Low Fat Plain Yogurt. Add 3 TBS drained Capers and and 2 TBS snipped Fresh Mint Leaves. Spoon sauce over warm salmon fillets.

Nutrition; 415 calories; 38gm protein; 19gm carbo.; 4gm fiber; 19gm total fats; 91mg choles.; 100mg calcium; 4mg iron; 134mg magnes.; 1078mg potass.; 231mg sodium; Vit. A 72 IU; Vit. C 39mg; Vit. E 9 IU.

SWORDFISH FILLETS in FRESH BASIL SAUCE

This recipe works for: Weight Control, Candida Healing, Women's Health
For 6 people: Preheat oven to 350°.

In a blender, whirl half a Lemon, coarsely peeled and seeded, and 6 TBS Olive Oil until blended. Pour into a hot skillet and let sizzle for 1 minute.

—Add 2 minced Shallots and $^1/_4$ cup minced Fresh Basil Leaves. Sauté 2 minutes. Add $1^1/_2$ cups Whole Grain Sourdough Bread Crumbs and $^1/_2$ cup chopped Toasted Almonds; stir until dry. Remove from heat; add $^2/_3$ cup Parmesan Cheese and $^1/_4$ teasp. Cracked Pepper.

—Oil a shallow baking dish and place 6 thick Swordfish Steaks (about 2 lbs.) in a single layer. Cover with the sauce and bake for 15 to 20 minutes, until fish whitens to opaque and sauce bubbles.

Nutrition; 382 calories; 35gm protein; 10gm carbo.; 2gm fiber; 22gm total fats; 62mg choles.; 201mg calcium; 2mg iron; 82mg magnesium; 541mg potassium; 157mg sodium; Vit. A 76 IU; Vit. C 5mg; Vit. E 6 IU.

MIXED SEAFOOD with BROWN RICE and GREENS

This recipe works for: Immune Power, Bone Building, Illness Recovery
For 6 hearty servings: Excellent hot or cold. Any seafood blend works.

Have ready 2 cups cooked Brown Rice.

—Sauté 1/2-lb peeled uncooked Shrimp and 1/2-lb Bay Scallops in 1 teasp. Chili Oil and 1 teasp. Toasted Sesame Oil until just opaque about 2 minutes. Remove from skillet with a slotted spoon and toss with the brown rice. Set aside.

—Add 1 teasp. Olive Oil to the skillet and sizzle 1/2 cup slivered Red Bell Pepper 3 minutes. Add 1 cup Frozen Green Peas and toss another 2 minutes until color changes to bright green. Mix veggies with seafood and grains. Mix in 1/4 cup Toasted Sunflower Seeds, 1/4 cup Raisins, 1 cup shredded Swiss Cheese or Rice Swiss Cheese. Set aside.

—Make the LEMON-YOGURT DRESSING. Mix 1 cup Plain Low Fat Yogurt, 3 TBS Lemon Juice, 1/4 cup snipped Green Onions, 1/4 cup diced Cucumber, 1 TB minced Crystallized Ginger, 1 TB Tamari and 1/2 teasp. Lemon-Pepper. Pour over seafood. Mix gently. Cover large salad plates with Baby Spinach Leaves. Mound on seafood rice salad.

Nutrition; 329 calories; 29gm protein; 37gm carbo.; 4gm fiber; 8gm total fats; 80mg choles.; 379mg calcium; 4mg iron; 141mg magnes.; 741mg potass.; 308mg sodium; Vit. A 365 IU; Vit. C 37mg; Vit. E 8 IU.

SESAME SEARED SALMON with GRILLED RADICCHIO

This recipe works for: Hair, Skin and Nails, Candida Healing, Bone Building
For 4 people: Preheat oven to 450°.

Coat 4 thick, skinned Salmon Fillets (about 2 lbs. total) with bottled Teriyaki Sauce.

—Toast 1/3 cup Sesame Seeds in a dry skillet until golden. Press salmon fillets onto seeds to coat both sides. Heat 1 TB Olive Oil in the skillet. Sear salmon fillets about 2 minutes each side. Place fillets in a baking pan and bake for about 6 to 8 minutes.

—Shred 3 small heads Radicchio. Heat 3 TBS Olive Oil and 2 TBS Lemon Juice in the skillet and sizzle radicchio for 3 minutes. Add 1 teasp. Garlic-Lemon Seasoning, 1 teasp. minced Ginger and 1/2 teasp. Cracked Pepper. Turn radicchio onto plates and top with a crusted salmon fillet.

EASY SOLE ROLLATINI

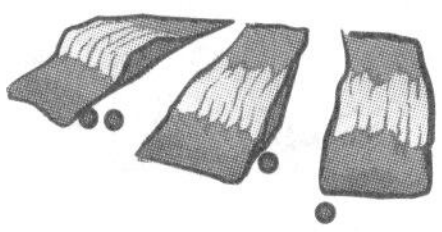

This recipe works for: Weight Control, Candida Healing
For 6 people: Preheat oven to 375°. Delicious with asparagus and brown rice.

Mix the filling: 1/2 cup grated Parmesan Cheese or Soy Parmesan, 1 TB snipped Fresh Basil, 1/2 cup chopped toasted Almonds, 1/2 cup snipped Fresh Parsley.

—Place two 16-oz. Sole or Flounder Fillets on a flat surface; spoon some filling on one end. Roll up. Place seam side down in an oiled baking dish. Mix 3 TBS Lemon Juice, 1/2 teasp. Lemon-Pepper and 3 TBS melted Butter; drizzle over. Spread remaining filling on top. Cover with foil and bake for 30 minutes until fish is opaque throughout.

GINGER POACHED SALMON with FRESH HERBS

This recipe works for: Heart Health, Sugar Imbalances, Addiction Recovery
For 4: Use a fish poacher for best results. Or a large wok with a steamer tray.

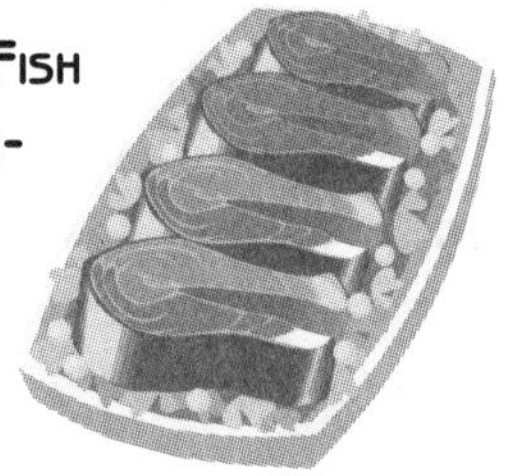

In the fish poacher or wok, simmer for 10 minutes 4 cups Fish Stock or Organic Chicken Broth, 4 cups Water and 2-oz. peeled Ginger Root, sliced thin. Season liquid with Sea Salt and Pepper.

—Simmer in a pan 3 minutes: 1 TB Butter, 2 minced Shallots, 2 TBS minced Crystallized Ginger, grated Zest of 1 Lemon. Add $^1/_4$ cup White Wine and 1 cup bottled Clam Juice. Simmer 5 minutes. Add 2 TBS Butter; stir til thickened; remove from heat. Whisk in 4 snipped Fresh Basil Leaves, 1 teasp. Fresh Thyme Leaves and Pepper to taste.

—Arrange 4 salmon filets on steaming rack and lower into liquid. Cover and cook for 5 minutes until opaque throughout. Separate leaves from 2 Heads Belgian Endive. Divide between plates and top with salmon. Spoon sauce over and serve immediately.

EARTH and OCEAN Very aromatic. You can taste the sea with your nose.

This recipe works for: Immune Power, Cancer Protection, Anti-Aging
For 6 servings:

Dry roast 1 cup Basmati Rice in a skillet for 5 minutes. Add 2 cups Water. Bring to a boil, cover, reduce heat and steam for 25 minutes until water is absorbed. Fluff, put in a serving bowl and set aside. Soak 5 dry Shiitake Mushrooms in water to cover until soft. Sliver mushrooms and discard woody stems. Save soaking water.

—Sauté in the skillet 2 minced Shallots in 3 TBS Olive Oil for 3 minutes. Add 1 cup sliced Brown Cremini Mushrooms, soaked Shiitake Mushrooms, 4 TBS soaking water, and 5 slivered Chanterelle Mushrooms. Sauté until brown and liquid almost evaporates, 8 minutes. Add and sauté until just opaque, 3 minutes: $^1/_2$ lb. Bay Scallops, $^1/_2$ lb. peeled Prawns, $^1/_4$ cup Sherry and $^1/_2$ teasp. Sweet Paprika. Add 2 minced Scallions and 2 TBS snipped Fresh Parsley. Heat 1 minute; serve over Basmati rice.

Nutrition; 300 calories; 23gm. protein; 8gm. carbo.; 2gm. fiber; 23gm total fats; 90mg choles.; 106mg calcium; 2mg iron; 88mg magnesium; 605mg potass.; 232mg sodium; Vit. A 156 IU; Vit. C 17mg; Vit. E 6 IU.

SALMON with SWEET BALSAMIC SAUCE

This recipe works for: Immune Power, Cancer Protection, Anti-Aging
For 2 servings:

Sizzle 1 Red Onion, thick sliced in 1 tsp. Olive Oil for 5 minutes. Add $^1/_2$ cup Orange Juice, 2 tsp. minced Crystallized Ginger and 4 TBS Balsamic Vinegar. Bring to a boil, reduce heat, cover and simmer 45 minutes. Add 1 teasp. Olive Oil and two 8-oz. Salmon Fillets. <u>Sear on each side 4 minutes</u>. Put salmon on plates and top with Balsamic-Onion sauce. Snip on 1 TB Cilantro Leaves.

SALMON BURGERS

This recipe works for: Women's Health, Healthy Pregnancy, Anti-Aging
For 4 servings: Preheat oven to 400°.

Make the burgers in a bowl: mix one 16-oz. can Red Salmon, 1 Egg, 2 TBS Dry Onion Flakes, $^1/_2$ teasp. Ginger Powder, $^1/_2$ teasp. dried Lemon Peel, $^1/_2$ teasp. Thyme, $^1/_2$ teasp. Lemon-Pepper. Let stand 15 minutes to blend flavors; then form into 4 burgers.

—Make the topping in a bowl: Dice 2 Roasted Red Peppers from a jar. Stir with 2 TBS Lime Juice, 4 drops Hot Pepper Sauce, 6 drops Toasted Sesame Oil, 1 TB Olive Oil, 4 minced Scallions, Sea Salt to taste and 1 TB snipped Fresh Mint. Chill 15 minutes.

—Cook salmon burgers in a heavy Lecithin-sprayed hot skillet, about 2 to 3 minutes on each side, til opaque throughout. Place a Boston Lettuce Leaf on half a Whole Grain Sourdough Bun, top with a burger and spoon on Red Pepper Sauce.

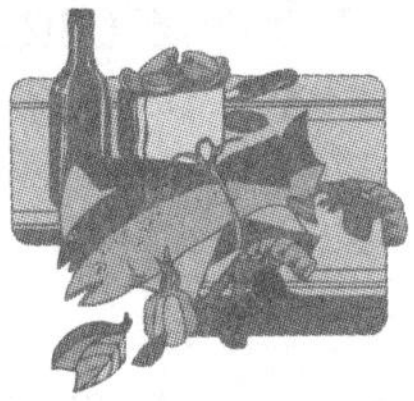

PESCADO CANCUN

This recipe works for: Liver and Organ Health
For 8 servings: Preheat oven to 350°.

In a bowl, sprinkle 2-lbs. thick Shark or Swordfish Filets with Lemon Juice; set aside.

—Sauté in 3 TBS Olive Oil for 5 minutes: 1 minced Clove Garlic, 1 cup diced Onion, 1 TB dry Chili Flakes, $^1/_4$ teasp. ground Cloves, $^1/_4$ teasp. ground Cumin, and $^1/_4$ teasp. ground Coriander. Add and simmer 15 minutes until bubbly: 3 cups diced Tomatoes, 1 cup chopped Black Olives, 3 TBS Lemon Juice, 1 TB Honey, $1^1/_2$ teasp. Lemon-Pepper.

—Pour over fish. Snip a generous amount of snipped Fresh Cilantro Leaves over top and bake for 20 minutes until tender and fish is white all the way through.

FRAGRANT RED SNAPPER with CAJUN SAUCE

This recipe works for: Immune Power, Cancer Protection, Brain Health
For 4 servings: Have ready four 8 x 12" rectangles of foil or baking parchment.

Wrap 1 lb. rinsed Red Snapper Filet in cheesecloth to maintain its shape. Poach in 1 quart Vegetable Broth for 3 minutes only. Remove and cut into 4 serving pieces.

—Reserve $^1/_2$ cup of the poaching broth and add to 2 TBS Butter in a pan; stir with 2 TBS Unbleached Flour, $^1/_4$ teasp. Sea Salt, $^1/_4$ teasp. White Pepper and a pinch Chervil until bubbly. Add $^1/_3$ cup Plain Yogurt and 2 TBS White Wine and stir until thickened. Remove from heat and set aside. Add 1 TB Butter to skillet and sizzle 24 peeled, large Shrimp until opaque. Remove and set aside. Sauté 1 TB Butter and 8 thin-sliced Mushrooms until just beginning to brown. Add mushrooms to the sauce.

—Make up the baking packets. Put 3 TBS sauce on bottom half of each rectangle. Lay on a piece of fish, and top with 6 shrimp. Spoon on more sauce. Fold the other half of rectangle over top, and seal all edges. Put in a shallow baking dish, and bake 15 minutes until fish is tender. Each person opens his own to savor the aroma.

Fish and Seafood on the Grill

I don't know any food I like any better, or that's better for you, than ocean foods barbecued outdoors on a grill. Since the Stone Age, on beach campfires, barbecued foods have tasted great. There's something about eating out-of-doors. The sunshine, fresh air, and surrounding green whet our appetites and increase our metabolisms to a healthy level. We breathe deeper, relax more, and feel better about almost everything. Almost everything tastes better barbecued, from fruits to vegetables to meats and especially sea foods. Does your family have picky eaters? Everybody shows up to a barbecue with bells on. Outdoor cooking is easy. Kids can help with everything.

Grill fish to perfection.

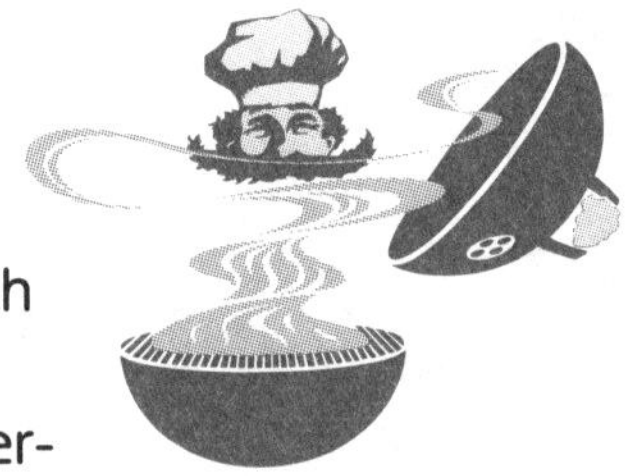

Heat grill while you prepare the fish.
Firm, dense fish can go directly on the grill: mackerel, mahi mahi, Hawaiian opah (moon-fish), orange roughy, salmon with skin, shark, sturgeon, swordfish, and tuna (aji).
Delicate flesh fish that need support: barracuda, bass, butterfish, catfish, Chilean seabass, cod, flounder, halibut, lingcod, rockfish, sablefish, salmon without skin, sand dab, snapper, sole, tilapia, and trout.

For direct heat-beneath the food:

1. For charcoal briquets, cover firegrate with a single, solid layer of ignited coals. Let briquets burn down to desired heat. For a gas barbecue, turn burners to high and close lid for 5 minutes. Adjust burners to desired heat. Note: Temperature varies from one grill to another. Exercise common sense and be careful to avoid burns! Set the barbecue grill in place and measure heat:
   —Very hot (you can hold your hand at grill level only 1 to 2 seconds)
   —Hot (you can hold your hand at grill level only 2 to 3 seconds)
   —Medium-hot (you can hold your hand at grill level 3 to 4 seconds)
   —Medium (you can hold your hand at grill level 4 to 5 seconds)
   —Medium-low (you can hold your hand at grill level 5 to 6 seconds)
   —Low (you can hold your hand at grill level only 6 to 7 seconds)
2. Oil grill first by brushing with salad oil. Lay food on grill, cook as recipe directs.
3. Cover gas barbecue for fish and seafood. Do not cover charcoal barbecue unless recipe specifies.

For indirect heat, on opposite side of the food:

1. For charcoal briquets, mound and ignite 60 briquets on the firegrate. Cover with lid. When briquets are dotted with gray ash, in 15 minutes, push equal amounts to opposite sides of firegrate. Add 5 more briquets to each mound of coals now and every 30 minutes while cooking. Set a drip pan on firegrate between coals.
   For a gas barbecue, turn burners to high and close lid for 5 minutes. Adjust burners for indirect cooking (no heat in center); keep on high unless recipe specifies other.
2. To oil grill, brush with salad oil. Lay food on grill, but not over heat source.
3. Cover grill (open vents for charcoal). BBQ according to recipe directions.

GRILLED SEA BASS with LEMON-TARRAGON SAUCE

This recipe works for: Overcoming Addictions, Liver - Organ Health, Men's Health
Makes 6 servings: Preheat barbecue.

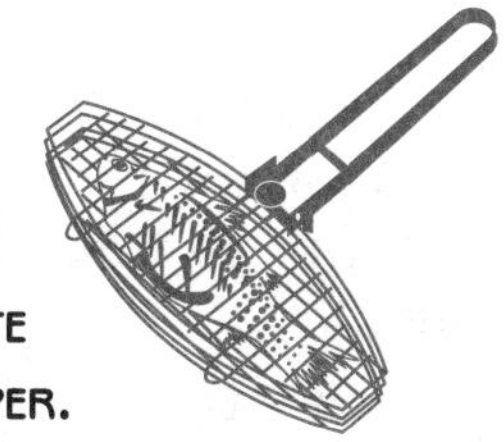

Simmer 1/2 cup bottled Clam Juice in a small saucepan until reduced to 2 TBS, about 5 minutes. Transfer to a blender. Add 3 TBS Lemon Juice and 3 TBS Tarragon Leaves. Blend briefly, and with machine running, gradually add 1/2 cup Olive Oil and 1/4 cup White Wine; blend well. Season sauce to taste with Sea Salt and White Pepper.
—Brush 6 Chilean Sea Bass Filets with Olive Oil; season with Lemon-Pepper. Place skin side down on barbecue. Grill until opaque in center (turn with tongs), about 3 minutes each side. Transfer to plates. Drizzle lemon sauce over.

AFRICAN SHORES GRILL The first BBQ may have come from Africa.

This recipe works for: Sports Nutrition, Liver - Organ Health, Men's Health
For 8 skewers: Heat your barbecue to high heat.

Warm 2 TBS Olive Oil in a pan. Stir in 2 minced Jalapeño Chilies, 2 teasp. minced Ginger and 1 minced Garlic Clove. Sizzle 5 minutes. Add 3/4 cup Sherry, 1/3 cup Tamari, 1/4 cup Honey and 2 teasp. Arrowroot Powder dissolved in 1 TB Lime Juice. Sizzle until mixture thickens slightly. Remove from heat. Add 1/4 cup snipped Fresh Cilantro.
—Divide 24 large peeled Shrimp and 24 large Sea Scallops on skewers. Brush with sauce. Grill for 3 minutes on each side. Serve hot with rest of sauce.

EASY GRILLED SHANGHAI PRAWNS

This recipe works for: Boosting Sexuality, Men's Health
For 4 appetizers: Heat your barbecue to high heat.

Soak 32 toothpicks in water while you make this recipe. Marinate 16 peeled butterflied Jumbo Prawns with 3 TBS bottled Teriyaki Sauce. Dust on 2 pinches Chili Powder. Set aside.
—Slice 2 to 3 large Japanese Eggplants in 1/4" slices on the diagonal so that each slice is about 2 inches long. You should have 32 slices. Toss Eggplant slices gently in a bowl with Olive Oil to lightly coat and Lemon-Pepper to taste.
—Assemble the appetizers: lay out eggplant slices on a flat surface. Top half of them with a prawn, a pinch of minced Green Onion and a sprinkle of Dulse Flakes. Top each with another eggplant slice and secure with 2 toothpicks. Chill.
—Using tongs, place each appetizer on the hot grill and cook until prawns are pink and eggplant is brown, about 4 minutes on each side. Watch closely.

Nutrition; 114 calories; 11gm protein; 9gm carbo.; 3gm fiber; 4gm total fats; 85mg choles.; 29mg calcium; 2mg iron; 40mg magnesium; 367mg potassium; 274mg sodium; Vit. A 39 IU; Vit. C 3mg; Vit. E 2 IU.

GRILLED SCALLOPS ASIAN STYLE

This recipe works for: Brain Power, Digestive Health, Men's Health
For 4 servings: Use long metal skewers for best results. Preheat grill to med. hot

Toast $^1/_2$ cup shredded, Unsweetened Coconut in a 250° oven until golden. Set aside. Peel, seed and chunk 2 Papayas and 2 Mangoes. Thread onto skewers for grilling. Thread 1 lb. rinsed large Sea Scallops on separate skewers for grilling. Lay skewers on a lightly oiled hot barbecue grill. Cook until fruit is hot and scallops are opaque, no more than 3 minutes per side. Watch closely... remove from heat; set aside.

—Make the dressing: Mix the toasted coconut with $^3/_4$ cup Orange Juice, 4 TBS Lime Juice, $1^1/_2$ tsp. Chinese 5-Spice Powder and 1 TB Olive Oil. Add 1 small package (8-oz.) Baby Spinach Leaves; toss to coat. Divide dressed greens on individual plates. Slide scallops and fruit from skewers to remaining dressing in the bowl. Stir to coat and spoon onto spinach. Sprinkle with granulated Dulse or crunchy Soy Bacon Bits.

FRESH AHI with ROSEMARY and THYME

This recipe works for: Boosting Sexuality, Brain Enhancement, Anti-Aging
For 4 servings: Preheat grill to hot and brush grill with oil.

Marinate 1-lb. thick Fresh Ahi Steaks for 1 hour in 2 TBS Lemon Juice, 3 TBS Olive Oil, 2 teasp. Fresh Rosemary Leaves, 2 teasp. fresh Thyme Leaves, $^1/_2$ teasp. Sea Salt, $^1/_2$ teasp. Cracked Pepper and 2 teasp. Sesame Seeds.

—Sear ahi for 2 minutes on each side until just pink in the center, squeezing with lemon juice during grilling. Garnish with Rosemary Sprigs.

Nutrition; 217 calories; 27gm. protein; 3gm. carbo.; 2gm. fiber; 10gm total fats; 43mg choles.; 81mg calcium; 2mg iron; 63mg magnesium; 304mg potassium; 179mg sodium; Vit. A 747 IU; Vit. C 2mg; Vit. E 4 IU.

MANGO SEAFOOD KEBABS

This recipe works for: Liver and Organ Health, Anti-Aging, Heart Health
For 4 people: Preheat grill and brush with oil.

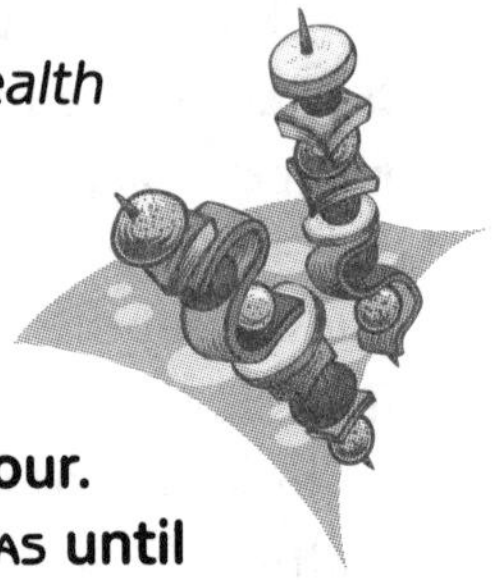

Cut 1 large, peeled Mango into 1" chunks. Rinse 1-lb. large fresh Sea Scallops; peel $^1/_2$-lb. large Shrimp. Lay in a shallow baking pan; marinate with 3 TBS Olive Oil, 3 TBS Lime Juice and 1 TB Tamari for one hour.

—Bring salted water to a boil and blanch 24 -30 trimmed Snow Peas until color changes to bright green. Rinse in cold water to set color.

—Thread snow peas, seafood and mango chunks onto skewers. Grill 4" from heat until seafood is opaque, about 2 minutes on each side, basting frequently. Squeeze on more Fresh Lime Juice to serve.

Nutrition; 254 calories; 33gm protein; 18gm carbo.; 3gm fiber; 5gm total fats; 124mg choles.; 100mg calcium; 2mg iron; 90mg magnesium; 567mg potass.; 304mg sodium; Vit. A 273 IU; Vit. C 27mg; Vit. E 4 IU.

BUTTERFLY SALMON with MUSTARD SAUCE

This recipe works for: Brain Power, Hair, Skin and Nails, Women's Health
For 18 servings: Have barbecue ready with indirect heat.

In a large skillet, combine $^1/_2$ cup diced Onion, 2 Green Onions, 1 cup Sake, 6 TBS Coarse-Grain Mustard, 2 TBS Honey, 1 TB Tamari and 2 tsp. dried Tarragon. Bring to a boil, stirring; cook for 7 minutes.

—Rinse a 7-lb. Whole Salmon, filleted but still attached down the back, with head removed; pat dry. Lay fish open skin down, on a sheet of foil (12 x 17 inch). Trim foil to fit fish. Spread onion mix over salmon. Set foil with salmon on grill but not over heat. Cover barbecue. Cook until fish is opaque throughout but moist-looking in thickest part, about 35 to 40 minutes. Slide a rimless baking sheet under salmon and foil, then slide-transfer fish onto a platter or board. Cut salmon and lift portions from skin with a wide spatula. Season to taste with Sea Salt and Lemon-Pepper.

Nutrition; 277 calories; 36gm protein; 3gm carbo.; 1gm fiber; 12gm total fats; 97mg choles.; 35mg calcium; 2mg iron; 55mg magnesium; 905mg potassium; 195mg sodium; Vit. A 24 IU; Vit. C 1mg; Vit. E 2 IU.

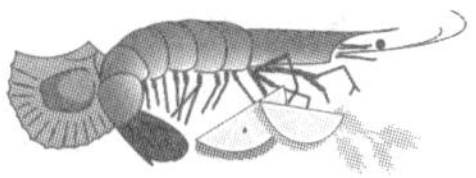

SHRIMP with LEMON PESTO

This recipe works for: Liver and Organ Health, Brain Enhancement, Heart Health
For 8 skewers: Heat the grill to hot. Brush the grill with oil.

Butterfly and flatten 32 jumbo size peeled Shrimp. Thread 4 shrimp onto each wooden skewer, sideways through the widest part.

—Make the pesto in the blender: $^1/_4$ cup Olive Oil, 2 TBS grated Lemon Peel, 1 TB Pine Nuts, 2 TBS grated Parmesan Cheese, 1 teasp. Garlic-Lemon Seasoning, and 1 teasp. Fructose; pour into a large flat pan. Roll skewered shrimp in the pesto marinade. Cover and chill. Cook on hot oiled grill for 5 minutes, basting often. Watch closely.

Marvelous Marinades and Sauces for Fish and Seafood

Fish and seafood is often so light that a tasty sauce or marinade can sometimes "make the dish." Mix and match these with almost any fish you buy.

HONEY MUSTARD SAUCE

Good for salmon, shrimp or a substantial fish like shark.

Mix together and chill: $^1/_4$ cup Dijon Mustard, $^3/_4$ cup Honey, $^1/_4$ cup Lemon Mayonnaise, 2 TBS Tamari, $^1/_4$ cup Plain Low Fat Yogurt, $^1/_2$ tsp. Sea Salt, and $^1/_4$ tsp. Pepper.

GREEN PEPPERCORN MARINADE and SAUCE

Good for swordfish, sea bass, monkfish, and halibut.

Whisk together: $^1/_4$ cup Tamari, $^1/_4$ cup Sherry, $^1/_4$ cup Sake, $^1/_4$ cup + 1 TB Brown Rice Vinegar, 2 TBS drained crushed Capers, 1 TB minced Ginger Root, 1 minced Clove Garlic, and $^1/_2$ cup Olive Oil.

MUSTARD MAYONNAISE

Good with salmon, scallops and ahi tuna.

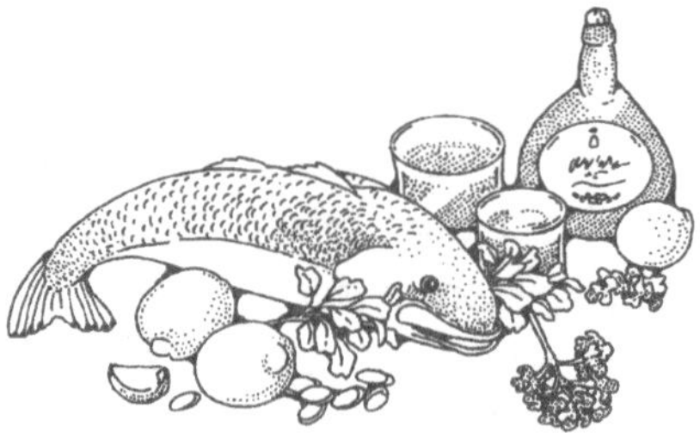

Blender blend: $^3/_4$ cup Coarse-Grain Mustard, 2 TBS Dry Mustard, $^1/_3$ cup Brown Sugar, 1 cup Lemon Mayonnaise, and $^1/_2$ cup snipped Fresh Dill Weed. Cover and chill until ready to use.

DILL TOPPING

Perfect for salmon, and for delicate white fish like sole, sand dabs or monkfish.

Mix together and chill: $^1/_4$ cup Plain Low Fat Yogurt, $^1/_4$ cup Light Mayonnaise, 1 TB Lemon Juice and $^1/_4$ teasp. dry Dill Weed.

MUSTARD DIP for SEAFOOD COCKTAIL

Good for shrimp, crab, oysters and clams.

Mix and chill: 2 TBS Lemon Mayonnaise, 2 teasp. Dijon Mustard, $^1/_2$ teasp. dry Thyme, $^1/_4$ teasp. Lemon-Pepper.

CHIPOTLE SAUCE

Good for shrimp, crab, oysters and clams. *For 4 servings:*

In a bowl combine $1^1/_2$-oz. Dried Chipotle Chilies and 2 cups Hot Water. Let stand 15 minutes to soften. Discard stems, seeds and veins and soaking water. In a pan sizzle 2 TBS chopped Leeks (whites part), 2 chopped Shallots and 2 TBS chopped Green Onion in 1 TB Butter for 1 minute. Add chipotles and 1 cup Organic Chicken Broth.

—Scrape into a blender and blend smooth. Return to pan, add 1 TB Butter and 1 TB Lemon Juice; simmer for 3 minutes. Season with Lemon-Pepper and spoon on fish.

Nutrition; 58 calories; 1gm protein; 3gm carbo.; 1gm fiber; 4gm total fats; 12mg choles.; 10mg calcium; trace iron; 4mg magnesium; 48mg potassium; 110mg sodium; Vit. A 43 IU; Vit. C 6mg; Vit. E trace.

GINGER-KETCHUP SAUCE

Enhancement for shellfish of all kinds

In a pan combine 1/2 cup Water, 4 TBS Sherry, 1/4 cup Tomato Paste, 2 TBS Maple Syrup, 2 TBS Lemon Juice, 1/2 teasp. Ginger Powder. Whisk until smooth, about 1 minute. Add 1 TB snipped Parsley, Garlic-Lemon Seasoning and drops Hot Pepper Sauce to taste.

FRESH TERIYAKI SAUCE

Enhancement for shellfish of all kinds.

Whisk in a bowl: 1 TB minced Ginger Root, 3 minced Cloves Garlic, 1 Jalapeño Pepper seeded and minced, 3 minced Scallions, 1/4 cup Tamari Sauce, 1/4 cup Sake, 2 TBS Maple Syrup, 1/2 teasp. Toasted Sesame Oil and 1 TB Olive Oil.

FRESH HERB MARINADE for FISH

Good for Sea Bass, Trout, Salmon and Monkfish.

Whisk in a bowl: 1/4 cup Lemon Juice, 1/4 cup dry Vermouth, 1/2 teasp. Sea Salt, 1/4 teasp. Cracked Pepper. Whisk in 2 TBS Olive Oil, 2 minced Shallots, 2 minced Cloves Garlic, 3 Jalapeño Peppers seeded and minced, 1/4 cup minced Green Bell Pepper, and 1/2 cup minced Red Bell Pepper.

—Stir in minced fresh herbs: 3 TBS Basil Leaves, 2 TBS Tarragon Leaves, 1 TB Rosemary Leaves, 3 TBS Parsley.

CRUMB SPRINKLE for BAKED FISH

Enhancement for light, white fish, such as sole, monkfish or sand dabs.

Mix in a bowl: 3 TBS melted Butter, 1/2 cup Whole Grain Bread Crumbs, 1 TB grated Parmesan Cheese, 3/4 teasp. Thyme, and 1/4 teasp. Lemon-Pepper. Coat fish before baking.

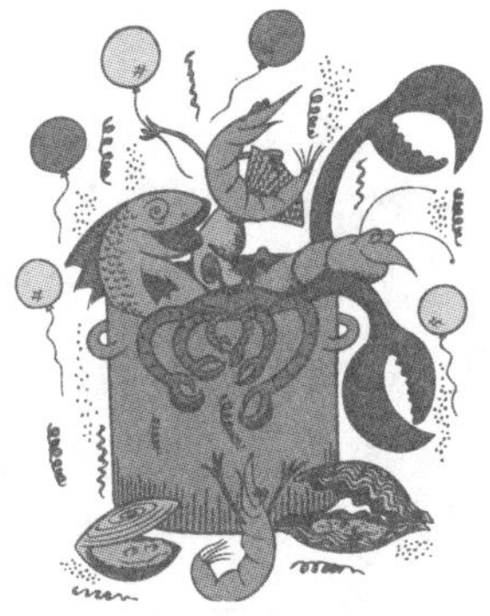

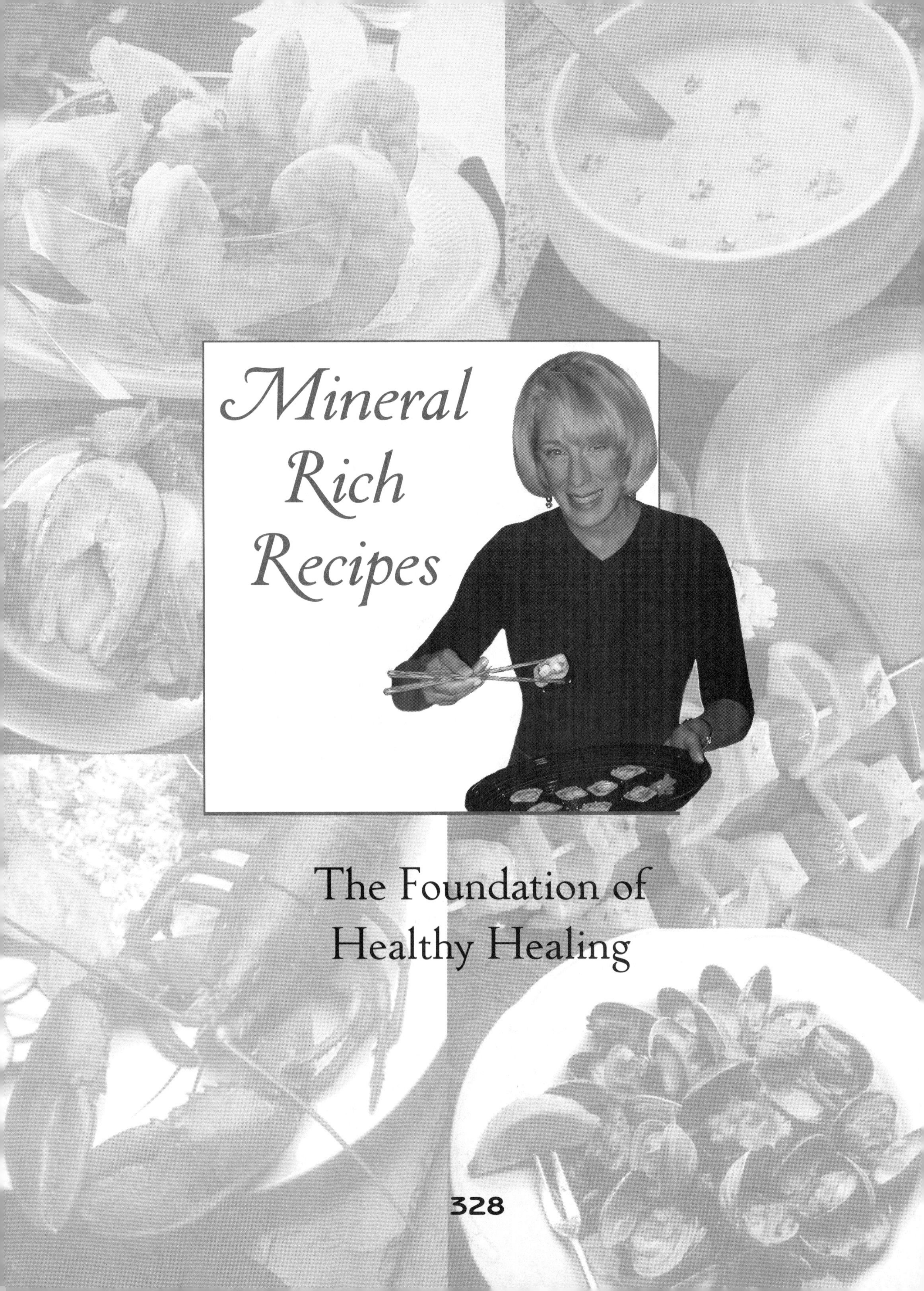

Mineral Rich Recipes

The Foundation of Healthy Healing

Boosting Your Minerals

Minerals are your body's building blocks.... critical for athletes, because you must have minerals to run. Minerals are needed by everybody for good health and an active life. **Hardly any of us get enough**.

Minerals are the most basic of nutrients. They are the bonding agents between you and your food. Without them, the body cannot absorb its nutrition.

Minerals are essential to bone formation and to your digestion. Minerals help keep your body pH balanced, alkaline instead of acid. They regulate nervous system electrical activity, and most metabolic actions, including nutrient flow between cells. They transport your body's oxygen, balance heart action, help you sleep, give you strength, and are keys to mental and spiritual balance.

Even small mineral deficiencies can cause severe depression, anxiety, P.M.S. and other menstrual disorders, hyperactivity in children, sugar imbalances like hypoglycemia or diabetes, nerve and emotional problems, heart disease, high blood pressure, osteoporosis, premature aging of skin and hair, and memory loss. Mineral deficiencies also reduce your ability to heal quickly.

Your body can't synthesize minerals; they must be obtained through your food, or mineral baths. Yet today, many minerals and trace minerals are no longer present in the foods we eat. They have been leached from the soil by the chemicals, sprays and other current practices of commercial farming. Even many foods that still show measurable amounts of mineral composition have less quality and quantity than we are led to believe. Most testing was done decades ago, when sprays, pesticides, fertilizers and chemicals were not as prolific as they are now.

To help you get more high mineral foods in your diet, I've listed on the next page the most important mineral rich foods. The recipes in this section will concentrate on the use of these foods.

Don't forget: Mineral content is higher and more absorbable in fresh foods. Organically grown fruits, vegetables and herbs are the best sources of both vitamins and minerals.

In these diets, high calcium recipes have more than 150mg, high magnesium more than 100mg, high potassium more than 400mg, and high iron more than 2mg per serving.

Get More Minerals in Your Diet!

Foods rich in calcium: sesame seeds, salmon, sea veggies, tofu, cheese, leafy greens, nuts and legumes, olives, broccoli, brown rice, wheat germ, figs, dates, raisins, onions, leeks and chives.

Foods rich in potassium: sea vegetables, brown rice, tofu and other soy foods, beans, nuts and seeds, most dried fruits, raisins, dates, bananas, broccoli, garlic, mushrooms, potatoes and yams.

Foods rich in iron: amaranth, wheat and wheat germ, millet, fish, molasses, chard, spinach and dark greens, pumpkin and sunflower seeds, turkey, black beans, raisins, prunes and peaches.

Foods rich in chromium: potatoes, bananas, turkey and chicken, green peppers, leafy greens, brewer's yeast, organ meats, mushrooms, corn, carrots, wheat germ and fish.

Foods rich in magnesium: poultry, organ meats, mushrooms, cheese, brewer's yeast, greens, celery, water chestnuts, tofu and soy foods, nuts, seeds, sea veggies, sea foods, grains and legumes.

Foods rich in zinc: nuts and seeds, sea veggies and sea foods, liver and organ meats, eggs, brewer's yeast, legumes, leafy greens, whole grains, mushrooms, maple syrup, onions and leeks.

Foods rich in chlorine: tomatoes, celery, lettuce, sea veggies, dark leafy greens, cabbage, radishes, eggplant, cucumber, potatoes and yams, carrots, cauliflower, leeks and onions.

Foods rich in copper: oysters, liver, nuts, legumes, mushrooms, avocados, leafy greens, grains, sea foods, blueberries, raisins.

Foods rich in phosphorus: yogurt, poultry, fish, nuts, brewer's yeast, cereals, peas and beans.

Mineral Rich Recipe Sections

High Mineral Drinks

Drinks are the quickest way to get more minerals... great for sports enhancement, for getting the edge on a high-stress day, or for energizing a tired afternoon.

SUGAR-FREE BANANA NOG

This recipe works for: Sports Nutrition, Liver and Organ Health, Kid's Health
Serves 3:

Blender blend to creamy smooth: 3 Bananas, 3 cups Vanilla Rice Milk, 2 TBS Rice Syrup, $^1/_2$ tsp. Vanilla and $^1/_2$ tsp. Cinnamon. Serve in frosty glasses with Nutmeg Sprinkles.

ORANGE CREAM SODA

This recipe works for: Overcoming Addictions, Sugar Imbalances, Kid's Health
Makes 3 servings:

Blender blend til smooth: 2 cups Low Fat Vanilla Rice Dream Frozen Dessert, 1 cup Orange Juice, 1 cup Lime Sparkling Juice, $^1/_4$ cup undiluted Orange Juice Concentrate.

Nutrition; 327 calories; 4gm protein; 47gm carbo.; 1gm fiber; 14gm total fats; 0mg choles.; 19mg calcium; trace iron; 18mg magnesium; 402mg potassium; 122mg sodium; Vit. A 23 IU; Vit. C 81mg; Vit. E 1 IU.

LEMON WHEEL CITRUS CIDER

This recipe works for: Bladder-Kidney Health, Sugar Imbalances, Arthritis
Makes 10 servings:

In a large pot: heat 1 quart Apple Juice, 2 cups Orange Juice, 2 TBS Lemon Juice, 2 Cinnamon Sticks, $^1/_3$ cup Maple Syrup and 6-oz. Cranberry Concentrate. Slice 1 Lemon in 10 wheels; stick centers with Whole Cloves and float on top of cider. Simmer 20 minutes. Remove cinnamon. Ladle into cups; top each with a lemon wheel.

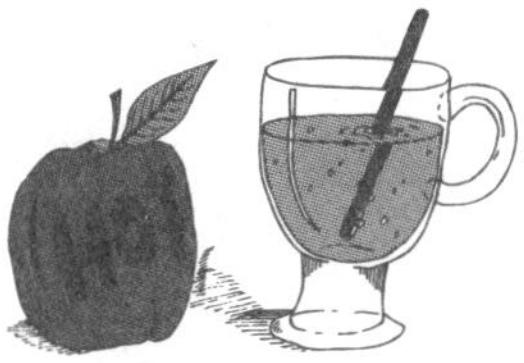

Nutrition; 104 calories; 1gm protein; 25gm carbo.; 1gm fiber; trace total fats; 0mg choles.; 35mg calcium; 2mg iron; 9mg magnesium; 257mg potassium; 8mg sodium; Vit. A 11 IU; Vit. C 219mg; Vit. E trace

ELECTROLYTE ENERGY DRINK

This recipe works for: Sports Nutrition, Men's Health, Fatigue Syndromes

Mix 1 part each in a storage jar: Nettles, Oatstraw, Alfalfa, Watercress or Dandelion Leaf, Rose Hips, Hibiscus, Green Tea. Use 1-oz. herbs for each drink. Okay hot or cold.

PIÑA COLADA MINERAL-ENZYME SMOOTHIE

This recipe works for: Men's Health, Digestive Problems, Arthritis, Kid's Health
Makes 2 servings: Peel and cube fruit before freezing.

Whirl in a blender: 1 cup Frozen Pineapple cubes, 1 Frozen Banana, $^3/_4$ cups Vanilla Rice Milk or Almond Milk, $^1/_2$ cup Frozen Vanilla Yogurt, $^1/_2$ cup Orange Juice, $^1/_2$ teasp. Vanilla Extract, and 3 TBS shredded Toasted Coconut. Serve while frosty.

HIGH MINERAL FRUIT and SOY SHAKE

This recipe works for: Women's Health, Bone Building, Arthritis, Cancer Protection
Makes 2 tall glasses:

Blender blend smooth: 1 cup Vanilla Lowfat Soy Milk, 1 Frozen Banana, 4 TBS Plain Low-Fat Yogurt, 2 diced Kiwi Fruits, 2 TBS Soy Protein Powder.

Nutrition; 210 calories; 12gm protein; 38gm carbo.; 3gm fiber; 1gm total fats; 1mg choles.; 320mg calcium; 7mg iron; 59mg magnesium; 598mg potassium; 99mg sodium; Vit. A 23 IU; Vit. C 80mg; Vit. E 2 IU.

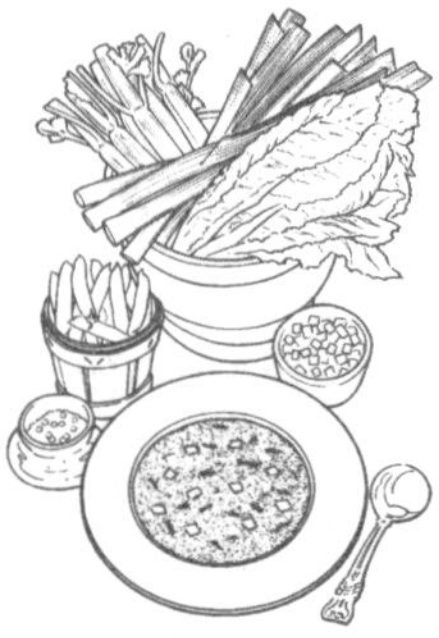

Mineral Soups and Salads

Use high mineral soups and salads to build (and rebuild) bone, muscle and connective tissue during a healing diet.

MISO BEAN SOUP Purifying, restorative, alkalizing, with healing protein.

This recipe works for: Recovery, Bone Building, Arthritis, Cancer Protection
For 10 servings, or for several healing days; freezes well: Use a large soup pot.

Soak 2 $^1/_2$ cups dry Black Beans in 10 cups Water overnight.

—Sauté 2 minced Cloves Garlic and 1 diced Onion in 2 TBS Olive Oil until brown. Add 1 cup Water, the soaked, drained Beans, 2 TBS Dark Miso Paste, 1 cup Red Wine and 9 cups Vegetable Broth; bring to a boil. Reduce heat. Simmer uncovered for 1$^1/_2$ to 2 hours stirring occasionally. Keep beans covered with liquid. Remove from heat to cool slightly. Purée soup in the blender in batches and return to the pot.

—Add $^1/_4$ cup Port or Marsala Wine, 1 tsp. Cracked Pepper and 1 tsp. Sea Salt. Heat through; ladle into shallow bowls. Top with crumbled hard boiled Egg and Lemon Slices

Nutrition; 233 calories; 14gm protein; 34gm carbo.; 12gm fiber; 3gm total fats; 42mg choles.; 55mg calcium; 3mg iron; 102mg magnes.; 540mg potassium; 280mg sodium; Vit. A 21 IU; Vit. C 4mg; Vit. E 1 IU.

RED ONION-RED WINE SOUP

Note: Research shows that the active anti-carcinogens in red wines work well with the high sulphur healing benefits of onions for Heart and Immune System Health.

For 12 servings: Use a large soup pot.

Make the healing soup broth fresh: 8 cups Water, 3 minced Cloves Garlic, 1 TB minced Ginger Root, 1 TB Fresh Thyme Leaves ($^1/_2$ teasp. dry), $^1/_4$ cup snipped Fresh Parsley Leaves (2 teasp. dry flakes), 1 TB dry Lemon Grass Leaves, $^1/_2$ teasp. Sea Salt, 3 Bay Leaves. Bring everything to a boil, and simmer for 25 minutes. Strain and discard solids; set broth aside while you prepare the soup.

—Sauté 2-lbs. sliced Red Onions, 4 minced Cloves Garlic and 4 TBS Olive Oil in the soup pot until translucent, 20 minutes. Add reserved broth, 1 cup Red Wine, 1-lb. diced Tomatoes, 1 cup Tomato Juice, $^1/_2$ teasp. Sea Salt and $^1/_2$ teasp. Black Pepper. Partially cover and simmer for 35 to 40 minutes.

—While soup is simmering, toast in the oven 2 cups Whole Grain Bread cubes drizzled with 4 TBS Olive Oil. Place toast in a serving tureen and pour hot soup over.

Nutrition; 139 calories; 3gm protein; 14gm carbo.; 2gm fiber; 7gm total fats; 0mg choles.; 35mg calcium; 2mg iron; 20mg magnesium; 294mg potassium; 160mg sodium; Vit. A 42 IU; Vit. C 19mg; Vit. E 2 IU.

MINERAL RICH SPINACH SOUP

This recipe works for: Respiratory Health, Bone Building, Allergy and Asthma

For 4 one cup servings:

Sauté $^1/_2$ cup sliced Scallions, $^1/_2$ cup sliced Celery, and 2 teasp. Anise Seeds in 1 TB Olive Oil for 8 minutes. Add 1 small bag Baby Spinach Leaves, $^1/_4$ tsp. Black Pepper, and 3 cups Organic Chicken Broth. Bring to a boil, reduce heat and simmer for 10 minutes. Pour into serving bowls; top with thin Lemon Wheels and Parmesan-Reggiano Cheese.

Nutrition; 114 calories; 8gm protein; 6gm carbo.; 3gm fiber; 4gm fats; 5mg cholest. 166mg calcium; 2mg iron; 50mg magnesium; 509mg potassium; 225mg sodium; Vit. A 302 IU; Vit. C 177mg; Vit. E 2 IU.

ITALIAN CIAMBOTTA

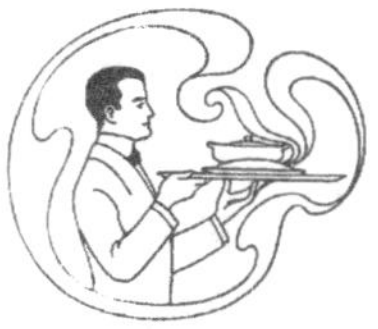

This recipe works for: Recovery, Men's Health, Sports Nutrition

For 6 people:

Sauté in 6 TBS Olive Oil, 3 minced Cloves Garlic, 3 diced Onions, and 1 cup <u>each</u> diced Red Bell Pepper, Yellow Bell Pepper and Orange Bell Pepper until fragrant, 10 minutes.

—Add 3 Red Potatoes in chunks and $^1/_2$ teasp. Sea Salt, and cook for 20 minutes. Add 1-lb. diced Plum Tomatoes and 1 cup Tomato Juice, (or a 28-oz. can Tomatoes with juice). Simmer for 20 more minutes. Add 2 sliced Zucchini and simmer for 5 minutes.

—Serve hot, topped with 6 sliced pitted Black Olives and $^1/_2$ teasp. Cracked Pepper.

MINERAL ONION ALMOND SOUP

This recipe works for: Heart Health, Anti-Aging, Allergy and Asthma
For 6 servings:

Sauté 4 diced Cloves Garlic and 4 diced Medium Onions in 3 TBS Olive Oil about 20 minutes. Add $1^1/_2$ cup chopped Almonds and sauté until browned, about 10 minutes.

—Puree in a blender until creamy. Pour into a soup pot and add 7 cups Vegetable Broth or Onion Broth (make from scratch or a natural mix) and 1 cup White Wine. Cover and cook over low heat for 20 minutes. Season with Sea Salt and Lemon-Pepper.

—Place a slice of Toast on the bottom of each soup plate. Sprinkle with grated Parmesan-Reggiano Cheese. Pour soup over and serve.

Nutrition; 330 calories; 14gm protein; 27gm carbo.; 6gm fiber; 20gm total fats; 6mg choles.; 246mg calcium; 3mg iron; 139mg magnes.; 450mg potassium; 217mg sodium; Vit. A 17 IU; Vit. C 4mg; Vit. E 14 IU.

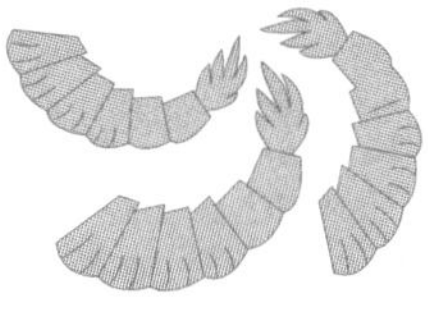

COOL CUCUMBER SHRIMP SOUP

This recipe works for: Hair, Skin and Nails, Women's Health
For 6 servings:

Peel and chop 2 large Cucumbers. Toss with $^1/_4$ cup Tarragon Vinegar, 1 teasp. Sea Salt and 1 TB Fructose. Let stand for 30 minutes to marinate. Then drain and purée in a blender until smooth. Add 1 cup Plain Yogurt and $^1/_2$ cup Water; blend again. Add $^3/_4$ cup, or 1 small bunch, Fresh Dill Weed; whirl again. Chill for 1 hour.

—Heat 2 TBS Olive Oil in a skillet, and toss 1-lb. small cooked Shrimp to coat. Remove and reserve. Add $^1/_4$ cup White Wine, and pinches of Sea Salt and Cracked Pepper to the pan; boil down until flavor is concentrated, about 3 minutes. Pour over shrimp and add the mixture to the soup. Chill again before serving.

Nutrition; 151 calories; 19gm protein; 8gm carbo.; 1gm fiber; 4gm total fats; 149mg choles.; 133mg calcium; 3mg iron; 46mg magnesium; 401mg potassium; 363mg sodium; Vit. A 88 IU; Vit. C 8mg; Vit. E 2 IU.

QUICK HOMEMADE VEGETABLE STEW

This recipe works for: Respiratory Recovery, Men's Health, Sports Nutrition
For 6 people: Make in a large soup pot.

Sauté 4 TBS Soy Bacon Bits and 3 minced Cloves Garlic in 2 teasp. Olive Oil until aromatic. Add 1-lb. chunked Potatoes and 2 sliced Carrots; toss for 5 minutes.

—Bring 4 cups Salted Water to a boil in soup pot. Add an 8-oz. package Frozen Baby Lima Beans, and a 16-oz. package French Cut Green Beans. When water returns to a boil, add sautéd veggies; simmer 15 minutes. Add 1 head shredded Green Cabbage; simmer for 10 more minutes. Add 1 TB Tamari, $^1/_2$ teasp. Black Pepper, and 1 teasp. Sea Salt. Turn into a serving dish and sprinkle with snipped Parsley.

AVOCADO CHICKEN SALAD

This recipe works for: Hair, Skin and Nails, Arthritis, Fatigue Syndromes
For 6 people:

Mix in a bowl: 2 cups diced cooked Organic Chicken, 1 large diced Avocado and 1 diced Rib Celery. Add 2 hard-cooked Eggs, crumbled. Mix in 4 TBS Raspberry Vinaigrette (Page 183) and season to taste with Lemon-Pepper. Serve in Boston Lettuce cups.

Nutrition; 213 calories; 28gm protein; 5gm carbo.; 2gm fiber; 9gm total fats; 126mg choles.; 32mg calcium; 2mg iron; 48mg magnesium; 465mg potassium; 88mg sodium; Vit. A 65 IU; Vit. C 4mg; Vit. E 2 IU.

HIGH MINERAL SPINACH SALAD

This recipe works for: Bone Building, Illness Recovery, Women's Health
For 6 people: Preheat oven to 400°.

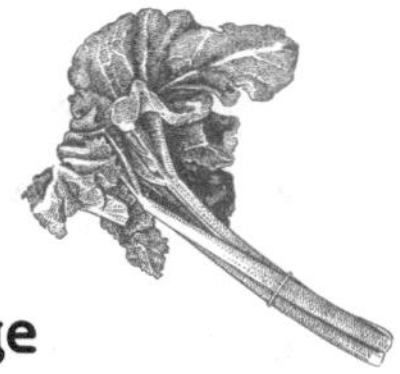

Toss together $1\frac{1}{2}$ cups Whole Wheat Bread Cubes, 1 TB Soy Bacon Bits, 2 TBS Balsamic Vinaigrette and 2 TBS Parmesan Cheese. Bake for 10 minutes until light brown. Set aside.

—Wash and tear 1 bag (6-oz.) Baby Spinach Leaves. Toss in a large salad bowl with 1 cup shredded Green Cabbage, 1 cup shredded Red Cabbage, 1 cup Tofu Cubes and 1 cup Water-Packed Artichoke Hearts, sliced. Pour on $\frac{1}{2}$ cup Balsamic Vinaigrette; marinate for 30 minutes. Toss with the toasted crouton blend and serve.

Nutrition; 134 calories; 9gm protein; 17gm carbo.; 4gm fiber; 3gm total fats; 3mg choles.; 176mg calcium; 4mg iron; 96mg magnesium; 407mg potassium; 95mg sodium; Vit. A 209 IU; Vit. C 27mg; Vit. E 2 IU.

MUSHROOM HEAVEN SALAD

This recipe works for: Cancer Protection, Immune Enhancement, Liver Health
For 4 people:

Wash a $\frac{1}{2}$ lb. blend of Fresh Chanterelle and Shiitake Mushrooms. Trim and discard bruised or tough stems. Slice mushrooms into matchsticks.

—In a large skillet over high heat, sizzle 3 TBS diced Shallots and the mushrooms in 2 TBS Olive Oil. Stir until juices evaporate and mushrooms begin to brown, 6 to 7 minutes. Add 2 TBS Sherry and stir to release browned bits, about 1 minute. Add 1 TB snipped Parsley, and Sea Salt and Cracked Pepper to taste.

—In a large bowl, mix remaining 2 TBS Olive Oil and 2 TBS Raspberry Vinegar. Toss 6 cups mixed Fresh Baby Asian Greens to blend. Divide onto plates and top with equal portions of mushroom mixture. Sprinkle with Parmesan-Reggiano Cheese.

Nutrition; 178 calories; 5gm protein; 13gm carbo.; 2gm fiber; 11gm total fats; 5mg choles.; 145mg calcium; 1mg iron; 34mg magnesium; 357mg potassium; 168mg sodium; Vit. A 99 IU; Vit. C 9mg; Vit. E 2 IU.

MINERAL-ENZYME SUMMER SALAD

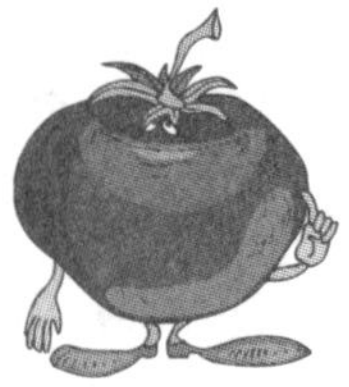

This recipe works for: Arthritis, Bone Building, Hair and Skin
Makes 4 servings:

Whisk dressing in a non-metallic bowl: 2 TBS Lime Juice and 1/2 tsp. of Sea Salt. Add and fold to combine: 4 diced Tomatoes, 3 diced Avocados, 3 thin-sliced Green Onions and 1/4 teasp. Garlic-Lemon Seasoning. Season with Lemon-Pepper and set aside.

—In a large bowl, whisk 1 TB Olive Oil, 1/4 tsp. ground Cumin, 1 TB Lime Juice. Toss with 1 package (6-oz.) Baby Spinach Leaves and 1 peeled diced Cucumber. Divide among plates. Mound on avocado mixture. Sprinkle with 2 TBS snipped Fresh Cilantro.

EASY MINERAL BREAD SALAD

This recipe works for: Sports Nutrition, Immune Breakdown, Men's Health
Makes 4 servings: Preheat oven broiler.

Rub 4 thick Wholewheat Sourdough Bread slices with Olive Oil and halves of 1 Garlic Clove. Toast bread, turning once, 4 minutes on each side. Cut bread into small cubes and put into serving bowl. Add 2 diced Beefsteak Tomatoes, 1 can (15-oz.) White Cannellini Beans, rinsed and drained, 1 thin sliced Red Bell Pepper and 1/4 cup snipped Fresh Basil.

—Make the ITALIAN DRESSING: In a bowl, whisk 4 teasp. Balsamic Vinegar, 1 tsp. Dijon Mustard, 3 TBS Olive Oil, 3 TBS Vegetable Broth (made from vegetable bouillon), Sea Salt and Cracked Black Pepper to taste. Pour dressing over salad and toss to coat. Let rest 5 to 10 minutes before serving.

MANY TREASURE RICE SALAD

This recipe works for: Weight Control, Heart Health, Liver and Organ Health
For 4 servings:

Toast 3/4 cup slivered Almonds in a 300° oven until golden. Set aside. Soak 6 dry Shiitake Mushrooms in water until soft. Slice and discard woody stems.

—Cook 1 cup Brown Basmati Rice in 2 cups Salted Water until tender. Add 1 TB Brown Rice Vinegar and let stand while you make the rest of the salad.

—Sauté in 2 TBS Olive Oil until aromatic: 1 TB grated Fresh Ginger, 2 thin sliced Leeks (white parts only), 3 sliced Green Onions, 1 thin sliced Red Bell Pepper. Add the shiitake mushrooms and 1 cup slivered Bamboo Shoots; sauté for 5 minutes. Add rice and almonds; heat through. Remove from heat and let rest.

—Make a large cup of Butter Lettuce Leaves, and fill with salad mixture; or roll up in 12 large Butter Lettuce Leaves and put 3 to 4 on each salad plate.

Nutrition; 368 calories; 11gm protein; 57gm carbo.; 7gm fiber; 14gm total fats; 0mg choles.; 129mg calcium; 3mg iron; 157mg magnes.; 767mg potass.; 240mg sodium; Vit. A 142 IU; Vit. C 49mg; Vit. E 9 IU.

Mineral Packed Seafoods

Ocean foods of all kinds are a primary source of nutritional minerals. Here are some delicious ways to add them to your diet.

SEAFOOD SALAD DELUXE

This recipe works for: Hair and Skin, Heart Health, Anti-Aging
For 8 servings:

Bring 4-qts. Salted Water to a boil. Drop in 1-lb. peeled Shrimp; then drop in 1-lb. Bay Scallops. Just before water returns to a boil, drop in 8-oz. Frozen Langoustinos or Surimi pieces and 1 cup Frozen Green Peas. Remove from heat; drain; pop in fridge.

—Make TARRAGON MAYONNAISE in the blender: 2 Eggs, $^1/_4$ cup Tarragon Vinegar, $^1/_3$ cup Dijon Mustard, 1 teasp. dry Tarragon, $^1/_4$ teasp. Cracked Black Pepper. Whirl briefly, then while blender is running, add $^1/_3$ cup Canola Oil and $^1/_3$ cup Olive Oil in a thin steady stream until mixture thickens.

—To serve, ring a large plate with 8 cups mixed Baby Spring Salad Greens. Spoon seafood in the middle; spoon Tarragon Mayonnaise over top.

POTATO-GREEN BEAN SALAD with DULSE FLAKES

This recipe works for: Men's Health, Sports Nutrition, Bone Building
For 4 servings: Dulse tastes a lot like bacon, great with beans and potatoes.

Steam 1-lb. thin sliced Red Potatoes for 10 minutes until just tender; add 8-oz. cooked Frozen French-Cut Green Beans. Cover, remove from heat and set aside.

—Heat 2 TBS Olive Oil in a skillet and sauté 2 TBS Sesame Seeds until golden. Add $^1/_2$ cup thin-sliced Scallions, 1 TB Lemon Juice, 1 TB Dulse Flakes, and $^1/_4$ teasp. Black Pepper; sauté until fragrant. Toss with potatoes and beans and serve hot.

Nutrition; 183 calories; 6gm protein; 34gm carbo.; 6gm fiber; 3gm total fats; 0mg choles.; 67mg calcium; 4mg iron; 106mg magnesium; 730mg potassium; 145mg sodium; Vit. A 34 IU; Vit. C 25mg; Vit. E 1 IU.

SPINACH - SHRIMP SALAD with MUSTARD DRESSING

This recipe works for: Weight Control, Heart Health, Bone Building
Makes 6 servings:

Place 2 packages Baby Spinach Leaves (12-oz.) in a large bowl. Toss with 1-lb. cooked Salad Shrimp.

—Make the dressing in a pan: mix 1 TB Honey and 1 tsp. Arrowroot Powder. Whisk in $^1/_3$ cup Dijon Mustard, 2 TBS Water, 2 TBS White Wine and 1 TB Balsamic Vinegar. Cook, stirring constantly, until dressing boils; stir in 2 TBS minced Fresh Dill or $1^1/_2$ tsp. dried Dill Weed. Pour dressing over salad. Mix well and serve at once.

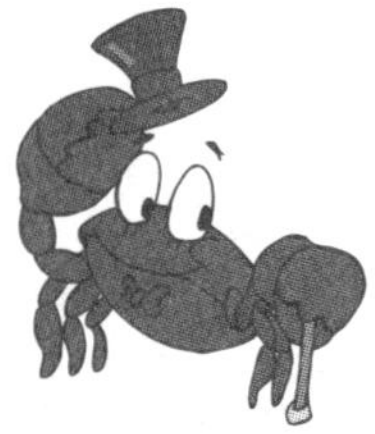

CRAB with TOMATO-CILANTRO SAUCE

This recipe works for: Weight Control, Heart Health, Bone Building
Makes 6 appetizer servings:

Sizzle 2 TBS Olive Oil, 2 minced Shallots and 2 teasp. minced Ginger for 5 minutes. Add 1/2 cup diced Zucchini, 1/2 cup diced Yellow Bell Pepper, 1/2 cup diced Red Bell Pepper, 1/2 cup diced Orange Bell Pepper and 1/4 cup diced Carrot. Remove from heat.

—Mix 8-oz. Crabmeat, 4 TBS Lemon Mayonnaise, 2 TBS snipped Chives and the sautéed vegetables in a large bowl. Season to taste with Garlic-Lemon Seasoning.

—Make the TOMATO-CILANTRO SAUCE in the blender: Combine 2 large diced Tomatoes, 1/3 cup snipped Fresh Cilantro, 2 TBS Tarragon Vinegar, 1 minced Garlic Clove, and 4 drops Hot Pepper Sauce; puree until almost smooth. Gradually add 1/2 cup Olive Oil and blend until sauce is thick. Transfer to a bowl. Season to taste.

—Arrange 2 separated heads Belgian Endive Spears on a large platter, tips toward platter edge. Spoon crab salad into center of platter. Drizzle sauce over endive. Garnish salad with snipped Fresh Chives and serve.

Nutrition; 240 calories; 9gm protein; 9gm carbo.; 2gm fiber; 18gm total fats; 33mg choles.; 69mg calcium; 2mg iron; 53mg magnesium; 476mg potassium; 157mg sodium; Vit. A 356 IU; Vit. C 67mg; Vit. E 5 IU.

BAKED SALMON LOAF with FRESH BASIL SAUCE

This recipe works for: Brain Boosting, Heart Health, Bone Building
For 4 servings: Preheat oven to 375°.

Mix together: 1 can (16-oz.) Red Salmon, 1/2 cup Whole Grain Granola, 1/2 cup White Wine, 2 TBS minced Shallots, 2 TBS Lemon Mayonnaise, 2 beaten Eggs, 2 TBS snipped Fresh Parsley, 1 teasp. Herbal Seasoning, and 1/2 teasp. Black Pepper; press into an oiled loaf pan. Bake for 50 to 60 minutes until set. Let rest for 10 minutes.

—Make the FRESH BASIL SAUCE in the blender: 1/3 cup packed Fresh Basil Leaves, 6 TBS Olive Oil, 2 TBS Parmesan Cheese, 1/2 teasp. Garlic-Lemon Seasoning. Pour over loaf before cutting; sprinkle with 2 TBS diced Black Olives and 2 TBS diced Walnuts.

MINT-BAKED SWORDFISH

This recipe works for: Weight Control, Heart Health, Women's Health
Makes 2 to 4 servings: Preheat the oven to 425°F.

Line bottom of a baking dish with 1/2 cup Fresh Mint Leaves in overlapping layers like fish scales. Slice half a Red Onion into rounds and place on top of the mint. Sprinkle with 1/2 teasp. Garlic-Lemon Seasoning. Rinse and pat dry 1-lb. Swordfish Steaks. Rub with Sea Salt and White Pepper. Place the fish on the onion.

—Make the sauce: combine 1 TB Tarragon Vinegar, 2 TBS Lemon Juice, 3 TBS White Wine and 1 TB Capers. Pour over fish. Bake for about 15 minutes.

MARYLAND CRAB CAKES

This recipe works for: Hair and Skin, Heart Health, Arthritis
For 6 servings:

Mix the crab cakes in a large bowl: $^{3}/_{4}$ lb. Fresh Lump Crabmeat, picked over and rinsed, $^{3}/_{4}$ cup grated Parmesan Cheese, $^{1}/_{4}$ cup Low Fat Cream Cheese, $^{1}/_{4}$ cup Whole Grain Cracker Crumbs, 1 Egg, 2 minced Green Onions, 2 TBS snipped Fresh Parsley, 1 teasp. Lemon-Garlic Seasoning, $^{1}/_{2}$ teasp dry Oregano.

—Add 2 teasp. Olive Oil to a hot skillet. Spoon in 3 to 4 TBS Crab Cake mix; mound and flatten into cakes. Cook 2 minutes until lightly browned. Turn with a spatula and cook 1 more minute. Remove and keep warm. Repeat until all are done.

—Peel and slice a large Avocado. Put Boston Lettuce cups on salad plates. Arrange avocado slices and crab cakes on top.

Nutrition; 247 calories; 21gm protein; 8gm carbo.; 2gm fiber; 11gm total fats; 102mg choles.; 265mg calcium; 2mg iron; 49mg magnesium; 502mg potass.; 286mg sodium; Vit. A 180 IU; Vit. C 8mg; Vit. E 3 IU.

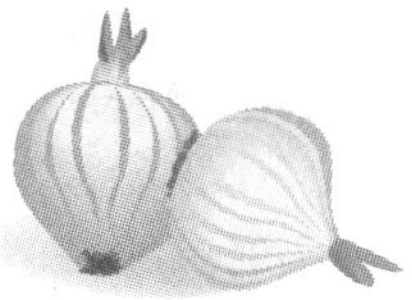

Prime Minerals from Onions

Onions, garlic, scallions, shallots, leeks and chives are long known for their antibiotic, anti-viral and anti-carcinogenic qualities. They make almost every savory recipe more delicious, too. Add the onion family to your nutritional healing program.

OVEN ROASTED RATATOUILLE in ONION SAUCE

This recipe works for: Bone Building, Liver-Organ Health, Addiction Recovery
For 6 people: Preheat oven to 450°F.

In a roasting pan, combine: 1 peeled Eggplant in 1-inch thick rounds, 1 thick-sliced Zucchini, 1 sliced Red Bell Pepper, 1 sliced Yellow Bell Pepper, 8 quartered Red Potatoes, 1 Yellow Onion cut in thick rings, and 10 minced Cloves Garlic. Scatter several Fresh Rosemary Sprigs over top. Drizzle with $^{1}/_{2}$ cup Olive Oil; season with Lemon-Pepper. Toss to coat. Roast vegetables, stirring every 5 minutes, for about 25 minutes. Add 6 quartered Plum Tomatoes. Continue roasting 10 to 12 minutes more.

—Make the ONION-BASIL SAUCE in a blender: combine $^{1}/_{2}$ cup packed Fresh Basil Leaves, 1 tsp. minced Garlic and 1 small chopped Onion. Add $^{1}/_{2}$ cup Lemon-Mayonnaise 1 TB. at a time, and a pinch of Sea Salt. Blend to smooth. Remove vegetables from oven and transfer to serving platter. Serve warm with sauce on the side.

Nutrition; 240 calories; 4gm protein; 36gm carbo.; 8gm fiber; 10gm total fats; 0mg choles.; 107mg calcium; 3mg iron; 54mg magnes.; 805mg potassium; 140mg sodium; Vit. A 205 IU; Vit. C 76mg; Vit. E 3 IU.

HIGH MINERAL LEEK TERRINE

This recipe works for: Men's Health, Allergies and Asthma, Cancer Protection
For 8 people: Preheat oven to 350°.

Soak 4 Shiitake Mushrooms in water until soft. Sliver and discard woody stems. Save soaking water.

—Sizzle 2 TBS Olive Oil, 3 minced Cloves Garlic, 1 sliced Yellow Onion, 4 diced Carrots and 8-oz. sliced Brown Cremini Mushrooms for 10 minutes until fragrant. Add 2 cups chopped Plum Tomatoes, the slivered Shiitake Mushrooms, 2 teasp. dry Thyme, 2 teasp. Italian Herbs and $^1/_2$ cup Sherry. Partially cover and simmer 30 minutes. Turn off heat and set aside.

—Trim and slice 12 Leeks (mostly white parts). Bring 4 cups Salted Water and the reserved mushroom soaking water to a boil. Simmer leeks for 15 minutes until tender. Drain and rinse in cool water to stop cooking. Set aside.

—Melt 4 TBS Butter in a pan. Add 6 TBS Whole Wheat Flour, stir for 1 minute. Add 1 cup Plain Low Fat Yogurt and 1 cup Organic Chicken Broth. Whisk to thick and smooth.

—Stir in 8-oz. Low Fat Cream Cheese and 8-oz. Low Fat Cottage Cheese. Re-season with Italian Herbs if necessary. Remove from heat and set aside.

—Assemble the terrine in a large buttered mold. Line mold with waxed paper, and spray paper with lecithin spray. Distribute leek slices to cover bottom of baking dish. Spoon on 1 cup of the tomato-vegetable mix. Top with another layer of leeks. Cover with yogurt-cheese sauce. Repeat layers until dish is filled, ending with the cheese sauce. Bake til bubbly and set, 45 minutes. Let sit for 30 minutes. Unmold onto a serving platter. Remove waxed paper and slice.

Nutrition; 370 calories; 14gm protein; 45gm carbo.; 8gm fiber; 9gm total fats; 30mg choles.; 254mg calcium; 6mg iron; 91mg magnesium; 945mg potass.; 198mg sodium; Vit. A 1189 IU; Vit. C 39mg; Vit. E 5 IU.

PASTA with ONION SAUCE

This recipe works for: Men's Health, Hair, Skin and Nails, Sports Nutrition
For 6 servings:

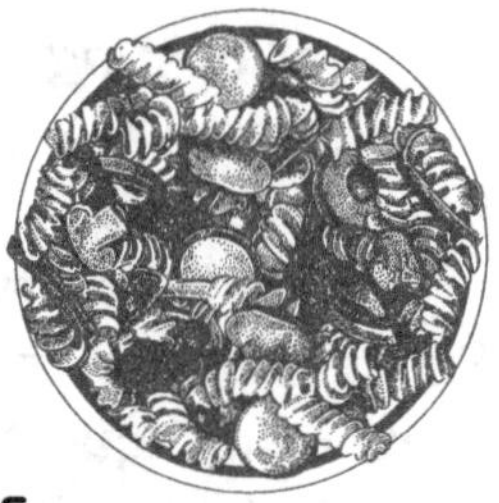

Bring a large pot of Salted Water to boil for the pasta.

—Sauté 6 cups thin-sliced Sweet Onions in 2 TBS Butter and 2 TBS Olive Oil in a large pot about 30 minutes. Stir occasionally so onions don't burn. Season with Sea Salt and Pepper.

—Dissolve 2 TBS Tomato Paste in 2 TBS Sherry and stir into onions. Add 1 cup Water and simmer uncovered for 10 minutes. Cover and remove from heat. Let cool slightly and stir in 2 beaten Eggs.

—Cook 12-oz. of your favorite pasta in the boiling water to al dente. Drain; put in a serving bowl. Top with onion sauce; sprinkle with $^2/_3$ cup Parmesan-Reggiano Cheese.

Nutrition; 370 calories; 16gm protein; 56gm carbo.; 9gm fiber; 6gm total fats; 15mg choles.; 245mg calcium; 2mg iron; 135mg magnes.; 533mg potass.; 257mg sodium; Vit. A 84 IU; Vit. C 13mg; Vit. E 2 IU.

HIGH MINERAL GRILLED RED ONIONS

This recipe works for: Respiratory Infection, Allergies - Asthma, Bone Building
Makes 6 servings: Heat a BBQ grill to hot.

In a large shallow dish whisk 2 teasp. dry Mint, 2 teasp. dry Oregano, 1 teasp. Honey, 1 teasp. Sea Salt, 4 TBS Balsamic Vinegar and 3 TBS Olive Oil together. Add 4 large Red Onions, sliced in thin rings; let marinate, covered and refrigerated overnight, turning once. Remove onions; discard marinade. Brush with Olive Oil; grill in a BBQ basket tuning once, for about 8 minutes or until tender. Salt and pepper to taste; serve hot.

CREAMY TOMATO ONION SOUP

This recipe works for: Men's Health, Heart and Artery Health
For 8 servings: Use a large soup pot.

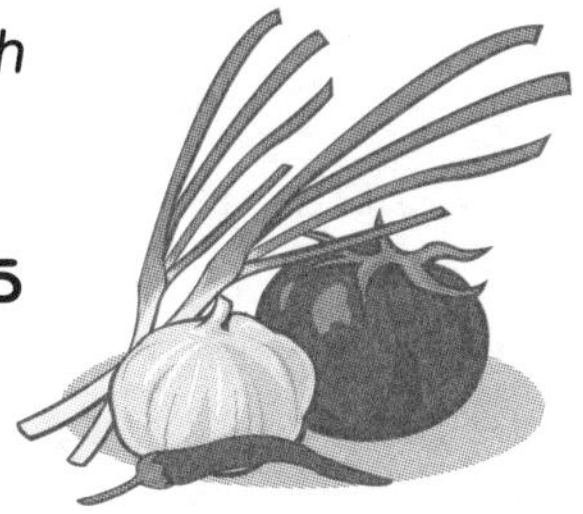

Sizzle 2 cups diced Yellow Onions in 2 TBS Olive Oil for 5 minutes until aromatic.

—Add 1 cup diced Carrots and 1 cup diced Celery; sauté for 5 more minutes. Turn mixture into a blender and whirl a few seconds with 1 cup Tomato Juice.

—Pour back into soup pot and add 3 more cups Tomato Juice, 1 cup White Wine, 1 cup Water, 3 TBS Dry Onion Soup Mix, 2 TBS Tamari and 4 TBS Almond Butter. Heat and stir occasionally about 10 to 15 minutes. Serve tasty hot.

Nutrition; 133 calories; 4gm protein; 14gm carbo.; 4gm fiber; 6gm total fats; 0mg choles.; 58mg calcium; 2mg iron; 55mg magnesium; 523mg potassium; 340mg sodium; Vit. A 460 IU; Vit. C 28mg; Vit. E 4 IU.

ONION PIE

This recipe works for: Hair, Skin and Nails, Men's Health, Heart and Artery Health
For 6 to 8 servings: Preheat oven to 350°.

Make a simple, quick crust by crushing 35 Whole Grain Crackers, mixing them with 5 TBS melted Butter and pressing into a 9" pie plate. Bake for 5 minutes to brown. Remove from oven and set aside.

—Sauté 5 sliced Yellow Onions in 3 TBS Butter until aromatic. Spread on the crust.

—Make the filling in the blender: 4 Eggs, 1-lb. Soft Fresh Tofu, 1 TB snipped Parsley, 1 tsp. dry Basil, 1 tsp. dry Thyme, 1 tsp. Sea Salt, 1/4 tsp. Pepper, 1/4 tsp. Nutmeg.

—Turn into a bowl and mix in 3 cups grated Low Fat Cheddar Cheese. Spread over onions. Dust with Paprika. Bake for 1 hour until set.

Nutrition; 437 calories; 31gm protein; 19gm carbo.; 3gm fiber; 25gm total fats; 198mg choles.; 640mg calcium; 6mg iron; 114mg magnesium; 453mg potass.; 484mg sodium; Vit. A 375 IU; Vit. C 7mg; Vit. E 2 IU.

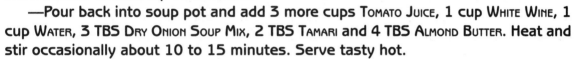

ROAST YORKSHIRE PUDDING

This recipe works for: Digestive Health, Allergies - Asthma, Men's Health
For 8 servings: Preheat oven to 500°.

In a shallow baking pan, roast 4 large Yellow Onions, quartered, in $^1/_4$ cup Balsamic Vinegar and 2 TBS Olive Oil until brown and fragrant, about 40 minutes. Baste with the marinade every 10 minutes to keep moist and flavorful.

—Remove from oven and let cool in the pan. Keep quarters intact. Dot with Butter. Reduce oven to 375°. Heat onions until sizzly - about 5 minutes.

—Whirl in a blender: 1 cup Whole Wheat Flour, $^1/_2$ cup Plain Yogurt, $^1/_2$ cup Water and 2 Eggs in the blender until smooth. Pour around onions, (not on top) and bake until well browned and puffy, about 35 to 40 minutes. Serve hot with dots of butter.

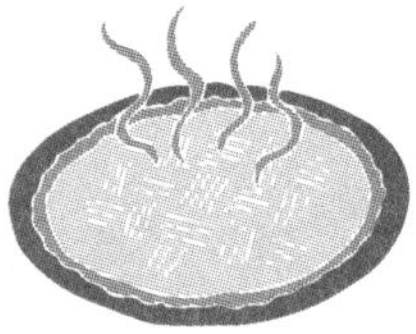

Mineral-Rich Veggie Pies

Vegetable pies are a delicious way to get your minerals. They are light, yet full of nutrition. They're easy to make, one-dish meals that just about everybody likes. You can eat just a small amount and feel satisfied. Each pie is enough for 8 servings.

VEGGIES and CHEESE in a PERFECTION CRUST

This recipe works for: Digestive Health, Waste Management, Men's Health
Preheat oven to 450° for the crust; 350° for the filled pie. Makes 8 servings:

Make the crust. Whisk until foamy: $^1/_3$ cup Plain Low Fat Yogurt, $^1/_3$ cup Water, 1 teasp. Baking Soda, 2 teasp. Cream of Tartar, $^1/_2$ teasp. Sea Salt. Mix in $^1/_3$ cup Olive Oil, 4 TBS melted Butter and $^1/_4$ cup Honey. Mix separately: $1^3/_4$ cup Unbleached Flour, $^1/_2$ cup Bran Flakes, $^1/_4$ cup Oat Flour and 2 TBS Toasted Sesame Seeds. Combine the 2 mixtures. Knead briefly on a floured surface, and roll or pat into a greased quiche pan. Prick bottom and bake for 5 minutes. Remove and cool for filling.

—Make the VEGETABLE-CHEESE filling: Bring 2-qts. Salted Water to a boil in a large pot. Add 6 cups mixed vegetables.... sliced Bell Peppers (any color), chopped Cauliflower, chopped Broccoli Florets, diced Carrots, sliced Brown or White Mushrooms, and sliced Water Chestnuts or Jicama. Blanch until color changes, about 5 minutes.

—Make the sauce: Mix 1 can (11-oz.) Cream of Mushroom Soup with $^1/_2$ cup White Wine. Add 3 TBS Butter, 2 TBS bottled Barbecue Sauce or Hickory Sauce, and 1 TB Tamari. Pour over veggies; cover with grated Low Fat Cheddar. Bake until brown and bubbly.

Nutrition; 387 calories; 9gm protein; 43gm carbo.; 4gm fiber; 19gm total fats; 26mg choles.; 126mg calcium; 3mg iron; 46mg magnes.; 502mg potass.; 514mg sodium; Vit. A 1010 IU; Vit. C 44mg; Vit. E 3 IU.

LOW FAT CLASSIC VEGGIE PIE

This recipe works for: Weight Control, Sugar Imbalances, Immune Boosting
Preheat oven to 375°F. Use a large Quiche baking dish. Reheat in a 325°F oven.

Make the crust in a bowl: mix $^1/_2$ cup Rolled Oats, $^1/_2$ cup Buckwheat Flour, $^1/_2$ cup Unbleached Flour, $^1/_4$ tsp. Sea Salt, $^1/_8$ tsp. Baking Powder. Drizzle on 4 or 5 TBS Canola Oil one tablespoon at a time until mixture looks like wet sand. Stir in 2 TBS Lemon Juice, 2 tsp. Honey and 2 TBS Cold Water. Mix lightly with a fork until dough forms a ball. Sprinkle 2 tsp. Sesame Seeds over bottom of a quiche pan, then pat in dough to cover top and sides. Prick sides and bottom of crust with a fork. Crimp edges. Bake for 10 minutes, remove from oven and reduce temperature to 350°F.

—Make the filling: in a skillet sizzle 1 cup diced Onion and 1 minced Clove Garlic in 1 TB Canola Oil and 1 TB White Wine for 5 minutes. Add garlic and sauté for 30 seconds. Add 3 cups small Broccoli Florets and 3 TBS Water; cover and steam until broccoli is bright green and slightly tender but not soft, about 2 minutes. Drain vegetables and spread evenly over crust.

—Make the sauce in a blender: whirl 3 Eggs until frothy. Add a 10-oz. package soft, Silken Tofu, 1 TB Dijon Mustard, 1 tsp. dry Basil, $^1/_4$ tsp. Nutmeg, $^1/_4$ tsp. Sea Salt, $^1/_4$ tsp. White Pepper and 2 TBS grated Parmesan Cheese. Blend until very smooth. Pour mixture over vegetables in pie crust. Arrange Red Bell Pepper strips and Black Olives in an attractive alternating pattern on top. Bake 40 minutes, until slightly puffy. Allow to cool 5 to 10 minutes before slicing.

Nutrition; 247 calories; 11gm protein; 24m carbo.; 4gm fiber; 12gm total fats; 70mg choles.; 140mg calcium; 4mg iron; 83mg magnes.; 412mg potassium; 245mg sodium; Vit. A 156 IU; Vit. C 52mg; Vit. E 4 IU.

TAMALE PIE

This recipe works for: Men's and Kid's Health, Allergies, Sports Nutrition
Preheat oven to 425°. Make in a heavy ceramic baking dish. Use leftover cornbead.

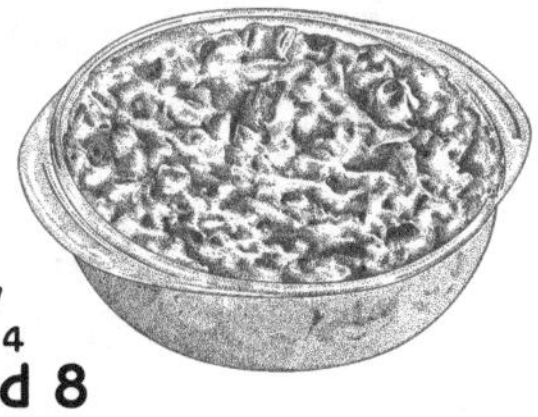

Have ready 1-lb. boned, skinned Chicken Breasts, cubed.

—Make the filling: in a pan, sizzle 1 diced large Yellow Onion in 2 TBS Olive Oil til fragrant. Blend in 2 TBS Cornmeal, 1$^1/_2$ cups Organic Chicken Broth, 2 TBS Chili Powder, 1 TB Balsamic Vinegar, $^1/_4$ tsp. Fennel Seed and $^1/_2$ cup chopped Green Chilies. Simmer covered 8 minutes. Stir in chicken and 1 cubed large Beefsteak Tomato; remove from heat.

—Make the dough in a bowl: mix 2 cups Cornmeal, 3 TBS Olive Oil, 1$^3/_4$ cups Organic Chicken Broth, $^1/_2$ teasp. Baking Powder and $^1/_2$ teasp. Sea Salt. Pat half the dough onto bottom of oiled baking dish. Add chicken mixture. Drop remaining dough on top of chicken mix in spoonfuls. Bake about 45 minutes until bubbly. Snip on Green Onions and Fresh Cilantro Leaves.

Nutrition; 290 calories;18gm protein; 29gm carbo.; 4gm fiber; 10gm total fats; 31mg choles.; 79mg calcium; 3mg iron; 79mg magnes.; 454mg potassium; 290mg sodium; Vit. A 102 IU; Vit. C 12mg; Vit. E 3 IU.

FRESH TOMATO BASIL CHEESE TART

This recipe works for: Men's and Kid's Health, Allergies, Sports Nutrition
Preheat oven to 325°. Pre-bake the crust given at the beginning of this section.

Sauté 1 diced Red Onion, 1 TB Soy Bacon Bits and 1 teasp. dry Oregano in 2 TBS Olive Oil until aromatic, about 7 to 8 minutes. Add and sauté briefly: 4 diced large Ripe Tomatoes, 1 teasp. mixed Italian Herbs, 1/4 cup snipped Fresh Basil, 1/4 cup White Wine, 2 teasp. crumbled Toasted Dulse, and 1/2 teasp. Cracked Pepper. Remove from heat; stir in 1/4 cup Parmesan Cheese, and 2 Eggs. Spoon into the pre-baked shell. Cover with 2 cups shredded Low-Fat Mozarrella Cheese. Bake 45 minutes until bubbly.

Nutrition; 307 calories; 6gm protein; 35gm carbo.; 2gm fiber; 15gm total fats; 24mg choles.; 128mg calcium; 2mg iron; 28mg magnesium; 264mg potassium; 208mg sodium; Vit. A 114 IU; Vit. C 3mg; Vit. E 2 IU.

THAI BROCCOLI PIE

This recipe works for: Cancer Protection, Women's Health, Fatigue Syndromes
Preheat oven to 375°. Use a deep ceramic baking dish.

Make the crust by spreading 2 cups cooked Brown Rice mixed with 2 TB Brown Rice Vinegar in a ceramic baking dish. Bake for 10 minutes until crusty on top.

—Make the filling in a pot: heat 1 TB Olive Oil and sizzle 1/2 cup diced Red Onion, 2 minced Garlic Cloves, 2 teasp. Wasabi Paste, 1/2 teasp. Sea Salt, 1/2 teasp. Cracked Pepper and 1/2 teasp. Cumin Powder. Stir in 2 TBS Whole Wheat Flour until bubbly. Add 4 cups Low Fat Chicken Broth; blend until smooth. Add 1/4 cup snipped Fresh Cilantro Leaves, 1 cup cubed Firm Tofu, 2 cups chopped Broccoli Florets and 1 diced Yellow Crookneck Squash. Spoon on top of rice and bake covered for 35-40 minutes.

DEEP GREENS PIE

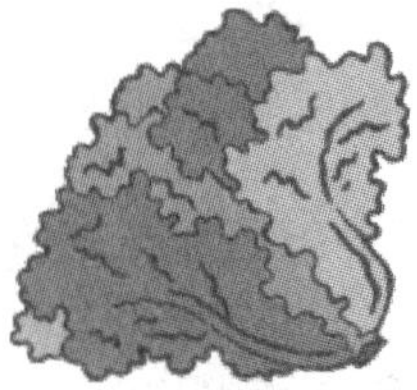

This recipe works for: Bone Building, Allergies, Immune Power
Preheat oven to 400°.

Prepare a pie crust. See our suggestions or use your own.

—Make the filling: Sauté 1 cup sliced Mushrooms in a skillet in 3 TBS Butter 5 minutes. Sprinkle on 1 TB Whole Wheat Flour and stir 1 minute. Spoon onto crust.

—Add 1 teasp. Butter to the skillet and sauté 2 TBS minced Shallots and 1/2 teasp. Herbs de Provence 3 minutes. Add 2 cups chopped mixed Greens (Spinach, Chard, Endive, etc.); simmer for only 1 minute. Puree in the blender until smooth. Pour greens over mushrooms. Sprinkle with 1 cup grated Low Fat Swiss Cheese.

—Make the sauce in the blender: 1 cup Plain Yogurt, 1/4 cup White Wine, 1/4 cup Water, 4 Eggs, 1/2 teasp. Honey, 1/2 teasp. Sea Salt, 1/4 teasp. Pepper, 1/4 teasp. Nutmeg and dashes Hot Pepper Sauce. Pour over pie and bake on the bottom oven rack for 15 minutes. Reduce heat to 325°; bake 30 minutes more, until puffy, brown and set.

DEEP DISH ITALIAN PIE

Like a mushroom pizza without the crust.

This recipe works for: Men's and Kid's Health, Allergies, Sports Nutrition

For one 9 x 13" pan: Preheat oven to 375°. Cut in 9 big squares to serve.

Have ready 1 (15-oz.) jar Natural Pizza Sauce, 1 small Eggplant peeled and sliced, and 1 1/2 cups grated Low Fat Mozarrella Cheese.

—Sauté 1 sliced Yellow Onion, 1 teasp. Italian Seasoning Herbs and 1/2 teasp. Anise Seed in 2 TBS Olive Oil for 5 minutes. Add 1 sliced Red Bell Pepper and 1-lb. sliced Mushrooms; toss until coated. Add 1-lb. chopped Fresh Tomatoes and toss to coat.

—Spread pizza sauce to cover bottom of the pan, and cover with the eggplant slices. Cover with Mozarrella. Top with the tomato/mushroom mixture. Pour on rest of Pizza Sauce. Sprinkle on 1/4 cup Red Wine. Scatter on top 2 TBS Parmesan-Reggiano Cheese. Bake covered for 20 minutes. Remove cover and bake for 20 more minutes.

Nutrition; 160 calories; 10gm protein; 14gm carbo.; 4gm fiber; 7gm total fats; 12mg choles.; 244mg calcium; 2mg iron; 37mg magnes.; 464mg potassium; 330mg sodium; Vit. A 128 IU; Vit. C 32mg; Vit. E 1 IU.

SWEET POTATO SUPPER PIE

This recipe works for: Women's Health, Anti-Aging, Overcoming Addictions

Preheat oven to 350°.

Toast 1 1/4 cups chopped Pecans in the oven for 5 to 7 minutes.

—Make the crust: mix 1/2 cup of the pecans with 4 TBS Butter and 1 1/4 cups Whole Wheat Pastry Flour; add 4 TBS Cold Water to form dough into a ball. Pat into a lecithin-sprayed baking pan. Chill.

—Make the filling: soak 6 Dried Apricots in water until soft. Slice thin. Reserve soaking water. Bake 2-lbs. Sweet Potatoes until soft. Peel and mash with rest of the Toasted Pecans, the sliced Apricots with 2 TBS reserved soaking water, 1/2 cup Plain Yogurt, 1 TB Butter, 1 TB Honey, 1/2 teasp. Cinnamon, 1/2 teasp. Sea Salt and 1/4 teasp. Nutmeg. Spread onto chilled crust. Sprinkle with 1/3 cup Toasted Wheat Germ and 1/2 cup grated Low Fat Cheddar Cheese. Bake for 50 minutes until browned and bubbly.

SHRIMP and SCALLION PIE

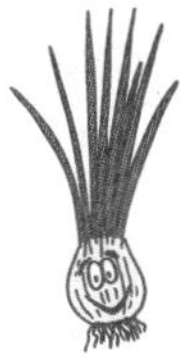

This recipe works for: Brain Health, Anti-Aging, Skin and Hair

Preheat oven to 375°. Have ready a prepared pie shell or crust.

Slice 1 Bunch Scallions crosswise. Separate green and white parts. Sauté white parts in 4 TBS Olive Oil with 1 TB chopped Fresh Ginger 5 minutes. Stir in 8-oz. small cooked Shrimp and green onion parts; turn into prepared pie shell. Add 3 TBS Whole Wheat Flour, 3 TBS Sherry, 1 tsp. Tamari and 1 tsp. Fructose to skillet; stir 5 minutes.

—Blender blend custard: 4 Eggs, 1 cup Plain Low Fat Yogurt, 1/2 cup Water, 1/2 cup Kefir Cheese, 3 TBS Sherry, 1/2 teasp. Sea Salt, and 1/4 teasp. Nutmeg. Pour over pie and bake for 45 minutes until set when shaken. Let set for 10 minutes. Serve hot.

LEEK and POTATO PIE

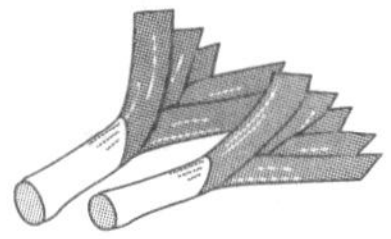

This recipe works for: Liver Health, Overcoming Addictions
Preheat oven to 450°. Use a round pie dish.

Make the crust: Have ready 1-lb. mashed Potatoes. Mix into a dough with 1 Egg, 1/3 cup Low Fat Cottage Cheese and 1 TB Whole Wheat Flour. Pat into pie dish. Bake until firm and springy, about 20 minutes. Remove and set aside.

—Sizzle for 12 minutes in 2 TBS Olive Oil and 1/2 tsp. Garlic-Lemon Seasoning, 3 thin-sliced Onions, 2 large thin sliced Leeks (white parts). Set aside. Blender blend custard: 1/2 cup Plain Low Fat Yogurt, 1/2 cup Water, 2 Eggs and 1 TB Whole Wheat Flour.

—Spread 1/2 cup Low Fat Cream Cheese over the potato crust. Cover with 2 TBS snipped Fresh Chives. Cover with leek mixture, and pour on egg custard. Bake until set, about 50 minutes. Cover with foil if top browns too fast.

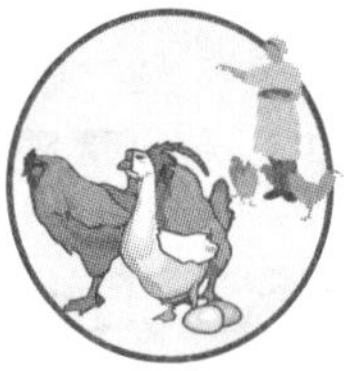

Chicken and Turkey are Full of Minerals

There's a big nutrition difference in poultry that is raised out of doors naturally, chemical-free. When domestic birds scratch and eat in a free-run environment, they don't need hormones or growth stimulants. The meat is lower in fat and cholesterol, higher in minerals, vitamins and proteins. The difference is reflected in full-flavored taste and juiciness. Free-run poultry nutrients are a good healing tool for people who need protein for body building, bone and tissue formation.

Roasting is one of the most wholesome ways to fix poultry. Roasting allows fat-free cooking, while still keeping the flavor and nutrition intact. The new boneless turkey roasts from natural growers are perfect for cooking in this way. Just roast for 25 minutes per pound at 325°F using the traditional oven method.

A brushed on glaze enhances the flavor of roast poultry. Here are two favorites:

HONEY GLAZE for ROAST TURKEY

Blend in a cup and brush on before and during roasting: 2 TBS Honey, 2 TBS Orange Juice, 1 TB Teriyaki Sauce, pinch Turmeric.

DARK BROWN GLAZE

Blend in a cup and brush on before and during roasting: 2 TBS Tamari, 2 TBS Molasses, 1 TB Honey, 1/4 teasp. Nutmeg.

ROAST TURKEY and BROWN RICE for RICH MINERALS

This recipe works for: Heart and Artery Health, Overcoming Addictions, Arthritis
For 6 servings: Preheat oven to 425°.

Make the ROASTING SAUCE: mince 6 Cloves Garlic and 4 TBS Fresh Ginger Root in a blender. Add 2 3/4 cups Low-Fat Organic Chicken Broth, 1 teasp. Sea Salt, 1 teasp. Pepper, and 1/4 teasp. Hot Pepper Sauce. Set aside. In a skillet, sizzle 3 small diced Onions, and 1 teasp. Cumin Powder in 2 TBS Canola Oil until onions brown.

—Place a 3-lb. Organic Turkey Breast on a rack in a roasting pan. Add 1 cup Brown Rice, the onions, the roasting sauce mix from the blender, and 1/2 cup Dried Tomato pieces. Cover, turn oven to 325° and bake for an hour and 15 minutes until tender. Remove from oven and add 1 cup Frozen Green Peas at the last minute. Let steam while you carve and remove turkey meat from the bone.

BAKED TURKEY SUPREME

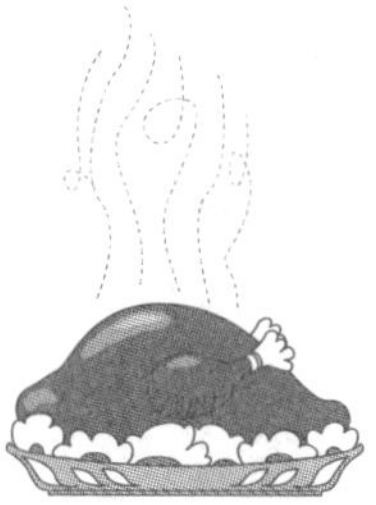

This recipe works for: Stress Reduction, Overcoming Addictions
For 8 servings: Preheat oven to 425°.

Have ready 4 cups diced cooked Turkey. Mix 1 (10-oz.) can Cream of Mushroom Soup with enough Water or White Wine to make 2 cups sauce.

—In a bowl, mix turkey and sauce with: 1 1/2 cups sliced Celery, 1 (7-oz.) can Sliced Waterchestuts, 1 cup shredded Low Fat Swiss Cheese, 1 cup chopped Pecans, 4 TBS minced Green Onions, 4 TBS Lemon Juice and 1/2 teasp. Lemon-Pepper.

—Turn into a casserole and cover with Crunchy Chinese Noodles and a scattering of toasted chopped Pecans. Bake for about 15 minutes, just to heat through.

Nutrition; 340 calories; 29gm protein; 12gm carbo.; 2gm fiber; 17gm total fats; 75mg choles.; 199mg calcium; 3mg iron; 65mg magnes.; 419mg potassium; 230mg sodium; Vit. A 49 IU; Vit. C 7mg; Vit. E 2 IU.

APPLE 'LASSES TURKEY LOAF Loaded with minerals.

This recipe works for: Liver-Organ Health, Overcoming Addictions, Heart Health
Enough for 8 servings: Preheat oven to 350°.

Mix ingredients in a large bowl: 2-lbs. ground Turkey, 1 cup crumbled Cornbread, 1 diced Tart Apple, 1/2 cup diced Onion, 1 Egg, 1/4 cup Molasses, 1/4 cup Plain Yogurt, 2 TBS Sherry, 1 1/2 teasp. Sea Salt, 1/4 teasp. Pepper. Place in an oiled loaf pan. Bake for 1 hour until crusty on top.

—Make a MOLASSES GLAZE: mix 2 TBS Molasses and 2 TBS Ketchup. Brush top and bake 20 more minutes to brown. Serve hot.

Nutrition; 259 calories; 36gm protein; 18gm carbo.; 1gm fiber; 5gm total fats; 134mg choles.; 146mg calcium; 4mg iron; 82mg magnes.; 685mg potassium; 440mg sodium; Vit. A 21 IU; Vit. C 2mg; Vit. E 1 IU.

LIGHT TURKEY MOUSSAKA

This recipe works for: Heart Health, Stress Reduction, Overcoming Addictions
For 9 servings with leftovers: Preheat oven to 450°.

Cut 2 large EGGPLANTS in $^1/_2$" slices. Brush eggplant slices with OLIVE OIL and lay in a single layer in 2 large baking pans. Bake for 20 minutes. Turn slices and bake for 10 more minutes until very soft. Lay slices from one pan in a single layer in a 9 x 13" shallow casserole. Set the other eggplant baking pan aside.

—Add 2 large sliced ONIONS to the empty pan. Scatter on 2 minced CLOVES GARLIC. Drizzle with 2 teasp. OLIVE OIL and $^1/_2$ cup WATER. Bake for 35 minutes, until moisture evaporates and onions are brown and fragrant. Stir to keep from burning. Remove from oven. Add $^1/_2$ cup SHERRY to deglaze; scrape up browned bits. Distribute $1^1/_2$ - lbs. ground TURKEY over the onions, and bake about 6 minutes. Remove from oven.

—Blend the sauce in a hot pan: 2 TBS WATER, $^1/_4$ tsp. FENNEL SEED, $^1/_4$ tsp. CARDAMOM POWDER, $^1/_4$ tsp. CINNAMON, $^1/_4$ tsp. CUMIN POWDER, 4 tsp. ARROWROOT POWDER, 1 tsp. SEA SALT. Add $1^1/_2$ cups ORGANIC CHICKEN BROTH. Heat to boiling, and pour over turkey and onions. Sprinkle generously with CRACKED PEPPER. Pour entire mixture over the eggplant slices in the casserole and smooth top. Cover with reserved EGGPLANT slices.

—Rinse sauce pan; make a smooth paste with 2 TBS ARROWROOT POWDER and 2 TBS WATER. Add half a carton of LOW FAT CREAM CHEESE (or KEFIR CHEESE) and $1^1/_2$ cups ORGANIC CHICKEN BROTH. Bring to a boil, stirring; spoon over eggplant. To serve, sprinkle with 2 TBS grated PARMESAN-REGGIANO CHEESE and bake at 350° until bubbly.

Nutrition; 258 calories; 29gm protein; 19gm carbo.; 5gm fiber; 4gm total fats; 72mg choles.; 108mg calcium; 3mg iron; 83mg magnesium; 816mg potassium; 305mg sodium; Vit. A 45 IU; Vit. C 5mg; Vit. E 1 IU.

HIGH MINERAL MU SHU CHICKEN

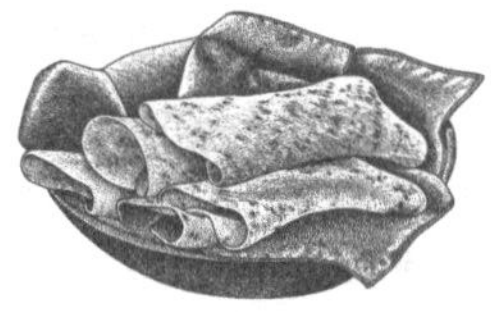

This recipe works for: Weight Control, Stress Reduction
For 8 servings:

Wrap 8 FLOUR TORTILLAS in foil; warm in a 250° oven for 15 minutes until soft.

Skin, bone and slice 2 CHICKEN BREASTS into strips. Marinate for 1 hour in $^1/_2$ cup SHERRY, 2 TBS TAMARI, 2 TBS SESAME OIL, 1 teasp. FRUCTOSE, 1 minced SHALLOT, and $^1/_2$ teasp. GINGER POWDER.

—Sauté in a skillet until fragrant: 2 TBS SESAME OIL, 1 teasp. TOASTED BROWN SESAME OIL, 1 sliced ONION, 6 large slivered SHIITAKE MUSHROOMS. Pour off marinade from chicken pieces and add to skillet. (Set chicken pieces aside.) Boil skillet liquid down to $^2/_3$ cup, about 2 minutes. Add chicken pieces and 2 cups chopped SPINACH LEAVES to mushroom mix. Add 2 EGGS and stir until eggs are just set.

Spoon some of the mixture over each tortilla. Top <u>each</u> with 1 teasp. HOISIN SAUCE, 1 TB minced GREEN ONION, 2 teasp. snipped TOASTED NORI. Roll up and serve hot.

Nutrition; 275 calories; 14gm. protein; 34gm. carbo.; 2gm. fiber; 7gm total fats; 60mg choles.; 156mg calcium; 4mg iron; 74mg magnes.; 501mg potassium; 328mg sodium; Vit. A 125 IU; Vit. C 5mg; Vit. E 2 IU.

FIVE MINUTE EASY CHICKEN, PEAS and BROWN RICE

This recipe works for: Illness Recovery, Stress Reduction, Sports Nutrition
For 6 servings: Preheat oven to 325°. Use a 9 x 13" baking pan.

Layer 3 cups diced cooked Organic Chicken Breasts in the oiled baking pan. Sprinkle with a layer of 2 cups cooked Basmati Rice. Dot with 2 TBS Butter. Layer on a 10-oz. box of Frozen Green Peas. Sprinkle on a 4-oz. can sliced Mushrooms with juice.

—Whisk together 2 cups Water, 1 Organic Chicken Bouillon Cube, 1 cup Plain Yogurt, 4 Eggs, $^{1}/_{2}$ teasp. Sea Salt, and 2 TBS snipped Fresh Parsley. Pour over casserole. Sprinkle with 3 TBS grated Romano Cheese and bake 45 minutes until set.

CHICKEN and VEGETABLES High in protein and minerals, low in fat.

This recipe works for: Weight Control, Men's Health, Respiratory Healing
Enough for 8 people: Preheat oven to 350°.

Bring 2 cups Low Fat Organic Chicken Broth to a boil. Stir in $1^{1}/_{2}$ cups mixed Whole Grains (or Kashi). Reduce heat. Cover and simmer for 10 minutes. Fluff and turn into a large Canola Oil-sprayed casserole.

—Skin, bone and slice 4 Organic Chicken Breasts into strips. Brown in 2 TBS Canola Oil until opaque, firm and tender. Arrange on top of grains in the casserole.

—Add 1 TB Canola Oil to the skillet and sauté for 5 minutes: 1 diced Red Onion, 2 diced Shallots, 1 sliced Red Bell Pepper. Add and sauté for 5 minutes more: 3 large diced Tomatoes, $^{1}/_{2}$ teasp. dry Basil, 1 teasp. Cumin, $^{1}/_{2}$ teasp. Oregano, and $^{1}/_{2}$ teasp. Pepper. Arrange vegetables over the chicken. Cover and bake for 30 minutes.

—Uncover, and stir in 2 cups trimmed Fresh Pea Pods. Cover again, turn off oven, and let peas steam until green, about 10 minutes. Delicious and fragrant with herbs.

Nutrition; 227 calories; 20gm protein; 37gm carbo.; 4gm fiber; 3gm total fats; 34mg choles.; 67mg calcium; 2mg iron; 89mg magnesium; 562mg potassium; 57mg sodium; Vit. A 121 IU; Vit. C 43mg; Vit. E 2 IU.

CHICKEN IN SESAME TAHINI SAUCE

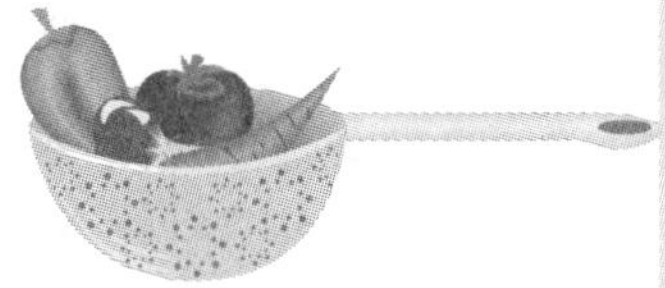

This recipe works for: Hair and Skin, Women's Health
For 6 servings:

Skin, bone and slice 4 Organic Chicken Breasts into strips. Brown in 4 TBS Canola Oil until opaque, firm and tender. Remove from heat and set aside.

—Add 2 TBS Sesame Oil to the skillet and sauté until aromatic: 2 diced Onions, 4 TBS snipped Fresh Cilantro, 1 chopped seeded Jalapeño Pepper, 1 teasp. Garlic-Lemon Seasoning. Add 2 cups Organic Chicken Broth, 6 TBS Sesame Tahini, 1 TB Herbs de Provence, $^{1}/_{2}$ teasp. Sea Salt and $^{1}/_{4}$ teasp. Pepper; bring to a boil. Add chicken strips. Cover and simmer over low heat for 30 minutes. Serve on a platter with cooked Basmati Rice.

Nutrition; 374 calories; 26gm protein; 30gm carbo.; 4gm fiber; 16gm total fats; 44mg choles.; 69mg calcium; 3mg iron; 146mg magnesium; 509mg potass.; 239mg sodium; Vit. A 12 IU; Vit. C 7mg; Vit. E 3 IU.

CHICKEN PESTO KIEV

This recipe works for: *Men's Health, Recovery from Illness, Fatigue Syndromes*
For 6 people: Preheat oven to 350°.

Split, bone, skin and pound flat 3 Whole Organic Chicken Breasts. Set aside and chill.

—Make the pesto in the blender: 1 cup packed Fresh Basil Leaves, $^3/_4$ cup Parmesan Cheese, $^1/_4$ cup Olive Oil and $^1/_2$ teasp. Lemon-Garlic Seasoning. Spoon some pesto over each chicken breast piece. Roll up and secure with a toothpick.

—Melt 6 TBS Butter in a shallow baking dish. Dip each roll in Seasoned Unbleached Flour, and place seam side down in a single layer in the dish. Bake for 40 minutes until chicken is opaque, steaming and fragrant.

—Make the RAISIN ALMOND SAUCE: in a small saucepan, sizzle 3 minutes, 2 minced Shallots, 2 TBS. Butter, $^1/_2$ teasp. Lemon-Garlic Seasoning and 1 TB Soy Bacon Bits. Add and simmer until fragrant: $^1/_2$ cup chopped Almonds, $^1/_4$ cup Raisins and $^1/_4$ teasp. Pepper. Pour over kiev rolls and serve immediately.

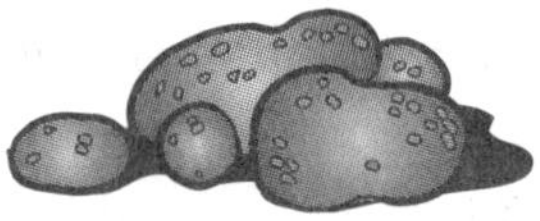

Potato Mineral Profits

The lowly potato may be one of Mother Nature's miracles. Potatoes are loaded with complex carbohydrates for long term energy. They are rich in fiber and minerals (with measureable potassium), and have virtually no fat and no cholesterol. They are a fine source of vitamin B_6 for nerve stability, and contain over 40% of the daily recommended amount of vitamin C. Boil 'em, bake 'em, chill 'em, fill 'em, broil 'em, or sauce 'em, but don't fry 'em. Potatoes are a delicious, nutritious, low-fat, vegetable.

ROASTED POTATOES with GINGER VINAIGRETTE

This recipe works for: Liver-Organ Health, Overcoming Addictions, Heart Health
For 12 servings: Preheat oven to 475°. Use a 12 x 15" baking pan.

Heat 3 TBS. Butter, 3 TBS. Olive Oil and 3 whole Garlic Cloves in baking pan.

—Peel 2-lbs. Yellow Dutch Potatoes and 2-lbs. Sweet Potatoes and cut in chunks. Roll chunks in the garlic butter to coat. Bake on the bottom rack of the oven for 30 minutes until tender. Stir frequently. Remove and let stand to absorb flavors. Sprinkle with $^1/_2$ cup chopped Walnuts and return to the oven for 15 more minutes.

—Mix the GINGER VINAIGRETTE: $^1/_4$ cup Tarragon Vinegar, $1^1/_2$ TBS Lime Juice, $^1/_2$ teasp. grated Fresh Ginger, $^1/_2$ teasp. Garlic-Lemon Seasoning, $^1/_2$ teasp. Tamari and 1 cup Canola Oil; pour over to serve.

Nutrition; 359 calories; 4gm protein; 35gm carbo.; 3gm fiber; 26gm total fats; 10mg choles.; 28mg calcium; 1mg iron; 39mg magnesium; 471mg potassium; 19mg sodium; Vit. A 1326 IU; Vit. C 26mg; Vit. E 8 IU.

VEGETABLE STUFFED BAKED POTATOES

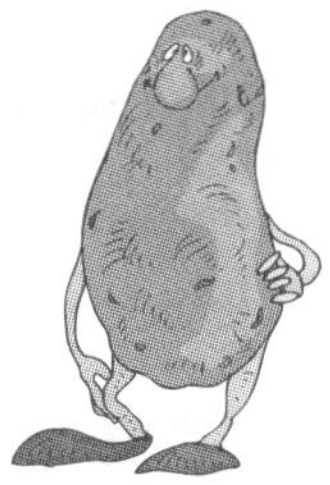

This recipe works for: Men's Health, Heart and Artery Health
For 4 servings: Preheat oven to 375°.

Steam 1 cup diced Broccoli til color changes to bright green. Drain and set aside.

Rub 4 large Russet Potatoes with Olive Oil and bake for 60 minutes until tender. Halve potatoes lengthwise. Scoop out meat into a bowl. Leave shell intact for filling. Arrange in a baking dish ready for stuffing.

—In the bowl, mix with the potato meat: add 1 cup Low Fat Cottage Cheese, $^1/_2$ cup Plain Low Fat Yogurt, 3 snipped Scallions, 1 diced Stalk Celery, 1 TB Tarragon Vinegar, 2 pinches Paprika. Fill potato shells. Top with broccoli and grated Parmesan Cheese. Sprinkle with Sea Salt and Pepper. Bake for 15 minutes until hot through and cheese is melted.

POTATO and ZUCCHINI GRATIN

This recipe works for: Liver-Organ Health, Immune Breakdown, Heart Health
Makes 6 servings: Preheat oven to 400°F. Position rack in upper third of oven.

Grease a shallow baking dish. Peel, thinly-slice and pat dry 2-lbs. Yellow Dutch Potatoes. Arrange half the potato slices in single layer over bottom of oil-sprayed baking dish, overlapping slightly. Sprinkle with Sea Salt, Cracked Pepper and dry mixed Italian Herbs. Sprinkle with half a finely chopped Onion.

—Arrange 1 thin-sliced Zucchini, slices overlapping slightly. Season with more Sea Salt, Cracked Pepper and dry mixed Italian Herbs; layer with remaining potato slices, overlapping slightly. Sprinkle with more Sea Salt, Cracked Pepper and dry mixed Italian Herbs. Top with another thinly sliced Zucchini, overlapping slightly. Mix $^1/_2$ cup Parmesan Cheese with Sea Salt, Cracked Pepper and dry mixed Italian Herbs, and cover top.

—Add $1^1/_2$ cups Organic Vegetable Broth to come three-quarters of the way up vegetables. Cover casserole with foil and bake until potatoes are almost tender, 30 minutes. Uncover and bake until potatoes are very tender, about 25 minutes more.

Nutrition; 206 calories; 8gm protein; 32gm carbo.; 3gm fiber; 3gm total fats; 6mg choles.; 151mg calcium; 1mg iron; 98mg magnesium; 629mg potassium; 226mg sodium; Vit. A 25 IU; Vit. C 14mg; Vit. E 1IU.

ROASTED POTATO and SWEET POTATO STICKS

This recipe works for: Food for Women, Kid's Nutrition, Recovery
Makes enough for 4 people: Preheat oven to 500°.

Oil a baking sheet. Cut 2 Yams and 2 Russet Potatoes in matchsticks. Toss with 1 to 2 TBS Canola Oil. Place side by side, not touching on baking sheet. Bake for 10 minutes til crusty. Season with Sea Salt, Pepper, Dulse Flakes and Herbal Seasoning Salt.

POTATO QUESADILLAS

This recipe works for: Food for Men, Sports Nutrition, Heart Health
Makes 8 servings: Preheat oven to 400°F.

In 1 TB Olive Oil in a nonstick skillet, sizzle 1 thinly sliced Onion, stirring often until golden brown, about 6 minutes. Stir in 1 large Russet Potato, peeled and cubed; cook for 1 minute. Stir in 1 cup Organic Chicken Broth and simmer until the potatoes are tender and liquid is absorbed, about 8 minutes. Season with Sea Salt and Pepper.

—Coat 2 nonstick baking sheets with Olive Oil Spray. Arrange 4 Flour Tortillas on sheets. Spread potato mixture among tortillas evenly. Top each with a tortilla. Coat tops of quesadillas with Olive Oil Spray. Bake, turning once, until light brown, about 10 minutes. Cut each quesadilla into 8 wedges. Put 1 cup Plain Yogurt, drained in a sieve for 30 minutes, 2 diced Tomatoes, 1 drained 4-oz. can Green Chilies and 1/2 cup snipped Green Onions in separate serving bowls. Serve as toppings.

Nutrition; 144 calories; 5gm protein; 19gm carbo.; 2gm fiber; 5gm total fats; 2mg choles.; 126mg calcium; 1mg iron; 23mg magnesium; 291mg potassium; 232mg sodium; Vit. A 27 IU; Vit. C 15mg; Vit. E 2 IU.

OVEN-BAKED ITALIAN POTATO WEDGES

This recipe works for: Food for Men, Sports Nutrition, Bone Building
Makes 4 servings: Heat oven to 475°F.

Coat baking sheet with Olive Oil Spray. In a large bowl, combine 3 snipped Scallions, 1/2 cup Reduced Fat Mayonnaise, 1/4 cup snipped Cilantro, 1 TB mixed Italian Herbs and 1/2 tsp. Sea Salt. Add 2-lbs. large Red Potatoes, cut into 1/2" wedges and toss to coat. Place potatoes, cut side-down, on baking sheet. Bake 20 minutes, turning once, or until tender. Sprinkle with 4-oz. shredded Low Fat Cheddar Cheese.

TWICE BAKED BROCCOLI POTATOES

This recipe works for: Cancer Protection, Overcoming Addictions, Immune Power
For 4 potato halves: Heat oven to 400°F.

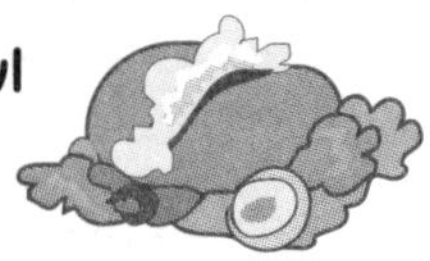

Bake 2 large Russet Potatoes until soft. Scoop insides into a bowl and mash. Put shells in a shallow baking dish and reserve meat. Steam 1 1/2 cups chopped Broccoli Florets and Upper Stems until color changes. Drain and divide between potato shells.

—Heat 2 TBS Canola Oil in a pan. Stir in 2 TBS Whole Wheat Flour until blended. Add: 3/4 cup Plain Low Fat Yogurt, 1/2 cup grated Cheddar Cheese, 1/4 cup Water, 1 teasp. Dijon Mustard, 1 teasp. Tamari, 1/2 teasp. Sea Salt, 1/4 teasp. Nutmeg, and dashes Sweet Paprika. Cook until thickened; mix with reserved potato meat for the filling.

—Spoon on top of broccoli, mounding high. Sprinkle with Parmesan Cheese; bake at 350° for 15 minutes. Run under the broiler for 30 seconds until brown and crusty.

Grilling Your Minerals

The sweetness of fresh garden vegetables is intensified on the grill. Aromatic wood chips, herb stems and leaves, or herb teas can be sprinkled over hot coals to impart unique, complex flavors. To use vegetable pieces larger than $^1/_4$" thick, like broccoli, cauliflower or potato chunks, blanch them first in boiling water, then plunge into cold water to stop cooking before bringing them to the grill. Precooking isn't needed for sliced vegetables like onions, bell pepper, tomatoes or eggplant. Use grilling baskets or flat skewers for vegetables. Remove all foods from the grill when they are golden, before they become charred, to avoid denaturing amino acids and DNA damage. Discard any charred portions to avoid dangerous hydro-carbons.

GRILLED VEGETABLES with BASIL RICE

This recipe works for: Respiratory Problems, Women's Health, Arthritis
Makes 6 servings: Preheat grill to hot.

Marinate vegetables in a shallow bowl: 1-lb. Fresh Asparagus, thick stems snapped off, 1 Red Onion, sliced in $^1/_2$-inch rings, 1 each, Orange, Red and Yellow Bell Peppers, sliced in quarters, 1 peeled Asian Eggplant thick sliced, 6 snipped Scallions, 3 Tomatoes, seeded and quartered. Pour on 3 TBS Olive Oil, $^1/_4$ cup Balsamic Vinegar, 1 tsp. Garlic Salt and 1 tsp. dried Oregano. Mix with hands to coat; marinate 20 minutes.

—Make the BASIL RICE: Heat 1 TB Olive Oil in a pan. Add 1 large cleaned Leek, green top cut off, white part sliced thin, 1 diced Carrot, 1 diced Stalk Celery, 1 tsp. Garlic Salt and $^1/_2$ teasp. Lemon-Pepper; heat 2 minutes. Add 1 cup Basmati Rice, stirring to coat. Add $1^1/_2$ cups Organic Vegetable Broth; bring to boil. Add 3 TBS snipped Fresh Basil, cover and reduce heat. Simmer until liquid is absorbed, 20 minutes.

—Grill marinated vegetables in a grilling basket until golden, turning once. Check veggies every 2 minutes as they cook at different rates. Asparagus is done in 4 minutes, then tomatoes, eggplant, peppers and finally onion in 15 minutes. Return vegetables to marinade as they are done and keep warm while rice finishes cooking. Fluff cooked rice and place on serving plates. Top rice with grilled vegetables.

GRILLED HIGH MINERAL VEGGIES and SEAFOOD

This recipe works for: Brain Boosting, Bone Building, Cancer Protection
Makes 6 servings: Preheat grill to hot.

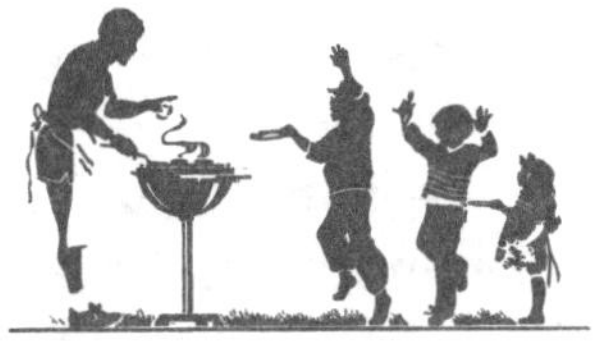

Thread on flat skewers: 6 large Sea Scallops, 6 butterflied Jumbo Prawns, 12 Broccoli Florets, 12 Red Bell Pepper Chunks, 12 Red Onion Wedges, 12 Orange Sections.

—Mix the PEPPER MARINADE: 2 tsp. Cracked Black Pepper, 1 tsp. Sweet-Hot Mustard, $^1/_4$ cup Olive Oil, $^1/_2$ tsp. Sea Salt, 2 TBS Raspberry Vinegar, 1 TB Sherry and pinches Rosemary Leaves. Pour over kebabs and marinate for 1 hour. Grill kebabs until golden, turning once - 5 to 10 minutes total.

HIGH MINERAL, HIGH ENZYME KEBABS

This recipe works for: Digestive Health, Liver and Organ Health, Hair and Skin
Makes 6 servings: Preheat grill to hot.

Thread on flat skewers: 6 large Sea Scallops, 6 butterflied Jumbo Prawns, 12 Cherry Tomatoes, 12 Red Bell Pepper Chunks, 12 Red Onion Wedges, 12 Fresh Pineapple Cubes.

—Mix the SHERRY MARINADE: $^1/_2$ cup Sherry, 2 TBS Sesame Oil, 2 teasp. Toasted Sesame Oil, 1 TB Sesame Seeds (Black if available), $^1/_2$ teasp. Garlic Salt, $^1/_4$ teasp. Pepper, 1 TB minced Crystallized Ginger. Pour over all kebabs and marinate for 1 hour.

—Grill kebabs until lightly browned, turning once, from 5 to 10 minutes total.

Nutrition; 137 calories; 8gm protein; 10gm carbo.; 2gm fiber; 6gm total fats; 38mg choles.; 49mg calcium; 2mg iron; 36mg magnesium; 372mg potassium; 160mg sodium; Vit. A 106 IU; Vit. C 36mg; Vit. E 1 IU.

CHILI HOT STICKS

This recipe works for: Men's and Kid's Health, Liver and Organ Health
Makes 24 appetizer skewers: Preheat grill to hot.

Soak 24 to 30 thin wood skewers in water at least 10 minutes.

—Cut 4 boneless, skinless Organic Chicken Breast Halves unto $^1/_2$" wide strips. Toss chicken with a blend of 4 tsp. Hot Chili Sauce, 2 TBS Olive Oil, $^1/_4$ cup Tamari and 2 TBS Cajun Seasoning Spice. Cover and let stand 10 minutes or chill up to 4 hours.

—Thread chicken strips onto skewers, dividing evenly. Grill 3 to 4 inches from heat, turning once, until chicken is lightly browned, 8 to 10 minutes. Serve hot.

Nutrition; 34 calories; 5gm protein; 1gm carbo.; trace fiber; 1gm total fats; 12mg choles.; 12mg calcium; 1mg iron; 8mg magnesium; 82mg potassium; 64mg sodium; Vit. A 22 IU; Vit. C 1mg; Vit. E trace.

FAST FIRE SWORDFISH STEAKS

This recipe works for: Brain Health, Women's Health, Anti-Aging
For 6 to 8 people: Heat the grill to hot. Brush the grill with oil.

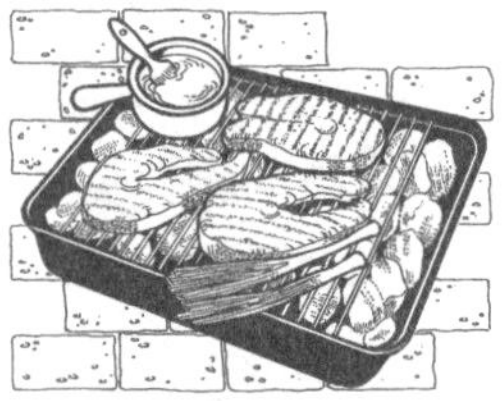

Have ready 6 to 8 rinsed thick Swordfish Steaks (about 2-lbs.)

—Mix the marinade in a large flat pan. Mix: $^1/_4$ cup Olive Oil, 2 TBS Lemon Juice, 1 TB Coarse-Grain Mustard, 2 tsp. Sherry, 1 tsp. Lemon-Garlic Seasoning, 1 tsp. Dijon Mustard. Marinate fish covered.

—Place swordfish in center of hot oiled grill and cover. Cook for 7 minutes. Uncover, slide a spatula under the fish and rotate for cross grilling marks. Cover again and cook 8 minutes. Turn fish and repeat. Check for doneness by removing fish with spatula and pressing with your fingers for firmness. (Cook for 3 minutes more if not firm.) Remove and let rest for 5 minutes before slicing against the grain to serve.

FRESH TUNA STEAKS with HERBS

This recipe works for: Brain Health, Hair and Skin, Bone Building
For 4 people:

Have ready 4 Fresh Ahi Steaks, 1 inch thick (1$^{1}/_{2}$-lbs.). Pour marinade over ahi in a bowl: $^{1}/_{2}$ cup Olive Oil, 4 crushed Sage Leaves, 2 minced Cloves Garlic, 2 crushed Sprigs Rosemary, 1 TB Lemon Juice, $^{1}/_{2}$ tsp. Italian Herbal Seasoning, $^{1}/_{4}$ tsp. Lemon-Pepper.

—Reserve marinade for the sauce. Grill steaks for 6 to 8 minutes, turning once, until barely cooked. Keep warm while you make the sauce. Strain herbs from the marinade. Put in a hot saucepan and add $^{1}/_{2}$ cup sliced Black Olives. Heat briefly until bubbly and add 4 TBS Capers. Pour over ahi.

Turkey and Chicken on the Grill

A whole turkey or chicken becomes an indescribable taste delight when it's roasted outdoors over a charcoal fire. With just a little attention and a few instructions, your barbecued poultry can be perfect. Pick your favorite marinade or basting sauce, and cover the whole bird. Place in a large plastic bag and chill in the fridge for 4 hours or overnight. Turn bag several times to marinate well.

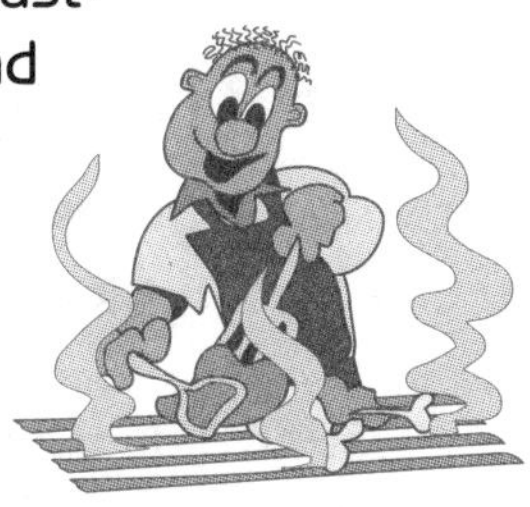

Follow poultry instructions for your barbecue grill, or use the following: on the firegrate in a covered barbecue, light 50 charcoal briquets. When coals are covered with grey ash, bank them on each side of the grate; put a drip pan in the middle. Add 10 briquets to the coals; add 10 more every 30 minutes during roasting to maintain heat. Place grill 6" above coals. Put turkey or chicken breast-side down with wings akimbo, directly above the drip pan. Baste with reserved marinade. Cover barbecue, open dampers, and roast for 45 minutes. Turn bird breast up and cook until meat at bone in thickest part of breast registers 160°. Baste bird often. Move to a platter, drape loosely with foil, and let sit 20 minutes before carving.

GRILLED TURKEY TENDERLOIN in CHARD WRAPS

This recipe works for: Brain Health, Hair and Skin, Bone Building
For 4 people: Preheat and oil the grill.

Have ready 1-lb. boned, skinned Turkey Tenderloin cut in 4 equal pieces. Have ready 4 large thin slices Smoked Salmon. Have ready 4 large Chard Leaves.

—Blender blend the sauce: $^{1}/_{3}$ cup Olive Oil, $^{1}/_{4}$ cup Balsamic Vinegar, 2 TBS minced Green Onions, 1 TB minced Fresh Parsley, 1 tsp. Sage Leaves and 1 tsp. Thyme Leaves.

—Plunge chard leaves in boiling water to wilt. Wrap each turkey piece in a smoked salmon slice, then in the chard leaf. Grill about 6" above coals for 20 to 25 minutes. Cut in 1" slices and arrange on plates cut side up. Season with Sea Salt and Cracked Pepper and top with sauce.

GRILLED, STUFFED TURKEY BURGER

This recipe works for: Stress Reactions, Fatigue Syndromes, Men's-Kid's Health
For 8 serving wedges:

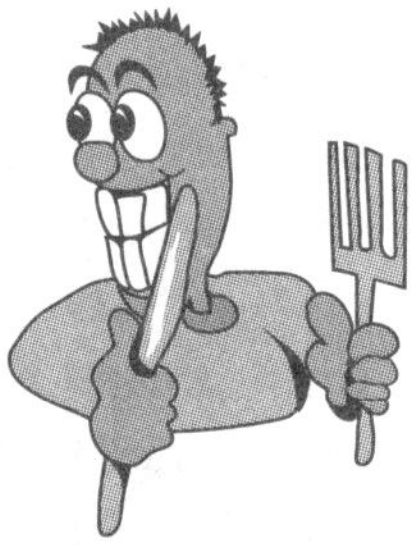

Mix the burger: $1^1/_4$ cup Cornbread Stuffing Mix, 1 can (4-oz.) drained Mushroom Pieces, $^1/_3$ cup Organic Chicken Broth, 1 teasp. Liquid Smoke or 1 TB Hickory Sauce, $^1/_4$ cup snipped Scallions, 1 Egg, $^1/_4$ cup chopped Almonds, 2 TBS Butter, 1 tsp. Lemon Juice, $^1/_4$ cup snipped Fresh Parsley.

—Mix 2-lbs. Ground Turkey with $1^1/_2$ teasp. Sea Salt. Divide in half, and pat into two 8" circles on waxed paper. Spoon stuffing mix onto 1 circle. Top with other circle and seal the edges with 1 Beaten Egg. Cook on foil or in a grill basket on an outside grill for 10 to 15 minutes.

—Serve with GOURMET BARBECUE SAUCE: Sauté in a pan until fragrant: 2 TBS Olive Oil, 1 diced Onion, $^1/_2$ diced Red Bell Pepper, $^1/_2$ teasp. Hot Pepper Sauce. Add and sauté 5 minutes: 1 large chopped Tomato, $^1/_4$ cup Red Wine Vinegar, and 3 TBS Honey.

—Remove from heat, cool slightly and put sauce in a blender with 6 ripe Plum Tomatoes. Whirl briefly so sauce is still chunky and spoon on Turkey Burger.

CHILI CHICKEN BURGERS on the GRILL

This recipe works for: Respiratory Healing, Fatigue Syndromes, Men's-Kid's Health
For 6 burgers: Preheat and oil the grill to hot.

Grind 1-lb. Organic Chicken Meat; mix with 2 TBS Cornmeal, 1 minced seeded Jalapeño Pepper, 1 TB Lime Juice, 2 teasp. Cumin Powder, 2 teasp. Chili Powder, 1 Egg, and $^1/_4$ teasp. Garlic Lemon Seasoning. Form into patties, and grill until no longer pink. Serve on grilled buns with all-natural Bottled Salsa and a squeeze of Lime.

Pizzas on the Grill

Pizza on the grill is incredible, totally different from the oven-baked variety.

PIZZA with SHRIMP and SUN-DRIED TOMATOES

This recipe works for: Brain Health, Anti-Aging, Men's Health
For 2 pizzas: Preheat the grill to hot. Watch carefully so bottom doesn't burn.

Place ready made Whole Grain Pizza Dough on foil and freeze for 10 minutes. Pinch up rims, so pizzas can hold sauce. Brush each with $1^1/_2$ teasp. Chili Oil.

—Oven roast 10 diced Shallots and 1 sliced Red Onion until fragrant. Divide veggies and 8-oz. chopped Raw Shrimp between pizzas. Sprinkle on $^1/_4$ cup snipped Fresh Basil. Cover with $^1/_2$ cup grated Parmesan Cheese and 1 cup chunked Low Fat Mozarrella Cheese. Top with 12 slivered, oil-packed Sun-Dried Tomatoes. Cover and cook for 6 to 8 minutes until heated through and cheese is melted.

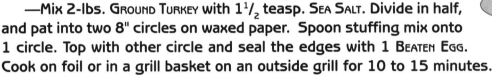

GRILLED TOMATO and MOZARRELLA PIZZA

This recipe works for: Men's Health, Immune Power, Allergies
For 2 big pizzas: Preheat and oil grill. Watch carefully so that bottom doesn't burn.

Have ready 2 large Whole Wheat Chapatis for the crusts. Top each, in order given, with crumbled Feta Cheese, diced Plum Tomatoes, snipped dry Dulse, snipped Fresh Basil Leaves, sliced Pitted Black Olives, Red Bell Pepper strips, pinches Italian Herbs, dollops of Tomato Sauce and toasted Walnut Pieces. Cover and cook for 6 to 8 minutes.

GRILLED QUESADILLAS (MEXICAN PIZZAS)

This recipe works for: Digestive Health, Liver and Organ Health, Kid's Health
Four flour tortillas: Preheat, oil grill.

Have ready 4 Whole Wheat Flour Tortillas. Make the CHILI SAUCE. Mix $^1/_4$ cup Low Fat Mayonnaise, 2 teasp. Red Wine Vinegar, 1 teasp. Chili Powder, $^1/_2$ teasp. Sea Salt and $^1/_4$ teasp. Cumin Powder. Spread each tortilla with some of the sauce and top with Tomato slivers, shredded Jalapeño Jack Cheese, diced Red Onion, and snipped Fresh Cilantro Leaves. Grill, covered on foil until cheese melts and veggies are fragrant. Fold in half and grill for 1 more minute.

GRILLED GOURMET PIZZA

This recipe works for: Anti-Aging, Bone Building, Sugar Imbalances
For 1 large pizza: Preheat and oil grill. Watch carefully so bottom doesn't burn.

Place ready made Whole Grain Pizza Dough on foil and freeze for 10 minutes. Pinch up rim so pizza can hold sauce. Brush with Olive Oil. Then invert on the hot grill. Peel off foil and grill for 3 minutes until bottom is light brown.

—Blender blend the sauce: 3 to 4 oil-packed Sun-Dried Tomatoes with a pinch Garlic Powder and enough oil from the jar to make a smooth paste. Make just enough to paint on the grilled side of the crust. Arrange chunked Mozarrella Cheese, sliced Green Onions, sliced Pitted Black Olives and Cherry Tomato Halves on top of the sauce. Sprinkle with grated Parmesan-Reggiano Cheese and return to the grill. Cover and cook for 6 to 8 minutes until heated through and cheese is melted.

Nutrition; 226 calories; 13gm. protein; 24gm. carbo.; 5gm. fiber; 7gm total fats; 15mg choles.; 269mg calcium; 2mg iron; 66mg magnes.; 256mg potassium; 201mg sodium; Vit. A 67 IU; Vit. C 7mg; Vit. E 2 IU.

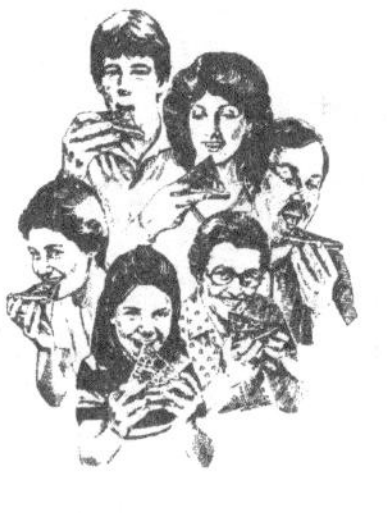

Mineral Rich Desserts

You might not expect to find high minerals in desserts, but in fact it's a very good place to find them. Desserts are a good way to get your minerals, especially for kids.... who hardly ever get enough.

RED GRAPE ICY GRANITA

This recipe works for: Liver and Organ Health, Anti-Aging, Weight Control
Makes 6 servings:

—Place a metal 13 x 9-inch baking pan and a metal spoon in the freezer.

—Stir 1 cup Water, 4 TBS Turbinado Sugar and 1 teasp. Stevia Powder in a saucepan. Bring to a simmer; cook for 5 minutes. Refrigerate until cold, 30 minutes.

—Puree 3 cups Red Seedless Grapes (1-lb.) in a blender. Strain puree through a fine-mesh sieve over a large bowl, pressing solids with a rubber spatula to extract juice; discard peels. Stir in $1^1/_2$ cups chilled White Grape Juice and the chilled syrup. Pour mixture into frozen pan. Freeze until ice crystals form around edges of pan, about 30 minutes. Stir ice crystals every 30 minutes with the frozen metal spoon into center of mixture until all liquid is frozen, about 2 hours. Scoop granita into 6 serving glasses; top with grape halves and mint sprigs.

Nutrition; 122 calories; 1gm. protein; 29gm. carbo.; trace fiber; trace total fats; 0mg choles.; 35mg calcium; 1mg iron; 7mg magnesium; 270mg potassium; 8mg sodium; Vit. A 6 IU; Vit. C 28mg; Vit. E 1 IU.

BLUEBERRY COBBLER

This recipe works for: Recovery from Illness, Anti-Aging, Waste Management
Makes 4 to 6 servings: Preheat oven to 325°. Use an 8-inch square baking pan.

Combine 3 cups Blueberries, $^1/_4$ cup Currants, 1 TB Brown Sugar, $^1/_4$ tsp. Cinnamon and $^1/_4$ tsp. Vanilla Extract in a medium bowl. Mix gently. Transfer to baking pan.

—Combine 1 cup Rolled Oats, 2 tsp. Brown Sugar, 3 TBS Whole Wheat Pastry Flour and $1^1/_2$ TBS soft Butter in the bowl. Mix with your fingers until mixture is crumbly. Spoon onto blueberry mixture. Bake 45 minutes until brown. Cool before serving.

SMOOTHY POPS

This recipe works for: Allergies- Asthma, Kid's Health, Heart Health
For 8 pops:

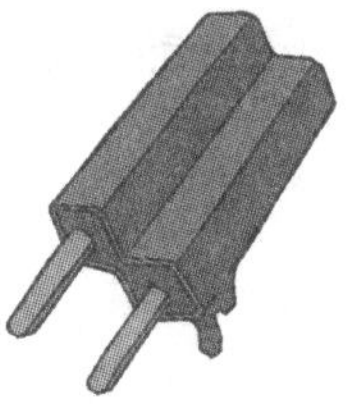

Blender blend 2 cups chilled, cut up Mixed Fruits until smooth. Add and blend $1^1/_2$ cups Vanilla Rice Milk, 1 cup Vanilla Yogurt, $^1/_2$ teasp. Nutmeg, $^1/_2$ teasp. Cinnamon and $^1/_3$ cup Honey or Maple Syrup. Pour into 8 paper-lined muffin cups; freeze for 1 hour. Insert a popsicle stick and freeze to firm.

SPICED PLUMS with YOGURT-HONEY CREAM

This recipe works for: Digestive Health, Anti-Aging, Men's Health
Makes 4 servings:

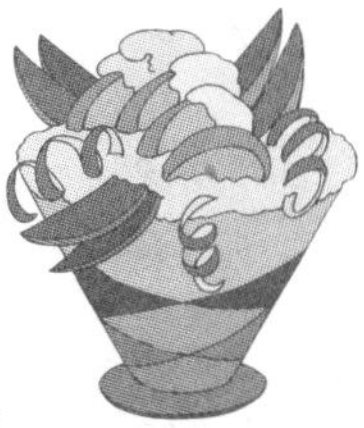

Whisk 1 cup Low Fat Cream Cheese and $^3/_4$ cup Vanilla Yogurt and 3 TBS Honey in a glass bowl to blend. Let stand, uncovered, in a warm place until thick, at least 6 hours or overnight. Chill until ready to serve.

—Heat a large skillet. Add 2-lbs. Ripe Plums, halved and cut into thick wedges, 1 teasp. minced Crystallized Ginger, 4 TBS Turbinado Sugar and 1 teasp. Stevia Powder; stir until sugar dissolves, forms glaze and plums are tender, about 8 minutes. Sprinkle plums with $^1/_2$ tsp. Cinnamon; spoon into bowls. Spoon on Yogurt Cream.

Nutrition; 372 calories; 11gm protein; 59gm carbo.; 5gm fiber; 7gm total fats; 36mg choles.; 178mg calcium; 2mg iron; 54mg magnesium; 641mg potass.; 37mg sodium; Vit. A 213 IU; Vit. C 22mg; Vit. E 3 IU.

AVOCADO CREAM Rich, creamy, good and nutritious. Don't miss it.

This recipe works for: Hair and Skin, Bone Building, Sugar Imbalances
For 4 servings:

Blender blend: 1 pint Vanilla Rice Dream Frozen Dessert, 1 peeled chunked Avocado, 2 TBS Orange Juice Concentrate. Whirl until smooth. Spoon into dessert glasses. Top with a Mint Leaf and freeze. Remove 5 minutes before you want to serve.

CHOCOLATE CHERRY PISTACHIO FRUITCAKE

This recipe works for: Recovery, Bone Building, Sports Nutrition
Makes 2 cake loaves (16 servings): Preheat oven to 300°F.

Lightly oil 2 cake loaf pans. In a large bowl, combine $^1/_2$ cup Unbleached Flour, $^1/_4$ cup Unsweetened Cocoa, $^1/_2$ cup Date Sugar or Turbinado Sugar, $^1/_4$ tsp. Baking Soda and $^1/_4$ tsp. Baking Powder. Stir in 1 cup Raisins, 3 cups Dried Cherries, $^1/_2$ cup chopped Walnuts, $^1/_2$ cup Dried Cranberries and 1 cup chopped Pistachios.

—Combine $^1/_4$ cup Arrowroot Powder, 2 tsp. Vanilla and $^1/_3$ cup Sherry in a small bowl, mixing smooth. Add to dry ingredients, mixing well with hands until fruit and nut pieces are completely coated. Press mixture into loaf pans and bake until batter is set, 45 to 50 minutes. Cool completely before removing from pans.

—Serve with APRICOT PINEAPPLE HONEY BUTTER: Puree 2-lbs. Fresh Apricots in the blender. Add 12-oz. cubed Fresh Pineapple. Turn into a bowl and mix with $^1/_2$ teasp. grated Orange Peel, 2 TBS Lemon Juice, $^3/_4$ cup Honey and $^1/_2$ cup Maple Syrup. Simmer uncovered, stirring until thick, about 2 hours. Spoon onto fruitcake.

Nutrition; 340 calories; 6gm protein; 77gm carbo.; 5gm fiber; 6gm total fats; 0mg choles.; 79mg calcium; 2mg iron; 57mg magnesium; 495mg potassium; 43mg sodium; Vit. A 317 IU; Vit. C 13mg; Vit. E 2 IU.

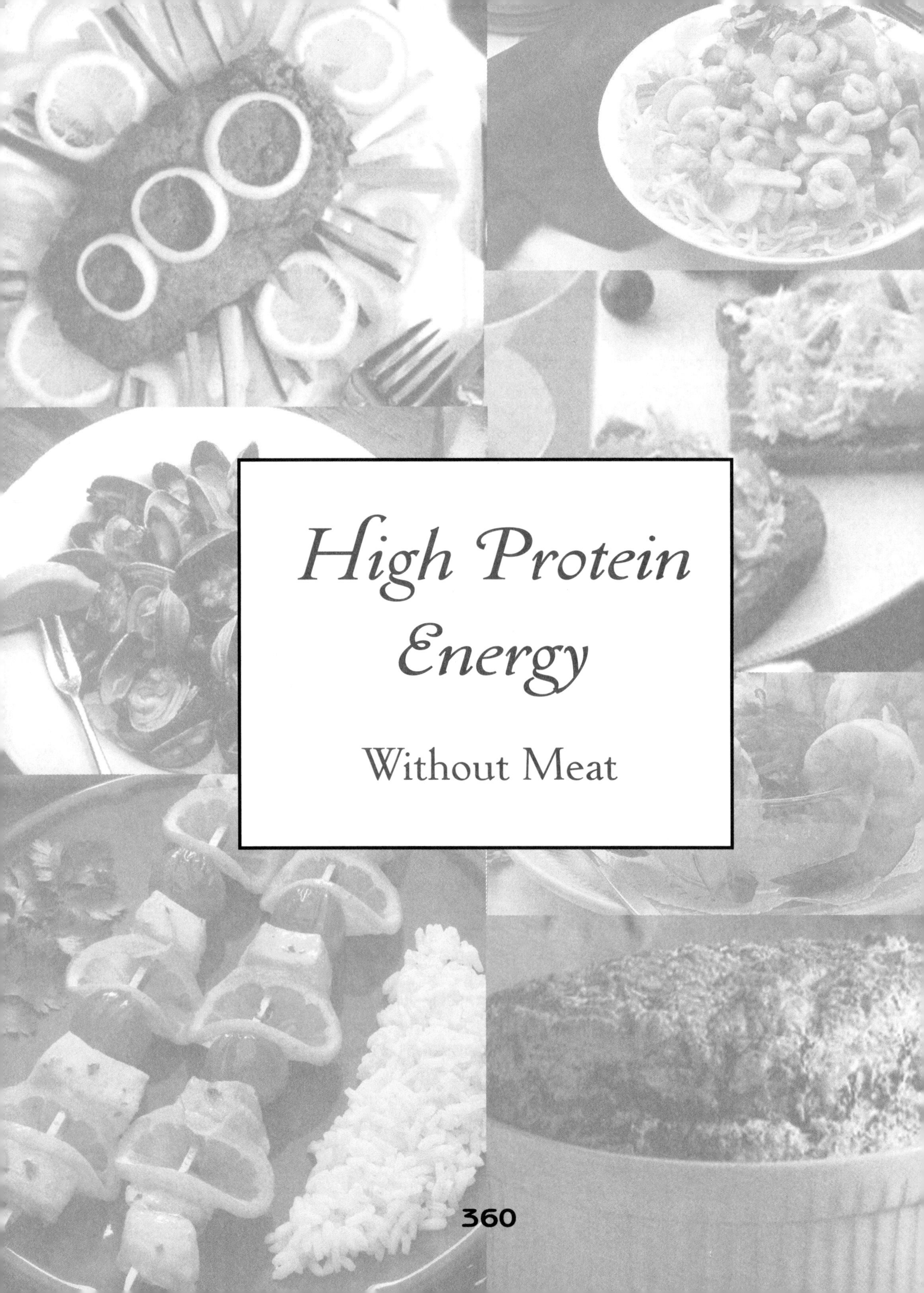

High Protein Energy

Without Meat

Protein Energy without Meat

You know you need protein for daily energy, body growth and general health. You may not know that protein is critical to successful healing from illness or injury, and to maintain immune resistance. When you suffer a wound or surgery trauma, your body loses protein, especially in skeletal muscle. You need extra high quality protein to recuperate and normalize your body functions.

After water, protein is the most plentiful substance in the body, the major constituent of every living cell and body fluid except for bile and urine. Protein regulates your acid-alkaline levels and body fluid balance. It helps to form enzymes, even some hormones.

Yet, except in its restore-and-repair mode, or for accelerated athletic performance, our bodies don't seem to need large amounts of protein to thrive.

Most of us have been taught that we need much more protein than we actually do. Americans, for instance, eat 2 to 4 times more protein than is needed for good nutrition or health. In developed countries, too much protein is a bigger health threat than too little. **If you eat enough healthy calories to maintain a reasonable weight, you will get more than enough protein automatically**. Even athletes, for whom "high protein" was once the only watchword, do not need an overabundance of protein. Muscle strength, power, and endurance grow from complex carbohydrates and unsaturated fats as well as from protein. (See Sports Nutrition & Healing Diets in the *Cooking For Healthy Healing Diet Book*.)

Most Americans think in terms of meat and animal foods for protein. But animal protein often comes loaded with saturated fat, calories and cholesterol. Overeating these foods adds unwanted weight **because excess protein turns into fat**. Too much protein impairs good kidney function, increases calcium loss in bones, and poses a clear health risk to heart and arteries.

Our most advanced research about human needs for protein shows that mankind is a part of the ecological system of the planet like everything else, putting the question about eating meat much more into perspective. (See About Red Meats in the *Cooking For Healthy Healing Diet Book*.)

Get the Right Kind of Protein in Your Diet

Experts agree that plant protein should furnish at least half, if not all of our protein intake. Vegetables high in protein are also rich in fiber and complex carbohydrates, and high in vitamins and minerals with little fat content. A vegetarian diet, even without dairy products can easily meet the RDA for protein. Vegetarians have lower cholesterol, denser bones and stronger teeth. Eating the majority of your protein from plant sources significantly increases your healing capability, and reduces your proneness to cancer and other diseases.

Where does plant protein come from? Soy foods, dried beans, nuts and seeds, potatoes, whole grains and pasta, brown rice, corn, bee pollen, bananas, sprouts, and nutritional yeast provide good plant protein. Complete vegetable protein, like that in tofu, tempeh, quinoa and nutritional yeast supplies all the necessary amino acids found in animal foods without the fat and cholesterol. Even plants that don't have "complete" protein in terms of amino acids, complement *other* vegetable protein foods (called protein complementarity), effectively boosting both quality and absorption of each food.

Examples of protein complementarity include rice with beans or tofu, and peas with potatoes or rice. Beyond complementarity we know a great deal about enzyme activity in relation to different foods today. It isn't even necessary to carefully match beans and grains, or dairy and nuts for protein complementarity any more.

Protein Rich Recipe Sections

For healing purposes, high protein is defined in this book as 12 grams or more per serving.

Your Non-Meat Protein Options

High quality vegetable protein sources to use in your meal and diet planning.

1: **Soy Foods:** Tofu, Tempeh, Miso, Soy Cheese and Soy Milk.
2: **Nuts:** Pine Nuts, Walnuts, Almonds, Cashews, Brazils and Hazelnuts.
3: **Seeds:** Pumpkin Seeds, Sesame Seeds, Sunflower Seeds.
4: **Beans and Legumes:** Peas, Peanuts, Lentils, Pintos, Limas, Mung Beans, Black Beans, White and Red Beans, Turtle Beans.
5: **Whole Grains:** Wheat and Wheat Germ, Brown, Basmati and Wild Rice, Millet, Barley, Bulgur, Buckwheat, Amaranth, Rye, Quinoa, and Amazake Rice Drink.
6: **Vegetables:** All Sprouts, Mushrooms.
7: **Sea Vegetables:** All
8: **Fruits:** Avocados, Coconuts, Prunes, Raisins, Apples, Figs and Dates.
9: **Bee Pollen:** Contains all the essential Amino Acids in one natural source.
10: **Nutritional Yeast:** Just 2 TBS contains as much protein as $^1/_4$ cup wheat germ, as much calcium as $^1/_2$ cup orange juice, as much phosphous as $^1/_4$ lb. haddock, as much iron as 1 cup spinach, as much thiamine as 1 cup wheat germ, as much niacin as $^1/_2$ cup brown rice, as much riboflavin as 4 eggs.
11: **Ginseng:** Increases protein content in the muscles.

About Amino Acids in Foods:

The body doesn't directly use the large protein molecules found in food for its protein needs. Proteins are made of amino acids coupled together into chains called peptides. These chains are protein building blocks, and they must be provided together in the diet for our bodies to use the protein energy we take in.

Twenty-three amino acids have been identified. The 8 essential amino acids must be supplied from food; the rest can be synthesized by the body. An adult man, for example, can produce about 300gms of new protein daily. Nine amino acids are essential to infants; eight are essential to adults. Amino acids help detoxify sediment crystals in the system, nourish vital organs and blood, release and eliminate acid-ash residues, and clear out metabolic sludge and excess mucous.

Your protein needs can be determined by your age and ideal body weight. An adult over 20 years of age should eat about 0.36 grams of protein *per pound* of body weight. For example: if you are a 40 year old woman, who weighs or should weigh, 120 pounds, you would multiply 120 x 0.36 giving you 43 grams of protein a day. Exceptions to this include pregnant and nursing women, and people recuperating from illness, injury or surgery.

Athletes have greater protein needs. The body's ability to produce protein decreases both during and after a workout. Protein needs are often 50% higher for endurance athletes than for the general population, and 3 to 6 times more for power lifters and strength athletes. Studies show that the higher the amount of lean body mass the more protein is needed for maintenance.

Perfect Protein from Eggs

Frittatas, Soufflés, Scrambles

Egg protein most closely approximates human protein, complete protein with all essential amino acids. Eggs are the standard for quality protein comparison. Regardless of one-sided publicity about eggs and cholesterol, they are in fact, still a perfect traditional food, balanced nourishment, with lecithin phosphatides to counterbalance cholesterol content. In addition, there are different types of cholesterol, some necessary to critical body functions, and we know that cholesterol behaves differently in the body when taken in as a food, rather than as a laboratory substance.

BROWN RICE PILAF with BAKED EGGS

This recipe works for: Men's Health, Bone Building, Immune Breakdown
For 4 servings: Preheat oven to 400°. Use a 10 to 12-inch ovenproof frying pan.

Make the pilaf: Sizzle 1 TB Butter and $^2/_3$ cup minced Shallots until golden, about 3 minutes. Add $1^1/_3$ cups Brown Basmati Rice and stir until grains are lightly toasted, 2 minutes. Add 2 cups Organic Low Fat Chicken Broth and $^3/_4$ tsp. Poultry Seasoning; stir, and bring to a boil. Cover, reduce heat and simmer until grains are tender to bite, about 12 minutes. Add $^1/_2$ cup shredded Swiss Cheese to pilaf.

—Using the back of a spoon, make 4 deep wells in rice. Slide 1 Egg into each well. Lay Plum Tomato slices around eggs. Bake until egg whites are opaque and yolks have desired texture, about 8 minutes, sprinkle mixture with $^1/_2$ cup shredded Parmesan-Reggiano Cheese. Use a wide spatula to scoop out pilaf and eggs, 1 at a time, and put on plates. Season with Sea Salt and Cracked Pepper to taste.

Nutrition; 437 calories; 23gm protein; 57gm carbo.; 4gm fiber; 14gm total fats; 234mg choles.; 375mg calcium; 2mg iron; 24mg magnes.; 186mg potassium; 350mg sodium; Vit. A 156 IU; Vit. C 3mg; Vit. E 1 IU.

HEALING MUSHROOM OMELETTE

This recipe works for: Cancer Protection, Skin, Hair and Nails, Immune Power
For 2 servings:

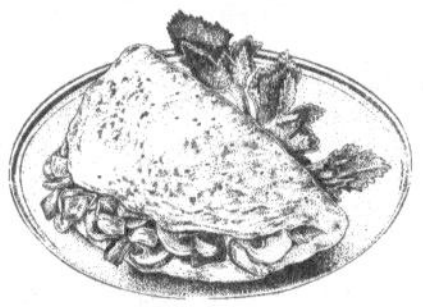

Heat 2 TBS Butter in a skillet. Sliver 6-oz. stemmed Fresh Shiitake Mushrooms and toss with butter and $^1/_4$ teasp. Lemon-Pepper for 4 minutes. Turn into a bowl, add 3 TBS snipped Green Onions and set aside.

—Heat 2 TBS Butter to foamy in the skillet. Add to pan 6 Eggs, beaten with 2 TBS Sherry; stir and shake pan to keep eggs moving. Cook until eggs have a creamy center. Spoon mushroom mixture across center of eggs. Tip pan forward and roll one-quarter of the omelette onto itself. Invert pan over a serving platter and roll omelette with folded part on the bottom. Serve immediately.

BABY ARTICHOKE QUICHES

This recipe works for: *Arthritis, Bone Building, Enhancing Sexuality*
For 12 servings: Preheat oven to 375°. Pan-spray 12 muffin cups.

Have ready 2 jars (11-oz.) Water-Packed Artichoke Hearts. Drain, chop, set aside.
—Blend in a blender til smooth: 2 cups Low Fat Cottage Cheese, 2 Eggs, 1/4 cup Low Fat Plain Yogurt, 1/4 cup Water, 1 cup grated Parmesan, 1/2 cup Fresh Parsley Leaves and 1 teasp. Garlic-Lemon Seasoning.
—Line muffin cups with Artichoke Leaves. Divide cheese mixture between cups. Sprinkle with Paprika. Bake for 30 minutes until puffy and brown. Serve warm.

Nutrition; 107 calories; 12gm protein; 7gm carbo.; 3gm fiber; 2gm total fats; 44mg choles.; 176mg calcium; 1mg iron; 30mg magnes.; 217mg potassium; 235mg sodium; Vit. A 58 IU; Vit. C 8mg; Vit. E 1 IU.

SPICY EGGS

This recipe works for: Men's Health, Skin, Hair and Nails, Fatigue Syndromes
For 6 servings:

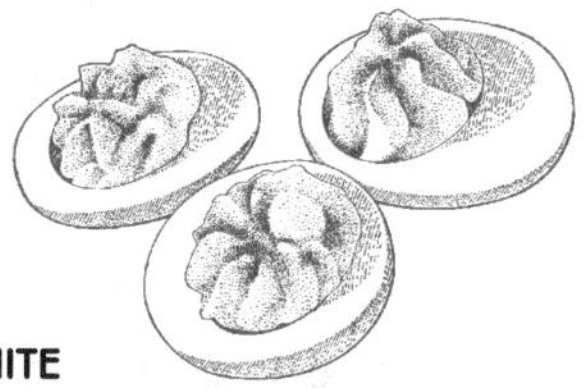

Have ready 6 Hard Boiled Eggs; remove the shells and cut lengthwise. Carefully remove the yolks, place in a basin and beat into a smooth paste with 1 TB Butter, 2 TBS grated Jalapeño Cheddar, 1 TB White Worcester Sauce, a pinch Sea Salt, a pinch White Pepper and a dash Cayenne for sharpness. Refill egg whites, leaving 1 TB of the paste for the sauce. Heat 1 TB Butter in a saucepan, mix with 1 TB Unbleached Flour, a pinch Sea Salt, 1/4 cup Low Fat Plain Yogurt, and 1/4 cup Water to make a sauce; let simmer 5 minutes stirring. Remove from heat; add remainder of the egg paste, 1/2 cup grated Low Fat Cheddar and 2 teasp. snipped Fresh Parsley. Place eggs on a serving plate and pour sauce carefully over eggs. Chill covered and serve cold.

PUFFY OVEN EGG CAKE

This recipe works for: Men's Health, Skin, Hair and Nails, Fatigue Syndromes
For 4 servings: Preheat oven to 425°F.

Mix in a bowl: 1 cup Unbleached Flour and 1 1/2 TBS Brown Sugar. Stir in 1 cup Rice Milk, 2 teasp. Canola Oil, 3 Eggs, 1/2 cup grated Low Fat Swiss Cheese and 1/2 tsp. Sea Salt. Coat an ovenproof nonstick skillet with Canola Oil Spray. Pour batter into skillet; bake egg cake until puffy and golden, 20 to 25 mintes. Slide cake from skillet onto serving platter; cut into 4 wedges. Serve hot with pinches Italian Herbs on top.

Nutrition; 256 calories; 14gm protein; 32gm carbo.; 1gm fiber; 7gm total fats; 166mg choles.; 285mg calcium; 3mg iron; 18mg magnes.; 114mg potassium; 354mg sodium; Vit. A 84 IU; Vit. C 1mg; Vit. E 2 IU.

PIZZA FRITTATA A command favorite for 20 years.

This recipe works for: Kid's Health, Stress Reactions, Overcoming Addictions
Enough for 4 hearty eaters: Preheat broiler to hot.

Beat 8 Eggs in a bowl with $^1/_2$ cup Low Fat Cottage Cheese, $^1/_2$ teasp. Sea Salt, $^1/_2$ teasp. Lemon-Pepper, and $^1/_2$ teasp. Tamari.

—Sizzle 2 TBS Butter in a large ovenproof skillet for 1 minute. Add eggs and cook, lifting the edges to let uncooked portion flow underneath til just soft set. Remove from heat, and sprinkle with $^1/_2$ cup grated Parmesan Cheese, $^3/_4$ cup Mozarrella Chunks, 4 sliced Mushrooms, $^1/_4$ cup minced Scallions and 4 thin slices Beefsteak Tomato. Sprinkle with 1 teasp. Pizza Seasoning or Italian Herb Blend. Run under the broiler for 45 seconds to melt cheese. Cut in wedges to serve.

Nutrition; 353 calories; 28gm protein; 6gm carbo.; 1gm fiber; 21gm total fats; 462mg choles.; 415mg calcium; 2mg iron; 35mg magnes.; 354mg potassium; 561mg sodium; Vit. A 338 IU; Vit. C 8mg; Vit. E 2 IU.

SPANISH TORTILLA FRITTATA

This recipe works for: Cancer Protection, Men's Health, Skin, Hair and Nails
Serves 6:

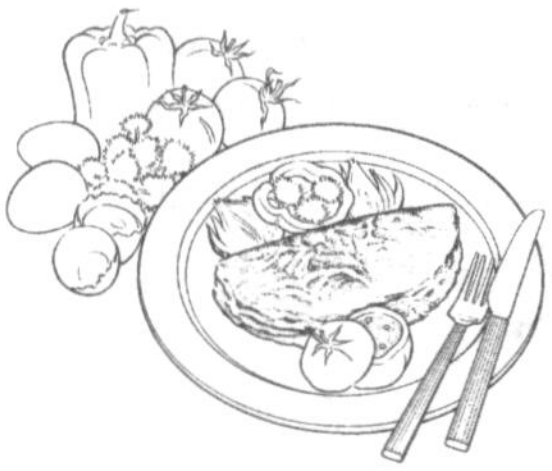

In a large skillet over high heat, sauté 1 chopped Onion and 2 minced Cloves Garlic in 3 TBS Olive Oil, about 5 minutes. Add 2 diced Red Potatoes tossing until golden and tender. Add 1 drained 7-oz. can chopped Olives and 1 drained 7-oz. jar Roasted Red Peppers, slivered. Sizzle 5 minutes.

—Reduce heat to low, and add 8 beaten Eggs. Cover pan and cook until eggs are set around the edges but still liquid in the center. Lift edges to let uncooked egg flow underneath. Cook 5 minutes more until egg is set on top but still moist. Ease a spatula down the sides to make sure egg isn't stuck to the pan. Place a large plate over the skillet; invert eggs onto the plate. Slide eggs back into pan cooked side up. Cook for 1 minute uncovered until set on the bottom. Slide out onto a serving plate.

—Serve hot with BLACK MUSHROOM WINE SAUCE: Soak 4 dried Shiitake Mushrooms in $^1/_2$ cup Sherry until soft. Sliver caps; discard woody stems. Reserve sherry for the sauce. Pureé 4 Plum Tomatoes in the blender for about 1 cup purée.

—Sauté in 1 TB Olive Oil until aromatic: $^1/_4$ cup chopped Green Onion, 1 teasp. Garlic-Lemon Seasoning, and pinches of Sea Salt and Pepper.

—Add 2 teasp. snipped Fresh Basil Leaves, 1 teasp. Fresh Oregano Leaves, $^1/_4$ teasp. dry Marjoram and 1 teasp. Tamari. Add the tomato purée, $^1/_2$ cup Organic Vegetable Broth and the mushroom soaking sherry. Simmer until sauce is reduced by half, about 20 minutes. Spoon over frittata.

Nutrition; 248 calories; 12gm protein; 16gm carbo.; 3gm fiber; 14gm total fats; 264mg choles.; 83mg calcium; 3mg iron; 32mg magnes.; 484mg potassium; 390mg sodium; Vit. A 295 IU; Vit. C 72mg; Vit. E 4 IU.

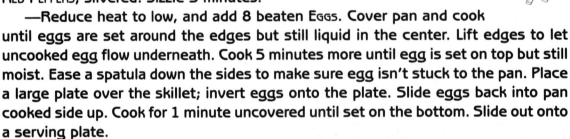

LOW FAT THREE VEGETABLE SOUFFLÉ

This recipe works for: Bone Building, Skin, Hair and Nails, Fatigue Syndromes
For 12 servings: Preheat oven to 400°.

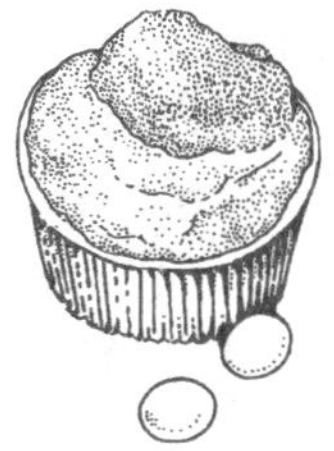

Make the SPINACH PURÉE. Steam 1 large Bunch Fresh Spinach for 1 minute to wilt. Drain in a colander. Squeeze liquid into a bowl. Purée spinach in a blender with 3 TBS reserved liquid, 2 Eggs, 1/4 cup Whole Wheat Pastry Flour, 1 teasp. Lemon Peel, 1/2 teasp. Garlic-Lemon Seasoning and 1/4 teasp. Sea Salt. Scrape into a bowl and set aside.

—Make the MUSHROOM PURÉE. Sauté 2 cups sliced Mushrooms and 1 small chopped Onion until fragrant. Purée in the blender with 2 Eggs, 1/4 cup Whole Wheat Pastry Flour and 1/4 teasp. Sea Salt. Scrape out into a bowl and set aside.

—Make the CARROT PURÉE. Boil 1 cup Salted Water. Add 3 chopped Carrots, 1 TB Fresh Thyme Leaves and 1 small chopped Onion. Cook for 15 minutes. Purée in the blender with 2 Eggs and 1/4 cup Whole Wheat Pastry Flour. Scrape into a bowl.

—Oil a 9" springform pan. Spread with the SPINACH PURÉE. Then spread with the MUSHROOM PURÉE. Then top with the CARROT PURÉE. Bake until top feels firm when pressed, about 45 minutes. Remove and cool; sprinkle with grated Parmesan-Reggiano Cheese and snipped Fresh Parsley. Remove sides of springform pan.

—Serve hot with LEMON SAUCE: Whisk 1 teasp. Dijon Mustard, 2 tsp. Garlic-Lemon Seasoning, 2 TBS Lemon Juice, 2 TBS Tomato Juice, 1 tsp. Tamari, 1/2 tsp. Cracked Pepper.

BABY SHRIMP SCRAMBLE

This recipe works for: Bone Building, Addiction Recovery, Illness Recovery
For 4 servings:

In a bowl mix 6 Eggs, 2 snipped Green Onions, pinches Sea Salt and Pepper.

—Sizzle 2 TBS Olive Oil and 1/4 cup chopped Onion for 5 minutes. Add egg mix and cook undisturbed until half set. Stir in 5-oz. cooked Baby Shrimp. Cook until set.

Nutrition; 213 calories; 17gm protein; 2gm carbo.; 1gm fiber; 14gm total fats; 379mg choles.; 57mg calcium; 2mg iron; 22mg magnes.; 189mg potassium; 131mg sodium; Vit. A 171 IU; Vit. C 5mg; Vit. E 3 IU.

EGG and TOMATO CUPS

This recipe works for: Men's Health, Liver-Organ Health, Anti-Aging
For 2 servings: Preheat oven to 325°.

Sauté 1/2 cup sliced Scallions and 1/4 cup sliced Mushrooms in 2 TBS Olive Oil until liquid evaporates. Sprinkle with 1 TB Whole Wheat Flour and stir until bubbly. Add 1 large chopped Tomato, 1 TB snipped Fresh Basil, 1/2 tsp. Lemon-Pepper. Stir until sauce bubbles. Blend in 3 TBS grated Parmesan. Divide between 2 baking cups. Break 1 Egg on top of each; bake 20 minutes. Sprinkle with snipped Parsley and serve hot.

Protein from Low Fat Cheeses

Cheeses are a good source of protein. The health problem has always been the fat that comes with them. The recipes here use only low fat cheeses so you can maximize your non-meat protein without high fats.

Important Note: Rice Cheese, Almond Cheese and Soy Cheeses may be used one-for-one in place of any low fat dairy cheese in these recipes.

CREAMY TOMATO CHEESECAKE

This recipe works for: Men's Health, Heart Health, Overcoming Addictions

For 16 appetizer servings: Preheat oven to 350°. Use a 10 x 15" baking pan.

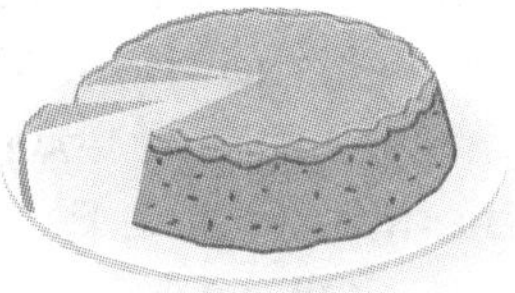

Make a press-in pastry base for the cheesecake: mix 6 TBS Canola Oil and $1^1/_4$ cups Whole Wheat Pastry Flour until crumbly. Mix in 1 Egg until dough holds together. Press into the oiled baking pan. Bake until light brown, about 10 minutes. Remove and cool before filling.

—Make the filling in the blender: $^1/_2$ cup Oil-Packed Dried Tomatoes, drained, plus 1 TB. oil from the jar, 1 teasp. dry Oregano, 6 minced Cloves Garlic and 3 Eggs. Blend very smooth. Add 2-lbs. Low Fat Cream Cheese in batches, blending each batch until very smooth. Turn into a bowl and stir in $^1/_2$ cup chopped Scallions and pinches Sea Salt and White Pepper. Spread filling onto pastry, and bake until puffy and brown, about 25 minutes. Cool, cover and chill for several hours. Cut in 2" squares; then cut squares diagonally into triangles.

Nutrition; 169 calories; 9gm protein; 10gm carbo.; 2gm fiber; 9gm total fats; 65mg choles.; 48mg calcium; 1mg iron; 23mg magnesium; 214mg potassium; 34mg sodium; Vit. A 92 IU; Vit. C 8mg; Vit. E 2 IU.

TOMATO CHEESE STRATA

This recipe works for: Men's Health, Heart Health, Hair, Skin and Nails

Serves 8: Preheat oven to 350°. Use an 8 x 11" baking pan.

Bring a large pot of Salted Water to boil. Add 1 teasp. Olive Oil so noodles won't stick, then add 12 to 16 Artichoke or Spinach Whole Wheat Lasagna Noodles. Cook only 10 minutes (they'll cook more later). Drain and set aside.

—Make the sauce while lasagna cooks: mix 5 Eggs, 1 cup Plain Yogurt, 1 cup Low-Fat Cottage Cheese, $^1/_2$ cup Red Wine, $^1/_2$ teasp. Lemon-Garlic Seasoning, $^1/_2$ teasp. Pepper.

—Assemble the strata. Line bottom of oiled baking pan with a layer of noodles. Sprinkle with 1 cup Low Fat Mozarrella Cheese. Scatter on half a 16-oz. jar Julienne-Cut, Oil-Packed Sun-Dried Tomatoes. Cover tomatoes with a scattering of chopped Black Olives. Cover olives with another layer of noodles, and repeat tomatoes. Pour sauce over and scatter chopped Walnuts on top. Bake uncovered until edges are light brown and center is firm, about 45 minutes. Cool slightly to set; then cut in squares.

CHEESE CUTLETS with SHRIMP and EGG SAUCE

This recipe works for: Women's Health, Liver and Organ Health, Brain Booster
For 6 servings: Preheat oven to 325°.

Toast 1/4 cup Sesame Seeds in the oven until golden.

Mix in a bowl: 2 cups Low Fat Cottage Cheese, 1 Egg, 2 minced Green Onions, 1/3 cup chopped Walnuts, 2 TBS Toasted Wheat Germ, 2 TBS snipped Fresh Parsley, 1/2 teasp. Sweet Paprika, 1/2 teasp. Sea Salt, 1/4 teasp. Nutmeg, and 1 1/2 cups Whole Wheat Bread Crumbs. Mix well with hands and shape into 6 round patties. Roll in Toasted Wheat Germ, and place on oiled baking sheets. Sprinkle with the sesame seeds and bake for 15 to 20 minutes until golden. Remove and set aside for saucing when done.

—Make SHRIMP - EGG SAUCE: have ready 2 Hard Boiled Eggs. Melt 2 TBS Butter and stir with 2 TBS Whole Wheat Flour until hot and bubbly. Stir in 1/2 cup Plain Low Fat Yogurt, 1/4 cup Sherry, 1/4 cup Water, 4 TBS snipped Fresh Parsley, 2 teasp. Herbs de Provence, 1/4 teasp. Sea Salt, 1/4 teasp. Dry Mustard and 1/4 teasp. White Pepper.

—Stir until thickened, about 7 minutes. Remove from heat and add 8-oz. small Salad Shrimp and the crumbled hard boiled eggs. Spoon over cutlets and serve.

Nutrition; 387 calories; 29gm protein; 28gm carbo.; 3gm fiber; 17gm total fats; 234mg choles.; 375mg calcium; 5mg iron; 88mg magnes.; 416mg potassium; 489mg sodium; Vit. A 167 IU; Vit. C 8mg; Vit. E 3 IU.

CHEESE QUESADILLAS with SALSA VERDE

This recipe works for: Kid's Health, Sports Nutrition, Overcoming Addictions
Makes 8 servings: Salsa Verde makes about 4 cups:

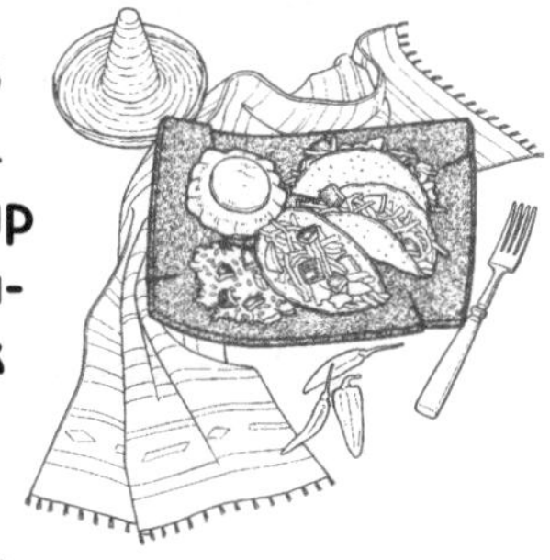

Have ready 16 (6-inch) Corn Tortillas. Have ready 2 cups shredded Low Fat Jack Cheese (about 8-oz.). Heat 1 tsp. Olive Oil in a nonstick skillet. Add 1 tortilla. Sprinkle tortilla with 1/4 cup shredded cheese, snips of Green Onion and dashes Nacho Seasoning. Top with another tortilla and press with spatula to stick tortillas together. Cook until cheese melts and tortillas are crisp and golden, about 2 minutes per side. Remove and drain on paper towels. Repeat with remaining tortillas and cheese, adding 2 teaspoonfuls oil as needed to keep from sticking. Cut quesadillas into quarters; place on serving platter.

—Serve with FRESH SALSA VERDE: combine in a pan, 2-lbs. husked, chopped Fresh Tomatillos, 2 small chopped Onions, and 1 cup Water. Cook stirring, until tomatillos are tender, about 5 minutes. Transfer mixture to a blender; blend to a chunky salsa texture. Chill about 1 hour. To serve, stir in 1 cup chopped Fresh Cilantro Leaves, 4 seeded, minced Jalapeño Chilies and 2 minced Garlic Cloves. Season to taste with Garlic-Lemon Seasoning.

Nutrition; 280 calories; 14gm protein; 37gm carbo.; 6gm fiber; 6gm total fats; 20mg choles.; 378mg calcium; 2mg iron; 69mg magnes.; 512mg potassium; 323mg sodium; Vit. A 302 IU; Vit. C 57mg; Vit. E 3 IU.

BROCCOLI and CHEESE

This recipe works for: Women's Health, Cancer Protection, Bone Building
For 8 servings: Preheat oven to 350°.

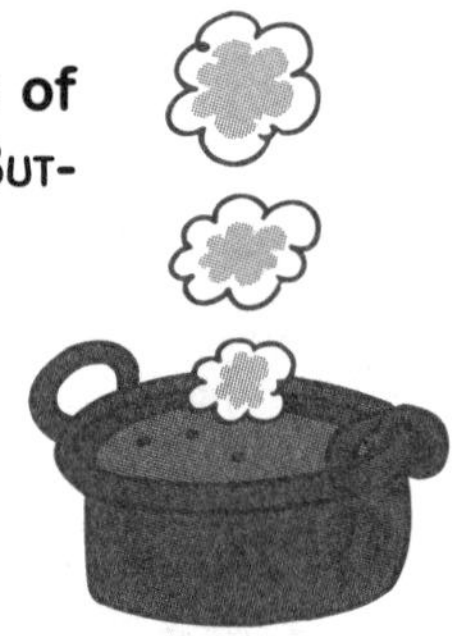

Spray a 9 x 13" baking pan with Canola Oil Spray and lay slices of Buttered Bread to fit in one layer. Have ready the same amount of Buttered Bread to fit on top.

—Have ready 1-lb. shredded Low Fat Cheddar Cheese.

—Sauté in 4 TBS Canola Oil 5 minutes, 1 large diced Onion and 8-oz. sliced Button Mushrooms. Heat a pot of Salted Water. Blanch 3 cups diced Broccoli until color changes to bright green. Remove with a slotted spoon and stir into onions and mushrooms. Add 3 TBS snipped Fresh Basil Leaves ($1^1/_2$ TBS dry) and 1 tsp. Lemon-Pepper.

—Mix $1^1/_2$ cups Low Fat Yogurt and $1^1/_2$ cups Water with 6 Eggs for the custard.

—Assemble the casserole: layer half the vegetable mix over the bread. Cover with half the cheese and the remaining bread layer. Repeat with remaining vegetables and cheese. Pour custard mix over. Cover with plastic wrap and chill. Bake uncovered about 45 minutes, until edges are light brown and the center is firm when jiggled. Let set for 15 minutes before cutting in serving rectangles.

Nutrition; 477 calories; 33gm protein; 34gm carbo.; 5gm fiber; 22gm total fats; 214mg choles.; 672mg calcium; 3mg iron; 88mg magnes.; 567mg potassium; 560mg sodium; Vit. A 361 IU; Vit. C 34mg; Vit. E 3 IU.

VEGGIES, BULGUR and CHEESE Full of minerals as well as protein.

This recipe works for: Women's Health, Hair and Skin, Stress Reactions
For 8 servings: Preheat oven to 350°. Use a 9" square baking dish.

Measure $^3/_4$ cup Bulgur Grain (Kasha) into a big bowl. Cover with $^3/_4$ cup Boiling Water and set aside to absorb.

—Sauté 2 cups diced Onion and 2 minced Cloves Garlic in 3 TBS Olive Oil for 10 minutes. In a food processor, shred 3 cups Zucchini; with a knife, thin slice 3 cups Fresh Spinach; add $1^1/_2$ tsp. Italian Herbs and $^1/_4$ tsp. Lemon-Pepper, and sauté 3 minutes.

—Mix in a bowl: 1 cup crumbled Feta Cheese (about 5-oz.), 1 cup Low Fat Cottage Cheese, $^3/_4$ cup snipped Fresh Parsley, 2 Eggs, 2 TBS Tomato Paste, and $^1/_4$ cup chopped Green Onions. Stir into bulgur.

—Assemble casserole. Layer bulgur mix on bottom of the baking dish. Cover with veggies. Top with cheese mix. Cover with 2 sliced Tomatoes; sprinkle with 1 cup grated Low Fat Cheddar Cheese. Top with $1^1/_2$ TBS Sesame Seeds; bake covered for 45 minutes; uncover and bake 15 minutes more. Let set 10 minutes out of the oven before serving.

Nutrition; 253 calories; 17gm protein; 20gm carbo.; 5gm fiber; 9gm total fats; 81mg choles.; 301mg calcium; 3mg iron; 79mg magnes.; 573mg potassium; 402mg sodium; Vit. A 322 IU; Vit. C 29mg; Vit. E 2 IU.

FANCY CHEESE NACHOS

This recipe works for: Kid's and Men's Health, Liver and Organ Health
Enough for a trayful:

Have ready 1-lb. of your favorite baked Nacho Chips toasted on a tray until crisp.
—Simmer in a pan over very low heat: 1/3 cup Plain Sparkling Water, 4-oz. Kefir Cheese (or Low Fat Cream Cheese), 8-oz. Low Fat Jalapeño Jack Cheese, 8-oz. Low Fat Cheddar Cheese, 1/2 cup shredded Spinach or Chard and 1/4 cup Natural Salsa until cheese melts smooth. Spoon over toasted chips, then briefly run under the broiler to brown.

Nutrition; 298 calories; 16gm protein; 28gm carbo.; 3gm fiber; 12gm total fats; 33mg choles.; 417mg calcium; 1mg iron; 45mg magnes.; 162mg potassium; 602mg sodium; Vit. A 193 IU; Vit. C 2mg; Vit. E trace

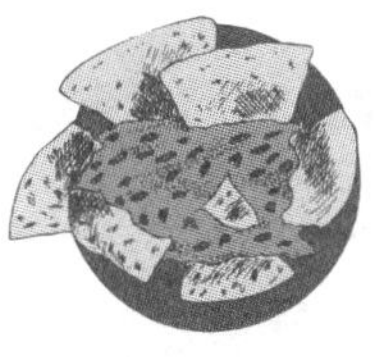

Protein from Soy Foods

Tofu, Tempeh, Miso and Soy Milk

Soy foods offer a complete, vegetarian source of protein. They also lend themselves to almost endless variations of taste and texture. The recipes in this section are only examples of the diversity of soy. See the chapter on **Cultured Foods** and other recipes throughout this book for more delicious ways to use soy foods.

TEXAS CHILI TOFU DOME

This recipe works for: Kid's and Men's Health, Liver - Organ Health, Stress
For 6 servings: Preheat oven to 350°.

Have ready 1-lb. Frozen Tofu, thawed, squeezed out and crumbled.
—Sauté in 2 TBS Olive Oil and 2 TBS Red Wine: 4 minced Garlic Cloves, and 1 diced Red Onion, 1 diced Red Bell Pepper for 10 minutes. Add 2 minced, seeded Jalapeño Peppers, 2 TBS Chili Powder, 1 teasp. Sea Salt, 2 teasp. dry Oregano, 2 teasp. Cumin Powder, 1/2 teasp. dry Thyme and simmer for 3 minutes until aromatic.
—Add a 28-oz. can drained Peeled Plum Tomatoes. Cook 10 minutes. Stir in the tofu and 1-lb. Ground Turkey. Add 1 cup Whole Wheat Bread Crumbs, 2 Eggs and 1 cup Corn Kernels. Put in a shallow baking dish and form into a dome. Bake for 1 hour. Remove, pour off excess juice, and grate on 8-oz. Soy Cheddar Cheese to cover dome.

Nutrition; 379 calories; 37gm protein; 34gm carbo.; 6gm fiber; 14gm total fats; 128mg choles.; 243mg calcium; 9mg iron; 146mg magnes.; 921mg potassium; 620mg sodium; Vit. A 452 IU; Vit. C 94mg; Vit. E 3 IU.

LIGHT, PUFFY TOFU POPOVERS

This recipe works for: Women's Health, Fatigue Syndromes, Healthy Pregnancy
Heat Pyrex custard cups or a popover pan in a hot oven first. Remove to fill only when batter is ready; immediately return to the hot oven. They will puff beautifully.
For 6 big popovers: Preheat oven to 400°F.

Put 1 TB Butter in each of 6 custard or popover cups. Put the cups on a baking sheet and heat in the oven while you make the batter. Cups must be very hot.

—Blender blend the batter: 3 Eggs, 1 teasp. Sea Salt, 2 TBS Sesame Seeds, 4 crumbled Cakes Tofu (1-lb.), $^3/_4$ cup Unbleached Flour. Pour the batter slowly over the butter in the cups. Do not stir. Bake for 20 minutes. Reduce heat to 350°F and bake for 15 more minutes. Fill with sauced veggies or just eat plain with a little Butter.

TOFU POTATO SALAD

This recipe works for: Sugar Imbalances, Allergies, Fatigue Syndromes
For 8 salads:

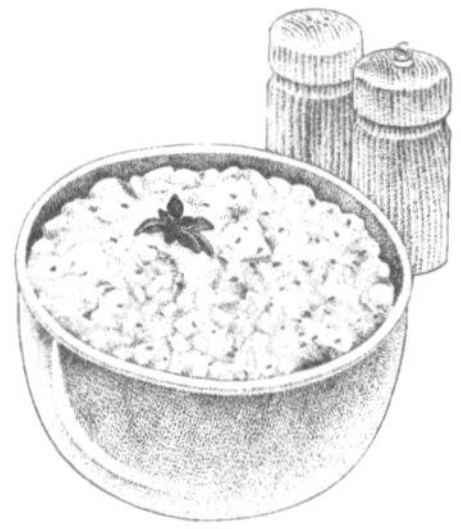

Steam $1^1/_2$-lb. Baby Red Potatoes til tender. Set aside.

—Have ready 1 (8-oz.) package Nature Burger or Falafel Mix. Mix with 1-lb. crumbled Tofu, $^1/_2$ cup Water, 1 TB Cider Vinegar, $^1/_4$ cup snipped Fresh Parsley and $^1/_4$ cup grated Parmesan Cheese.

—Sauté in a skillet until aromatic: 1 TB Olive Oil, $^1/_2$ cup diced Onion, $^1/_2$ cup diced Celery and 2 TBS Pimentos. Add burger mixture and simmer for 15 minutes until browned. Add potatoes, toss and chill.

—Mix the dressing while salad is chilling: $^1/_3$ cup Cider Vinegar, $^1/_3$ cup Walnut Oil, $^1/_4$ cup Ketchup and 1 TB Tamari. Pour over potato salad and sprinkle with more snipped Fresh Parsley.

Nutrition; 398 calories; 19gm protein; 37gm carbo.; 4gm fiber; 21gm total fats; 4mg choles.; 223mg calcium; 8mg iron; 116mg magnes.; 773mg potassium; 290mg sodium; Vit. A 46 IU; Vit. C 14mg; Vit. E 6 IU.

NUTTY TOFU SPREAD Good with dunkers or by itself.

This recipe works for: Heart Health, Hair and Skin, Women's Balance
About $1^1/_2$ cups, for 4 servings:

Mix in the blender: $^1/_2$ carton Kefir Cheese (or Low Fat Cream Cheese), 8-oz. Silken Tofu, $^1/_3$ cup Sesame Tahini, 1 TB Honey, 1 TB minced Green Onion, and 1 TB snipped Parsley. Pack into individual oiled scalloped shells and chill. Serve in the shell with crackers or toast, or unmold onto large Boston Lettuce Leaves; cover with 2 TBS Toasted Sesame Seeds.

Nutrition; 296 calories; 17gm protein; 14gm carbo.; 3gm fiber; 20gm total fats; 16mg choles.; 226mg calcium; 9mg iron; 143mg magnesium; 335mg potassium; 11mg sodium; Vit. A 90 IU; Vit. C 3mg; Vit. E 1 IU.

SOY PROTEIN POWER SHAKE

This recipe works for: Heart Health, Anti-Aging, Liver and Organ Health
For 2 shakes:

Blender blend until smooth: 2 cups Honey-Vanilla Soy Milk, 2 Frozen Bananas, 4 TBS Vanilla Soy Protein Powder, 3 TBS Nutritional Yeast Flakes, 2 TBS Bee Pollen, 2 TBS Toasted Wheat Germ, 2 TBS Cocoa Powder, 1 TB Lecithin Granules, 1 teasp. Cinnamon.

Nutrition; 437 calories; 29gm protein; 72gm carbo.; 11gm fiber; 10gm total fats; 0mg choles.; 558mg calcium; 18mg iron; 120mg magnes.; 946mg potassium; 195mg sodium; Vit. A 10 IU; Vit. C 11mg; Vit. E 5 IU.

CALIFORNIA FALAFEL SALAD

This recipe works for: Heart Health, Arthritis, Men's and Kid's Health
For 6 salads:

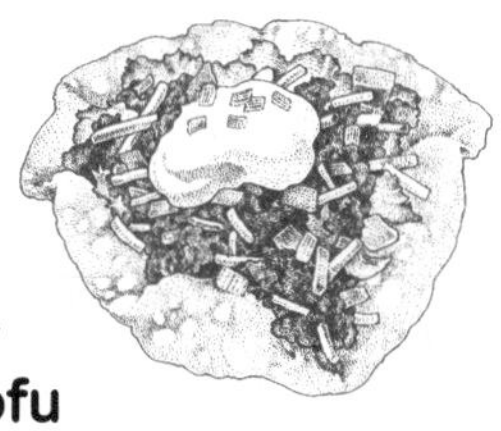

Boil 1-lb. cubed Extra Firm Tofu in 1 cup Boiling Water for 5 minutes. Drain. Toss with 8-oz. Falafel Mix or Sesame Burger Mix from the health food store; set aside.

—Sauté 1/2 cup minced Green Onion in 1 TB Olive Oil for 2 minutes. Add 1/2 cup Water and let bubble. Remove from heat. Add tofu and falafel mix. Toss to coat and set aside to absorb water.

—Add 2 crumbled Hard Boiled Eggs, 1 cup thin-sliced Celery, 1 TB Sweet Hot Mustard, 1/2 cup Lemon Mayonnaise and 1/2 cup Sweet Pickle Relish. Stir just lightly to moisten. Chill for 1 hour and serve over shredded Romaine Lettuce on toast.

Nutrition; 397 calories; 21gm protein; 33gm carbo.; 4gm fiber; 19gm total fats; 71mg choles.; 219mg calcium; 11mg iron; 124mg magnes.; 617mg potassium; 422mg sodium; Vit. A 80 IU; Vit. C 8mg; Vit. E 1 IU.

TOFU TAMALE PIE

This recipe works for: Heart Health, Immune Power, Bone Building
Serves 6 to 8: Preheat oven to 350°.

In a large wok, sauté in 3 TBS Olive Oil, 2 minced Cloves Garlic, 1 diced Onion, 1-lb. crumbled Firm Tofu and 1 diced Red Bell Pepper until brown.

—Remove from heat and stir in 1 cup cooked Brown Rice, 6 to 8 chopped Tomatoes, 1 (4-oz.) can chopped Green Chilies, 1 cup Corn Kernels, 1/2 cup Vegetable Broth, 1 cup Yellow Cornmeal, 1/4 cup Red Wine, 2 TBS Chili Powder, 1/2 teasp. Cumin Powder and 1/2 teasp. Pepper.

—Bake for 45 minutes. Remove from oven; sprinkle on grated Low Fat Jack Cheese and 2 TBS minced Green Olives to cover top. Bake for 15 more minutes until bubbly.

Nutrition; 287 calories; 16gm protein; 33gm carbo.; 5gm fiber; 11gm total fats; 5mg choles.; 222mg calcium; 8mg iron; 110mg magnes.; 586mg potassium; 240mg sodium; Vit. A 229 IU; Vit. C 45mg; Vit. E 2 IU.

TOFU MUSHROOM STIR FRY

This recipe works for: Circulatory Health, Liver - Organ Health, Cancer Protection
For 4 servings: Use a large wok.

Combine in a bowl: 3 TBS Lemon Juice, 3 TBS Tamari, 2 minced Cloves Garlic and 2 TBS grated Ginger and 2 teasp. Honey. Add 2 Tofu Cakes, cut into strips. Toss to coat.
—Dissolve 2 teasp. Arrowroot Powder in 1/3 cup Organic Chicken Broth; set aside.
—Heat 2 TBS Olive Oil to sizzling. Add 2 cups sliced Mushrooms and the tofu strips; toss for 3 minutes. Add 1 1/2 cups trimmed Pea Pods and 3 sliced Green Onions; toss 3 minutes. Stir in arrowroot mixture; stir until thickened. Sprinkle with 2 TBS Toasted Sesame Seeds and 2 TBS minced Crystallized Ginger. Serve hot over Brown Rice.

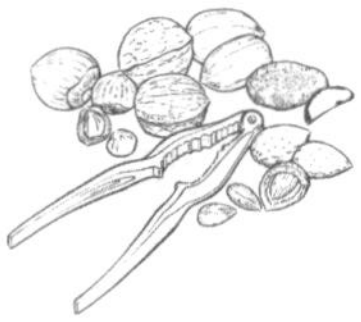

Protein from Nuts, Seeds and Sprouts

Nuts, seeds and sprouts are high energy foods, full of rich, nutritious vegetarian protein for healing. Eat them with grains, beans and low fat dairy foods to complete the amino acid profile for protein synthesis. Nuts, seeds and sprouts are rich in essential fatty acids, vitamin E, potassium, magnesium, iron, zinc, B vitamins and fiber.

NUT and SEED GRANOLA

This recipe works for: Sports Nutrition, Men's and Kid's Health, Heart Health
Makes about 8 cups: Preheat oven to 300°F. Refrigerate in air-tight container.

Mix 3 cups old-fashioned Oats, 1 cup shredded Coconut, 1/2 cup Wheat Germ, 1/2 cup shelled Sunflower Seeds (about 3-oz.), 1/2 cup chopped Walnuts and 1/2 cup Pumpkin Seeds on a heavy large baking sheet
—Stir in a pan until honey melts: 6 TBS Honey, 4 TBS Canola Oil, 2 TBS Fructose, 1 1/2 teasp. Vanilla Extract and 1/2 teasp. Cinnamon. Remove from heat and stir in 2 TBS Bee Pollen Granules. Pour over oat mixture baking sheet and toss to coat. Bake mixture until golden brown, stirring occasionally, about 30 minutes. Crumble mixture into a big bowl. Stir in 3/4 cup Raisins and 1/2 cup Banana Chips.

SKILLET SPROUTS and SEEDS

This recipe works for: Fatigue Syndromes, Immune Breakdown, Candida
For 2 servings: Use a large skillet.

Heat 1 TB Canola Oil. Add 1/2 cup snipped Green Onions and 1 cup grated Carrots. Sauté 3 minutes only. Add 4 cups Bean Sprouts, 4 TBS Onion Broth, 1 TB Sesame Seeds and 1 teasp. Lemon-Pepper. Toss over high heat for 30 seconds until sprouts are hot.

CHEESY TOMATO NUT ROAST

This recipe works for: Men's Health, Sugar Imbalances, Cancer Protection
For 4 people: Preheat oven to 350°. Use an oil-sprayed loaf pan.

Sauté 1 chopped Onion, 1 teasp. Herbal Seasoning Salt and $^1/_4$ teasp. Hot Pepper Sauce in 2 TBS Olive Oil for 5 minutes. Add 1 cup Miso Broth (2 TBS Miso Paste to 1 cup Water) to onions. Heat until bubbly, and remove pan from heat.

—Add $1^1/_2$ cups chopped Walnuts ground in the blender with 3 crumbled slices Whole Grain Bread and 6 TBS Toasted Wheat Germ. Turn half the mixture into oiled loaf pan and press in. Top with 2 sliced Tomatoes. Top tomatoes with a covering of shredded Mozarrella Cheese. Top with other half of nut mix and smooth top. Bake for 30 minutes. Cover with grated Parmesan Cheese during last few minutes of baking.

Nutrition; 493 calories; 23gm protein; 32gm carbo.; 7gm fiber; 33gm total fats; 7mg choles.; 186mg calcium; 4mg iron; 171mg magnes.; 638mg potassium; 427mg sodium; Vit. A 77 IU; Vit. C 17mg; Vit. E 7 IU.

PEANUT TOFU PITA FILLING

This recipe works for: Fatigue Syndromes, Liver - Organ Health, Stress Reactions
For 2 cups:

Make it in the blender: 1 teasp. Garlic-Lemon Seasoning, 1 (16-oz.) can Chickpeas, rinsed and drained, 4-oz. Silken Tofu, 4 TBS Lemon Juice, 2 TBS Crunchy Peanut Butter, 1 TB Olive Oil. Scrape out; season with Lemon-Pepper and stuff pitas.

WHEAT GERM and WALNUT LOAF

This recipe works for: Men's Health, Liver - Organ Health, Sports Nutrition
For 6 servings: Preheat oven to 350°.

Toast 1 cup chopped Walnuts and 1 cup Wheat Germ on a tray until brown.

—Sauté 1 large chopped Onion, 1 teasp. Thyme and $^1/_4$ teasp. Marjoram in 2 TBS Butter for 5 minutes. Turn into a bowl and mix with walnuts and wheat germ. Mix in 3 Eggs, 2 TBS Sesame Seeds, 1 teasp. Sea Salt, $^1/_2$ teasp. Pepper, $^3/_4$ cup Tomato Juice and 1 cup grated Cheddar. Pack into a Canola Oil sprayed loaf pan and bake for 45 minutes until moist but firm. Let rest before slicing.

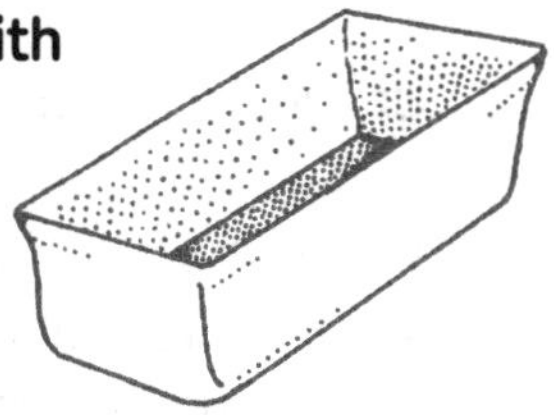

—Serve with FRESH TOMATO SAUCE: Brown $^1/_2$ diced Onion and 2 minced Cloves Garlic in 2 TBS Olive Oil for 5 minutes. Add 1 grated Carrot, 2 TBS diced Red Bell Pepper, 4 cups chopped Tomatoes, 1 teasp. Oregano, $^1/_2$ teasp. Thyme, $^1/_2$ teasp. dry Basil, $^1/_2$ teasp. Sea Salt, $^1/_2$ teasp. Fructose, and $^1/_2$ teasp. Lemon-Pepper. Simmer for 30 minutes to reduce liquid and spoon over loaf.

Nutrition; 422 calories; 19gm protein; 25gm carbo.; 6gm fiber; 30gm total fats; 136mg choles.; 230mg calcium; 5mg iron; 126mg magnes.; 767mg potassium; 412mg sodium; Vit. A 588 IU; Vit. C 37mg; Vit. E 8 IU.

SPROUT - SHIITAKE SALAD

This recipe works for: Cancer Protection, Immune Power, Overcoming Addictions
For 4 salads:

Rinse, drain and toss: 1 (4-oz.) Tub Alfalfa Sprouts, 1 cup Bean Sprouts and 1 cup Sunflower Sprouts. Place in a salad bowl. Thin slice 8-oz. Fresh Shiitake Mushroom Caps and add to bowl.

—Mix the dressing: $^1/_3$ cup Sherry, $^1/_4$ cup Tamari, 1 TB minced Crystallized Ginger and 1 teasp. Honey. Pour over salad and toss to coat.

Nutrition; 93 calories; 7gm protein; 17gm carbo.; 3gm fiber; 0 total fats; 0mg choles.; 23mg calcium; 2mg iron; 35mg magnesium; 210mg potassium; 276mg sodium; Vit. A 6 IU; Vit. C 10mg; Vit. E trace

HIGH ENERGY SPROUT and SEED SALAD

This recipe works for: Illness Recovery, Bone Building, Men's Health
For 3 salads:

Mix in a bowl just to moisten: $^1/_2$ cup Oriental Snack Mix (available in most health food stores; or use your favorite crunchy snack mix), 2 TBS Toasted Sesame Seeds, 2 TBS Sunflower Seeds, 2 TBS Almond Granola, 1 Carrot, cut in matchsticks, 3 TBS snipped Fresh Cilantro Leaves, 1 (8-oz.) carton Lemon-Lime Yogurt and $^1/_4$ teasp. Pepper.

–Mound onto Boston Lettuce cups and top with crumbled Hard Boiled Egg, grated Parmesan Cheese and a handful Alfalfa Sprouts.

Nutrition; 374 calories; 19gm protein; 24gm carbo.; 6gm fiber; 22gm total fats; 81mg choles.; 371mg calcium; 3mg iron; 117mg magnes.; 579mg potassium; 354mg sodium; Vit. A 756 IU; Vit. C 5mg; Vit. E 6 IU.

THAI NOODLE STIR FRY

This recipe works for: Weight Control, Bone Building, Men's Health
For 6 servings:

Bring 4 qts. Salted Water to a boil. Add 1-lb. dry Linguine and cook just to al dente, about 3 minutes. Drain. Toss with 1 TB Olive Oil and set aside in a serving bowl.

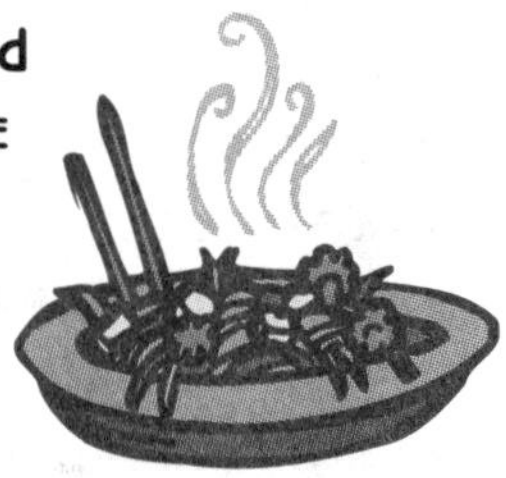

—Heat wok over high heat for 1 minute. Stir-fry 2 minced Cloves Garlic, 3 sliced Scallions, 4 TBS Tamari, 3 TBS Lime Juice, 1 teasp. Brown Sugar and $^1/_4$ teasp. Hot Pepper Sauce for 1 minute until fragrant. Turn off heat and add 2 cups Bean Sprouts. Toss and pour over noodles. Serve hot.

Nutrition; 249 calories; 12gm protein; 46gm carbo.; 3gm fiber; 4gm total fats; 0mg choles.; 145mg calcium; 3mg iron; 40mg magnesium; 242mg potassium; 326mg sodium; Vit. A 6 IU; Vit. C 9mg; Vit. E 1 IU.

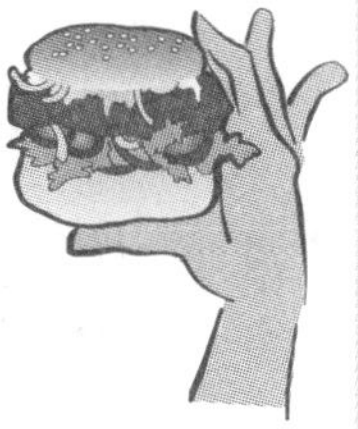

ZUCCHINI SUN SEED BURGERS

This recipe works for: Hair and Skin, Immune Power, Women's Health
For 6 burgers:

Split 3 Whole Grain English Muffins. Run under the broiler to brown tops; set aside.
—Shred $1^1/_2$ lbs. Zucchini into a colander. Salt and let drain for 30 minutes.
—In a skillet, sauté 1 large diced Onion in 1 TB Olive Oil 10 minutes. Return into a bowl and add the zucchini, $^1/_4$ cup Wheat Germ, 2 Eggs, pinches Sea Salt and Pepper, and $^1/_4$ cup Parmesan Cheese.
—In the skillet, sizzle 1 TB Olive Oil, and 1 TB Soy Bacon Bits. Ladle 3 mounds of zucchini mix into pan and form into 3" cakes. Cook until bottoms are light brown, about 3 minutes. Turn and cook for 3 more minutes. Repeat for 3 more cakes.
—Spread muffin halves with spoonfuls of LIGHT CHEESE SAUCE: stir 1 TB Butter and 1 TB Whole Wheat Flour until bubbly. Add $^1/_4$ cup diced Onion; sauté for 5 minutes. Add $^1/_4$ cup Plain Low Fat Yogurt and $^1/_4$ cup White Wine. Reduce heat and simmer until thickened. Season with 2 pinches each, Nutmeg, Sea Salt and Pepper. Turn off heat. Add $^1/_2$ cup shredded Mozarrella Cheese and let melt. Top burgers with Tomato slices and a dollop of Cheese Sauce. Run under broiler for 30 seconds; serve hot.

Nutrition; 230 calories; 14gm. protein; 22gm. carbo.; 6gm. fiber; 9gm total fats; 84mg choles.; 258mg calcium; 2mg iron; 79mg magnes.; 591mg potassium; 320mg sodium; Vit. A 129 IU; Vit. C 16mg; Vit. E 3 IU.

Protein from Whole Grains

Whole grains are protein packed, but most whole grains are not "complete proteins" because their lysine content is too low. I recommend eating whole grains with legumes, higher in lysine, for protein balance. The ancient grain quinoa is the only exception. Quinoa is a rich source of lysine and a good source of healing protein because its amino acid profile closely resembles the pattern usable by the body.

OATS and ALMONDS PILAF

This recipe works for: Heart / Cholesterol Health, Bone Building, Arthritis
For 3 servings:

Toast 1 cup sliced Almonds for 10 minutes at 325°. Stir and shake often.
—Sauté 1 diced Onion and 2 minced Cloves Garlic in 2 teasp. Olive Oil. Add 1 cup Oats and sauté until fragrant, 5 minutes. Add $1^3/_4$ cup Onion Broth; bring to a boil. Cover and simmer 15 to 20 minutes until liquid is absorbed. Remove from heat. Fluff and mix in 3 TBS snipped Fresh Parsley and half of the toasted nuts. Top with 3 TBS snipped Fresh Parsley and the rest of the almonds.

Nutrition; 427 calories; 15gm protein; 32gm carbo.; 8gm fiber; 31gm total fats; 0mg choles.; 155mg calcium; 4mg iron; 186mg magnes.; 566mg potassium; 13mg sodium; Vit. A 42 IU; Vit. C 13mg; Vit. E 6 IU.

WHOLE GRAIN STUFFING BAKE

This recipe works for: Cancer Protection, Kid's-Men's Health, Sports Nutrition
For 6 servings: Preheat oven to 350°.

Toast 4 cups WHOLE GRAIN BREAD CUBES until dry and crisp. Remove; leave oven on.
—Sauté in 2 TBS OLIVE OIL, 1 cup diced ONION, $^1/_2$ teasp. SEA SALT and $^1/_2$ teasp. PEPPER for 10 minutes. Stir in 2 diced RIBS CELERY, 2 cups chopped MUSHROOMS, 1 TB DIJON MUSTARD and 1 teasp. HERBAL POULTRY SEASONING. Add 2 TBS WHOLE WHEAT FLOUR and stir 5 minutes until flour blends in. Add 4 TBS SHERRY and cook for 5 minutes more.
—Toss with bread cubes, and spread into a shallow buttered baking casserole.
—Sprinkle with 1 cup diced WALNUTS, with $^1/_2$ cup grated LOW FAT CHEDDAR.
—Beat 4 EGGS with $^1/_3$ cup PLAIN LOW FAT YOGURT and 2 TBS WATER. Pour on stuffing. Dust with NUTMEG and PAPRIKA; bake for 45 minutes until firm and brown.

BROCCOLI and HIGH PROTEIN GRAINS

This recipe works for: Stress, Anti-Aging, Women's Health
For 5 servings:

Blanch 4 cups BROCCOLI FLORETS in a large pot of boiling SALTED WATER until color changes to bright green. Drain and rinse immediately with cold water. Set aside.
—Sizzle in a skillet, 2 TBS CANOLA OIL and 2 TBS BUTTER, $^1/_4$ teasp. NUTMEG and 4 dashes HOT PEPPER SAUCE 2 minutes. Add 2 cups cooked BROWN BASMATI RICE, $^1/_2$ cup cooked AMARANTH, and $^1/_2$ cup TOASTED SUNFLOWER SEEDS; toss to coat. Remove from heat and add $^1/_2$ cup diced LOW FAT SWISS CHEESE, $^1/_4$ cup PLAIN LOW FAT YOGURT, $^1/_4$ cup KEFIR CHEESE and $^1/_4$ cup LEMON MAYONNAISE. Add broccoli and toss briefly. Return to heat; toss until cheese melts. Serve right away.

Nutrition; 385 calories; 15gm protein; 35gm carbo.; 6gm fiber; 19gm total fats; 24mg choles.; 237mg calcium; 3mg iron; 137mg magnes.; 491mg potassium; 89mg sodium; Vit. A 189 IU; Vit. C 66mg; Vit. E 13 IU.

BROWN RICE WITH CHEESE

This recipe works for: Bone Building, Weight Control, Women's Health
For 6 servings: Preheat oven to 350°.

Have ready 3 cups cooked BROWN BASMATI RICE. Blanch 2 cups BROCCOLI FLORETS in a large pot of boiling SALTED WATER until color changes to bright green.
—Mix rice and broccoli together with: 1 cup shredded LOW FAT SWISS CHEESE, $^1/_3$ cup PLAIN LOW FAT YOGURT, $^3/_4$ cup ORGANIC LOW FAT CHICKEN BROTH, $^1/_2$ cup minced GREEN ONIONS, $^1/_4$ cup snipped PARSLEY, 3 TBS LOW-FAT MAYONNAISE, 2 TBS DIJON MUSTARD, and $^1/_2$ teasp. LEMON-PEPPER. Turn into a CANOLA OIL sprayed casserole; sprinkle with $^1/_4$ cup chopped ALMONDS and $^1/_4$ cup WHEAT GERM. Bake for 20 minutes until hot and brown.

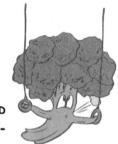

WHOLE GRAIN PASTA SALAD

This recipe works for: Illness Recovery, Sports Nutrition, Men's Health
For 8 servings:

Bring 2-qts. Salted Water to a boil; cook 1-lb. Whole Grain Pasta to al dente. Drain, toss with 1 teasp. Olive Oil to keep separated, and place in a large mixing bowl.

—Mix the salad: 1 diced Red Bell Pepper, 1 chopped Tomato, 1 sliced Avocado, 1 peeled diced Cucumber, 3 snipped Green Onions, $^1/_4$ cup snipped Fresh Parsley, 1 small can sliced Black Olives, drained, 6 thin-sliced Mushroom Caps (reserve stems), 3 TBS snipped Fresh Basil. Toss with the pasta. Cover with grated Parmesan Cheese.

—Serve with MUSHROOM LEMON VINAIGRETTE: Sauté the Mushroom Stems in 2 teasp. Olive Oil for 5 minutes. Add 1 cup Water and simmer 10 minutes to extract mushroom flavor. Strain and discard mushrooms. Boil liquid over high heat for 3 minutes until reduced to 3 TBS. Whisk mushroom essence with 2 TBS Tamari, 2 TBS Lemon Juice, $^1/_2$ cup Olive Oil, $^1/_2$ teasp. Sea Salt and $^1/_4$ teasp. Lemon-Pepper. Chill and pour over pasta salad at serving. Sprinkle with 2 TBS Toasted Sesame Seeds.

Nutrition; 387 calories; 13gm protein; 38gm carbo.; 8gm fiber; 22gm total fats; 5mg choles.; 156mg calcium; 3mg iron; 79mg magnes.; 416mg potassium; 437mg sodium; Vit. A 128 IU; Vit. C 31mg; Vit. E 5 IU.

POLENTA MILANESE

This recipe works for: Illness Recovery, Fatigue Syndromes, Sugar Imbalances
For 10 people: Preheat oven to 350°.

Bring 6 cups Water to a boil and add 2 cups Polenta in a thin stream, stirring. Add 4 TBS Butter, 1 teasp. Sea Salt and $^1/_2$ teasp. Pepper; simmer for 20 minutes. Stir occasionally to prevent sticking. When thickened, remove from heat and stir in $^3/_4$ cup Parmesan Cheese. Pour mixture into a large oiled casserole. Chill.

—Make the VEGETABLE SAUCE: Sauté 2 minced Cloves Garlic and 4 cups diced Onion in 3 TBS Olive Oil for 10 minutes. Add 3 Ribs Celery, 3 TBS dry Basil, 2 teasp. dry Oregano, 1 teasp. Sea Salt and $^1/_4$ teasp. White Pepper; sauté 5 minutes. Add 1 large peeled Eggplant in cubes, 1 Red Bell Pepper in squares, and $1^1/_2$ cups sliced Zucchini for 5 minutes more. Add and simmer until blended: $1^1/_2$ cups White Wine, 3 TBS Tomato Paste, and $1^1/_2$ cups chopped Fresh Tomatoes. Remove from heat and stir in $^1/_2$ cup grated Parmesan-Reggiano Cheese.

—Pour vegetable mix on top of polenta. Top with 3 cups cubed Mozarrella Cheese, and bake 45 minutes until cheese browns and bubbles.

Nutrition; 437 calories; 22gm protein; 47gm carbo.; 5gm fiber; 17gm total fats; 43mg choles.; 529mg calcium; 2mg iron; 71mg magnes.; 630mg potassium; 535mg sodium; Vit. A 244 IU; Vit. C 30mg; Vit. E 2 IU.

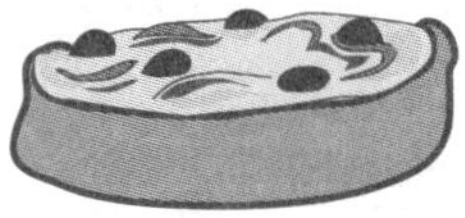

Protein from Beans and Legumes

Beans and legumes are outstanding protein sources, yielding over 20% protein, and under 20% fat. They include black, kidney, lima and navy beans, split peas, soybeans, wheat germ, black-eyed peas, and lentils.

PASTITSIO

This recipe works for: Illness Recovery, Sports Nutrition, Arthritis
For 8 people: Preheat oven to 400°.

Cover $^3/_4$ cups Lentils with 3 cups Water in a kettle and let soak for a few hours. Add 1 teasp. Sea Salt and 1 TB Olive Oil and let cook til water is almost evaporated, about 30 minutes.

—Sauté in a large skillet until fragrant: 3 TBS Olive Oil, 2 TBS Butter, 2 minced Cloves Garlic, 2 large diced Onions, 1 large peeled Eggplant in cubes, 1 teasp. Sea Salt, $^1/_2$ teasp. Cinnamon, $^1/_2$ teasp. Oregano, $^1/_2$ teasp. Pepper and $^1/_4$ teasp. Anise Seed. Cover and simmer 10 minutes. Add 8 chopped Tomatoes, the cooked Lentils and remaining liquid. Cook until thick, stirring occasionally. Stir in 1 small can Tomato Paste.

—Meanwhile, bring Salted Water to a boil for 1 lb. Artichoke or Spinach Pasta. Cook for 10 minutes to al dente. Toss with a little Olive Oil to separate. Set aside.

—Spray a large casserole with Olive Oil Spray; cover the bottom with a layer of noodles. Sprinkle with Parmesan Cheese to cover. Top with a layer of lentil mixture. Repeat until all ingredients are used, ending with the lentils.

—Make the sauce: melt 3 TBS Butter in a pan. Stir in 3 TBS Whole Wheat Flour until bubbly. Whisk in $1^1/_2$ cups Plain Yogurt, 1 cup Water, and $^1/_2$ cup White Wine. Remove from heat and whisk in 3 Eggs. Pour over casserole. Sprinkle with $^1/_2$ cup Parmesan and $^1/_2$ cup Romano Cheese and bake for 1 hour. Serve very hot.

BLACK BEAN CHILI with BUTTERNUT SQUASH

This recipe works for: Illness Recovery, Immune Power, Men's Health
Makes 6 servings: Preheat oven to 375°.

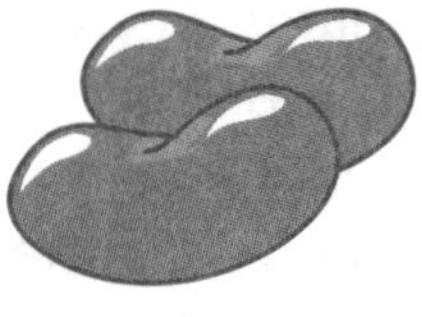

Cut 1 large Butternut Squash in half, scoop out seeds, and place halves cut side down in a baking dish with $^1/_4$-inch of water. Cover and bake until tender, about 30 minutes. Peel, cut into chunks and set aside.

—In large pot, heat 1 TB Olive Oil; sizzle 2 large diced Onions and 3 minced Cloves Garlic for 5 minutes. Mix in 1 diced Red Bell Pepper, 1 (16-oz.) can Black Beans, drained and rinsed, 1 (28-oz.) can Tomatoes diced, 1 (4-oz.) can chopped Mild Green Chilies, 1 tsp. Ground Cumin, and $^1/_2$ tsp. dried Oregano. Bring to a boil. Reduce heat and simmer 15 minutes. Stir in squash and season to taste with Sea Salt. Serve warm.

Nutrition; 236 calories; 12gm protein; 44gm carbo.; 14gm fiber; 3gm total fats; 0mg choles.; 171mg calcium; 4mg iron; 131mg magnes.; 1105mg potass.; 470mg sodium; Vit. A 1210 IU; Vit. C 75mg; Vit. E 2 IU.

CREAMY SESAME BEANS

This recipe works for: Immune Enhancement, Anti-Aging, Hair and Skin
For 4 servings: Preheat oven to 350°F.

Toast 1/4 cup Sesame Seeds in the oven until golden, 2 minutes. Leave oven on.
—Blanch 3 cups Frozen French-Cut Green Beans and 1/2 Yellow Onion sliced in rings, in 1 cup Vegetable Broth for 8 minutes. Drain and mix in 1 cup sliced Celery, 2 TBS Whole Wheat Flour, 1 cup Plain Low Fat Yogurt and 1 teasp. Sesame Salt.
—Turn into a deep casserole. Stir in 1/2 cup Low Fat Cottage Cheese, 1/2 teasp. Oregano, 1/2 teasp. Pepper and 1/4 teasp. Garlic-Lemon Seasoning. Sprinkle with sesame seeds and 1/2 cup Whole Wheat Bread Crumbs; bake for 30 minutes.

CHEESE and RICE ENCHILADAS

This recipe works for: Asthma and Allergies, Men's and Kid's Health
For 8 enchiladas: Preheat oven to 350°F.

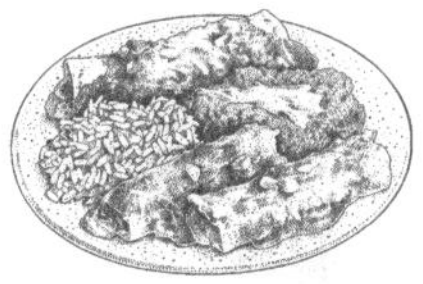

Have ready 8 Corn Tortillas. Oil a 9 x 13" baking dish.
—Make the filling: mix 1 cup cooked Brown Rice with 1 cup grated Low Fat Cheddar Cheese, 1/2 cup diced Black Olives, 1/4 cup diced Walnuts, 2 TBS Toasted Sunflower Seeds, dashes Hot Pepper Sauce.
—Make the sauce: sauté in 3 TBS Olive Oil, 2 minced Cloves Garlic, 1 diced Onion and 2 seeded, minced Jalapeño Chilies for 10 minutes. Add 4 cups chopped Tomatoes and 1/2 teasp. Nacho Seasoning; sauté for 10 minutes more.
—Assemble enchiladas: dip a tortilla into the hot sauce until soft. Lay flat and line 1/8 of the filling down the center. Roll up and lay seam side down in the baking dish. Fill all and lay side by side. Top with grated Cheddar Cheese and crushed Tortilla Chips. Bake for 10 -15 minutes until cheese bubbles, and chips are toasty.

Nutrition; 273 calories; 13gm protein; 27gm carbo.; 4gm fiber; 13gm total fats; 15mg choles.; 267mg calcium; 2mg iron; 67mg magnes.; 356mg potassium; 254mg sodium; Vit. A 145 IU; Vit. C 20mg; Vit. E 5 IU.

HEALTHY CHILI CHEESE TOSTADAS

This recipe works for: Kid's Health, Heart Health, Men's Health
For 6 tostadas: Preheat oven to 450°F.

Toast 6 Whole Wheat Tortillas for 7 minutes until golden. Set aside.
—Sauté in 1 TB Olive Oil 10 minutes: 1 diced Onion, 1 can (4-oz.) diced Green Chilies, 1 tsp. Oregano. Stir in 1 cup diced Red Bell Pepper, 4-oz. cooked Salad Shrimp.
—Assemble the tostadas: Leave a small circle in the center of each tostada for an egg. Spread vegetable mixture over the rest. Sprinkle with shredded Low Fat Jack Cheese to cover. Bake for 3 minutes until cheese melts. Remove and top each tostada with slivered Tomato. Break an Egg in the center of each and bake until eggs are set.

GOURMET BLACK BEAN PESTO

This recipe works for: Immune Power, Men's Health, Bone-Muscle Building
For 4 cups:

Soak for 2 hours, $1^{2}/_{3}$ cups Dry Black Beans in a pot with 6 cups Organic Chicken Broth and $1^{1}/_{2}$ teasp. Cumin Powder. Bring to a boil. Cover and simmer, about 2 hours. Drain. Mash 1 cup of beans and mix with rest of the whole beans. Set aside.

—Mince 1 jar Roasted Red Bell Peppers. Mix with 4-oz. crumbled Feta Cheese.

—Blender blend the CILANTRO PESTO: 4 teasp. Olive Oil, 3 cups packed Fresh Cilantro Leaves, $^{1}/_{2}$ cup oven-toasted Pine Nuts, 1 teasp. Garlic-Lemon Seasoning.

—Assemble the pesto layers. Line a loaf pan with plastic wrap, leave lots of excess drape over the sides. Spoon in $^{1}/_{3}$ of the bean mix. Press down and smooth. Cover with Cilantro Pesto. Cover pesto with all but 2 TBS of roasted peppers. Cover with feta cheese. Top cheese with remaining beans. Press down and smooth. Fold draped plastic wrap over and chill until firm. Invert on a plate or shallow dish. Top with the reserved minced peppers and serve with cocktail rye toasts.

LENTIL NUT ROAST

This recipe works for: Sugar Imbalances, Overcoming Addictions, Men's Health
Enough for 8 people: Preheat oven to 350°.

Have ready 4 cups cooked Lentils.

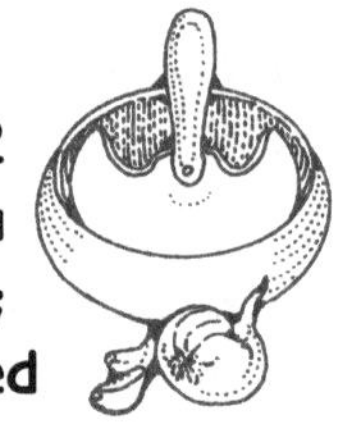

—Sauté in 3 TBS Olive Oil for 5 minutes, 3 minced Cloves Garlic, 2 chopped Onions and 3 large Ribs Celery with Leaves. Add 1 cup Whole Grain Bread Crumbs, $^{1}/_{2}$ cup Toasted Wheat Germ, 2 teasp. Thyme and 2 teasp. Sage; toss to coat. Remove from heat; mix in cooked lentils, $^{1}/_{4}$ cup snipped Fresh Parsley and 1 cup chopped Walnuts.

—Press into a 9 x 13" baking dish. Sprinkle with $^{1}/_{2}$ cup Whole Grain Bread Crumbs. Cover and bake for 40 minutes. Uncover and bake for 5 more minutes to brown and crisp. Let rest for 10 minutes before slicing. Serve with spicy tomato sauce, or:

—Blender blend a LEMON CHEESE SAUCE: 1 cup Low Fat Cottage Cheese, 4 TBS Lemon Mayonnaise, $^{1}/_{4}$ cup Low Fat Yogurt, 2 TBS Lemon Juice, 2 TBS snipped Chives, $^{1}/_{2}$ tsp. Sea Salt, $^{1}/_{2}$ tsp. Pepper and $^{1}/_{4}$ tsp. Tarragon. Serve in dollops on nut roast slices.

BLACK BEAN SOPES

This recipe works for: Sugar Imbalances, Overcoming Addictions. Men's-Kid's Health
Makes about 24 sopes: Preheat oven to 400°F.

Make shells: Fit 6-inch Corn Tortillas into large muffin tins or 3-inch baking cups. Crisp in the oven for 3 minutes. Remove and spoon 2 cups cooked Black Beans into each shell; crumble 3-oz. Feta Cheese or Goat Cheese on top, dust with 1 tsp. Nacho Seasoning and sprinkle with Cilantro Leaves.

EASY BARBECUED BEANS

This recipe works for: Cancer Protection, Overcoming Addictions, Hair -Skin
Makes 4 servings: Preheat oven to 350°F.

Drain 4 cups any combination canned White Beans, Kidney Beans and Pinto Beans.
—In a large oven-ready skillet, sauté in 2 TBS Olive Oil for 5 minutes, 2 minced Cloves Garlic, and 1 chopped Onion. Stir in the beans, 1 can (16-oz.) chopped Plum Tomatoes with juice, $^1/_2$-lb. Ground Turkey (optional), $^1/_4$ cup Molasses, 2 TBS Sweet Hot Mustard, 1 TB Soy Bacon Bits, 1 TB snipped Dry Dulse and 1 cup Mesquite Barbecue Sauce. Simmer 3 minutes to blend and bake in the oven for 1 hour.

PORTABELLA-RED LENTIL SALAD

This recipe works for: Fatigue Syndromes, Overcoming Addictions, Anti-Aging
Makes 4 servings:

In a pan, stir $^1/_2$ cup minced Shallots in 1 tsp. Olive Oil until limp, about 3 minutes. Add 1 cup Red Lentils, 3 cups Organic Chicken Broth, and 2 tsp. Thyme. Bring to a boil, cover, reduce heat, and simmer about 10 minutes. Drain and set aside.
—Trim and rinse 4 Portabella Mushroom Caps. Sliver, then sizzle in a small skillet with 2 TBS Olive Oil 2 TBS Balsamic Vinegar and half a slivered Red Bell Pepper until soft and fragrant. Sprinkle with Garlic-Lemon Seasoning to taste and 1 TB Lemon Zest.
—Mound 4 cups Frisée Greens or mixed greens equally on salad plates; divide lentil mix on top, then mushroom-pepper mix. Spoon about 1 TB Lemon Mayonnaise onto each salad.

Nutrition; 307 calories; 19gm protein; 42gm carbo.; 9gm fiber; 7gm total fats; 0mg choles.; 77mg calcium; 6mg iron; 76mg magnes.; 874mg potassium; 39mg sodium; Vit. A 113 IU; Vit. C 27mg; Vit. E 2 IU.

BLACK BEAN SOUP

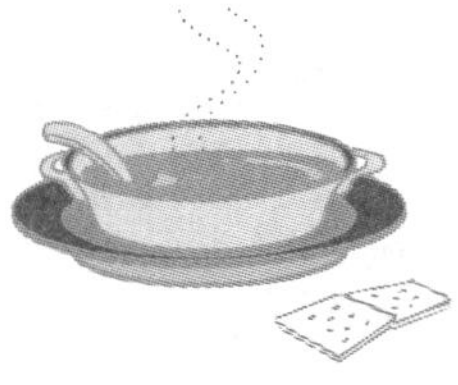

This recipe works for: Illness Recovery, Cancer Protection
For 6 to 8 servings:

Soak 1-lb. Black Turtle Beans overnight in a pot. Drain, rinse, and just cover with cold water. Bring to a boil, and cook until soft.
—As beans cook, sauté in 2 TBS Olive Oil for 8 minutes: 2 minced Cloves Garlic, 1 diced Onion, 2 diced Ribs Celery and 2 diced Carrots. Add to cooking beans; cover and cook until tender along with the beans. Remove from heat to slightly cool. Purée in the blender briefly.
—Return to the pot, and add 3 cups Organic Vegetable Broth, $^1/_2$ cup Red Wine, $^1/_4$ cup Lemon Juice, 1 teasp. Sea Salt, $^1/_2$ teasp. Pepper, $^1/_2$ teasp. Allspice. Pour into soup bowls and float a thin Lemon slice on top of each bowl.

Nutrition; 211 calories; 12gm protein; 32gm carbo.; 11gm fiber; 4gm total fats; 0mg choles.; 48mg calcium; 3mg iron; 88mg magnes.; 551mg potassium; 287mg sodium; Vit. A 509 IU; Vit. C 8mg; Vit. E 1 IU.

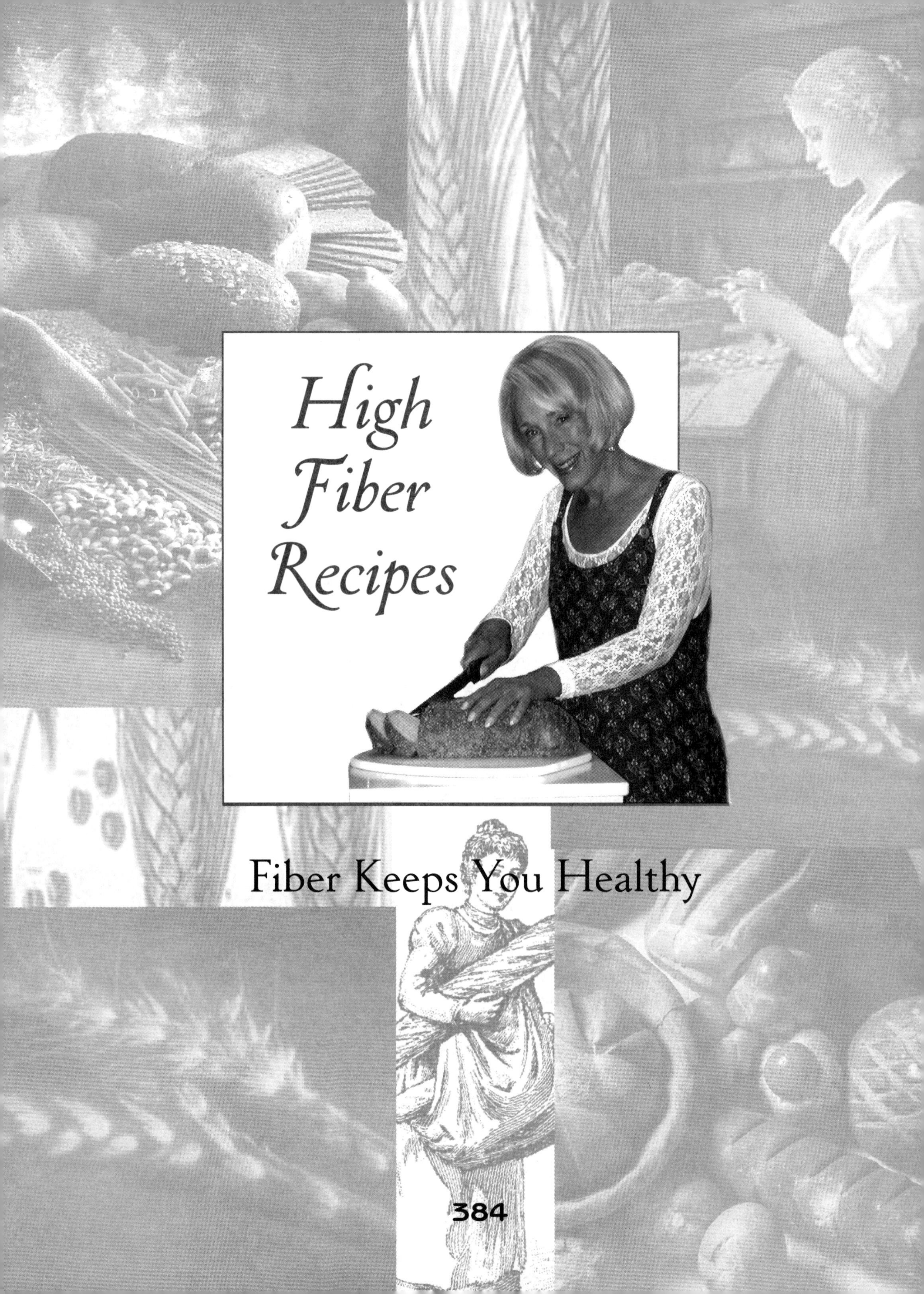

High Fiber Recipes

Fiber Keeps You Healthy

High Fiber Makes Your Day

Fiber from whole foods is the "mover and shaker" in your diet.... the metabolic companion of healthy complex carbohydrates.

Fiber foods are one of the few things in this world that give you something for nothing. Without adding calories or bulk, fiber helps control your weight, eases and regulates elimination, helps prevent cardiovascular problems, and acts as a colon and fat cleanser.

Fiber promotes healthy bacteria in your colon, and enhances body functions that keep harmful cholesterol and fat levels low.

Fiber foods slow down calorie absorption for weight control; they take up space in your stomach, making you feel full. Plant fiber also absorbs water in your small intestine, then passes through the colon acting as a "sweep," to help your body eliminate wastes.

Fiber helps you heal and protects against disease. Cancer, heart disease, gout, gallstones, high blood pressure, diabetes, anemia, elimination problems like Crohn's disease, colitis, diverticulitis, varicose veins, hemorrhoids, ulcers, chronic constipation and irritable bowel syndrome all respond to an increase in dietary fiber.

Fiber helps triglycerides, cholesterol, and blood sugar fluctuations. Adding high fiber foods helps control the moods swings, irritability and energy drops from these problems, and builds a feeling of well being for your emotions.

Fiber comes in several forms in food: cellulose, hemicellulose and lignan from brans and grains; pectin from fruits and vegetables; gums from legumes and some herbs; mucilages from seeds.

—Vegetable fiber sources include spinach, corn, peas, sweet potatoes, cucumbers, squashes, broccoli, cabbage, carrots, celery, potatoes and onions.

—Fruit fiber sources include strawberries, bananas, raisins, figs, pears, prunes, apples and avocados.

—Whole grain fiber sources include brown rice, oats, barley, and wild rice.

—Bean and legume fiber sources include lentils, split peas, pinto beans, and green beans.

More About Fiber and Cholesterol

Our bodies have two kinds of cholesterol. 1: High density lipo-protein (HDL - good cholesterol) is internally manufactured in the intestinal tract and liver. It serves as raw material for cell membranes, protects nerve sheathing, plays a role in the creation of vitamin D and sex hormones, and helps our circulatory systems transport cholesterol to the liver for removal as bile. 2: Low density lipo-protein (LDL - bad cholesterol), is a diet problem, usually from too much saturated fat, and low fiber, refined foods. Bad cholesterol causes harmful deposits that lodge in the blood vessels and become arterial plaque. For good health, the idea is to lower your body's LDL, and increase HDL. Still, while the ratio of HDL to LDL is important, the lower your total cholesterol level, the better. Every one percent increase in total blood cholesterol translates into a two percent increase in heart disease risk.

The strongest influence on blood cholesterol levels is saturated fat, especially from red meats. Saturated fats affect cholesterol levels <u>five times more</u> than bad dietary cholesterol (LDL). The second greatest influence is an excess of total fat calories.

High fiber foods help reduce harmful cholesterol. Boost your whole grains and brans, beans and legumes, fruits, leafy greens, and sea greens. Natural plant lipids (phytosterols), like those from olive, flax and canola oils also emulsify and lower harmful blood fats. High chlorophyll foods, like spirulina, chlorella, and dark leafy greens metabolize fats better. A glass or two of wine with dinner reduces stress and encourages good HDL production.

Fiber Rich Recipe Sections

For a health maintenance diet, a high fiber portion contains 2 or more grams of fiber. Add fiber to your diet gradually, to allow your body to adapt to more "roughage" easily. Low cholesterol means 100mg or less. Very low cholesterol means 30mg or less.

Fiber For Breakfast.... Make Your Day

My favorite fiber sources for breakfast? Fruits and whole grains. Fruits like prunes, apples, figs, dates, papaya and mangos, are well-known for their fiber. Grains for breakfast may sound bland when compared with meals loaded with butter and sugar, but replacing nutrition-poor additives with spices and herbs give grains both flavor and health benefits. Both herbs and spices contain powerful antioxidants or other phytochemicals that aid digestion, regulate cholesterol and blood sugar.

A.M.- P.M. FIBER DRINK An excellent drink for daily regularity.

This recipe works for: Waste Management, Better Digestion, Men's Health
Take 1 heaping tablespoon in juice in the morning and at bedtime.

Mix in the blender: 3 parts Oat Bran, 2 parts Flax Seed, 1 part Psyllium Husk Powder, 1/2 part Acidophilus Powder, 1/4 part Fennel Seed. May be stored in an airtight container.
—To make 1 drink in the blender: add 1 heaping tablespoon fiber mix, about 8-oz. Juice, 1 Banana, Honey to taste.

Nutrition per tablespoon; 40 calories; 2gm protein; 9gm carbohydrate; 4gm fiber; 1gm fat; 0 choles.; 66mg calcium; 2mg iron; 41mg magnesium; 137mg potass.; 5mg sodium; Vit. A 21 IU; Vit. C trace; Vit. E trace

PRUNE-APPLE SMOOTHIE for FIBER

This recipe works for: Waste Management, Liver-Organ Health, Kid's-Men's Health
Makes 2 drinks:

In a bowl, cover 6 - 8 Pitted Prunes with hot water and let stand until plump, about 15 minutes. Put prunes in the blender and reserve soaking water.
—Add to prunes and blend smooth: 1 cup Apple Juice, 1/2 cup Nonfat Vanilla Yogurt, 1/4 tsp. Cinnamon, 1/2 to 1 tsp. Vanilla Extract, 1/4 teasp. Nutmeg, 4 TBS Reserved Prune Water and 1 Banana, or 1/2 cup Crushed Ice.

PERFECT FIBER CEREAL

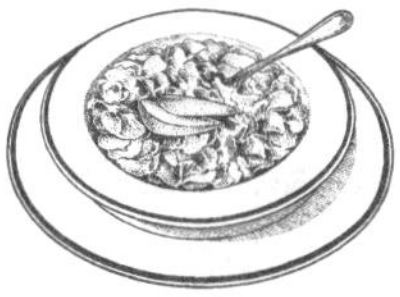

This recipe works for: Regularity, Cancer Protection
Makes about 3 cups:

Oven toast a nut and seed mix: 1/4 cup sliced Almonds, 1/4 cup Pumpkin Seeds, 1/4 cup Sunflower Seeds, 1/4 cup chopped Walnuts, pinches Cinnamon and Cardamom Powder.
—Soak 4-oz. Pitted Prunes, 4-oz. dried Apricots and 4-oz. dried Papaya in water to cover. Simmer over low heat to reduce liquid by half. Stir in 2 TBS Honey. Stir in 2 sectioned Oranges, 1 sliced Banana and nut mix. Serve warm or cold.

Nutrition; 55 calories; 1gm protein; 8gm carbo.; 3gm fiber; 2gm total fats; 0 choles.; 13mg calcium; 1mg iron; 22mg magnesium; 148mg potass.; 1mg sodium; Vit. A 36 IU; Vit. C 6mg; Vit. E 3 IU.

SWEET COUSCOUS with NUTS and DATES

This recipe works for: Men's Health, Allergies - Asthma, Illness Recovery
Makes 8 servings: Preheat oven to 350°F. Use a 13 x 9-inch baking dish.

Oven toast a nut and seed mix: 1/4 cup sliced Almonds, 1/4 cup Pumpkin Seeds, 1/4 cup Pine Nuts, 1/4 cup Sunflower Seeds, 1/4 cup Blanched Hazelnuts, 1/4 cup chopped Walnuts, 2 TBS Fructose, and pinches Cinnamon, Sea Salt and Cardamom Powder.

–Place 2 2/3 cups Couscous (about 1-lb.) in a large bowl. Bring 2 2/3 cups Water, 1/4 cup Fructose and 4 TBS Canola Oil to boil in a large saucepan, stirring to blend. Pour mixture over couscous and stir. Cover and let stand 10 minutes. Fluff with a fork. –Mix nuts and 8-oz. chopped Pitted Dates into couscous. Transfer couscous to baking dish. Cool and cover with foil. Bake couscous about 20 minutes. Spoon into bowls. Pass hot Vanilla Almond Milk or Vanilla Rice Milk at serving.

CARROT and RAISIN OATMEAL

This recipe works for: Kid's Health, Bone Building, Waste Management
For 4 servings:

Shred 2 Carrots in a food processor. Toss with 1/2 teasp. Sea Salt. Add to 4 cups Water. Bring to a rapid boil. Reduce heat to a simmer and cook for 4 minutes. Add 1/2 cup Raisins and cook for 3 minutes. Stir in 2/3 cup Oat Bran, 1 1/3 cups Rolled Oats, and 1/2 teasp. Cinnamon. Cook stirring until thick, about 5 minutes. Serve at once.

Nutrition; 220 calories; 8gm protein; 47gm carbo.; 7gm fiber; 2gm total fats; 0 choles.; 47mg calcium; 3mg iron; 58mg magnesium; 455mg potass.; 283mg sodium; Vit. A 1015 IU; Vit. C 5mg; Vit. E 1 IU.

PUMPKIN MUFFINS A special treat.

This recipe works for: Men's Health, Women's Balance, Heart Health
Makes 12 muffins: Preheat the oven to 350°F.

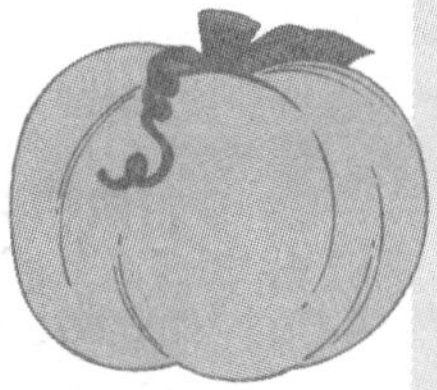

Dice the meat of a small Pumpkin (or Butternut Squash). You'll need 1 cup cooked Pumpkin Puree for the muffins. Cook in Salted Water. Then drain and puree in a blender til smooth. Set aside. Brush muffins tins with Canola Oil or line with paper muffin cups.

—Combine dry ingredients in a bowl: 2 cups Unbleached Flour, 1 1/2 cups Whole Wheat Pastry Flour, 2 TBS non-aluminum Baking Powder and 1/2 tsp. Sea Salt.

—In another bowl, whisk wet ingredients: 1/2 cup Canola Oil, 1 cup Maple Syrup, 1 cup Apple Juice, 1/2 cup Vanilla Almond Milk and the pumpkin puree. Turn the wet mixture into the dry mixture; combine them gently until just mixed.

—Divide between muffin cups. Bake for 50 minutes to 1 hour, until edges of muffins are golden brown. Let the muffins sit in a pan until cool.

RAISIN GRAPENUTS MUFFINS

This recipe works for: Men's Health, Digestive Health, Sports Nutrition

For 6 big deli-style Sunday breakfast muffins: Preheat oven to 375°. Use oiled pyrex custard cups. For 8 regular-size muffins: Preheat oven to 400°. Use paper-lined muffin cups in a muffin tin.

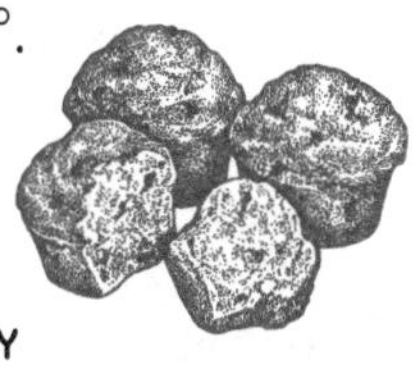

Mix dry ingredients: 1 cup Unbleached Flour, 1/2 cup Whole Wheat Pastry Flour, 1 cup Grapenuts, 1 cup Rolled Oats, 1 1/2 teasp. Baking Soda. Form a well in the center and pour in: 1 cup Plain Yogurt, 1/2 cup Honey, 1 Egg, 1/4 cup Canola Oil, 1/2 cup Raisins. Stir until lumpy and bake for 30 minutes until springy when touched.

Nutrition; 272 calories; 7gm protein; 50gm carbo.; 4gm fiber; 6gm total fats; 19 choles.; 51mg calcium; 7mg iron; 48mg magnesium; 219mg potass.; 270mg sodium; Vit. A 176 IU; Vit. C 2mg; Vit. E 2 IU.

OAT BRAN BANANA PANCAKES A treat for kids of all ages.

This recipe works for: Men's Health, Bone Building, Waste Management

For 18 pancakes: Preheat griddle until a drop of water skitters on the surface.

Toss together: 1 cup Oat Bran, 1 teasp. Baking Soda, 2 teasp. Fructose. Add 1 very ripe Banana, mashed, 1 1/2 cups Plain Yogurt and 2 teasp. Vanilla.

—Beat 4 Egg Whites to soft peaks. Fold into batter, and stir in 2 TBS melted Butter. Ladle 2 to 3 pancakes onto griddle or skillet, and spread into circles. Cook until bubbles appear on the surface, about 1 minute. Flip and cook until bottoms are brown, about 1 minute more. Serve hot with Maple Syrup or Honey.

Nutrition; 78 calories; 4gm protein; 14gm carbo.; 2gm fiber; 2gm total fats; 4choles.; 44mg calcium; 1mg iron; 32mg magnesium; 147mg potass.; 98mg sodium; Vit. A 16 IU; Vit. C 8mg; Vit. E trace

DRIED CHERRY-BANANA BREAD

This recipe works for: Men's and Kid's Health, Arthritis, Circulatory Health

Makes 2 medium loaves: Preheat oven to 350°F.

Soak 1/2 cup Dried Cherries in warm water for 30 minutes. Spray 2 medium loaf pans with Canola Oil Spray. In a large bowl, blend: 1/2 cup Unbleached Flour, 1/2 cup plus 2 TBS Whole Wheat Flour, 2 TBS Coarse Cornmeal, 1 tsp. Cinnamon, 1/2 tsp. Baking Powder, 1/4 tsp. Baking Soda, 1/4 tsp. Sea Salt and 1/4 tsp. Allspice.

—Blender blend until smooth: 1 very ripe Banana, 1/4 cup Turbinado Sugar, 3 TBS Honey, 1 Egg, 1 TB Canola Oil, 1/2 cup Vanilla Yogurt, 1/4 cup Orange Juice and 1 TB grated Orange Zest.

—Make a well in the dry ingredients, add wet ingredients to well; gently stir just until no specks of flour remain. Drain cherries and fold into batter. Spoon into the loaf pans. Bake until a toothpick inserted into center comes out clean, 45 minutes.

HONEY APPLE PANCAKES

This recipe works for: Men's - Kid's Health, Immune Power, Illness Recovery
For 8 pancakes: Preheat a griddle to hot.

Mix in a bowl: $1^1/_4$ cups WHOLE WHEAT PASTRY FLOUR, 1 teasp. BAKING POWDER, $^1/_4$ teasp. APPLE PIE SPICE, $^1/_4$ teasp. SEA SALT and $^1/_4$ teasp. BAKING SODA. Combine in another bowl: 1 EGG, $^3/_4$ cup APPLE JUICE, 2 TBS HONEY, 1 TB CANOLA OIL.

—Stir the two mixtures together until slightly lumpy. Ladle onto hot oiled griddle, turn when bubbles appear and cook for 1 more minute.

MOLASSES CORN MUFFINS

This recipe works for: Hair, Skin and Nails, Bone Building, Waste Management
For 12 muffins: Preheat oven to 400°.

Mix together gently: 1 cup YELLOW CORNMEAL, $1^1/_2$ cups UNBLEACHED FLOUR, 2 teasp. BAKING POWDER, $^1/_2$ teasp. BAKING SODA, 1 EGG, 1 cup PLAIN LOW FAT YOGURT, $^1/_2$ cup SPARKLING WATER, 2 TBS CANOLA OIL, 4 TBS UNSULPHURED MOLASSES, $^1/_2$ teasp. CINNAMON, pinch SEA SALT. Bake for 25 minutes until a toothpick inserted in a muffin comes out clean. Serve with MAPLE SYRUP.

Nutrition; 151 calories; 4gm protein; 25gm carbo.; 2gm fiber; 3gm total fats; 19choles.; 160mg calcium; 2mg iron; 36mg magnesium; 271mg potass.; 185mg sodium; Vit. A 17 IU; Vit. C 1mg; Vit. E 1 IU.

ORANGE FRENCH TOAST

This recipe works for: Men's Health, Bone Building, Illness Recovery
Makes 6 slices:

Whisk in a bowl: 3 EGGS, $^3/_4$ cup ORANGE JUICE, 1 tsp. grated ORANGE ZEST, $^1/_2$ tsp. CINNAMON and 2 TBS HONEY. Arrange bread slices in a 9 x 13-inch baking dish. Pour egg mixture over 6 slices WHOLE WHEAT SOURDOUGH BREAD, cover and refrigerate for at least 30 minutes.

—Heat a large nonstick skillet or griddle. Spray with CANOLA OIL. Add bread slices to pan in batches, cooking about 3 minutes on each side, until golden brown. Serve with MAPLE SYRUP.

Nutrition; 177 calories; 7gm protein; 30gm carbo.; 3gm fiber; 4gm total fats; 105 choles.; 49mg calcium; 2mg iron; 38mg magnesium; 201mg potass.; 217mg sodium; Vit. A 55 IU; Vit. C 16mg; Vit. E 1 IU.

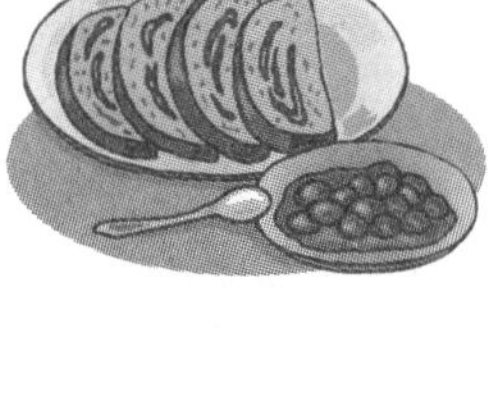

Vegetable Fiber Lowers Cholesterol

The medical world rule of thumb has been 180mg. or less of cholesterol for people under thirty, and 200mg. or less for people over thirty. Vegetarians find these levels easy to achieve, since most saturated fat and cholesterol comes from animal products. Total vegans average around 125mg; lacto-vegetarians average around 150 to 160mg.

HIGHLY SAVORY EGGPLANT

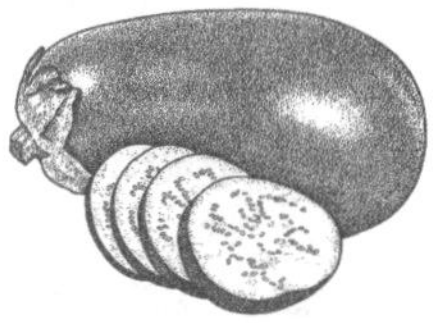

This recipe works for: Heart and Circulatory Health, Liver Health
Makes 4 servings: Preheat broiler.

Peel and cut 2-lbs. EGGPLANT into strips. Salt, sprinkle with 2 TBS chopped dried ONION, and set in a colander to drain for 30 minutes. Rinse, then place strips on OLIVE OIL sprayed baking sheets. Broil 3 to 4 inches from heat until browned. Turn strips over and brown other side, watching carefully. Insides should be soft.

—Heat a large OLIVE OIL sprayed wok. Add 2 TBS minced GINGER, 1 TB minced GARLIC and stir-fry for a few seconds, adding 4 to 6 drops TOASTED SESAME OIL to keep from sticking. Add broiled eggplant strips, 1 cup ORGANIC VEGETABLE BROTH, $^1/_4$ cup minced SCALLIONS, 2 TBS TAMARI, 2 TBS BALSAMIC VINEGAR, 1 TB SHERRY, $^1/_2$ TBS HOISIN SAUCE and 1 tsp. FRUCTOSE. Toss over high heat for 2 minutes. Stir in 1 TB ARROWROOT POWDER dissolved in 2 TBS WATER and stir until thickened. Drizzle with $^1/_2$ teasp. TOASTED SESAME OIL, toss briefly and transfer to warm serving dish.

Nutrition; 136 calories; 4gm protein; 23gm carbo.; 6gm fiber; 4gm total fats; 0 choles.; 33mg calcium; 1mg iron; 40mg magnesium; 578mg potass.; 482mg sodium; Vit. A 22 IU; Vit. C 7mg; Vit. E 1 IU.

FAST GOURMET RATATOUILLE

This recipe works for: Men's Health, Waste Management, Heart Health
Makes 6 servings:

Place 6 cups EGGPLANT cubes (about 3 small) in a colander in the sink. Sprinkle with 1 teasp. SEA SALT and 2 teasp. BALSAMIC VINEGAR; toss to mix. Let stand 15 minutes, then rinse under cold running water. Drain well. Pat dry with paper towels.

—In a large, wide skillet, heat 1 TB OLIVE OIL. Sizzle eggplant until golden at edges, about 6 to 7 minutes. Add 2 thin sliced ONIONS, 1 thin sliced RED BELL PEPPER, and 2 minced CLOVES GARLIC; cook, stirring occasionally, until golden, about 5 minutes. Add 2 cubed ZUCCHINI and stir about 5 minutes. Stir in one can (28-oz.) crushed TOMATOES with juice, $^1/_4$ cup RED WINE, $^1/_2$ tsp. CRACKED PEPPER, $^1/_4$ cup snipped FRESH BASIL and $^1/_4$ tsp. HERBS DE PROVENCE and bring to a boil. Reduce heat and simmer briskly until vegetables are tender and sauce has thickened slightly, about 7 minutes. Remove from heat and stir in basil. Serve hot or at room temperature.

Nutrition; 98 calories; 3gm protein; 16gm carbo.; 5gm fiber; 3gm total fats; 0 choles.; 61mg calcium; 2mg iron; 44mg magnesium; 665mg potass.; 257mg sodium; Vit. A 180 IU; Vit. C 51mg; Vit. E 2 IU.

GRILLED ONIONS and RADICCHIO

This recipe works for: Hair, Skin and Nails, Bone Building, Waste Management
For 4 people: Preheat and oil grill.

Separate segments from 4 Navel Oranges and set aside. Squeeze out as much juice as possible from peel into a bowl; grate about 1 tsp. Orange Zest from the peel.

—Mix the small amount of juice and the zest with 4 teasp. Sherry, 2 teasp. Olive Oil, and 1 teasp. Lemon-Pepper. Toss half with 1 large head separated Radicchio Leaves. Toss half with the orange segments and arrange them on a serving platter.

—Brush slices of 1 large Red Onion with 1 teasp. Olive Oil, and sprinkle with Sea Salt and Pepper. Roast about 4" from coals until soft and just beginning to blacken. Turn onto serving platter. Grill radicchio leaves from 2 to 4 minutes until softened, slightly brown and fragrant. Arrange on platter with the rest and serve hot.

Nutrition; 118 calories; 2gm protein; 21gm carbo.; 3gm fiber; 4gm total fats; 0 choles.; 72mg calcium; 1mg iron; 23mg magnesium; 402mg potass.; 142mg sodium; Vit. A 27 IU; Vit. C 86mg; Vit. E 1 IU.

HIGH FIBER HASH BROWNS

This recipe works for: Sports Nutrition, Men's Health
For 8 servings:

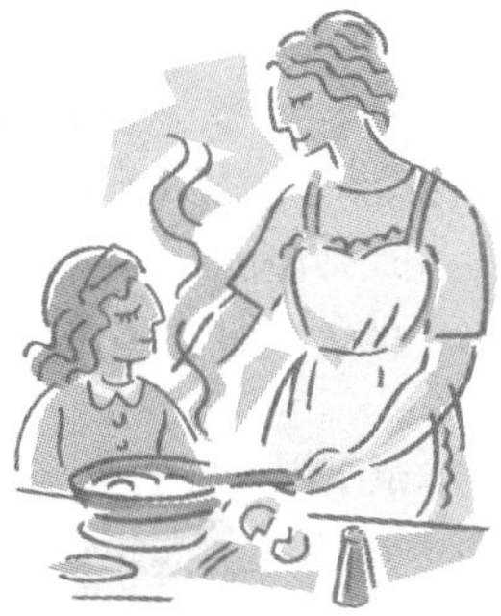

Boil 5 Red Potatoes in water over high heat for 5 minutes. Drain and set aside. —Dry toast 2 TBS Soy Bacon Bits in a large skillet about 5 minutes. Add 2 TBS Olive Oil and 2 large thin sliced Onions; sauté for 25 minutes; set aside.

—Grate potatoes in a food processor; season with $^1/_2$ tsp. Sea Salt, $^1/_2$ tsp. Fructose, and $^1/_4$ tsp. Pepper. Add 2 TBS Olive Oil and the potatoes to the skillet. Press against bottom and sides to form a crust. Cook for 15 minutes until brown on the bottom. Drizzle on 1 TB Olive Oil, $^1/_2$ tsp. Garlic-Lemon Seasoning and 1 teasp. Rosemary. Mix in onions, and run under the broiler for 1 minute to brown and crisp. Serve hot.

SWEET CARROT CRUNCH

This recipe works for: Cancer Protection, Sugar Imbalances, Respiratory Health
For 4 servings:

Cut 6 to 8 medium Carrots in matchsticks. Cook covered in Salted Water until just barely tender. Drain, remove from pan and set aside.

—Melt $1^1/_2$ TBS Butter in the pan. Add $1^1/_2$ TBS Maple Syrup, $1^1/_2$ TBS grated Orange Zest, and 4 TBS slivered Almonds or chopped Walnuts. Simmer until a fragrant sauce forms. Return carrots to pan and toss to heat through, about 3 minutes.

Nutrition; 141 calories; 2gm protein; 18gm carbo.; 4gm fiber; 8gm total fats; 12 choles.; 55mg calcium; 1mg iron; 35mg magnesium; 424mg potass.; 93mg sodium; Vit. A 3079 IU; Vit. C 13mg; Vit. E 3 IU.

POTLUCK VEGETABLE BAKE

This recipe works for: Women's Health, Bone Building, Immune Power
For 6 people: Preheat oven to 350°. Use a 9 x 13" shallow baking dish.

In a large skillet, sauté 2 sliced Yellow Onions in 2 TBS Olive Oil for 3 minutes. Add and stir briefly: 2 Carrots sliced in thin matchsticks, $^1/_2$ head Green Cabbage thin sliced, 2 cakes (8-oz.) cubed Firm Tofu, 1 TB Tamari, $^1/_4$ cup White Wine, $^1/_4$ cup Water. Add 1 small head thin sliced Swiss Chard; toss to coat.

—Mix the topping in a bowl: 1 cup Whole Grain Bread Crumbs, $^1/_4$ cup Olive Oil, $^1/_2$ cup grated Parmesan Cheese, 1 TB dry Basil, $^1/_2$ teasp. dry Oregano, 1 teasp. Paprika and $^1/_2$ teasp. Pepper. Spoon veggies into the baking dish. Sprinkle with topping, and bake for 15 to 20 minutes until brown and bubbly.

Nutrition; 258 calories; 13gm protein; 17gm carbo.; 4gm fiber; 16gm total fats; 6 choles.; 270mg calcium; 6mg iron; 102mg magnesium; 545mg potass.; 289mg sodium; Vit. A 856 IU; Vit. C 27mg; Vit. E 4 IU.

SWEET ANNA YAMS

This recipe works for: Men's - Women's Health, Bone Building, Sugar Imbalances
For 6 people: Preheat oven to 425°. Use a 9-inch cake pan.

Cut 2-lbs. Yams in paper thin slices. Heat 4 TBS Butter and 4 TBS Canola Oil with 1 teasp. Nutmeg, $^1/_2$ teasp. Sea Salt and $^1/_4$ teasp. White Pepper. Drizzle some on the bottom of cake pan. Arrange $^1/_6$ of the yam slices in overlapping rounds to cover bottom. Drizzle with butter mix, and sprinkle with 1 TB Parmesan Cheese. Repeat layers until ingredients are used. Cover pan with foil and press down to compress.

—Bake on the lowest oven rack for 30 minutes. Uncover and bake 45 minutes longer, until edges are crisp and brown. Let stand for a few minutes to concentrate texture. Drain off butter. Loosen yams around the edges. Place a round plate on top of the pan, invert and remove pan. Cut in wedges to serve.

FIBER VEGGIE TOSS

This recipe works for: Men's - Women's Health, Immune Power, Heart Health
For 4 people as a main dish:

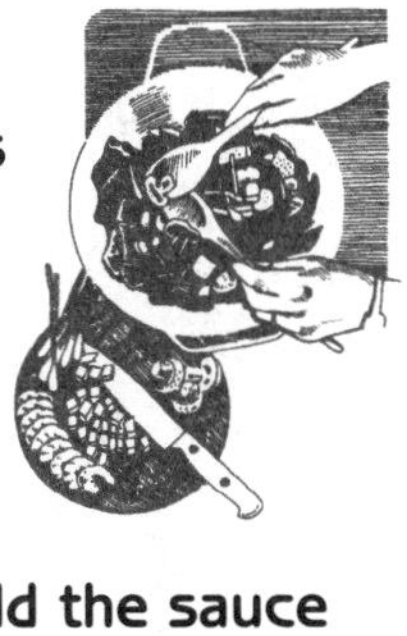

Have ready: 4 cups sliced Celery, 1 cup trimmed Snow Peas, $2^1/_2$ cups sliced Mushrooms, 1 cup thin sliced Onions, 1 slivered Red Bell Pepper,

—Mix the sauce: 1 TB Tamari, 2 TBS Arrowroot Powder, 1 teasp. Sherry, 1 teasp. Fructose and $^1/_2$ teasp. Hot Chili Oil.

—Heat a wok for 1 minute. Add 1 TB Canola Oil and 1 teasp. Toasted Sesame Oil. Heat briefly. Add celery, bell pepper and onions. Sizzle for 3 minutes. Add mushrooms and snow peas and $1^3/_4$ cups Miso Broth. Add the sauce and bring to a boil. Let bubble until thickened. Serve over crispy Chinese Noodles.

Fiber from Rice, Pasta and Whole Grains

Fiber from whole grains, pasta and rice helps regulate blood sugar, prevents constipation, protects the heart by lowering cholesterol, and fights many cancers. Fiber helps you lose weight by helping you to feel full longer. Attention pasta lovers! Just one cup of cooked whole grain pasta contains the same amount of fiber as $^1/_2$ cup of oat bran- 6 grams. My personal favorite choice is brown rice because it goes well with almost everything and is also high in insoluble fiber, recently shown to protect women's heart health as they age.

COUNTRY CORN BREAD STUFFING

This recipe works for: Women's Health, Heart Health, Bladder-Kidney Health
For 8 servings: Preheat oven to 350°.

Heat 1 cup Cranberries in a pan until they pop. Toast $^3/_4$ cup chopped Walnuts.
—Sauté 1 large chopped Onion in 2 TB Olive Oil for 10 minutes. Add 8-oz. sliced Tofu Hotdogs; sauté 5 more minutes. Turn into a large baking bowl. Add 1 TB Butter and let sizzle 1 minute. Then add 3 cups crumbled Whole Grain Bread, 2 chopped Tart Apples, the cooked cranberries, the toasted walnuts, 1 teasp. crumbled Sage Leaves or Poultry Seasoning, $^1/_4$ cup snipped Fresh Parsley and $1^1/_2$ cups crumbled Cornbread; toss to coat. Turn into the baking bowl with onions and tofu. Pour on $^1/_2$ cup Organic Chicken Broth, $^1/_4$ cup Sherry and $^1/_4$ cup Plain Yogurt. Bake 30 minutes until golden.

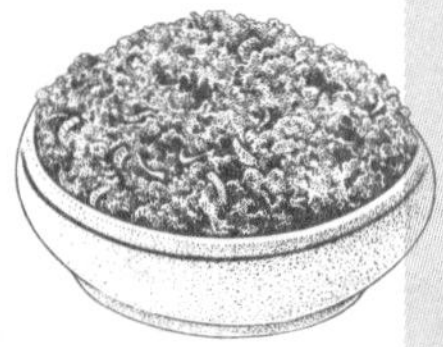

Nutrition; 364 calories; 13gm protein; 35gm carbo.; 5gm fiber; 21gm total fats; 17 choles.; 176mg calcium; 3mg iron; 77mg magnesium; 315mg potass.; 331mg sodium; Vit. A 42 IU; Vit. C 8mg; Vit. E 3 IU.

PRUNE WALNUT MUFFINS

This recipe works for: Waste Management, Sugar Imbalances, Heart Health
For 18 muffins: Preheat oven to 350°.

Mix the dry ingredients in a large bowl: 1 cup Whole Wheat Pastry Flour, $^1/_2$ cup Toasted Wheat Germ, $^1/_2$ cup Grapenuts, 1 TB Baking Powder and $^1/_4$ teasp. Baking Soda. Add fruits, nuts and spices: 1 cup diced Prunes, $1^1/_2$ teasp. Cinnamon, $^1/_2$ cup diced Walnuts, $^1/_2$ teasp. Powdered Ginger and $^1/_4$ teasp. Nutmeg.
—Mix the wet ingredients in a large pan and heat until syrupy: $^1/_2$ cup Plain Yogurt, $^1/_2$ cup Water, 2 Eggs, 2 TBS Frozen Orange Juice Concentrate, 3 TBS soft Butter and 3 TBS Honey. Add to dry ingredients in the bowl and combine until just gently moistened. Pour into Canola Oil sprayed muffin tins or paper-lined muffin cups and bake for 20 to 25 minutes until a toohpick inserted in the center comes out clean.

Nutrition; 154 calories; 5gm protein; 25gm carbo.; 3gm fiber; 5gm total fats; 28 choles.; 89mg calcium; 3mg iron; 41mg magnesium; 225mg potass.; 122mg sodium; Vit. A 112 IU; Vit. C 4mg; Vit. E 2 IU.

BROWN RICE SPOONBREAD

I call it yeast free bread without density.

This recipe works for: Men's Health, Heart Health, Weight Control
For 6 servings: Preheat oven to 375°.

Have ready 2 cups Cooked Brown Rice.
—Combine 1 cup Yellow Cornmeal and 1 cup Boiling Water; let stand for an hour.
—Separate 2 Eggs. Combine the Egg Yolks with $^1/_2$ cup Plain Yogurt, $^1/_2$ cup Water, 3 TBS Canola Oil, 1 teasp. Honey and $^1/_2$ teasp. Sea Salt. Pour over cornmeal and mix well. Mix in the brown rice.
—Beat the Egg Whites to stiff peaks and fold in gently (very important for lightness). Pour into a 9" square pan and bake for 40 to 45 minutes until puffed and golden; shrinking slightly from the sides of the pan. Let cool for 5 minutes.

IRON SKILLET CORN BREAD

This recipe works for: Women's Health, Heart Health, Bladder-Kidney Health
For a 9 x 9" pan or cast iron skillet; 9 pieces: Preheat oven to 425°.

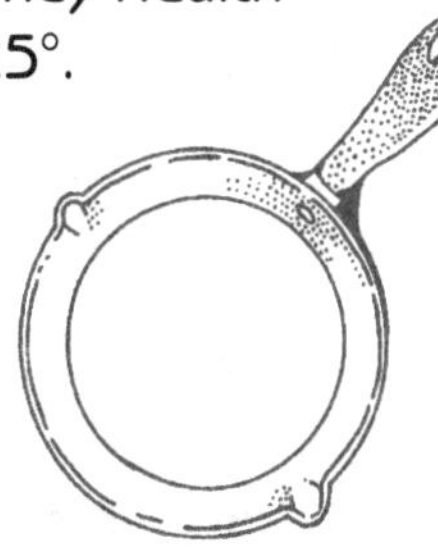

Combine dry ingredients: 1 cup Unbleached Flour, $1^1/_2$ cups Yellow Cornmeal, 2 TBS Toasted Wheat Germ, 2 TBS Fructose, 4 teasp. Baking Powder and $^1/_2$ teasp. Sea Salt.
—Blender blend the wet ingredients: 2 Eggs, 1 cup Plain Yogurt, $^1/_2$ cup Water, $^1/_4$ cup Canola Oil and 2 TBS Maple Syrup.
—Stir the two together just to moisten. Pour into cast iron skillet, or an oil sprayed 9 x 9" pan and bake for 20 minutes until springy and golden.

HARVEST GRAIN and VEGGIE BAKE

This recipe works for: Men's Health, Heart Health, Cancer Protection
For 8 people: Preheat oven to 425°.

Slice 6 small Zucchini into rounds. Salt and place in a colander to drain.
—Bring 2 cups Organic Vegetable Broth to a boil. Add 1 cup Brown Basmati Rice. Cover, reduce heat and steam for 25 minutes until water is absorbed. Toss rice with 2 TBS Parmesan Cheese and 2 TBS snipped Fresh Cilantro. Set aside.
—Sauté for 2 minutes in a skillet: 1 minced Clove Garlic and 1 diced Onion, 2 TBS Butter and 2 TBS Olive Oil. Add $^1/_2$ diced Yellow Bell Pepper, 1-lb. chopped Tomatoes and the Zucchini. Reduce heat; simmer until most of the tomato juice is evaporated. Mix with the cooked rice, and put in a Olive Oil sprayed baking dish. Sprinkle with Whole Grain Bread Crumbs, Sunflower Seeds, Parmesan Cheese, and Lemon-Pepper to taste. Bake for 30 minutes. Cool slightly to set and serve.

Nutrition; 209 calories; 5gm protein; 31gm carbo.; 4gm fiber; 8gm total fats; 9 choles.; 61mg calcium; 1mg iron; 33mg magnesium; 389mg potass.; 79mg sodium; Vit. A 123 IU; Vit. C 29mg; Vit. E 2 IU.

QUICK COUSCOUS & BROCCOLI FRITTATA

This recipe works for: Women's Health, Heart Health, Bladder-Kidney Health
For 4 people: Preheat oven to 350°.

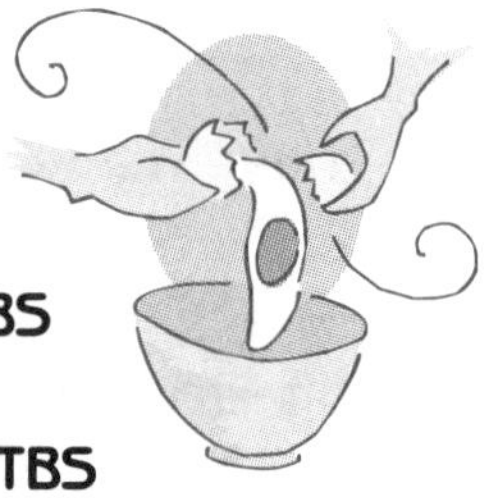

Have ready 2 cups cooked Couscous.

—Blanch 1 cup diced Broccoli in boiling Salted Water until color changes to bright green. Drain and remove from heat. Sauté 4 TBS diced Onion in 2 teasp. Olive Oil for 5 minutes.

—Mix couscous, broccoli and onion together in a bowl with 3 TBS Parmesan Cheese, 2 beaten Eggs, 2 TBS Lemon Mayonnaise, 2 TBS Plain Yogurt, 1/2 teasp. Sea Salt and 1/4 teasp. Pepper. Turn into an Olive Oil-sprayed casserole dish. Sprinkle with 1/3 cup shredded Low Fat Mozarrella Cheese and bake for 25 minutes until set.

BROWN RICE SALAD

This recipe works for: Bladder-Kidney Health, Sexual Health, Weight Control
For 6 servings:

Have ready 3 cups cooked Short Grain Brown Rice. Toss rice in a bowl with 3/4 cup Low Fat Italian Vinaigrette Dressing, the sliced kernels from 3 Ears Steamed Corn (or a 16-oz. can), 1 cup steamed French Cut Green Beans, 2 sliced Red Radishes, 2 TBS snipped Fresh Parsley, 3/4 cup crumbled Feta Cheese, and 1 small, peeled, cubed Cucumber. Sprinkle on pinches Italian Herbs to taste. Serve in Boston Lettuce cups.

Nutrition; 257 calories; 8gm protein; 48gm carbo.; 4gm fiber; 4gm total fats; 12 choles.; 113mg calcium; 2mg iron; 72mg magnesium; 392mg potass.; 364mg sodium; Vit. A 67 IU; Vit. C 14mg; Vit. E 1 IU.

RICE LAYERS

This recipe works for: Women's Health, Heart Health, Weight Control
For 6 people: Preheat the oven to 350°. Use an olive oiled 8 x 8" square pan.

Mix and toss 3 cups cooked Brown Basmati Rice with 1 teasp. Tamari, 1 teasp. dry Basil, 1/2 cup minced Fresh Parsley, and 1/3 cup sliced Almonds.

—Sauté 3 large diced Onions and 3 minced Shallots in 2 TBS Olive Oil 10 minutes. Add 1 Red Bell Pepper in thin strips and sauté for 3 minutes.

—Assemble layers in the baking pan. Spoon a layer of rice over the bottom. Cover with a layer of Low Fat Ricotta Cheese. Cover with a layer of onions and peppers. Repeat layers. Cover top with grated Parmesan-Reggiano Cheese. Bake for 20 to 25 minutes to warm through, and run under the broiler for 30 seconds to brown top.

—Try it: Just as good.... broccoli-zucchini or mushroom and sliced turkey layers instead of onions and peppers.

Nutrition; 306 calories; 11gm protein; 35gm carbo.; 4gm fiber; 13gm total fats; 22 choles.; 267mg calcium; 2mg iron; 76mg magnesium; 345mg potass.; 272mg sodium; Vit. A 146 IU; Vit. C 36mg; Vit. E 4 IU.

CARROT OAT BRAN MUFFINS

This recipe works for: Waste Management, Heart Health, Bone Building
For 12 big muffins: Preheat oven to 325°.

Mix dry ingredients: 1/2 cup Whole Wheat Pastry Flour, 1/2 cup Unbleached Flour, 1/2 cup Oat Bran, 1 teasp. Baking Soda, 1 teasp. Baking Powder, 1/2 teasp. Sea Salt, 1 teasp. Allspice and 1/2 teasp. Cardamom Powder.

—Mix wet ingredients; 2/3 cup Canola Oil, 2/3 cup Honey, 2 TBS Maple Syrup, 2 Eggs and 1 1/2 cups grated Carrots. Mix gently to moisten, spoon into paper muffin cups or greased muffin tins, and bake for about 30 minutes until springy when touched.

Nutrition; 236 calories; 3gm protein; 29gm carbo.; 3gm fiber; 13gm total fats; 35 choles.; 47mg calcium; 1mg iron; 22mg magnesium; 121mg potass.; 240mg sodium; Vit. A 403 IU; Vit. C 2mg; Vit. E 5 IU.

HONEY of a PASTA SALAD

This recipe works for: Women's Health, Heart Health, Bladder-Kidney Health
For 4 to 6 servings:

Bring 2 qts. Salted Water to a boil; cook 2 cups Vegetable Rotelli Spirals for 9 minutes. Rinse in cold water and drain. Toss with 1 teasp. Olive Oil. Set aside.

—Sauté 3 TBS Soy Bacon Bits and 3 TBS chopped Walnuts in 1 TB Olive Oil for 6 minutes until fragrant and brown. Add to pasta and set aside.

—Mix the sauce in a bowl: 1/2 cup diced Celery, 1/2 cup shredded Carrot, 1 sliced Green Onion, 1/3 cup Low Fat Mayonnaise, 1 TB Honey and 1/2 teasp. Cracked Pepper. Add to pasta and toss together. Serve on mounded Baby Spinach Leaves.

Fiber from Beans and Legumes

Beans and legumes are loaded with friendly fiber. A 3" piece of any sea vegetable added to bean cooking water increases assimilation and digestibility.

BUTTERY BEANS and PINE NUTS

This recipe works for: Men's Health, Heart Health, Arthritis
For 4 servings:

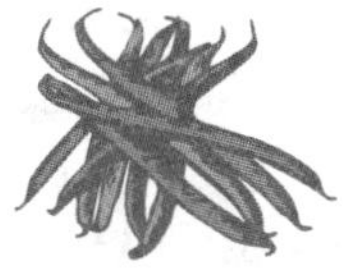

Blanch a 20-oz. package Italian Green Beans in boiling water for 3 minutes. Drain.

—Sizzle BUTTER SAUCE in a small pan until golden: 3 TBS Butter, 1 teasp. Sea Salt, 1 TB Sesame Seeds, 1/4 cup snipped Parsley, 1/2 teasp. Lemon-Pepper, 1 cup Pine Nuts and a pinch Thyme Leaves. Toss with beans and serve hot.

HOT CINNAMON-LEMON LENTILS

This recipe works for: Detoxification, Heart Health, Men's Health
For 6 servings:

Sauté 1 large sliced Onion and 1 minced Clove Garlic in 2 TBS Canola Oil until transparent. Add and sauté until fragrant: 1 TB minced Crystallized Ginger, 1-lb. rinsed Lentils, $^1/_4$ teasp. Hot Pepper Sauce, $^1/_4$ teasp. Sweet Paprika, 2 Bay Leaves and 2 broken Cinnamon Sticks. Add $3^1/_2$ cups Organic Chicken Broth. Lower heat, cover and cook for 15 to 20 minutes until lentils are tender. Add 2 TBS Lemon Juice and 1 teasp. Lemon-Pepper. Remove bay leaves and cinnamon sticks. Serve hot.

Nutrition; 335 calories; 25gm protein; 48gm carbo.; 11gm fiber; 6gm total fats; 0 choles.; 61mg calcium; 7mg iron; 86mg magnesium; 844mg potassium; 390mg sodium; Vit. A 11 IU; Vit. C 9mg; Vit. E 2 IU.

FANCY FIBER BEANS

This recipe works for: Illness Recovery, Reproductive Health, Men's Health
For 6 servings: Mayacamas Mushroom Soup Mix is available at health food stores.

Blanch 1 pkg. (16-oz.) Frozen French-Cut Green Beans in hot water for 3 minutes.

—Make the <u>sauce recipe</u> of 1 package Mayacamas Mushroom Soup Mix. Combine with drained green beans in a mixing bowl. Add $^1/_4$ cup Sherry, 1 can (7-oz.) Sliced Water Chestnuts, 1 teasp. Sweet Hot Mustard, $^1/_2$ teasp. Herbal Seasoning Salt, $^1/_4$ teasp. Thyme, $^1/_4$ teasp. Lemon-Pepper, $^1/_2$ cup grated Low Fat Cheddar Cheese and $^1/_4$ cup Low Fat Cream Cheese. Turn into a shallow casserole. Sprinkle with more grated Cheddar to cover, and scatter with Crunchy Chinese Noodles. Bake 30 minutes to heat and crisp.

FIBER BEANS and ARTICHOKES BAKE

This recipe works for: Sexuality, Osteoporosis, Arthritis, Overcoming Addictions
Makes 8 servings:

In a large pot, heat 2 TBS Olive Oil; stir in 1 minute until fragrant: 2 TBS minced Crystallized Ginger Root, $^1/_4$ teasp. Coriander Powder and $1^1/_2$ teasp. Cumin Seeds. Add 2 diced Carrots, 2 diced Ribs Celery, 1 diced Red Bell Pepper, and stir 5 minutes.

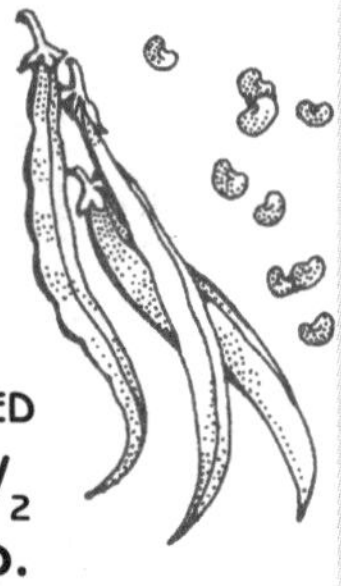

—Add 1 can ready-to-eat Fava Beans, or 10-oz. package Lima Beans. Add 1 jar (11-oz.) Water-Packed Artichoke Hearts, $^1/_4$ cup slivered Sun-Dried Tomatoes, $1^1/_2$ cups Organic Low-Fat Chicken Broth, $^3/_4$ teasp. Sea Salt, $^1/_2$ teasp. Turmeric, $^1/_2$ teasp. Sweet Paprika, $^1/_4$ teasp. Saffron Threads, $^1/_2$ teasp. Nutmeg, 1 TB Lime Juice. Simmer 15 minutes. Add 8-oz. Frozen French-Cut Green Beans; let steam until green, 3 minutes. Remove from heat and serve over cooked Cous-Cous and top with $^2/_3$ cup snipped Fresh Cilantro Leaves.

MILD MIXED VEGETABLE CHILI

This recipe works for: Sports Nutrition, Men's-Kid's Health, Liver-Organ Health
For 8 to 10 servings, (left-overs for another delicious meal).

Combine ingredients in a large pot: 2 cups cooked Black Beans, 32-oz. canned chopped Tomatoes, 2 diced Onions, 1 cubed, peeled Eggplant, 2 cubed Zucchini, 1 chopped Red Bell Pepper, $1^1/_2$ cups Corn Kernels, $^1/_3$ cup snipped Fresh Parsley, 2 TBS Chili Powder, 2 TBS dry Basil, 2 TBS dry Oregano, 1 TB dry Dill Weed, $1^1/_2$ TB Cumin Powder, 2 teasp. Garlic-Lemon Seasoning and 1 cup Organic Chicken Broth. Cook about $1^1/_2$ hours.

BAKED BEANS with VEGETABLES

This recipe works for: Men's Health, Sports Nutrition, Waste Management
For 6 servings: Preheat oven to 375°F.

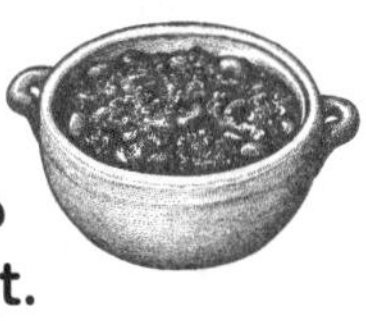

Put 2 cups dry Navy Beans in a pot with 6 cups Water and 1 teasp. Sea Salt. Simmer covered, about two hours. Drain and mix with 1 diced Red Bell Pepper, $^3/_4$ cup Molasses, 2 diced Red Onions, 2 TBS Coarse Ground Mustard, $^1/_2$ teasp. Garlic Powder and $^1/_2$ teasp. Cinnamon. Turn into a 3-qt. baking dish and bake covered for 1 hour.

Nutrition; 380 calories; 16gm protein; 77gm carbo.; 7gm fiber; 2gm total fats; 0 choles.; 473mg calcium; 12mg iron; 236mg magnesium; 2165mg potass.; 283mg sodium; Vit. A 71 IU; Vit. C 26mg; Vit. E 1 IU.

BEAN BURGERS very digestible with a delicate sweet-hot flavor.

This recipe works for: Candida Healing, Weight Control, Overcoming Allergies
For 10 patties: Preheat oven to 350°.

Have ready $1^1/_2$ cups cooked Short Grain Brown Rice.

—Soak 1 cup dry Azuki Beans overnight in water to cover. Drain soaking water; add 3 cups Salted Water to a large pot. Cook beans for about 1 hour until tender.

—Mix cooked beans with the cooked rice in a bowl; mix in 1 teasp. Sesame Seeds, $^1/_2$ cup Whole Wheat Bread Crumbs, 1 diced Red Bell Pepper, $^1/_2$ cup snipped Scallions, 1 TB Chinese 5-Spice Powder, 2 TBS Tamari, 1 TB minced Crystallized Ginger, $^1/_2$ teasp. Sea Salt and $^1/_4$ teasp. Hot Pepper Sauce.

—Form into 10 patties. Roll in Toasted Sesame Seeds, and put on Olive Oil-sprayed baking sheets. Bake until piping hot in the center, 15 to 20 minutes. Serve on toasted rice cakes or buns with Sunflower Sprouts and....

—QUICK HOT and SOUR SAUCE: heat and stir for 5 minutes, $1^1/_2$ TBS Sherry, 2 TBS Tamari, 1 TB Toasted Sesame Oil, 1 pinch Stevia Powder, $^1/_2$ teasp. Hot Pepper Sauce, 1 TB Brown Rice Vinegar and 1 snipped Green Onion.

Nutrition; 178calories; 7gm protein; 33gm carbo.; 2gm fiber; 2gm total fats; 0 choles.; 35mg calcium; 2mg iron; 6mg magnesium; 418mg potass.; 474mg sodium; Vit. A 49 IU; Vit. C 16mg; Vit. E trace.

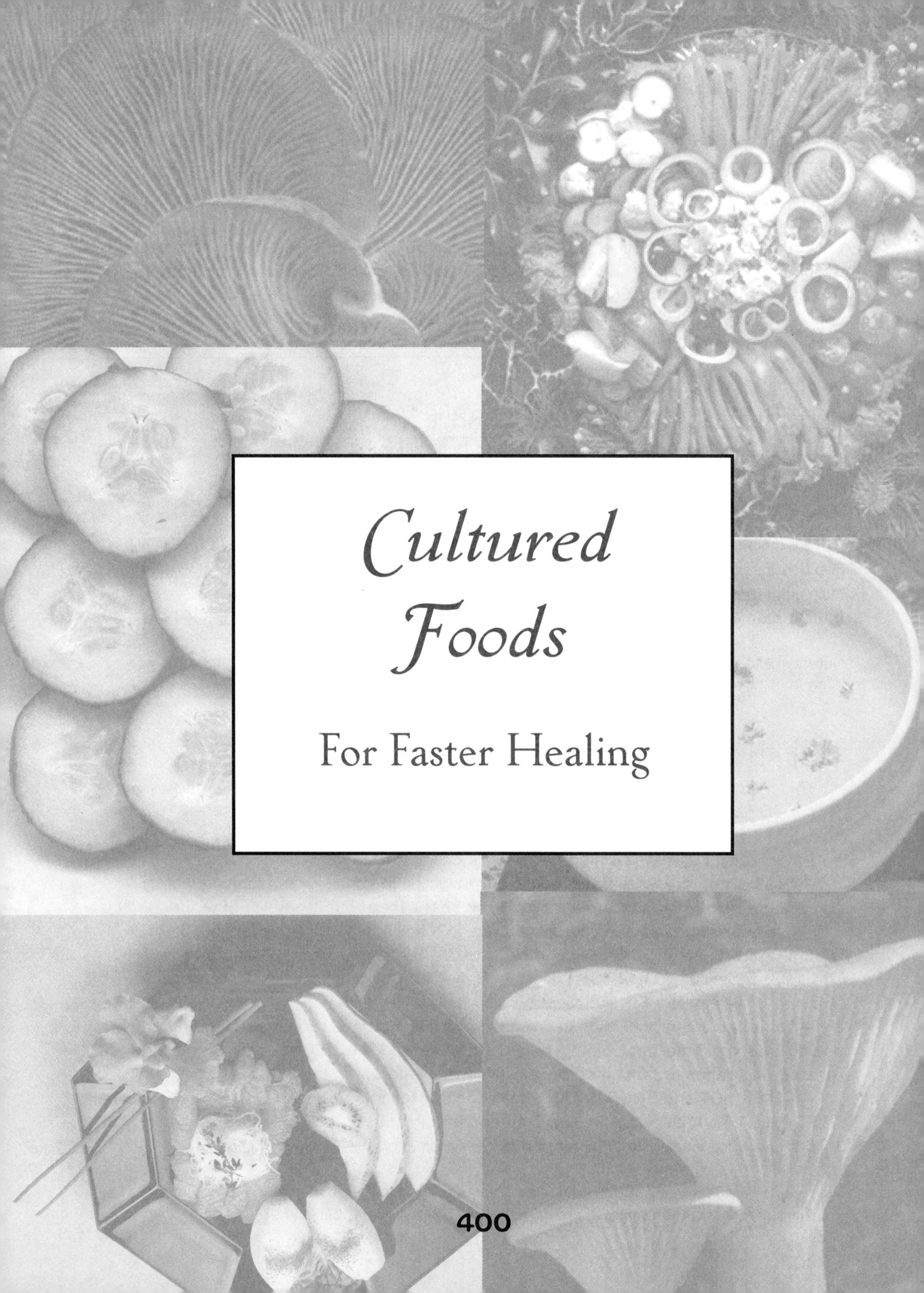

Cultured Foods

For Faster Healing

Cultured Foods For Healing

Cultured foods can be an important, even critical, part of your healing program. Cultured foods promote acid-alkaline balance (important for disease prevention), strengthen the digestive system with enzymes that inhibit pathogens, and build immune response. They are a specific for *Candida Albicans*, lactose intolerance and all malabsorption problems. For more information on adding "culture" to your healing diet, see *Cultured Foods Offer Healing Probiotics*, pages 58-66 in my **Cooking For Healthy Healing Diet Book.**

My favorite cultured foods for healing:

Yogurt: a cultured dairy food, is a key immune response stimulant. Studies show people who eat yogurt with active cultures produce four times more *gamma interferon*, a natural immune booster with anti-viral action. Yogurt can fight diarrhea caused by antibiotic overload, and lower cholesterol. Yogurt even normalizes vaginal pH against *Candida* overgrowth. Research shows that eating just one cup of yogurt daily reduces *Candida Albicans* yeast living in the vagina by three times. Note: Full-fat yogurt products should be avoided by people with bladder infections and dairy intolerance. Low fat and non-fat yogurt are better tolerated.

Kefir: thought by many experts to be a better cultured dairy choice than yogurt because it contains twice as much friendly bacteria and has substantially more nutrients. Kefir is easier to digest for babies, invalids and the elderly. Kefir, like yogurt, is an immune boosting food, and is used with success by naturopaths to help HIV, herpes, cancer and chronic fatigue syndrome. A natural tranquilizer, kefir is a good food for children with ADD, too.

Acidophilus:, a "friendly bacteria," can be used directly on foods (including pet foods) for health. Just sprinkle a teaspoon of powder, or the contents of one capsule, on your favorite foods. Acidophilus helps your body produce B vitamins, enzymes and natural antibiotics. Like all cultured foods, it counters the side effects of antibiotic therapy like diarrhea, upset stomach, and *Candida* infections. (I've used it successfully for years in a vaginal suppository for yeast infections.) Note: Don't cook with acidophilus. It negates its healing properties.

Cultured Soy Foods are full of benefits for health. Soy bean products help protect the heart by lowering cholesterol and supporting the vascular system. Further, research shows soy plays an important role in the natural treatment of osteoporosis, and hormone-related cancers like breast and prostate cancer. A rich source of phytoestrogens, soy enhances female vitality during menopause, too.

My favorite cultured soy foods:

Tofu: made from fermented soy milk, tofu adds richness to recipes while safeguarding you against disease. New studies show tofu even helps fight prostate cancer; research on 8,000 Hawaiian men (who traditionally have high rates of prostate cancer) shows that the men who eat the most tofu have the lowest rates of prostate cancer. Tofu is high in protein and lower in fat and calories than meat or poultry.

Tempeh: a delicious, protein-packed cultured soy food, tempeh is made from whole soybeans fermented with a grain like rice or millet. It's a good choice for meat eaters evolving into vegetarians, because it's so hearty and filling. I especially like tempeh squares pre-marinated in teriyaki or Szechwan sauce.

Miso: made from fermented soybean paste, unpasteurized miso (pasteurization kills its active cultures), found in the refrigerated section of Asian food stores and health food stores is the best choice. A true superfood for health, miso is an immune system enhancer that helps neutralize toxins and repress carcinogens. I like miso in tonic broths and sauces with vegetables and immune boosting herbs.

Soy Milk: made from soaked, ground and cooked whole soybeans, soy milk is the basis for most soy foods... tofu, soy yogurt, soy frozen desserts, soy cheeses and cream cheese, and soy yuba sheets for tacos or tamalas. Almost everyone likes soy milk. Some picky kids actually favor soy milk over commercial dairy milk. Soy milk is rich and creamy, and is available plain or in flavors like vanilla or chocolate. Use it in desserts, smoothies and on whole grain cereals.

Cautions: Eaten in excess (more than 4 servings a day), soy foods may disrupt thyroid function and deplete minerals like zinc, calcium and iron. Soy beans are also routinely genetically engineered. Choose organic soy products whenever possible.

Vinegar: used since ancient times as a preservative to extend the freshness of foods, and as an elixir for health. The Japanese folk remedy Tamago-su (egg vinegar) was consumed by the Samurai as a source of strength and power. Aged wine vinegar, balsamic vinegar, brown rice vinegar, apple cider vinegar, raspberry vinegar and herbal vinegars like tarragon vinegar are all good choices in a healing diet. Vinegar, like other cultured foods, helps digestive problems like heartburn and gas. It has also been effectively used in vaginal douches for feminine problems for decades. Just add 2 teasp. of apple cider vinegar to one cup of warm water for the best results.

Apple cider vinegar: well known for health benefits since ancient times, apple cider vinegar is a source of over 30 important nutrients. It contains natural antibiotics and antifungals that fight ear infections, dandruff and athlete's foot, even when used externally. It soothes sore throats in a gargle or diluted drink mix. Cider vinegar enhances memory, fights arthritis and promotes weight loss.

Raw Sauerkraut: one of the richest sources of enzymes and *lactobacillus*; successfully used by natural healers to treat *Candida* yeast disorders. Sauerkraut regenerates the blood, improves digestion and boosts metabolism. Use it in salads, on sandwiches, rice cakes, pizzas and omelettes. Commercial sauerkrauts are heated which degrades their life-giving enzymes. A raw sauerkraut food like Rejuvenative Foods VEGI-DELITE offers the best healing results.

Wine: used since ancient times for its pain-relieving, antiseptic and relaxing properties, wine is six times more effective than Pepto-Bismol in killing the bacteria linked to traveler's diarrhea. Wine aids circulation, protects the heart, even helps the eyes! Studies show just 2 glasses of wine per day cuts heart disease risk by 50%. As little as 2 glasses a month may cut the risk of macular generation in half. Research in the journal Epidemiology reveals that 2 glasses of wine a day reduces death rates from all causes by up to 30%! Resveratrol, a wine component, may even help prevent cancer.

Cautionary note: research shows resveratrol has mild estrogenic effects that may aggravate hormone dependent tumors, or add to high estrogen stores in women using HRT drugs.

The key to using wine wisely is moderation. I recommend a glass with dinner or lightly cooking with it for the best results.

Sadly, the grapes which produce our wines are one of the most heavily sprayed fruits in America. And, grape skins have a high affinity for fluoride, a highly toxic substance used in pesticides and regularly added to the water supply. (For more, see my chapter on *"Water,"* pages 58-63 in my **Cooking For Healthy Healing Diet Book.**) Choose organic wines for your healing diet. Organic wines have no added sulfites which may cause allergy reactions like congestion or stuffy nose for many people.

Cultured Foods Recipe Sections

The recipes in this chapter show you how to use cultured foods for healing.

Cultured Basics

Drinks, Marinades, Sauces

Fresh cultured foods like tofu and yogurt have a light delicate flavor that enhances almost any type of recipe or cuisine. Marinating tofu in a sauce or dressing is the essence of successful cooking with this food. Cut tofu into strips or cubes before marinating for best results. Chill while marinating for best blending of flavors.

PEACHY YOGURT SMOOTHIE

This recipe works for: Sports Nutrition, Men's-Kid's Health, Waste Management
Makes 2 servings:

Peel, pit and slice 2 Peaches; freeze solid. Freeze 1 peeled Banana. Then blender blend fruit with 1 cup Low Fat Vanilla Yogurt, $^1/_4$ cup Orange Juice, 2 TBS Lemon Juice and $^1/_4$ cup Orange Honey. Pour into chilled tall glasses and serve.

CULTURED FRUIT SHAKE

This recipe works for: Digestive Health, Immune Breakdown, Liver-Organ Health
Makes 2 servings:

Blender blend: $^1/_2$ cup Strawberry Soy Protein Powder, $^1/_2$ cup Pineapple Juice, $^1/_2$ cup Orange Juice, 1 cup brewed Green Tea, $^1/_2$ cup Strawberries or Orange Segments, 2 TBS Lemon Juice, 2 tsp. Acidophilus Powder. Add $^1/_2$ cup Vanilla Yogurt or 1 Banana if desired.

GREEN TEA FROSTY with ACIDOPHILUS

This recipe works for: Liver-Organ Health, Weight Control, Respiratory Health
Makes 1 pitcher; eight 8-oz. servings:

Slice and freeze 1 peeled Lemon and 1 peeled Orange. Blender blend with $^1/_2$ cup Honey, 2 cups brewed Green Tea, 2 cups brewed Raspberry Tea, 2 cups brewed Hibiscus Tea, 2 cups White Grape Juice and 1 TB Acidophilus Powder. Decorate with Orange and Lemon Peels.

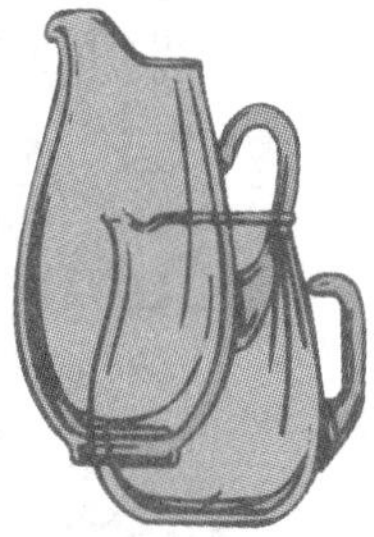

STEVIA FROST with ACIDOPHILUS

This recipe works for: Anti-Aging, Sugar Imbalances, Respiratory Health
Makes 1 pitcher; eight 8-oz. servings:

Slice and freeze $^1/_2$ pint Raspberries and $^1/_2$ pint Strawberries and 1 peeled Kiwi. Just before serving, blender blend the fruit with 4 cups brewed Green Tea, $^3/_4$ tsp. loose Stevia Leaf, 2 tsp. Acidophilus Powder, and $^1/_2$ cup lightly packed Fresh Mint Leaves; use about 1 cup fruit, $^3/_4$ cup tea and 2 TBS mint at a time. Garnish with mint sprigs.

MARINATED TOFU for SNACKS, SALADS, SANDWICHES

This recipe works for: Bone Building, Women's Health, Hair, Skin and Nails
Enough for 6 servings:

Blanch 1-lb. Extra Firm Tofu in boiling water for 5 minutes. Slice or cube as needed. —Whisk the marinade: $^{1}/_{4}$ cup Tamari, 2 TBS Brown Rice Vinegar, 1 TB fresh grated Ginger, 2 TBS Toasted Sesame Seeds, 2 TBS Sherry, 2 teasp. snipped Sea Veggies, 1 teasp. Toasted Sesame Oil, $^{1}/_{2}$ teasp. Fructose or 1 pinch Stevia Powder and dashes Hot Pepper Sauce or Hoisin Sauce. Marinate tofu for 1 hour or more in the fridge.

Nutrition; 146 calories; 14gm protein; 4gm carbo.; 1gm fiber; 9gm total fats; 0 choles.; 164mg calcium; 8mg iron; 87mg magnesium; 224mg potassium; 460mg sodium; Vit. A 14 IU; Vit. C trace; Vit. E trace

MISO SAUCE

This recipe works for: Immune Power, Fatigue Syndromes, Illness Recovery
For $^{3}/_{4}$ cup:

Sauté 1 TB Olive Oil, 1 minced Clove Garlic, $^{1}/_{2}$ cup minced Shallots, and 1 teasp. grated Ginger in a saucepan until fragrant. Add and bring to a gentle boil: 2 TBS Tamari, 1 teasp. Honey, 2 TBS Chickpea Miso dissolved in 2 TBS Water, and $1^{1}/_{2}$ TBS Kuzu Chunks or Arrowroot Powder dissolved in 3 TBS Water. Stir one minute and remove from heat.

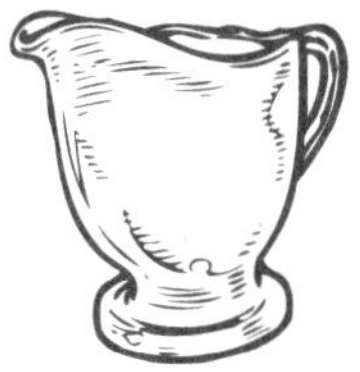

SESAME MISO DIPPING SAUCE Great for all kinds of sushi-sashimi.

This recipe works for: Liver-Organ Health, Immune Health, Hair, Skin and Nails
Makes 1 cup:

Mix $^{1}/_{2}$ cup Brown Rice Vinegar, $^{1}/_{4}$ cup Organic Vegetable Broth, 2 TBS Miso, 1 TB Fructose, 2 slivered Green Onions and 2 TBS Toasted Sesame Seeds.

MISO MARINADE Marinate fish, vegetables, tofu, potatoes, or chicken.

This recipe works for: Disease recovery, Women's Health, Heart and Artery Health
Makes $^{1}/_{2}$ cup (4 servings): It keeps beautifully. A little goes a long way.

Shake together in a jar and chill: $^{1}/_{2}$ cup Chickpea Miso Paste, $1^{1}/_{2}$ TBS Honey, $^{1}/_{2}$ cup Sake or Sherry, 1 TB minced Crystallized Ginger, $^{1}/_{3}$ cup Tamari, $^{1}/_{2}$ teasp. Garlic-Lemon Seasoning.

Nutrition; 134 calories; 6gm protein; 19gm carbo.; 2gm fiber; 2gm total fats; 0 choles.; 30mg calcium; 2mg iron; 26mg magnesium; 141mg potassium; 1329mg sodium; Vit. A 3 IU; Vit. C trace; Vit. E trace

GINGER MISO MARINADE Great for baked salmon, tofu or tempeh.

This recipe works for: Heart - Artery Health, Arthritis, Respiratory Illness
For about 2 cups (8 servings):

Blender blend: 4 TBS Light Chickpea Miso Paste, 1/2 cup Water, 2 teasp. grated Fresh Ginger, 2 teasp. Brown Sugar, 1/4 cup White Wine, 1/4 cup Brown Rice Vinegar, 2 teasp. Toasted Sesame Oil. Whirl briefly just to mix and add 1/2 cup Canola Oil very slowly while blending, to form an emulsion. Spread on tofu or salmon and bake or grill.

Nutrition; 156 calories; 1gm protein; 3gm carbo.; 1gm fiber; 12gm total fats; 0 choles.; 6mg calcium; trace iron; 4mg magnesium; 19mg potassium; 247mg sodium; Vit. A 1 IU; Vit. C trace; Vit. E 5 IU.

HONEY and SPICE TOFU SAUCE

This recipe works for: Sugar Imbalances, Men's Health, Hair, Skin and Nails

Sauté briefly to blend flavors: 3 TBS Tamari, 3 TBS Honey, 3 TBS Toasted Walnuts, 3 TBS Lemon Juice, 3 TBS Mild Sesame Oil, 1/2 teasp. Sweet Hot Mustard, 1/2 teasp. Worcestershire Sauce, 1/4 teasp. Lemon-Pepper. Pour over tofu and steamed veggies.

EASY TAMARI MARINADE for TOFU

This recipe works for: Digestive Health, Weight Control, Anti-Aging
Makes 1/2 cup (2 servings):

Whisk in a bowl and pour over tofu: 2 teasp. Tamari, 2 teasp. Balsamic Vinegar, 2 teasp. Soy Bacon Bits, 1/2 teasp. Dry Mustard, 1/2 teasp. Cracked Pepper, 1 teasp. Italian Herbs and 4 TBS Olive Oil. Chill for 30 minutes. For baking tofu, and for tofu salads.

Nutrition; 287 calories; 6gm protein; 6gm carbo.; 2gm fiber; 26gm total fats; 0 choles.; 47mg calcium; 2mg iron; 31mg magnesium; 185mg potassium; 273mg sodium; Vit. A 5 IU; Vit. C 1mg; Vit. E 5 IU.

BALSAMIC-LIME VINAIGRETTE for TOFU

This recipe works for: Liver and Organ Health, Digestive Health
For 12-oz. tofu (4 servings):

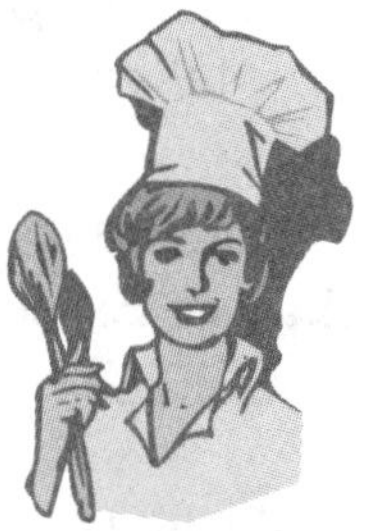

Shake together in a jar; pour over tofu and chill: 1/4 cup Canola Oil, 2 TBS Balsamic Vinegar, 1/4 teasp. Fructose, 1/4 teasp. Dry Mustard, 1/4 teasp. Cracked Pepper, 1/4 teasp. Sea Salt, Juice of 1 Lime, grated Zest of 1 Lime, pinch Sweet Paprika.

Nutrition; 256 calories; 14gm protein; 6 gm carbo.; 1gm fiber; 21gm total fats; 0 choles.; 178mg calcium; 9mg iron; 80mg magnesium; 212mg potassium; 147mg sodium; Vit. A 14 IU; Vit. C 3mg; Vit. E 5 IU.

MILD TOFU SALSA

This recipe works for: Women's Health, Weight Control, Anti-Aging
Serves 6:

Have ready 8-oz. Frozen Firm Tofu, thawed, liquid squeezed out by hand, and crumbled into a bowl. Dry toast 1/2 cup Pumpkin Seeds in a skillet for 3 minutes. Remove from skillet, sprinkle with Sea Salt to taste and set aside.

—Add 1 TB Olive Oil to the skillet and heat to hot. Add 1 TB Cumin Seeds, 1 teasp. Sea Salt and 1 TB Lemon Zest and toss for 2 minutes. Add tofu and toss for 1 minute. Add 1/2 cup Organic Vegetable Broth and bring to a boil. Simmer briefly to blend flavors. Then transfer to a bowl and set aside.

—Add 1 TB Olive Oil to the wok; add 4 minced Cloves Garlic, 1 seeded minced Jalapeño Pepper and 2 diced Red Onions. Sizzle for 2 minutes til fragrant. Add 2 TBS crumbled dry Dulse, 1 diced Red Bell Pepper and 1 diced Yellow Bell Pepper, 3 cups Corn Kernels, 1/2 cup diced Jicama and 1 teasp. Garlic-Lemon Seasoning. Sizzle 2 minutes. Remove from heat. Add 2 diced Tomatoes and 2 cups snipped Cilantro or Watercress Leaves. Serve hot sprinkled with the pumpkin seeds.

Nutrition; 267 calories; 13gm protein; 29gm carbo.; 6gm fiber; 14gm total fats; 0 choles.; 117mg calcium; 7mg iron; 130mg magnesium; 565mg potassium; 557mg sodium; Vit. A 217 IU; Vit. C 70mg; Vit. E 3 IU.

You can also: Marinate tofu in bottled Italian dressing; or Bragg's Liquid Aminos or Red Star Yeast Broth; or bottled hickory, mesquite or barbecue sauce; or natural liquid smoke with a little water and wine for a grilled flavor.

Using Acidophilus as a Cultured Recipe Ingredient

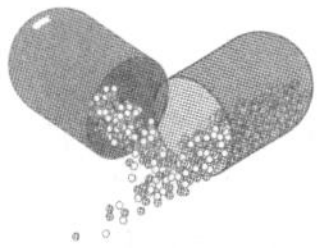

One of the best ways to get the healing benefits of probiotics is by sprinkling a few pinches of acidophilus powder on foods. It works well for the elderly (often deficient in "friendly flora"), people with weakened immune systems who aren't absorbing nutrients properly, and people whose digestive tracts have been damaged by candida, ulcers, diverticulosis or celiac disease. For them, processing acidophilus gelatin caps or even vegicaps can be too difficult. It is good for children with diarrhea who may not take it in any other way.

Adding acidophilus powder to cold drinks is well tolerated by most people, even babies! In fact, John Hopkins research shows babies fed formulas with acidophilus have less diarrhea and diaper rash. (Use child dosage.) I highly recommend it for thrush (oral Candida) to help reduce symptoms and prevent recurrence.

Cooking with acidophilus negates its healing ability. For better healing results, sprinkle it on cold or lukewarm foods. Or, add a teaspoon to your favorite smoothie. Use acidophilus right away for the best probiotic viability. Leaving it out on foods or drinks for too long can dramatically reduce the amount of active "friendly" bacteria.

Cultured Starters

Appetizers, Soups, Salads

Add versatile cultured foods to your diet anytime. Miso, Tofu, Tempeh, and pickled vegetables are perfect at the start of a meal because they enhance digestion.

GREEN GODDESS TOFU DIP and DRESSING

This recipe works for: Bone Building, Candida Healing, Women's Health
Makes 2 1/2 cups:

Pulse in a food processor: 3 chopped Shallots, 1/4 cup Parsley, 1/2 cup Watercress and 1/3 cup Cilantro Leaves. Turn into a bowl and combine with 1 (12-oz.) package Soft Silken Tofu, 1/2 cup Soy Mayonnaise, 1/2 cup Kefir Cheese or Soy Cream Cheese, 2 TBS Lemon Juice and 1 teasp. Lemon-Pepper. Sprinkle with 1 teasp. Dulse Flakes. (Optional: add 1 diced drained Cucumber.)

COTTAGE CHEESE - VEGGIE SPREAD

This recipe works for: Immune Health, Candida, Women's Health
Makes 3 cups:

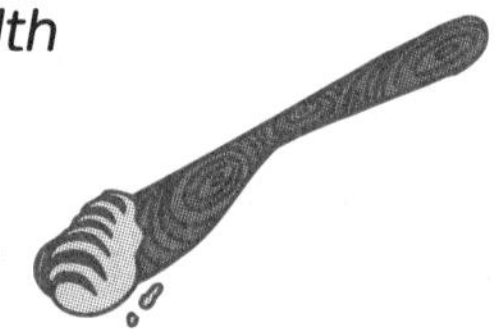

Whisk together: 8-oz. Low Fat Cottage Cheese, 8-oz. Plain Low Fat Yogurt, 2 teasp. Lemon-Pepper. Stir in 1/4 cup <u>each</u>: grated Carrot, diced, drained Cucumber, minced Red Bell Pepper and minced Red Onion or Olives.

WATERCRESS-TOFU TAPENADE

This recipe works for: Liver - Organ Health, Sugar Imbalances, Bone Building
Makes 2 cups:

Pulse in a food processor until pasty: 2 chopped Shallots, 2 TBS Olive Oil, 1/2 cup chopped Toasted Walnuts, 1/2 cup packed Basil Leaves, 2 chopped Scallions and 3 cups stemmed Watercress. Scrape into a bowl and stir in 1/2 cup Parmesan-Reggiano Cheese, 1/2 cup Soft Silken Tofu, 2 TBS White Wine and 1/2 teasp. Garlic-Lemon Seasoning.

SWEET-HOT TOFU CURRY DIP

This recipe works for: Digestive Health, Candida Healing, Liver-Organ Health
Makes 2 cups:

Heat in a pan: 2 TBS Honey, 2 TBS Water, 2 TBS Sherry. Stir in 1 TB Curry Powder, 1 teasp. Ground Coriander, 1/4 teasp. Pepper. Simmer 3 minutes. Cool 15 minutes. Add 2 TBS Dijon Mustard, 4 TBS Soy Mayonnaise and 1 (12-oz.) pkg. Soft Silken Tofu.

FROM SCRATCH TOFU TORTILLAS

Light, low fat and elastic, use these tender tortillas as chapati dippers, as wrappers for fajitas, burritos or egg rolls, as pastries or crepes, or as light crusts for pizzas and quiches. The dough freezes well, and the recipe can be cut down easily.

Enough for 16 tortillas:

Blender blend: 1-lb. Very Fresh Soft Tofu, 6 TBS Soft Butter, 2 TBS Olive Oil, 2 TBS Baking Powder and $1^1/_2$ teasp. Sea Salt. Turn into a mixing bowl. Add 3 cups Unbleached Flour. Mix until smooth and elastic. Chill.

—Divide into 16 parts and form into balls. Roll out each one into an 8" circle. Bake on a preheated ungreased skillet or griddle over medium high heat, until done but not brown. Stack with waxed paper between each layer for storing or freezing.

Nutrition; 181 calories; 7gm protein; 19gm carbo.; 1 gm fiber; 8gm total fats; 11 choles.; 134mg calcium; 4mg iron; 32mg magnesium; 257mg potassium; 250mg sodium; Vit. A 45 IU; Vit. C trace; Vit. E 1 IU.

Use the tortillas to make MUSHROOM FAJITAS.

—Soak 2 large dry Shiitake Mushrooms in water until soft in a big bowl. Sliver, chop, and discard woody stems and soaking water. Add 4-oz. chopped Button Mushrooms, $^1/_2$ cup slivered Jicama, 1 diced Carrot, $^1/_4$ cup diced Celery, 3 minced Shallots and 3 minced Green Onions.

—Sizzle in a skillet in 2 TBS Olive Oil for 3 minutes: half a sliced Red Onion, 2 minced Cloves Garlic, 1 TB minced Crystallized Ginger, 1 TB Tamari, $^1/_2$ teasp. Cumin Seeds, $^1/_2$ teasp. dry Oregano, $^1/_4$ teasp. Sweet Paprika, and 1 TB Sherry. Add the veggie mix and toss for 5 minutes. Remove from heat; add 1 cup chopped Baby Spinach Leaves and $^3/_4$ cup shredded Soy Cheddar.

Fajitas

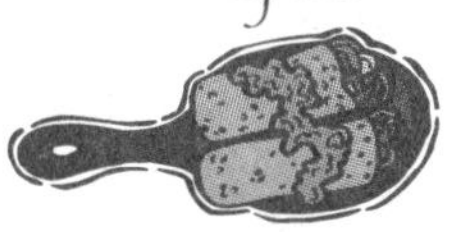

—Preheat a broiler. Divide mixture between 6 tortillas; roll and wrap, tucking in bottom end and sides. Divide 1 handful Sunflower Sprouts or Bean Sprouts between fajitas. Broil for 1 minute; serve hot.

Nutrition; 269 calories; 10gm protein; 29gm carbo.; 3gm fiber; 13 gm total fats; 11 choles.; 189mg calcium; 6mg iron; 55mg magnesium; 556mg potassium; 406mg sodium; Vit. A 454 IU; Vit. C 11mg; Vit. E 3 IU.

Dip the fajitas in DOUBLE CULTURED LEMON SOUR CREAM.

For six 2 oz. servings:

Blender blend until creamy: 1 cup Low Fat Cottage Cheese, 2 TBS Lemon Juice, 2 TBS Lemon Mayonnaise or Soy Mayonnaise, $^1/_4$ cup Plain, Low-Fat Yogurt, 1 tsp. Lemon Zest, $^1/_2$ tsp. Lemon-Pepper.

Nutrition; 71 calories; 6gm protein; 3gm carbo.; trace fiber; 4gm total fats; 6 choles.; 74mg calcium; 1mg iron; 2mg magnesium; 97mg potassium; 139mg sodium; Vit. A 6 IU; Vit. C 3mg; Vit. E 2 IU.

Try the tofu tortillas above as the crust for the following TOFU APPETIZER PIZZA.

TOFU APPETIZER PIZZA

Tofu balls freeze well if you have too many.

This recipe works for: Men's and Kid's Health, Sports Nutrition, Heart Health
For 35 to 40 small balls (12 servings): Preheat oven to 400°F.

Make the tofu balls in a big mixing bowl. Mash 1 package Tofu Burger Mix with 1-lb. Soft Tofu. Add 1 Egg, 1/4 cup grated Parmesan Cheese, 1/4 cup snipped Fresh Parsley, 2 TBS Olive Oil and 1 TB Red Wine Vinegar. Roll into balls and place on an Olive Oil sprayed baking sheet. Bake for 18 to 20 minutes until brown and crusty.

—Make the PIZZA SAUCE. Sauté in a skillet about 5 minutes: 3 TBS Olive Oil, 1 cup diced Onion, 1 cup diced Green Bell Pepper, and 1/2 teasp. Anise Seed or Fennel Seed. Add 1 (15-oz.) jar Natural Pizza Sauce; stir until bubbly. Reduce heat; simmer 20 minutes.

—Fit a tofu tortilla (previous page) on a pizza pan, or put 2 on a 15 x 11" baking sheet. Spoon on sauce to cover. Top with chunks of Mozarrella Cheese, and arrange tofu balls around the pizza. Bake for 30 minutes on the bottom rack of the oven.

Nutrition; 177 calories; 11gm protein; 12gm carbo.; 3gm fiber; 11gm total fats; 18 choles.; 142mg calcium; 5mg iron; 61mg magnesium; 266mg potassium; 269mg sodium; Vit. A 74 IU; Vit. C 12mg; Vit. E 1 IU.

TOFU DIPPING STICKS

Good dunkers for creamy dips.

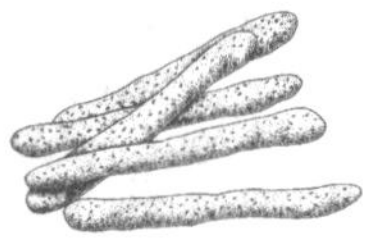

This recipe works for: Women's Health, Allergy-Asthma
For about 30 sticks: Preheat oven to 375°.

Blender blend: 1-lb. Soft Tofu, 3/4 cup Soft Butter, 1 teasp. Sea Salt, 2 1/2 teasp. Baking Powder. Pour into a mixing bowl and beat with 2 1/4 cups Unbleached Flour, 1/2 cup Poppy Seeds or grated Parmesan Cheese. Beat until elastic and smooth. Divide into 30 parts and roll between your palms into 4" sticks. Place on Olive Oil sprayed baking sheets and bake for 35 minutes. Serve warm, with ONION TOFU DIP.

—Sauté half a small diced Onion and 1 minced Clove Garlic in 2 TBS Olive Oil until brown. Add 1/3 cup grated Carrot, and dashes of Hot Pepper Sauce. Sauté for 3 minutes. Blender blend until smooth with 2 TBS Raspberry Vinegar, 2 cakes Soft Tofu, 2 TBS snipped Chives, 1 TB Tamari and 1/4 teasp. Cracked Pepper.

BAKED TOFU KABOBS

This recipe works for: Illness Recovery, Allergy-Asthma Healing, Fatigue Syndromes
For 6 skewers: Run skewers under a broiler for 30 seconds to "charcoal" kabobs.

Blanch 1-lb. Extra Firm Tofu in boiling water for 5 minutes. Cut in large cubes. Marinate tofu cubes for 1 hour in your favorite marinade. (See previous pages for suggestions.) Marinate 1 peeled cubed Eggplant, 1 Red Bell Pepper, 8 whole Button Mushrooms, and 1 chunked Red Onion for 1 hour in 4 TBS Italian Vinaigrette, 3 TBS Sherry, 2 TBS Tamari and 1 TB Dijon Mustard. Alternate Tofu cubes with the veggie cubes on the skewers. Bake on oiled sheets, or on a barbecue grill until tender.

TOFU BASIL BITES with TOMATO OLIVE SAUCE

This recipe works for: Infection Protection, Men's Health, Sugar Imbalances
For 18 bites: Preheat oven to 325°F. Serve on toothpicks around sauce bowl.

Make the sauce first. Sauté for 10 minutes: 3 TBS Olive Oil, 1 diced Onion, 1 teasp. Lemon-Garlic Seasoning, $^1/_2$ teasp. Oregano, $^1/_2$ teasp. Thyme, $^1/_2$ teasp. Hot Pepper Sauce and 1 TB snipped Fresh Basil. Add 1 can (28-oz.) chopped Tomatoes and simmer uncovered about 45 minutes. Let cool slightly, pureé in the blender; add back to the pot. Stir in $^1/_3$ cup Cilantro Leaves and 12 diced Black Olives. Pour into a serving bowl.

—Make tofu bites: prepare $^1/_2$ package Tofu Burger Mix as directed with 2 cakes (8-oz.) Soft Tofu. Add 2 TBS Parmesan Cheese and 2 TBS snipped Fresh Basil (2 teasp. dry). Roll into 18 balls; place on oiled sheets. Bake 15 minutes turning until golden.

TOFU FALAFELS with GINGER TAHINI SAUCE

This recipe works for: Men's and Kid's Health, Arthritis, Immune Power
For 36 homemade falafel bites: Preheat oven to 350°F.

Mix in a bowl and form into 1" balls: 3 caked mashed Soft Tofu, 1 small diced Yellow Onion, 2 minced Green Onions, 4 TBS Sesame Tahini, 4 TBS Lemon Juice, 3 TBS Olive Oil, 2 teasp. Toasted Sesame Oil, 3 TBS Tamari, 1 cup Whole Grain Bread Crumbs, $^1/_4$ cup snipped Fresh Parsley, 2 teasp. ground Turmeric, 1 teasp. ground Cumin and $^1/_2$ teasp. Lemon-Pepper. Roll in Sesame Seeds to completely coat. Place on Olive Oil sprayed baking sheets. Chill for an hour before baking until crusty.

—Serve with GINGER TAHINI SAUCE. Blender blend: 2 cakes crumbled Soft Tofu, 2 TBS Sesame Tahini, 2 teasp. Chickpea Miso Paste, 1 teasp. Honey, 2 teasp. grated Ginger and a pinch Curry Powder. Add 2 TBS Yogurt Sour Cream or Soy Mayonnaise for creaminess if desired. Serve bites on toothpicks surrounding sauce bowl.

Nutrition; 47 calories; 2gm protein; 3gm carbo.; 1gm fiber; 4gm total fats; 0 choles.; 19mg calcium; 1mg iron; 23mg magnesium; 49mg potassium; 99mg sodium; Vit. A 4 IU; Vit. C 2mg; Vit. E 1 IU.

FRUIT and TOFU BITES with GINGER DRIZZLE

This recipe works for: Heart Health, Weight Control, Waste Management
For 8 long, flat metal skewers: Preheat a barbecue grill to hot.

Press liquid from a 16-oz. block Firm Tofu. Place it under a cutting board with a heavy jar on top for 30 minutes. Cut into large cubes. Have ready 1-lb. soaked, plumped Pitted Prunes, and 1 peeled chunked Pineapple. Thread tofu and fruit on skewers.

—Make the GINGER DRIZZLE: Simmer $^1/_2$ cup Orange Marmalade, $^1/_2$ cup Tamari, 2 TBS minced Crystallized Ginger, $^1/_2$ tsp. Garlic Powder and 2 tsp. Toasted Sesame Oil for 5 minutes. Marinate kebabs for 30 minutes; baste during grilling. Serve hot.

INCREDIBLY HEALTHY MISO SOUP

This recipe works for: Detoxification, Immune Breakdown, Cancer Protection

Soak Wakame or Dulse Sea Vegetable (about $1^1/_2$-inch piece per person) in water to cover for 5 minutes; then cut into small pieces. Add to a pot of cold water (1 cup per person plus 1 cup "for the pot") and bring to a boil.

—Dice 1 small Daikon Radish, 3 Fresh Shiitake Mushroom Caps; add to the boiling broth and simmer 2 to 4 minutes until vegetables are soft. Add Miso ($^1/_2$ to 1 flat tsp. per cup broth plus 1 tsp. "for the pot"), and simmer for 3 to 4 minutes. Remove from heat; add 1 bunch Baby Bok Choy or 1 small bag Baby Spinach Leaves (7-oz.).

Nutrition (4 servings); 62 calories; 7gm protein; 9gm carbo.; 3gm fiber; 1gm total fats; 0 choles.; 91mg calcium; 4mg iron; 71mg magnesium; 581mg potassium; 291mg sodium; Vit. A 390 IU; Vit. C 32mg; Vit. E 2 IU.

HEALING TOFU SOUP

This recipe works for: Men's and Women's Health, Immune Breakdown, Arthritis
Makes 6 servings:

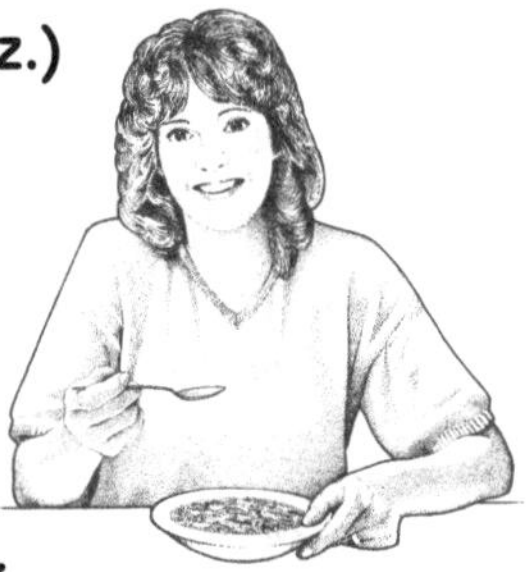

Drain and press under a heavy skillet for 45 minutes, 1 (12-oz.) box Extra Firm Tofu. Cut pressed tofu into small cubes.

—In a large pot, heat to hot 2 TBS Canola Oil. Add 1 TB Hoisin Sauce, 2 TBS minced Crystallized Ginger, $^1/_2$ tsp. Anise Seed, 1 tsp. White Pepper and the tofu cubes. Stir until they brown around the edges, about 5 minutes. Add $^1/_2$ cup chopped Onion, 1 Whole Bulb Garlic peeled and minced, 3 slivered Fresh Shiitake Mushroom Caps, 1 large diced Plum Tomato, 2 seeded minced Jalapeño Peppers and 3 TBS Sake. Cook, stirring, about 10 minutes.

—Add 1-qt. Organic Chicken Broth, 3 cups Water, $^1/_4$ cup Tamari, drops Sambal Hot Sauce and 2 TBS Lime Juice; stir to mix. Simmer to blend flavors, about 20 minutes.

MISO-TOFU SOUP with SHRIMP

This recipe works for: Immune Health, Brain Enhancement, Cancer Protection
For 4 servings: Use a large wok.

Toss in a bowl: 8-oz. small peeled Shrimp and 8-oz. sliced Extra Firm Tofu in a bowl with 1 teasp. Arrowroot Powder and 1 teasp. Sea Salt. Set aside. In another bowl, stir 3 TBS Arrowroot Powder in 3 TBS Sake and 2 teasp. Tamari. Set aside.

—Swirl 1 TB Canola Oil in a wok. Heat and sizzle 1 TB minced Ginger. Add shrimp and tofu; toss for 1 minute only. Add 4 cups Organic Chicken Broth, $^1/_2$ cup slivered Shiitake Mushroom Caps, $^1/_2$ cup sliced Brown Cremini Mushrooms and $^1/_2$ cup trimmed Pea Pods. Toss 2 minutes. Reduce heat to low; stir in Arrowroot mix. Remove from heat; drizzle in 1 beaten Egg White, stirring until it sets. Serve with Fresh Cilantro on top.

SWEET MISO GUMBO with SEA VEGGIES

This recipe works for: Cancer Protection, Immune Breakdown, Weight Control
Serves 4-6: Pass extra Balsamic Vinegar for seasoning.

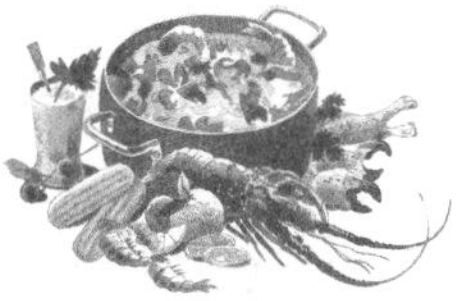

Mix the gumbo seasoning in a bowl: 1 teasp. <u>each</u>: Paprika, Ground Cumin, Dry Mustard, Dry Thyme, Dry Oregano, Dry Basil, and Sea Salt; add $^{1}/_{2}$ teasp. Lemon Zest, $^{1}/_{4}$ teasp. White Pepper and $^{1}/_{4}$ teasp. Black Pepper.

—Soak about $^{1}/_{2}$ cup dry Sea Veggies (like Wakame, Sea Palm or Arame) in water to cover. Then finely snip with kitchen shears and set aside.

—In a large skillet, heat 1 TB Toasted Sesame Oil and 1 TB Canola Oil. Add gumbo seasoning and sizzle with 2 minced Cloves Garlic, 1 diced Onion, 1 diced Red Bell Pepper, the sea veggies and 2 tsp. Filé Powder. Cook partially covered for 30 minutes.

—In a soup pot bring 1-qt. Salted Water to a boil. Add 1-lb. thin-sliced Carrots and 1 Bay Leaf. Cook 15 minutes. Drain; reserve cooking water, discard bay leaf.

—Blender blend the gumbo puree: the carrots, 2 cups reserved cooking water, 2 TBS Miso, 2 tsp. Balsamic Vinegar and $^{1}/_{4}$ tsp. Hot Pepper Sauce. Return to soup pot. Add the gumbo veggies. Add 1 package (16-oz.) peeled, cooked Frozen Langoustinos, 4 thin-sliced Green Onions and 4 TBS Lemon Juice. Let stand, covered for 10 minutes.

GOLDEN SOUP

This recipe works for: Cancer Protection, Immune Breakdown, Weight Control
For 8 servings:

In a soup pot, sauté 1 chopped Yellow Onion in 2 TBS Olive Oil for 10 minutes. Add 2 chopped Tomatoes, 4 medium Yellow Crookneck Squash, and 1 cup diced Carrots. Sauté for 5 more minutes. Add 3 cups Organic Chicken Broth; bring to a boil and simmer until tender, about 15 minutes. Remove from heat and cool slightly.

—Blender blend in batches <u>with</u> $^{1}/_{2}$ cup Plain Yogurt, $^{1}/_{4}$ cup White Wine, $^{1}/_{4}$ cup Water and $^{1}/_{4}$ cup snipped Fresh Basil Leaves. Serve warm topped with Tomato slices.

VEGETABLE HERB STEW

This recipe works for: Cancer Protection, Bone Building, Respiratory Problems
For 6 to 8 servings:

Chunk 1 Red Potato, and cook until tender in 4 cups Organic Vegetable Broth.

—Sauté 1 chopped Onion and 1 minced Clove Garlic in 3 TBS Olive Oil 5 minutes. Add and sauté for 5 minutes: 1 diced Carrot, 1 diced Rib Celery, 8-oz. sliced Mushrooms, $^{1}/_{2}$ teasp. Thyme, $^{1}/_{2}$ teasp. Dill Weed, $^{1}/_{2}$ teasp. dry Basil, $^{1}/_{2}$ teasp. Herbal Seasoning and $^{1}/_{2}$ teasp. Pepper. Add mixture to the potato stock; simmer 20 minutes.

Add and heat: 1 cake cubed Tofu, $^{3}/_{4}$ cup White Wine, 2 TBS Sherry and 1 TB Tamari. Remove from heat; add 1 cup Frozen Peas and let sit for 5 minutes while peas warm.

REFRESHING CUCUMBER TOFU SALAD

This recipe works for: Bladder-Kidney Problems, Hair, Skin and Nails
Makes 6 servings:

Blanch 1-lb. cubed Extra Firm Tofu and 3 Whole Shallots in boiling water for 5 minutes. Remove from heat and add $^1/_3$ cup snipped Dry Arame Sea Vegetable. Drain, mince the shallots then put the pot with tofu and veggies in the fridge to chill.

—In a large salad bowl, toss 1 long cubed European Cucumber, 1 diced Apple, 4 Ribs Celery, and $^3/_4$ cup Toasted Walnut Pieces. Snip on 1 TB Fresh Dill, 1 TB Fresh Cilantro and 1 TB Fresh Mint.

—Blender blend the MISO DRESSING: $^1/_4$ cup Flax Oil, 3 TBS Chickpea Miso, 3 TBS Lemon Juice, 1 TB Crystallized Ginger, $^1/_2$ cup Water, $^1/_4$ cup Sake, $^1/_4$ cup Sesame Tahini.

—Add the chilled tofu and veggies to the salad bowl. Toss with dressing and serve in Boston Lettuce cups.

TOFU TACO SALAD with CHILI-LIME CREAM

This recipe works for: Men's and Kid's Health, Sports Nutrition, Stress Protection
Makes 6 servings: Preheat oven to 350°F.

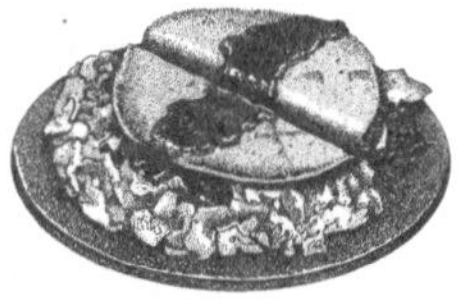

Have ready 6 Whole Wheat Tortillas. Place tortillas on oven racks and bake until crispy and golden, 10 minutes. Place 1 tortilla on each of 6 salad plates.

—Have ready 1 head shredded Romaine Lettuce or 1 small bag (6-oz.) Baby Spinach Leaves. Have ready 1 Bunch Cilantro, stemmed with leaves snipped. Have ready 8-oz. Frozen Firm Tofu, thawed, liquid squeezed out by hand, and crumbled into a bowl.

—In a large bowl, mix 1 drained can (15-oz.) Corn Kernels, 1 drained can (15-oz.) Black Beans, 1 cup peeled cubed Jicama, 1 diced Red Bell Pepper and $^1/_2$ cup snipped Fresh Cilantro Leaves. Chill.

—Make the taco filling: sizzle 2 TBS Olive Oil, 1 diced Onion, 1 seeded minced Jalapeño Chili and 2 minced Cloves Garlic for 5 minutes. Add the crumbled tofu. Cook 5 minutes. Stir in 1 can (15-oz.) chopped Tomatoes with liquid, 1 tsp. ground Cumin, 1 teasp. Chili Powder, and 1 teasp. Garlic-Lemon Seasoning. Cook, stirring occasionally, for 5 minutes. Remove from heat.

—Make the CHILI-LIME CREAM: Blend $^2/_3$ cup Yogurt Sour Cream (page 426), $^1/_4$ tsp. Garlic Salt, 2 TBS Lime Juice, 1 tsp. Chili Sauce and 2 TBS snipped Fresh Cilantro.

—Assemble salad. Divide romaine or spinach over tortillas. Drizzle on a little of the chili-lime cream. Blend rest of cream with the corn and black bean mixture. Divide over romain or spinach. Divide mounds of tofu filling on top of beans and corn. Sprinkle Roasted Salted Pumpkin Seeds and snipped Scallions on top of each salad.

Nutrition; 389 calories; 22gm protein; 66gm carbo.; 15gm fiber; 9gm total fats; 1mg choles.; 218mg calcium; 9mg iron; 190mg magnesium; 1173mg potassium; 507mg sod.; Vit. A 452 IU; Vit. C 82mg; Vit. E 6 IU.

CRUNCHY TOP TOFU SALAD

This recipe works for: Women's Health, Digestive Health, Fatigue Syndromes
For 6 people:

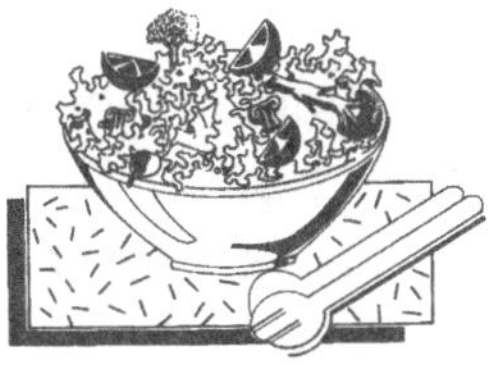

Blanch 2 cakes cubed Extra Firm Tofu in boiling Salted Water for 10 minutes. Drain. Add 1/2 cup bottled Natural French Dressing. Chill in the fridge for 30 minutes.

—Assemble the rest of the salad in a baking dish. Mix 1/2 cup Soy Mayonnaise, 1/2 cup Yogurt Sour Cream (page 426) or Kefir Cheese, 1 1/2 cups diced Celery, 1/2 cup toasted sliced Almonds and 1 cup crisp Chinese Noodles.

—Mix salad with the marinated tofu. Sprinkle with 1 more cup crisp Chinese Noodles and 1 cup Low Fat Cheddar Cheese. Serve cold or run under a broiler for 30 seconds until the top is brown and crunchy.

Nutrition; 325 calories; 14gm protein; 23gm carbo.; 2gm fiber; 21gm total fats; 20m choles.; 304mg calcium; 4mg iron; 77mg magnes.; 325mg potassium; 450mg sodium; Vit. A 72 IU; Vit. C 2mg; Vit. E 3 IU.

TOASTED PITA-TOFU SALAD

This recipe works for: Candida Healing, Liver-Organ Health, Fatigue Syndromes
Makes 4 servings: Preheat oven to 375°F.

Brush 3 Pita Bread Rounds with 2 TBS Olive Oil; sprinkle with Garlic-Lemon Seasoning. Cut into bite-size pieces and arrange on a large baking sheet. Bake until golden, stirring occasionally, about 12 minutes. Remove and set aside to cool.

—Mix 3 diced Tomatoes, 6 cups Baby Spinach Leaves (1 small bag), 3 sliced Green Onions, 1/2 cup snipped Fresh Parsley, 1/2 cup snipped Fresh Mint, 1/2 cup sliced Red Onion, 1 diced European Cucumber, and toasted pita bread in large bowl. Whisk 1/3 cup Lemon Juice, 1/2 teasp. Lemon-Pepper and 1/3 cup Olive Oil in a small bowl to blend. Pour over salad and toss to coat. Season with Sea Salt and Cracked Pepper if needed.

Nutrition; 371 calories; 10gm protein; 37gm carbo.; 10gm fiber; 23gm total fats; 0 choles.; 253mg calcium; 18mg iron; 120mg magnesium; 998mg potass.; 421mg sodium; Vit. A 685 IU; Vit. C 70mg; Vit. E 8 IU.

TOFU "EGG" SALAD

This recipe works for: Candida Healing, Cholesterol Health, Fatigue Syndromes
Serves 4: Serve in boston lettuce cups, on a mixed sprout bed or in pita pockets.

Mash together in a bowl: 1 box (12-oz.) Firm Light Tofu, 1 TB Lemon Juice, 2 teasp. Yellow Mustard, 1 diced Rib Celery, 3 minced Scallions, 1 teasp. Fructose, 1/2 teasp. Turmeric, 1/2 teasp. Tamari, 1/2 teasp. Sea Salt, 1/2 teasp. White Pepper, 1/2 minced Green Bell Pepper or 3 TBS Sweet Pickle Relish, 2 TBS snipped Fresh Parsley, 1/3 cup Soy Mayonnaise and a pinch Paprika.

RAINBOW TOFU SALAD

Vary this salad with any fresh vegetables.

This recipe works for: Candida Healing, Men's Health, Sugar Imbalances
For 2 large or 4 medium salads:

Blanch 1-lb. Extra Firm Tofu in boiling water for 5 minutes. Cut in cubes. Marinate cubes in: 1 TB Honey, 1/4 cup Sweet Pickle Relish, 1 TB Olive Oil, 1 teasp. Chickpea Miso, 1 TB Sherry and 1 1/2 teasp. Sweet Hot Mustard while you make the rest of the salad.

Toss in a mixing bowl: 1/2 cup shredded Red Cabbage, 2 sliced Scallions, 1 chopped Tomato, 1 diced Rib Celery, 1 diced Carrot, 1/2 sliced European Cucumber, 2 TBS Toasted Almonds, 2 TBS Toasted Sunflower Seeds and 2 TBS Roasted Pumpkin Seeds. Serve in a salad bowl lined with large overlapping Boston Lettuce Leaves.

Serve with TOFU MAYONNAISE - a low-fat, no cholesterol, dairy-free mayonnaise. (also great as a sandwich spread or add 4 TBS Plain Yogurt and 1/2 teasp. Tarragon Vinegar to use in place of sour cream.)

—Blend in the blender to mayonnaise consistency: 8-oz. Silken Tofu, 2 TBS Olive Oil, 1 1/2 TBS Lemon Juice, 1/2 teasp. Sea Salt, 1/2 teasp. Dijon Mustard.

DELICIOUS CULTURED VEGETABLE PICKLES

This recipe works for: Candida Healing, Detoxification, Liver-Organ Health
For 8 servings:

Mix veggies in a bowl: 1/2 cup thin-sliced Red Radishes, 1 cup matchstick-sliced Daikon White Radish, 1 thin-sliced European Cucumber, 1 thin-sliced Carrot, 1 slivered Red or Orange Bell Pepper, 1 TB shredded Fresh Ginger and 1 teasp. Sea Salt. Let marinate for 2 hours, then press excess liquid out through a colander.

—In a pan, bring 1/3 cup Umeboshi Vinegar or Raspberry Vinegar and 2/3 cup Water to a boil. Pour over veggies and chill in the fridge overnight.

Fresh, raw sauerkraut is available in many health food stores. If you can't find it, here's how to make your own:

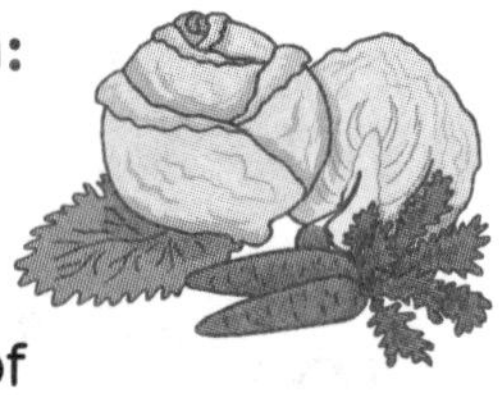

Cabbage is the main element of sauerkraut. You can use green cabbage alone, or make a half-and-half blend of green and red. Use a food processor to chop or shred 1 small head of Green Cabbage and 1 2-inch piece Fresh Ginger; set aside. Chop a blend of other vegetables — like 1 Beet, 2 Carrots and 1 Green Bell Pepper. Or make a Kim Chee blend of Carrots, Onions, Red or Yellow Bell Pepper, fresh grated Ginger and a little Chili Pepper. Place the veggies in a sanitary glass or stainless steel pot (never use plastic) and let sit for about 7 days at a moderate room temperature (59° to 71°). The naturally present enzymes, lactobacillus acidophilus, lactobacillus plantarum, and lactobacillus brevi in the vegetables proliferate, transforming the sugars and starches in the vegetables into lactic and acetic acids.

Refrigerate your cultured vegetables and eat them within six months. They'll hold their flavor, enzymes and lactobacillus cultures.

Tofu-Tempeh Burgers and Sandwiches

Tofu burgers put tofu on the American map - low-fat, no cholesterol burgers without the beef. Taste tip: Even though it's an extra step, freezing tofu <u>first</u> gives it a chewy, meaty, yet tender taste, perfect for burgers or sandwiches. Squeeze out excess liquid and crumble the tofu to leave more facets for soaking up seasonings.

TOFU BURGER SUPREME

This recipe works for: Men's and Kid's Health, Heart Health, Sports Nutrition
For 8 burgers: Preheat oven to 375°.

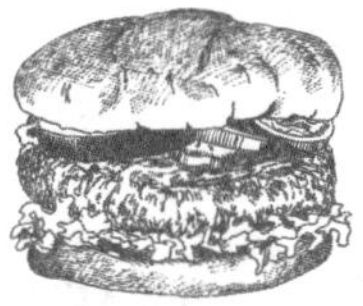

Freeze 2 (12-oz.) packages Extra Firm Tofu. Thaw, squeeze out water and crumble in a bowl. Mix in 2 Eggs and $^3/_4$ cup Almond Butter.

—Sauté in 1 TB Butter and 1 TB Olive Oil: 1 chopped Onion, 1 TB Coarse Grain Mustard and $^1/_2$ teasp. Herbal Seasoning 5 minutes. Mix in the tofu, $^1/_2$ cup Granola, $^1/_2$ cup Ketchup, $^3/_4$ cup Bean Sprouts or shredded Carrots, $^1/_2$ teasp. Lemon-Pepper; form into patties. Roll in Wheat Germ, Sesame Seeds or crushed Granola. Bake on greased sheets until brown outside and moist inside, about 25 minutes.

Nutrition; 395 calories; 22gm protein; 22gm carbo.; 4gm fiber; 28gm total fats; 57 choles.; 264mg calcium; 11mg iron; 182mg magnesium; 594mg potass.; 261mg sodium; Vit. A 68 IU; Vit. C 6mg; Vit. E 10 IU.

QUICK BARBECUE TEMPEH SANDWICHES

This recipe works for: Men's and Kid's Health, Heart Health, Sports Nutrition
For 6 sandwiches: The sauce makes the difference.

Slather bottled Hickory Barbecue Sauce over 2 (8-oz.) packages Baked Tempeh Slices. Broil for 3 minutes on each side. Serve open face on Whole Grain Bread with shredded Lettuce, Tomato slices and dollops of TAHINI SAUCE: Blender blend $^1/_2$ cup Sesame Tahini, 1 TB Lemon Juice, $^1/_2$ cup Kefir Cheese or Low Fat Cream Cheese, $^1/_4$ cup Sweet Pickle Relish, $^1/_2$ teasp. Herbal Seasoning Salt. Add 2 TBS Water if needed for consistency.

HEARTY TEMPEH HERO PITAS

This recipe works for: Men's - Kid's Health, Fatigue Syndromes, Sports Nutrition
Serves 4:

Cut 1 package (8-oz.) Baked Tempeh into strips. Sizzle 1 small Red Onion in 1 TB Olive Oil 5 minutes. Add 3 TBS Tamari, 3 TBS Red Wine, 2 TBS Lemon Juice, 4 TBS Cilantro Leaves, 1 tsp. dry Mint, 1 tsp. dry Oregano, $^1/_2$ tsp. dry Basil and $^1/_2$ tsp. Cracked Pepper. Add tempeh strips and coat. Stuff into pitas. Make a sauce with 1 chopped Cucumber mixed with 1 cup Plain Yogurt, $^1/_2$ teasp. Lemon-Pepper and 2 TBS Lemon Juice. Spoon on top.

SOUTHWEST TOFU SANDWICH

This recipe works for: Men's and Kid's Health, Heart Health, Sports Nutrition
For 4 sandwiches:

Have ready 4 slices Whole Grain Toast.

—Blanch 1-lb. Extra Firm Tofu in boiling water 5 minutes. Slice; brush with Tamari.

—Make the filling in a skillet: Sizzle 1 small diced Red Onion and 1 small diced Red Bell Pepper in 1 TB Olive Oil 5 minutes. Turn off heat and mix in 1 diced Tomato, $^3/_4$ cup crushed Tortilla Chips, $^3/_4$ cup shredded Soy Cheddar, 4 TBS Soy Mayonnaise or Yogurt Sour Cream, 2 TBS Lemon Juice, $^1/_2$ tsp. Chili Powder, $^1/_2$ tsp. dry Oregano, $^1/_2$ tsp. Cumin, $^1/_4$ tsp. Paprika and $^1/_4$ tsp. Sea Salt. Pile on toast. Top with Sunflower Sprouts.

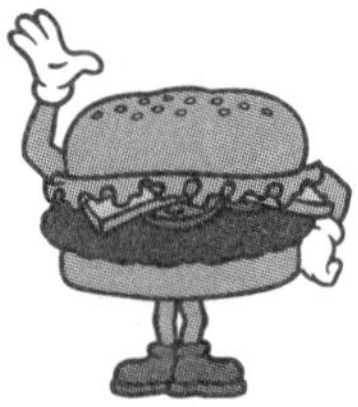

TOFU NUT BURGERS

This recipe works for: Heart and Artery Health, Fatigue Syndromes
For 6 burgers: Preheat grill to hot.

Freeze 1 package (16-oz.) Extra Firm Tofu. Thaw, squeeze out water and crumble in a bowl. Mash with 1 Egg and Sea Salt and Pepper to taste.

—Saute 1 diced Onion and 3 minced Cloves Garlic in 1 TB Olive Oil for 10 minutes until brown. Add 3 TBS Barbecue Sauce, the mashed Tofu mix, $^1/_4$ cup Toasted Wheat Germ and 1 cup ground Walnuts or Hazelnuts. Chill for 10 minutes. Then form into 6 patties, and grill for 3 to 4 minutes on each side.

(Great alternative: heat 2 TBS Olive Oil to hot in a heavy skillet and sizzle 8-oz. sliced Mushrooms for 5 minutes. Then add burger patties to the skillet and sizzle until light brown on both sides. Roll in Sesame Seeds; serve with mushrooms. Yum.)

TOFU SLOPPY JOES with VEGGIES nutrient rich.

This recipe works for: Illness Recovery, Kid's Health, Stress and Exhaustion
Serves 4: Preheat oven to 425°F.

Toast and have ready 4 Whole Wheat Hamburger Buns.

—Freeze 16-oz. Extra Firm Tofu. Thaw, squeeze out water and crumble in a bowl.

—Mix with 1 Yellow Bell Pepper and 1 Red Bell Pepper, thinly sliced, 2 thinly sliced Carrots, 1 cubed Zucchini and 1 cup of your favorite Barbecue Sauce. (I like Mesquite for a real southwestern taste.) Set aside to marinate

—In a skillet, sizzle 1 large ring-sliced Onion in 2 TBS Olive Oil until translucent. Add Tofu-Veggie mix and toss to coat, 5 minutes. Turn mixture into a baking dish, and bake 30 minutes until brown and bubbly. Serve over toasted buns.

Nutrition; 420 calories; 27gm protein; 53gm carbo.; 10gm fiber; 15gm total fats; 0 choles.; 288mg calcium; 16mg iron; 200mg magnesium; 915mg potassium; 711mg sodium; Vit. A 1218 IU; Vit. C 67mg; Vit. E 8 IU.

TOFU SALAD PITAS

This recipe works for: Illness Recovery, Kid's Health, Stress and Exhaustion
For 4 servings:

Have ready 4 sandwich size Pita Pocket Breads. Blanch 1-lb. Extra Firm Tofu in boiling water 5 minutes. Crumble in a bowl and mix with 1/2 cup Lemon Mayonnaise, 1 1/2 cups shredded Carrots, 1/2 cup diced Celery, 1/4 cup minced Red Onion, 2 teasp. Dijon Mustard, 1/2 teasp. Honey, 1/2 teasp. Lemon-Pepper and 2 pinches Turmeric, 1 cup Alfalfa or Sunflower Sprouts. Stuff into pita pockets.

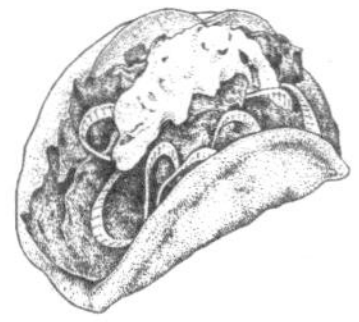

TOFU GARBANZO PITAS

This recipe works for: Weight Control, Allergies-Asthma, Heart Health
For 4 pitas:

Have ready 4 sandwich size Pita Pocket Breads. Mash the filling in a bowl: 1 can (15-oz.) drained rinsed Garbanzo Beans, 8-oz. drained crumbled Firm Tofu, 1 tsp. Ground Cumin, 1 tsp. Sweet Paprika, 1/2 tsp. Lemon-Pepper, 2 TBS Lemon Juice. Mix in 1 diced European Cucumber and 2 cups Baby Spinach or Watercress. Stuff into pita pockets.

TEMPEH BURRITO WRAPS

This recipe works for: Weight Control, Allergies-Asthma, Men's and Kid's Health
For 4 servings: Preheat a broiler.

Have ready 4 soft Whole Wheat Tortillas. Place in a baking dish, 8-oz. Tempeh, cut in strips, and 2 sliced Red Onions. Slather with a natural barbecue sauce, marinate for 10 minutes, then barbecue or run under a broiler until brown. Assemble wraps: spread 1 cup Baby Spinach Leaves down center of each tortilla. Divide tempeh mix on top of spinach; roll up tucking in sides as you roll to form a bundle. Slice in half.

SEED-Y HUMMUS PITAS

This recipe works for: Hormone Health, Hair and Skin, Men's and Kid's Health
For 4 pitas:

Pan roast 2 TBS White Sesame Seeds, 4 TBS Pumpkin Seeds and 1 teasp. Lemon-Garlic Seasoning for 5 minutes. (To make BLACK HUMMUS PITAS with a totally different taste, use black sesame seeds.)

—Blender blend seed mix with 2 TBS Olive Oil, 1 can (15-oz.) Garbanzo Beans, 3 TBS Lemon Juice, 2 TBS Plain Yogurt, 1/2 tsp. Ground Cumin and Sea Salt to taste. Blend smooth. Turn into a bowl; mix with 8-oz. drained crumbled Firm Tofu, 1 slivered Red Bell Pepper and 1/4 cup sliced Black Olives. Stuff pitas and sprinkle with snipped Cilantro.

SPICY ASIAN SLAW WRAPS

This recipe works for: Digestive Health, Liver Health, Anti-Aging
For 4 servings: Slice in half to eat.

Have ready 4 soft Whole Wheat Tortillas. Shred half a small Red Cabbage and half a small Green Cabbage. Boil 16-oz. Tofu in Salted Water 10 minutes. Drain, blot dry, cut in cubes; set aside in a mixing bowl. Make the slaw: Sizzle 1 TB Olive Oil, 4 TBS diced Onion and 1 teasp. Wasabi Paste in a large skillet. Add tofu and toss 5 minutes. Add cabbage and toss 2 minutes. Add 2 TBS Brown Rice Vinegar, 2 TBS Tamari, 2 TBS Sake, $^1/_4$ tsp. Paprika, $^1/_4$ tsp. Oregano, $^1/_4$ tsp. White Pepper and $^1/_4$ tsp. Black Pepper.

—Assemble wraps: Divide slaw down the center of each tortilla. Divide tofu on top of slaw; roll up tucking in sides as you roll to form a bundle.

CULTURED SAUERKRAUT REUBEN

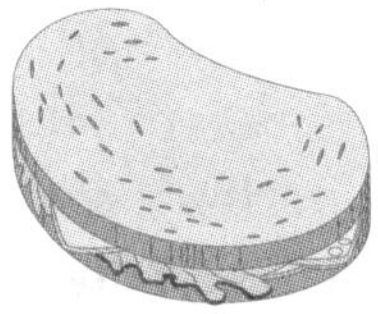

This recipe works for: Digestive Health, Liver and Organ Health
For 4 sandwiches: Preheat oven to 350°F.

Have ready 8 slices Whole Grain Rye Bread. Bake 16 slices Tempeh Bacon (in health food stores) on Olive Oil sprayed baking sheets for 20 minutes, or use strips of Dulse, a sea vegetable that tastes deliciously like smoky bacon. Have ready $1^1/_2$ cups drained Sauerkraut (cultured vegetables). Have ready Thousand Island Dressing.

—Build sandwiches: Lay bread slices flat. Spread with Thousand Island Dressing. Top 4 slices with 2 strips tempeh or 2 strips dulse, a slice of Swiss Cheese or Soy Swiss Cheese, and more Thousand Island Dressing. Divide sauerkraut between sandwiches. Top with a cheese slice, 2 more strips tempeh or dulse and another bread slice. Bake sandwiches until cheese melts, about 15 minutes. Slice and serve hot.

Nutrition; 423 calories; 25gm protein; 45gm carbo.; 6gm fiber; 17gm total fats; 8 choles.; 178mg calcium; 8mg iron; 96mg magnesium; 610mg potassium; 764mg sodium; Vit. A 79 IU; Vit. C 10mg; Vit. E 3 IU.

BUBBLE TOP TOFU-MUSHROOM SANDWICH

This recipe works for: Immune Power, Liver Health, Anti-Aging
For 4 sandwiches: Preheat oven to 400°F; or preheat a broiler to hot.

Freeze 1 package (16-oz.) Firm Tofu. Thaw, squeeze out water and crumble. Sauté with 2 TBS Butter and 1 diced Onion for 10 minutes. Add $^1/_4$ cup minced Celery, and 2 cups thin-sliced Mushrooms. Sprinkle on 4 TBS Unbleached Flour; stir until bubbly.

—Blender blend the sauce: 1 cup plain Yogurt, 8-oz. Low Fat Cream Cheese, $^1/_2$ cup Soy Mayonnaise, $^1/_4$ cup White Wine, $^1/_2$ teasp. Sea Salt, $^1/_4$ teasp. Pepper and 2 Vegetable Bouilion Cubes. Pour into skillet and bring to a boil. Simmer stirring constantly until thickened, and sauce is reduced by about 25% to concentrate flavors. Put Whole Grain Toast slices on a baking sheet. Top with sauce, and bake or broil until bubbly.

Grains and Vegetables with Culture

Cultured foods like tofu and tempeh provide protein complementarity with all types of whole grains. When eaten together, they yield a complete protein. Culturing makes assimilation of both grains and vegetables even greater - a case of one and one making three for healing.

GIANT TOFU VEGETABLE BALL

This recipe works for: Stress - Exhaustion, Sports Nutrition, Men's and Kid's Health
For 6 servings: Preheat oven to 350°F.

Freeze 2 packages (24-oz.) FIRM TOFU. Thaw, squeeze out water; crumble in a large mixing bowl.

—Sauté in a skillet in 3 TBS CANOLA OIL for 15 minutes: 2 minced CLOVES GARLIC, 1 chopped ONION, 2 teasp. ITALIAN HERBS, $^1/_4$ teasp. HOT PEPPER SAUCE. Finely chop 1 bunch SPINACH or CHARD. Add to skillet; remove pan from heat and let greens wilt.

—Turn into bowl with tofu and add: $^1/_2$ cup WHOLE GRAIN BREAD CRUMBS or CORN BREAD CRUMBS, 2 EGGS, 1 teasp. SEA SALT and $^1/_4$ cup PARMESAN CHEESE. Turn mixture into a Canola Oil sprayed shallow baking dish and form into a big, rounded, smooth hemisphere. Bake for $1^1/_2$ hours until well browned. Let stand for 10 minutes to set. Serve in wedges with a FRESH TOMATO SAUCE. (See index for choices.)

Nutrition; 284 calories; 24gm protein; 13gm carbo.; 3gm fiber; 17gm total fats; 72mg choles.; 356mg calcium; 14mg iron; 152mg magnes.; 628mg potass.; 523mg sodium; Vit. A 332 IU; Vit. C 16mg; Vit. E 3 IU.

TOFU GADO GADO

This recipe works for: Stress Reactions, Women's Health, Overcoming Addictions
For 4 people:

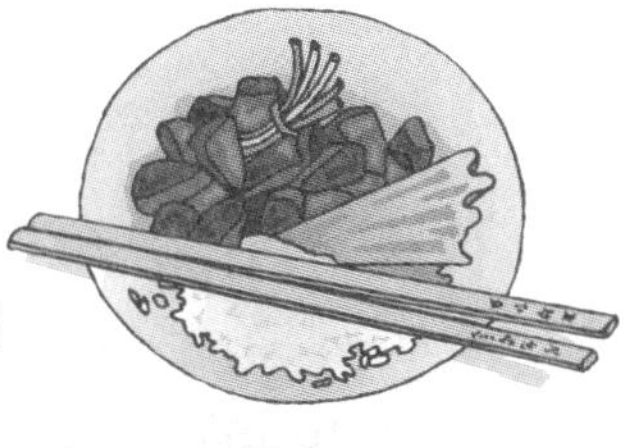

Steam in a wok steamer for 8 or 9 minutes: 2 CARROTS cut in matchsticks and 2 cakes TOFU, cut in strips.

—Add and steam 5 more minutes; 1 small ZUCCHINI cut in matchsticks, 1 cup FRENCH-CUT GREEN BEANS and 1 cup thin-sliced GREEN CABBAGE.

—Make the sauce as veggies steam: mix $^1/_2$ cup BLACK TEA, $^1/_4$ cup CHUNKY PEANUT BUTTER, 2 minced SHALLOTS, 2 minced GREEN ONIONS, 2 TBS HONEY, $^1/_2$ small jar ROASTED RED BELL PEPPERS slivered, 1 TB LEMON JUICE, 1 TB TAMARI, $^1/_4$ tsp. HOT PEPPER SAUCE.

—Lift steaming rack with the veggies off the hot water. Set aside for a minute. Drain out water, and put wok back on heat. Pour sauce into the hot wok. Let it come to a bubble for 5 minutes. Add more black tea if needed. Add vegetables back to wok with 1 cup BEAN SPROUTS. Heat through, about 3 minutes. Serve over BROWN RICE.

Nutrition; 340 calories; 13gm protein; 52gm carbo.; 7gm fiber; 11gm total fats; 0 choles.; 104mg calcium; 4mg iron; 154mg magnesium; 682mg potassium; 230mg sodium; Vit. A 1130 IU; Vit. C 60mg; Vit. E 3 IU.

VEGGIE CAKES with SWEET and SOUR SAUCE

This recipe works for: Digestive and Liver Health, Arthritis, Anti-Aging
For about 24 small cakes: Preheat a griddle to hot.

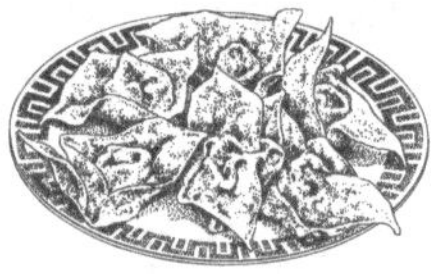

Make the CULTURED BALSAMIC VEGGIES. Mix the pickling spice: 4 cups Cold Water, 1/2 cup Balsamic Vinegar, 3 TBS Sea Salt, 1 TB minced Garlic, 2 teasp. ground Turmeric, 2 teasp. Cumin Seeds, 2 teasp. minced Ginger, and 1 seeded minced Jalapeño Pepper. Bring to a boil and simmer for 5 minutes. Let cool.

—In a large bowl mix the pickling vegetables: 1 cup slivered Daikon Radish, 1 cup thin-sliced Cauliflower, 1 cup thin-sliced Carrots, 1 cup slivered Beets, 1 cup shredded Green Cabbage, 1 cup Green Beans, 1 cup diced Parsnips, 1 cup diced Baby Turnips. Toss with pickling spice. Add sprigs of Fresh Dill and Thyme. Cover bowl and culture for 3 to 5 days. Add 3 cups Bean Sprouts, and 1-lb. cooked Salad Shrimp (or 1-lb. Tofu, excess water pressed out and diced).

—Make the batter: whisk 2 cups Rice Flour and 2 1/2 cups Cold Water until smooth. Add 3/4 cup Canola Oil and 1/2 teasp. Ginger Powder; set aside.

—Make the pancakes on the hot oiled griddle. Dab spoonfuls of the shrimp mixture around the griddle, and pour about 1/4 cup of the batter over top of each. Smooth out and cook until edges turn a deep brown and curl up, about 5 minutes. Drain on towels. Repeat to use all batter and veggies. Turn out onto a serving plate.

—Serve with a SWEET and SOUR BARBECUE DIPPING SAUCE: Sauté 1 diced Onion and 2 minced Cloves Garlic in 2 TBS Canola Oil until very brown. Add 1 cup Ketchup, 3/4 cup Pineapple Juice, 1/4 cup Pineapple Chunks, 3 TBS Molasses, 1 TB Sweet-Hot Mustard, 1 TB minced Crystallized Ginger and 1 TB Miso Paste. Reduce heat, and simmmer for 15 minutes until thick. Stack vegetable patties with a little sauce in between reach, or fold them over, and dip them in the sauce with your fingers.

Nutrition; 193 calories; 17gm protein; 22gm carbo.; 2gm fiber; 9gm total fats; 32mg choles.; 65mg calcium; 2mg iron; 44mg magnesium; 360mg potassium; 889mg sodium; Vit. A 156 IU; Vit. C 15mg; Vit. E 4 IU.

ZUCCHINI TOFU STUFFING PUFF

This recipe works for: Hormone Health, Anti-Aging, Sugar Imbalances
For 4 people: Preheat oven to 350°F.

Steam 2 to 3 small Zucchini until just barely tender. Drain and set aside.

—Mix in a bowl: 1 cup grated Soy Cheddar, 12-oz. mashed Firm Tofu, 3/4 teasp. Dill Weed, 3 Eggs, 1 teasp. Herbal Seasoning Salt and 1/2 cup Bread Cubes. Mix in zucchini.

—Turn into a shallow lecithin-sprayed baking dish, and top with Crunchy Chinese Noodles or crushed Corn Chips. Bake for 30 minutes to blend flavors.

Nutrition; 313 calories; 23gm protein; 24gm carbo.; 2gm fiber; 15gm total fats; 160mg choles.; 265mg calcium; 11mg iron; 115mg magnes.; 523mg potass.; 664mg sodium; Vit. A 119 IU; Vit. C 8mg; Vit. E 1 IU.

TOFU SHEPHERD'S PIE

This recipe works for: Men's Health, Sports Nutrition, Waste Management
For 10 servings: Preheat oven to 375°F. Use a round casserole or 9 x 13" baker.

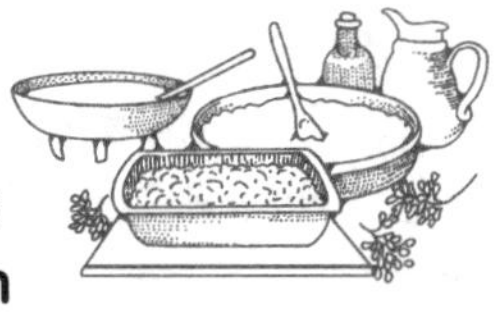

Freeze 2 packages (24-oz.) Firm Tofu. Thaw, squeeze out water; crumble in a large mixing bowl.

—Make the mashed potato topping: bake 6 large Yellow Dutch Potatoes until soft. Mash in a large bowl; then beat until fluffy with $^{1}/_{2}$ cup Plain Yogurt, $^{1}/_{2}$ cup Cottage Cheese, 3 TBS Butter, $^{1}/_{2}$ tsp. White Pepper, $^{1}/_{2}$ tsp. Sea Salt and 1 TB Tamari. Set aside.

—Make the filling: sauté 1 large sliced Yellow Onion and the crumbled tofu in 2 TBS Olive Oil for 15 minutes. Add 6 sliced Mushrooms, $^{1}/_{2}$ tsp. dry Basil, $^{1}/_{2}$ tsp. dry Thyme and 2 teasp. Herbal Seasoning Salt; sauté for 5 more minutes. Place in the bottom of the oiled baker. Dilute 1 can Condensed Mushroom Soup with White Wine to make 2 cups, or make 2 cups of your favorite mushroom sauce or gravy. Spoon on top of the veggies. Scatter on 1 cup Frozen Peas right from the freezer. Spread on the mashed potato top. Bake for 35 minutes to heat and brown the potato crust.

Nutrition; 284 calories; 17gm protein; 30gm carbo.; 3gm fiber; 12gm total fats; 11mg choles.; 202mg calcium; 8mg iron; 99mg magnes.; 701mg potassium; 530mg sodium; Vit. A 60 IU; Vit. C 6mg; Vit. E 1 IU.

SEA GREENS and TOFU STIR FRY

This recipe works for: Women's Health, Hair, Skin and Nails, Bone Building
Serves 6:

In a bowl, combine 1 cup mixed snipped Dry Sea Greens... good choices, Arame, Wakame and Sea Palm Crunchies, and 3 cups water. Let stand to soften, about 10 minutes. Drain and set aside.

—Blanch 1-lb. Extra Firm Tofu in boiling water for 5 minutes. Press out excess water; cut in cubes. Blanch 4 cups Broccoli Florets in Salted Water for 30 seconds until bright green. Drain and set aside in a large bowl.

—Set a large wok over high heat. Sizzle 1 TB Canola Oil, 4 minced Cloves Garlic and 1 tsp. Garlic-Lemon Seasoning for 2 minutes. Add 3 cups slivered Fresh Shiitake Mushroom Caps and tofu. Toss 3 minutes. Remove from heat; add to broccoli bowl.

—Return wok to heat; sizzle 1 TB Canola Oil and 1 teasp. Chinese 5-Spice Powder. Add 1 large Carrot cut in matchsticks, and 2 cups trimmed Snow Peas. Toss for 1 minute. Add 4 cups shredded Chinese Nappa Cabbage and 4 cups sliced Bok Choy. Toss for 1 minute. Add $^{1}/_{4}$ cup Sherry and let bubble for 1 minute. Turn into broccoli bowl.

—Return wok to heat; sizzle 1 TB Canola Oil, 2 TBS minced Crystallized Ginger and 1 tsp. Garlic-Lemon Seasoning. Add 4 sliced Green Onions, 1 cup Orange Juice, 1 TB Light Miso, 3 TBS Tamari, and 2 tsp. Arrowroot Powder dissolved in 2 teasp. Sherry. Whisk 2 minutes, then add all veggies, the sea greens, 1 tsp. Toasted Sesame Oil and 4 TBS Sesame Seeds. Toss for 2 minutes to heat and blend flavors. Serve immediately.

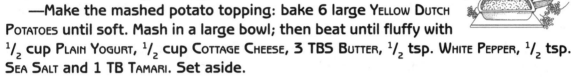

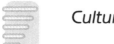

TOFU - BROCCOLI SIZZLE

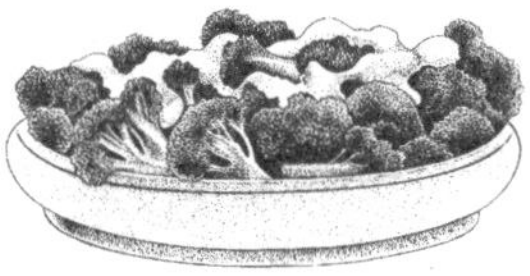

This recipe works for: Weight Control, Cancer Protection
Serves 4: Use a large wok.

Blanch 1-lb. Extra Firm Tofu in boiling water for 5 minutes. Drain, pat dry with paper towels and cube. Marinate 10 minutes in a large bowl with 2 TBS Tamari, 2 TBS Lime Juice, 2 TBS Sake and 1 teasp. Toasted Sesame Oil. In a small bowl stir 2 teasp. Arrowroot Powder into 2 TBS Sake.

—Heat 1 TB Canola Oil in the wok. Sizzle 1 thinly sliced Red Onion, 1 TB minced Ginger and 2 minced Cloves Garlic for 5 minutes. Add tofu and marinade, and 1/2 cup Organic Vegetable Broth. Add 4 cups Broccoli Florets and toss for 2 minutes until color turns bright greeen. Add arrowroot mixture and stir for 1 minute until thickened. Turn onto a serving plate. Sprinkle with Toasted Sesame Seeds and serve hot.

TOFU, not MEAT, LOAF

This recipe works for: Weight Control, Men's and Kid's health, Candida Healing
Serves 8: Preheat oven to 350°F. Spray a loaf pan with Olive Oil spray.

Freeze 1 package (16-oz.) Extra Firm Tofu. Thaw, squeeze out water; crumble in a large mixing bowl. Have ready 2 cups cooked Lentils, and 2 cups Short Grain Brown Rice. Combine with the tofu.

—Sizzle 1 large diced Onion, 1 teasp. Onion Salt, 2 minced Cloves Garlic and 1 teasp. Garlic Salt in 2 TBS Olive Oil for 5 minutes. Add 1 cup diced Mushrooms and 2 TBS Tamari; sizzle 5 minutes. Add the tofu mix and sizzle 5 minutes more.

—Blender blend smooth: 2 Eggs, 1/2 cup Ketchup, 1/4 cup slivered Oil-Packed Sun-Dried Tomatoes, 1/4 cup Tamari. Turn into a large bowl; add tofu mixture, 1 cup Rolled Oats, 1 cup grated Carrot, 1/2 cup Toasted Wheat Germ and 1/2 teasp. Cracked Pepper.

—Turn into prepared pan. Mix 1/4 cup Ketchup with 1 TB snipped Fresh Basil. Spread on top of loaf. Bake until firm, about 1 1/2 hours. Let stand for 30 minutes to cool and firm; then invert onto a serving plate or slice right from the baking pan.

TOFU-WALNUT PEPERONATA for PASTA

This recipe works for: Weight Control, Men's and Kid's health, Candida Healing
Serves 4:

Have ready 1-lb. cooked Capellini or Bowtie Pasta.

—Sizzle in a skillet: 1 TB Olive Oil and 1/2 cup Walnuts until fragrant. Remove and set aside. Add 4 TBS Olive Oil, and sizzle 1 sliced Onion, 1 small peeled, cubed Eggplant, 12-oz. cubed Firm Tofu and 4 TBS jarred slivered Oil-Packed Sun-Dried Tomatoes for 10 more minutes. Add 1 slivered Red Bell Pepper, 1 cubed Zucchini and 1 diced Tomato; sizzle 10 minutes. Make capellini nests in 4 pasta bowls. Fill with peperonata and sprinkle with Parmesan Cheese. Or mix bowties with peperonata and Parmesan.

EASY TOFU TETRAZZINI

This recipe works for: Women's Health, Hair, Skin and Nails, Hormone Balance
Enough for 4 people: Preheat oven to 350°F.

Freeze 16-oz. Firm Tofu. Thaw, squeeze out water; crumble in a bowl.

—Cook 6-oz. Egg or Sesame Noodles to al dente in 2-qts. Salted Water. Pour into an Olive Oil-sprayed baking dish, cover to keep warm.

—In a large skillet, sauté 2 TBS Olive Oil, 1 diced Onion, the crumbled tofu and $1^1/_2$ teasp. Italian Seasoning Herbs until pungent, about 10 minutes. Add 1-lb diced Tomatoes. Remove from heat; stir in 1 cup Cottage Cheese, $^1/_2$ cup snipped Fresh Parsley and $^1/_2$ cup shredded Mozarrella Cheese. Spoon over noodles. Sprinkle with more cheese, and bake for 30 minutes until bubbling.

Nutrition; 465 calories; 36gm protein; 37gm carbo.; 3gm fiber; 22gm total fats; 42mg choles.; 444mg calcium; 15mg iron; 151mg magnes.; 705mg potass.; 356mg sodium; Vit. A 183 IU; Vit. C 34mg; Vit. E 3 IU.

LOW FAT TOFU LASAGNA WITH FRESH HERBS

This recipe works for: Liver - Organ Health, Men's - Kid's Health, Sports Nutrition
12 servings: Preheat oven to 350°F. Spray a lasagna baker with Olive Oil spray.

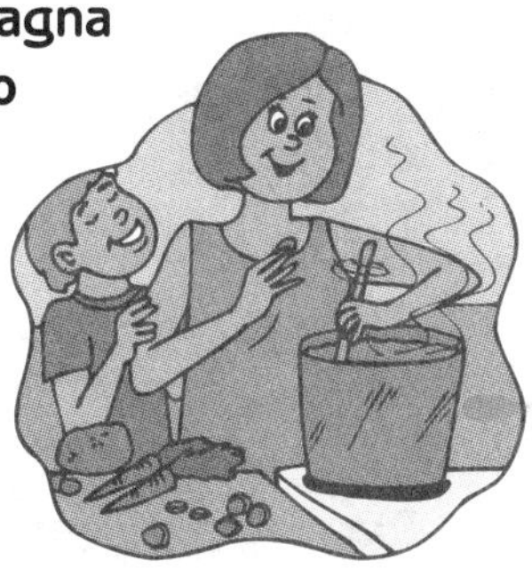

Use 2 packages (24-oz.) Extra Firm Frozen Tofu for the "lasagna noodles" in this recipe. Thaw, squeeze out water, and slice into very thin slabs. Set aside.

—Make the LASAGNA SAUCE: sauté 1 large chopped Onion and 2 minced Cloves Garlic in 4 TBS Olive Oil until aromatic, 10 minutes. Add 1 chopped Yellow Bell Pepper, 2-lbs. chopped Plum Tomatoes, 1 cup sliced Mushrooms, 2 TBS snipped Parsley, 2 teasp. Tamari, 1 teasp. grated Lemon Zest, $^1/_2$ teasp. Fresh Basil ($^1/_4$ teasp. dry), $^1/_2$ teasp. Fresh Oregano ($^1/_4$ teasp. dry), $^1/_2$ teasp. Fresh Rosemary ($^1/_4$ teasp. dry), $^1/_2$ teasp. Fresh Thyme ($^1/_4$ teasp. dry), $^1/_2$ teasp. Lemon-Pepper, $^1/_4$ teasp. Nutmeg; sizzle for 5 minutes. Add $^1/_2$ cup Red Wine and $^1/_2$ cup Organic Vegetable Broth; simmer on low heat for 15 minutes. Remove from heat; mix in 2-lbs. Low Fat Ricotta or Cottage Cheese and 1 Egg.

—Assemble the lasagna. Slice 4 large Tomatoes. Cover bottom of the lasagna baker with half the tofu slices Spread with half the lasagna sauce. Top with half the tomato slices and cover with the rest of the lasagna sauce.

—Mix $^1/_2$ cup snipped Fresh Basil with $^1/_2$ cup Feta Cheese and sprinkle over sauce. Repeat layers, topping the whole thing with the rest of the tomato slices. Bake covered with foil until bubbling, about 20 to 25 minutes. Sprinkle with more Feta Cheese. Let rest 10 minutes before cutting to serve.

Nutrition; 301 calories; 22gm protein; 15gm carbo.; 2gm fiber; 17gm total fats; 50mg choles.; 391mg calcium; 7mg iron; 87mg magnesium; 618mg potass.; 282mg sodium; Vit. A 247 IU; Vit. C 41mg; Vit. E 3 IU.

TEMPEH - GREEN BEAN STROGANOFF

This recipe works for: Men's Health, Hair, Skin and Nails, Libido Health
For 6 servings:

Bring 2-qts. Salted Water to a boil for 8-oz. Egg Noodles, and cook until just barely tender. Drain and toss with 1 teasp. Canola Oil to separate. Place in a serving bowl.

—Cube 1 package (12-oz.) Baked Tempeh. Marinate for 30 minutes in $^1/_4$ cup Chickpea Miso dissolved in 2 TBS Sherry and 2 TBS Water.

—Sauté 2 sliced Onions in 3 TBS Canola Oil until very brown, 15 minutes. Add 1 package French Cut Green Beans; sauté 5 minutes. Toss with noodles and set aside.

—Add marinade and tempeh to the hot skillet. Sprinkle with $^1/_2$ teasp. Dry Oregano, 1 teasp. Dry Basil and 1 TB Arrowroot Powder dissolved in 1 TB Tamari. Toss to coat and add 1 cup Plain Yogurt. Heat gently and serve over green beans and noodles.

Nutrition; 365 calories; 20gm protein; 43gm carbo.; 4gm fiber; 13gm total fats; 27 choles.; 182mg calcium; 4mg iron; 83mg magnesium; 510mg potassium; 565mg sodium; Vit. A 75 IU; Vit. C 8mg; Vit. E 3 IU.

Desserts with Culture

Tofu can take the heaviness out of desserts. It is a smooth, non-dairy, low fat substitute for cream cheese, or ricotta cheese, or just to lighten texture.

TOFU LEMON RICE PUDDING

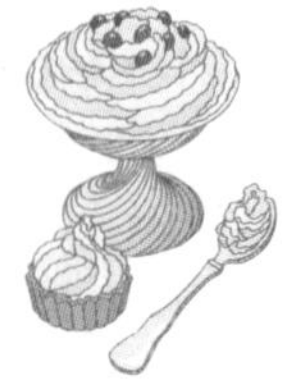

This recipe works for: Kid's and Men's Health, Stress-Fatigue
For 8 servings: This is a good kid's treat. Preheat oven to 350°F.

Toast 1 cup Shredded Coconut until light gold.

—Blender blend until very light: $1^1/_2$ packages (12-oz.) Soft Silken Tofu, 4 TBS Maple Syrup, $^1/_2$ cup Honey, 3 Eggs, $^1/_4$ cup Lemon Yogurt, 2 TBS Lemon Juice, $^1/_2$ teasp. Lemon Peel, $1^1/_2$ teasp. Vanilla, $^1/_2$ teasp. Cinnamon, and $^1/_2$ teasp. Nutmeg.

—Turn out into a large bowl and mix with 1 cup cooked Short Green Brown Rice, the toasted coconut and $^3/_4$ cup Raisins. Put in a Canola Oil sprayed casserole and bake for 1 hour until fragrant and set.

YOGURT SOUR CREAM for FRESH FRUIT

This recipe works for: Liver and Organ Health, Heart Health, Women's Health
For 8 servings:

Line a strainer with cheesecloth. Put 2 cups Plain Yogurt (gelatin free only) in cheesecloth; suspend over a bowl (save whey for an immune boosting soup) or over the kitchen sink faucet. Let drain overnight and voila! Serve over sliced Fresh Fruits.

CULTURED FRUITS

This recipe works for: Waste Management, Heart Health, Weight Control
Serves 6:

In a large pan, place 2 cored, sliced Pears, 2 cored, sliced Apples, $^1/_2$ cup dried, pitted Apricot Halves, $^1/_2$ cup Raisins, $^1/_4$ cup Maple Syrup, 2 TBS minced Crystallized Ginger, $^1/_4$ teasp. Cinnamon, 1 teasp. Vanilla and 3 cups Red Grape Juice. Bring to a boil, cover and simmer for 15 minutes. Remove from heat. To serve, divide between individual bowls and top each with 2 dollops Vanilla Low Fat Yogurt.

CREAMY TOFU CHEESECAKE A custard cheesecake.

This recipe works for: Waste Management, Heart Health, Weight Control
For 8 servings. Use a crumb crust, or no crust at all. Preheat oven to 350°F.

Mix the cake in the blender: 2 Eggs, 16-oz. Soft Silken Tofu, $^2/_3$ cup Honey, 2 TBS Maple Syrup, 2 TBS Fructose, 8-oz. Kefir Cheese or Low Fat Cream Cheese, 3 TBS Lemon Juice and $1^1/_2$ teasp. Vanilla. Turn into a Graham Cracker Crust or a Canola Oil sprayed 8 x 8" square pan. Bake for 1 hour. Remove, dust with Nutmeg, cool and chill. Scatter sweet chopped fruits over the top before serving for a fresh touch.

Nutrition; 241 calories; 10gm protein; 33gm carbo.; 2gm fiber; 9gm total fats; 68mg choles.; 103mg calcium; 4mg iron; 83mg magnesium; 164mg potassium; 104mg sodium; Vit. A 93 IU; Vit. C 4mg; Vit. E trace.

SWEET POTATO TRIFLE with SOY NUT CREAM

This recipe works for: Men's Health, Hormones and Sexuality, Kid's Health
For 8 servings: Preheat the oven to 350°F. Use tall parfait glasses.

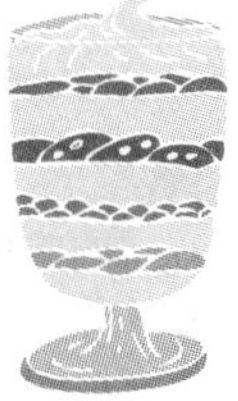

Roast 2 large Sweet Potatoes in the oven until goo-ey about 25 minutes. Turn off oven and put in a shallow pan with $^1/_2$ cup chopped Walnuts and $^1/_2$ cup chopped Hazelnuts. Toast while the oven cools, about 10 minutes. Remove and set aside.

—Make the SPICE SYRUP: in a pan, combine 2 TBS Tapioca Pearls with $^1/_2$ cup Water and $^1/_4$ cup Apple Juice. Let stand 10 minutes. Then heat while whisking in $^1/_2$ cup Maple Syrup, $^1/_2$ cup Honey, 1 TB Vanilla, $^1/_2$ teasp. Ginger Powder, $^1/_2$ teasp. Cinnamon, $^1/_4$ teasp. Nutmeg, $^1/_4$ teasp. Sea Salt and $^1/_4$ teasp. Lemon Peel Powder. Whisk in 2 TBS Arrowroot Powder in 3 TBS Sherry; mixture will thicken. Set aside.

—Blender blend sweet potatoes with 1 TB Vanilla. Add spice syrup and puree. Chill in the blender.

—Make the SOY NUT CREAM: oven toast 2 cups Soy Nuts for 10 minutes. Whisk in a bowl, $^1/_2$ cup Soy Milk, 2 teasp. Vanilla and $^1/_4$ Maple Syrup.

—Assemble the dessert: alternate layers of cold sweet potato-spice puree and soy milk cream. Sprinkle toasted soy nuts between each layer.

TOFU RAISIN NUT PUDDING

This recipe works for: Allergies - Asthma, Cholesterol Health, Kid's Health
For 10 servings: Preheat the oven to 350°F.

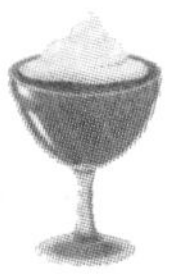

Blender blend the pudding: 16-oz. Soft Silken Tofu, 2 Eggs, 4 TBS melted Butter, 4 TBS Canola Oil, 1 cup Maple Syrup, 1 cup Honey, $^1/_2$ cup Rice Flour and $^1/_2$ tsp. Baking Soda. Turn into a Canola Oil sprayed baking dish. Stir in 1 cup chopped Walnuts and 1 cup Raisins. Bake for 45 minutes until set and firm.

Nutrition; 240 calories; 19gm protein; 35gm carbo.; 2gm fiber; 12gm total fats; 269mg choles.; 233mg calcium; 14mg iron; 163mg magnes.; 554mg potass.; 205mg sodium; Vit. A 193 IU; Vit. C 23mg; Vit. E 4 IU.

BLUEBERRY TOFU CHEESECAKE

This recipe works for: Hair, Skin and Eyes, Hormone Health, Respiratory Health
Serves 8: Preheat oven to 350°F. Use a springform pan or 10-inch pie plate.

Make the crust: mix 2 cups Whole Wheat Graham Cracker Crumbs, 2 TBS Maple Syrup, 1 TB Canola Oil and 3 to 4 TBS Water. Press into Canola Oil sprayed baking pan and bake for 5 minutes. Remove and cool.

—Make the filling: blender blend to smooth, 16-oz. Firm Tofu, 16-oz. Low Fat Cream Cheese, 1 (8-oz.) carton Kefir Cheese, 1 cup Maple Syrup, $^1/_2$ cup Honey, 2 TBS Lemon Juice, $^1/_2$ teasp. Cinnamon and 2 teasp. Vanilla. Pour into crust, and bake for 20 minutes only. Remove from oven; cool for 10 minutes while you make the topping.

—Make the topping: blender blend to smooth, 2 TBS Maple Syrup, 2 TBS Honey, 1 teasp. Lemon Zest, 2 teasp. Lemon Juice, 2 TBS Arrowroot Powder, 2 TBS Sherry and 1 teasp. Vanilla. Pour over the cake and bake for 10 to 15 more minutes. Remove, cool and chill until ready to serve. Cover top with 2 cups (1 pint) drained Blueberries.

GINGER SHORTCAKE with HONEY-YOGURT CREAM

This recipe works for: Heart and Artery Health, Allergies - Asthma, Arthritis
Serves 6: Preheat oven to 450°F. Use a non-stick baking sheet.

Mix 3 to 4 cups mixed Raspberries and sliced Strawberries sweetened with Honey to taste. Sprinkle with 1 TB minced Crystallized Ginger. Chill in the fridge.

—Make the shortcake: Mix in a bowl, $^1/_2$ cup Soy Milk or Rice Milk, 1 TB Lemon Juice, 2 teasp. Lemon Zest, 1 TB minced Crystallized Ginger, 2 TBS Maple Syrup. Mix in another bowl: $1^1/_2$ cups Whole Wheat Pastry Flour, $^1/_4$ tsp. Sea Salt, $^1/_2$ tsp. Baking Soda, 1 tsp. Baking Powder, $^1/_4$ cup Canola Oil. Make a well in the center, pour in liquid mixture; stir to blend into a dough. Turn onto a floured board; knead several times. Pat, divide and shape into 6 rounds. Bake 10 minutes, until a toothpick comes out clean. Cool on a rack at least 15 minutes. To serve, split shortcakes horizontally; place bottom halves on 6 dessert plates. Mix berries with 2 cups Vanilla Yogurt; sprinkle with more minced Crystallized Ginger.

ALMOND TOFU CREAM PIE

Make this a day ahead for best results.

This recipe works for: Hair, Skin and Nails, Sugar Imbalanced, Men's Health

Serves 8: Preheat oven to 350°F. Use a springform pan or 10-inch pie plate.

Make the crust: mix 2 cups Whole Wheat Graham Cracker Crumbs, 4 TBS Honey, 1 TB Canola Oil, $^1/_2$ teasp. Almond Extract and 3 TBS Water. Press into Canola Oil sprayed baking pan and bake for 5 minutes. Remove and cool.

—Make the filling: blender blend to smooth, 16-oz. Firm Silken Tofu, 16-oz. Kefir Cheese, 4 TBS Fructose, 4 TBS Almond Butter, $^1/_2$ teasp. Sea Salt, 1 teasp. Almond Extract, 1 teasp. Orange Zest, 2 TBS Orange Juice, 2 TBS Arrowroot Powder, 2 TBS Sherry. Pour into crust; bake 35 more minutes. Remove and chill until serving.

RASPBERRY TOFU MOUSSE

This recipe works for: Allergies - Asthma, Weight Control, Kid's Health

For 8 servings: Blueberries are great, too.

Heat $^1/_2$ cup Apple Juice with 2 TBS Tapioca Pearls and $^1/_4$ cup Water for 10 minutes. Then blender blend with 1 package (12-oz.) Soft Silken Tofu and 3 cups Raspberries, 3 TBS Honey, 1 TB Maple Syrup and 1 teasp. Vanilla. Chill in dessert cups; serve cold.

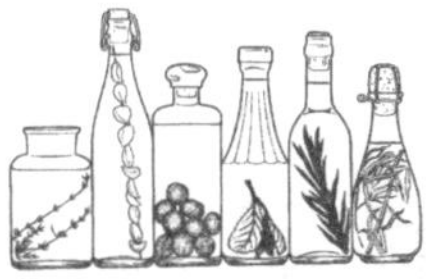

Healing Vinegars

The essence of cultured healing foods, vinegar promotes smooth digestion, helps flush the gallbladder and improves metabolism for weight control. Although slightly acidic itself, vinegar promotes the production of bicarbonate which helps normalize over-acid body conditions.

HERB GARDEN HEALING VINEGAR

This recipe works for: Digestive Health, Liver - Organ Health, Heart - Artery Health

For 1 gallon: Keeps well for 8 months or more.

Make this vinegar in a gallon jar: combine 5 cups White Wine or Red Wine Vinegar, 1 Onion quartered, 4 Cloves Garlic peeled, 4 pieces Crystallized Ginger Root peeled, 10 multicolored Peppercorns, and 5 to 10 sprigs each of the following fresh herbs: Rosemary, Sage, Thyme, Tarragon, Basil, Parsley, and Mint.

Let vinegar sit in a kitchen cupboard for 3 to 4 weeks; shake occasionally to reblend. Then strain through a fine sieve and bottle in colored glass bottles to keep. Close tight to store.

HIGH MINERAL CARROT and RADISH VINEGAR

This recipe works for: Digestive Health, Liver - Organ Health, Bone Health
For 2 quarts: Keeps well for 1 to 2 weeks if covered with vinegar-spice.

In a large pot, combine 2 cups Brown Rice Vinegar, 2 cups Water, 4 TBS Sea Salt, 3 TBS Honey, 2 dried Red Chili Peppers and 2 big chunks Crystallized Ginger. Add 3 to 4 sprigs fresh herbs <u>each</u>: Dill Weed, Rosemary and Basil; 2 teasp. Mustard Seed, 2 teasp. Coriander Seeds, 2 teasp. Anise Seeds and 2 TBS Cardamom Pods and 6 Peppercorns.

—Cut 6 Carrots, 4 Red Radishes and 2 Daikon White Radishes into decorative shapes. Put in a large glass container and cover with pickling sauce mix. Refrigerate for 2 to 3 days. Remove desired number of pickles and leave the rest in the pickling spice.

CRANBERRY VINEGAR

This recipe works for: Women's Health, Liver - Organ Health, Bladder-Kidney Health
For 2 quarts: Keeps well covered with vinegar-spice for up to 3 months.

In a large jar combine 6 to 8 cups Fresh or Frozen Cranberries. Dissolve $^1/_2$ cup Honey, 4 chunks Crystallized Ginger, 1 sliced Lemon with peel, and 8 to 10 Cardamom Pods in 4 cups Apple Cider Vinegar and pour over cranberries. Make sure cranberries are covered by liquid. Let stand about 2 weeks to pickle. Then strain through a fine sieve and bottle in colored glass bottles to keep. Close tight to store.

RASPBERRY VINEGAR Set aside 8 of the berries for the bottle.

This recipe works for: Women's - Men's Health, Heart Health
For 4 cups:

Combine 4 cups Fresh Raspberries in a saucepan with 3 cups White Wine Vinegar, and 2 TBS Honey. Cover and bring to a boil over high heat. Remove and let stand, covered, until cool. Then pour liquid into a bottle through a fine strainer. Discard solid residue. Add reserved berries to the bottle and seal.

APPLE CIDER VINEGAR for HEALING

This recipe works for: Detoxification, Liver Health, Immune Power
For 4 cups: Rich in malic acid for healing energy.

Pare and core 4 large tart Apples. Combine with 3 cups Cider Vinegar, 4 chunks Crystallized Ginger and 2 TBS Honey. Cover and bring to a boil over high heat. Remove and let stand covered, until cool. Then pour liquid into a bottle through a fine strainer. Discard solid residue.

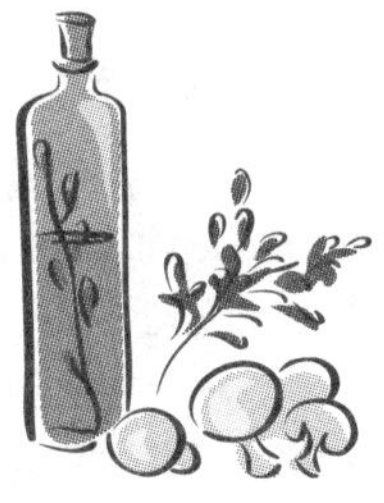

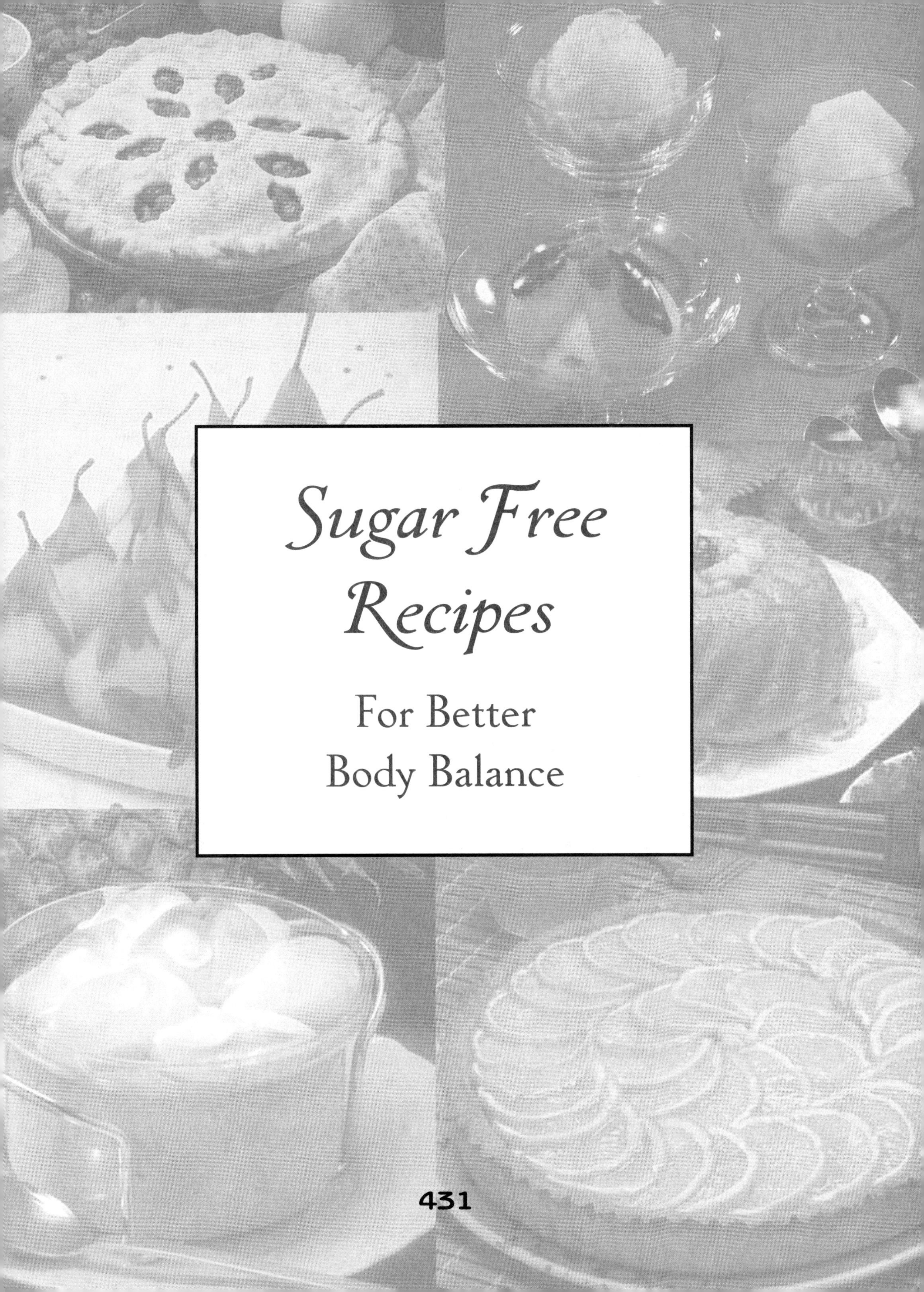

Sugar Free Recipes

For Better Body Balance

Sugar Free Sweet Treats

Sugar in America is synonymous with fun and good times. Our culture instills the powerful urge for sugary foods at an early age. While Americans have been cutting back on fat, sugar consumption is at an all-time high, and rising, increasing 28% since 1983. Sugar has become its own food group, counting for an astounding 20% of total calories for adult Americans each day.

The news is even worse for our kids who are regularly overdosed on sugar. Today's kids eat enough sugar to make up fully half of their daily calories! Sugar especially attacks energy levels and mood. Hyperactivity and Attention Deficit Disorder (ADD), affecting up to 10% of America's children, are aggravated by a high sugar diet. The problem is so out of control that over 46 health advocacy groups signed a letter to the U.S. Department of Health in 1998, urging it to commission funds for studies on sugar before the problem gets worse.

Sugar has so infiltrated our food supply that we hardly notice it's there. As our lives move faster, and become more stressful, sugar often plays a bigger part and becomes harder to avoid, especially as we turn to more convenience foods. Almost all snack foods and pre-prepared foods have added sugar to enhance their flavor. Sugars like high fructose corn syrup are in most commercial juices and sodas, and are no good for health. In August of 1999, the *Center For Science in the Public Interest* filed a petition to the U.S. FDA to require more explicit labeling of added sugar in foods.

There is already evidence that American sugar intake is implicated in scores of American health problems.... like diabetes, kidney stones, heart disease, and chronic dental problems. Nearsightedness, eczema, psoriasis, dermatitis, gout, indigestion, yeast infections, even the development of staph infections are related to our excessive sugar consumption.

Research shows sugar causes changes in cellular proteins and nucleic acids related to premature aging. Studies reveal that rats fed a high fructose diet age faster and demonstrate changes in collagen related to premature skin wrinkling and sagging.

Too much sugar triggers the overproduction of insulin, stressing the pancreas, the organ responsible for blood sugar regulation. Pancreas exhaustion leads to sugar disorders, inviting diabetes and hypoglycemia to take hold. Experts even speculate that the rise in pancreatic cancer correlates with the excessive rise in sugar consumption.

Clearly, a high sugar diet is a major factor in the U.S. rise in weight gain and obesity. Sugar requires insulin production for metabolism - a process that promotes the storage of fat. Metabolized sugar is transformed into fat globules, and distributed over the body where the muscles are not very active - on the stomach, hips and chin. Every time you eat sugar, some of those calories become body fat instead of energy.

Sugar also plays a part in many psychological reactions. It is a food that we eat to "cope" in times of stress, to satisfy a hole in both our palates and our psyches. As a physically addictive substance, it affects the brain first, offering a false energy lift that eventually lets you down lower than when you started. In reality, it produces an over-acid condition in the body, stripping out stabilizing B vitamins.

Sugar can be a major interference in your healing program.

Too much sugar leads to nutritional deficiencies, particularly upsetting mineral balances. It drains away calcium, overloading the body with acid-ash residues responsible for much of the stiffening of joints and limbs in arthritic conditions. Sugar robs the body of B vitamins in the digestive tract, so that they cannot act. Skin, nerve and digestive problems result. Sodas, sweetened with high fructose corn syrup, cause mineral loss, especially phosphorous and calcium, which may contribute to osteoporosis, a crippling bone disease! Most of us are familiar with the energy drop after a sugar binge. New studies show too much sugar is also linked to more serious depression.

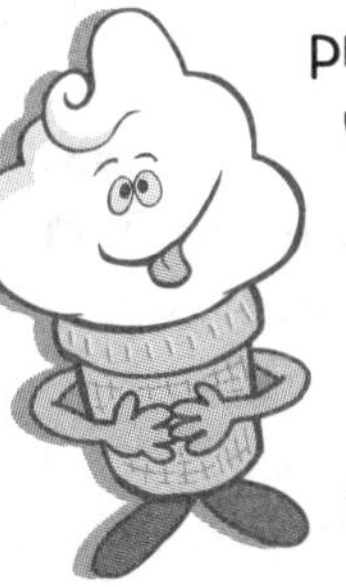

Finally, a high sugar diet suppresses immune response because refined sugar destroys the ability of white blood cells to kill germs for up to 5 hours after consumption. In addition, sugar feeds candida yeast and cancer, and disrupts hormonal health by inhibiting the release of growth hormone. It also lowers disease control, a proven fact for those with diabetes and hypoglycemia, and now becoming known as well for people with high triglycerides and blood pressure.

We need some sugar. Without sugar, in the form of "glucose" or blood sugar, we would die. But, our bodies get enough glucose when we eat complex carbohydrates from vegetables, whole grains and legumes.

Incredibly, in America, our "off-the-charts" refined sugar consumption (coupled with our lack of fresh fruits and vegetables) may be the foundation of almost all of our new susceptibility to degenerative disease. It is certainly a factor in our low overall health. Refined sugar is the ultimate naked carbohydrate, stripped of all nutritional benefits. If you think that too much sugar plays a part in your health problems, the sugar-free recipes in this section are a good choice for you.

Your Sugar-Free Options

See *in the Diet Book "Sugar"* pg. 91 and the "Food Digest," pg. 476 for more.

What's left after you've eliminated sugar? Just because you follow a sugar free diet doesn't mean you have to give up good taste or sweet comforts. The recipes in this section offer satisfying help and health, with honey, maple syrup, fruit juices, stevia, rice syrup and barley malt.... naturally sweet foods that your normal body processes handle correctly..... without extra stress or abnormal reactions.

The following list can help you easily convert to these natural sweeteners:

Note: If you have serious blood sugar problems, like diabetes or hypoglycemia, consult the appropriate pages in the Diet Book or your healing professional, about the kind and amount of sweets your body can handle.

• **HONEY: use $^1/_2$ cup honey to replace 1 cup of sugar; reduce the liquid in your recipe by $^1/_4$ cup.**

• **FRUCTOSE:** a commercially produced sugar with the same molecular structure as that found in fruit, fructose has a low glycemic index, meaning that it releases glucose into the bloodstream slowly. Fructose is almost twice as sweet as sugar, so less is needed for the same sweetening power. **Use $^1/_3$ to to $^2/_3$ cup to replace 1 cup of sugar.**

• **STEVIA:** *(an all natural sweet herb)*, is available as either a powdered or liquid extract in America. Experts say that stevia may soon be regarded as one of the most good-for-you sweeteners on earth. Unlike other sweeteners, stevia can actually regulate blood sugar, significantly increasing glucose tolerance. It is effective for weight control because it contains no calories, and may even block fat absorption. Stevia is 25 times sweeter than sugar when made as a tea with 1 tsp. leaves to 1 cup of water.

—Two drops of liquid infusion equal 1 teaspoon of sugar in sweetness. In baking, 1 teaspoon of stevia powder is equal to 1 cup of sugar. Use $^1/_4$ teasp. powdered stevia extract or 8 drops liquid extract to replace 1 tablespoon sweetness; 1 pinch powdered extract or 2 to 4 drops liquid extract to replace 1 teaspoon sweetness.

• **BARLEY MALT and BROWN RICE SYRUP-** are mild, natural sweeteners made from barley sprouts, or cultured rice and water cooked to a syrup. Only 40% as sweet as sugar, barley malt's blood sugar activity is a slow, complex carbohydrate release that does not upset insulin levels. **Use $1^1/_4$ cups syrup to replace 1 cup of sugar; reduce the liquid in your recipe by $^1/_4$ cup.**

• **BLACKSTRAP MOLASSES- use $^1/_2$ cup molasses to replace 1 cup of sugar; reduce the liquid in your recipe by $^1/_4$ cup.**

• **MAPLE SYRUP - use $^1/_2$ to $^2/_3$ cup maple syrup to replace 1 cup of sugar; reduce the liquid in your recipe by $^1/_4$ cup.**

• **DATE SUGAR-** ground, dried dates, the least refined, most natural sweetener, with a high sucrose concentration. It can be used much like brown sugar. **Use $1^1/_4$ cups date sugar to replace 1 cup of sugar.** To use in baking, mix with water before adding to the recipe to prevent burning, or add as a sweet topping after removing your dish from the oven.

• **FRUIT JUICE-** apple and pear juices seem to work the best in recipes. **Use 1 cup juice to replace 1 cup of sugar; reduce the liquid in your recipe by $^1/_3$ cup.**

• **SUCANAT-** *(an acronym from sugar cane natural)* is the trade name for a sweetener made from dried granulated cane juice, available in health food stores. Its average sugar content is 85%, with complex sugars, vitamins, minerals, amino acids and molasses retained. **Use 1 to 1 in place of sugar.** It is still a concentrated sweetener; use carefully if you have sugar balance problems.

• **TURBINADO SUGAR-** although a refined sugar, it is less refined than white table sugar. **Use 1 to 1 in place of sugar.**

• **SPICES- (Vanilla, Cinnamon, Cardamom, Ginger)-** use to replace sugary toppings, and in sauces instead of sugar for sweetness.

Sugar Free Recipe Sections

Sugar free baking is easy today. There are many natural sweeteners with health benefits in addition to their sweetening power. The sugar free recipes in this chapter focus on areas where sugar use is usually considered necessary.

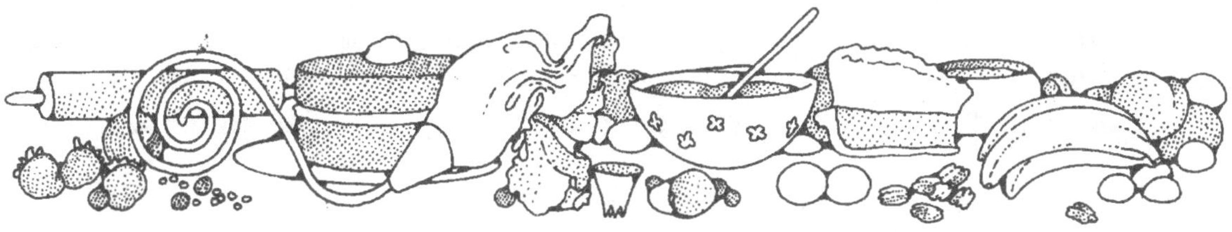

Sugar Free Cookies and Bars

Everybody loves cookies... they're the ultimate comfort food. You don't have to deprive yourself of cookies to be healthy. Try these sugar free recipes.

TRAIL MIX BARS

This recipe works for: Men's and Kid's Health, Sports Nutrition, Heart Health
For 12 bars: Preheat oven to 350°.

Toast on a baking sheet: 1 cup shredded Coconut, 1 cup chopped Walnuts, 1/2 cup Wheat Germ, 1/4 cup Rolled Oats. Remove and combine in a bowl with: 1/2 cup Date Sugar, 3 Eggs, 1 cup chopped Dates, 1/2 cup Molasses, 1/4 cup Honey, and 1/2 cup Whole Wheat Pastry Flour. Press into an oiled square baking pan and bake for 20 minutes.

—Sprinkle top with a mix of 2 TBS Date Sugar and 1/2 teasp. Allspice. Cut in bars.

Nutrition; 282 calories; 7gm protein; 40gm carbo.; 4gm fiber; 12gm total fats; 52mg choles.; 146mg calcium; 4mg iron; 90mg magnesium; 654mg potass.; 28mg sodium; Vit. A 29 IU; Vit. C 1mg; Vit. E 2 IU.

BEE POLLEN NUT BARS

This recipe works for: Hormone Health, Immune Power, Sports Nutrition
Makes 16 to 24 bars:

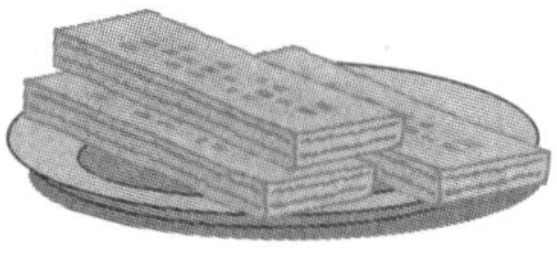

Mix in a large bowl: 3 cups Peanut Butter, 3/4 cup Almond Butter, 2 cups Honey, 1/2 cup Date Sugar, 1 cup Carob Chips, 3/4 cup Grapenuts Cereal, 3/4 cup Crispy Rice Cereal, 3/4 cup Toasted Shredded Coconut, 1/2 teasp. Cinnamon, 1/4 cup Bee Pollen Granules.

Fill a baking sheet. Press down and roll with a rolling pin to flatten evenly. Cover with plastic wrap and chill overnight. Cut into bars.

BREAKFAST ENERGY BARS

This recipe works for: Anti-Aging, Sugar Imbalances, Waste Management
Makes 12 bars: Preheat oven to 350°F.

Toast on a baking sheet: 1/2 cup chopped Almonds, 1/2 cup chopped Walnuts, 1/4 cup Wheat Germ, 1 cup Quick-Cook Oats, 1 cup Grapenuts, and 1 cup Bran Cereal about 5 minutes. Remove, grind together in a food processor and turn into a large bowl.

—Add: 4 TBS Honey, 2 teasp. Date Sugar, 1 teasp. grated Orange Zest, 1 teasp. Cinnamon and 1/4 teasp. Sea Salt. Stir in 1 cup Vanilla Almond Milk, 1 Egg, 1/4 cup Canola Oil and 1/2 cup dried, diced Mixed Fruit. Spray an 8" square pan with Canola Oil spray.

—Pack mixture into pan and bake for 20 to 30 minutes. Cool, cut in bars.

Nutrition; 251 calories; 8gm protein; 32gm carbo.; 6gm fiber; 12gm total fats; 17mg choles.; 68mg calcium; 6mg iron; 89mg magnesium; 259mg potass.; 203mg sodium; Vit. A 228 IU; Vit. C 5mg; Vit. E 3 IU.

FRESH GINGER-COCONUT COOKIES

This recipe works for: Heart and Artery Health, Men's Health, Weight Control
Makes 42 ball cookies:

Toast 16-oz. shredded Unsweetened Coconut and 1/4 cup Sesame Seeds in the oven until golden. Save about 1/2 cup for rolling cookies in.

—Turn rest into a double boiler over simmering water and warm with 3 TBS peeled grated Fresh Ginger (or 3 TBS minced Honey Crystallized Ginger), 1/2 cup Red Grape Juice or Cranberry Juice, 3 TBS Crunchy Peanut Butter and 1 pinch Sea Salt.

—In another pan, melt 1/2 cup Date Sugar, 1 TB Unsweetened Cocoa Powder and 2 TBS Honey. Blend in coconut-juice mixture. Chill in the fridge. Roll 42 small balls. Mix 2 TBS Date Sugar with reserved coconut-sesame mix and roll cookies in the mix.

Nutrition; 96 calories; 1gm protein; 7gm carbo.; 2gm fiber; 8gm total fats; 0mg choles.; 14mg calcium; 1mg iron; 17mg magnesium; 87mg potass.; 18mg sodium; Vit. A 1 IU; Vit. C trace; Vit. E trace.

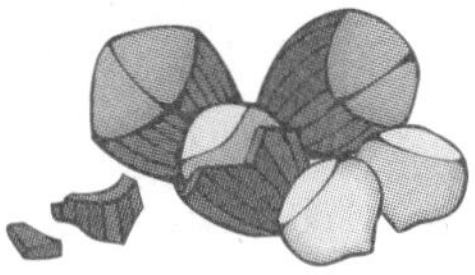

SPICED NUT BALLS

This recipe works for: Hair, Skin and Nails, Heart Health, Digestion
For 60 balls: Preheat oven to 350°F. Spray baking sheets with Canola Oil spray.

Mix dry ingredients: 1 cup Unbleached Flour, 1 cup Whole Wheat Pastry Flour, 1/2 tsp. each: Baking Powder and Baking Soda, 1 tsp. each: Ginger Powder, Cinnamon, Cardamom Powder and 1/4 tsp. each: Nutmeg. and Sea Salt.

—Cream the dough in another large bowl: 1 stick Butter, 1 Egg, 1 cup Date Sugar, 1/2 tsp. Stevia Powder, 2 TBS Molasses and 1/2 cup chopped Walnuts.

—Combine both mixtures, then turn out on a floured surface and knead briefly. Wrap in plastic and chill. Roll into balls and bake for 15 minutes. Cool on racks.

PINEAPPLE-CRANBERRY BARS

This recipe works for: Liver-Organ Health, Immune Health, Hair, Skin and Nails
For 24 bars: Preheat oven to 350°F. Use a Canola Oil sprayed 9 x 13" baking pan.

Heat 1 1/2 cups Cranberries and 1 1/2 cups Orange Juice until cranberries pop.

—Beat in a bowl: 4 TBS Butter, 2 TBS Maple Syrup, 1 teasp. grated Orange Zest, 2 Eggs and cranberry-orange juice mix.

—In another bowl, stir together: 2 1/2 cups Whole Wheat Pastry Flour, 2 teasp. Baking Powder, 1 teasp. Baking Soda, 1/2 teasp. Cinnamon and 1/2 teasp. Nutmeg.

—Mix both together and stir in 1 cup chopped Walnuts. Spoon into baking pan. Top with a mixture of 3/4 cup shredded Coconut and 3/4 cup crushed drained Pineapple.

—Bake for 20 to 25 minutes until a toothpick comes out clean. Cool and cut.

Nutrition; 131 calories; 4gm protein; 15gm carbo.; 2gm fiber; 7gm total fats; 23mg choles.; 43mg calcium; 1mg iron; 34mg magnesium; 142mg potass.; 90mg sodium; Vit. A 31 IU; Vit. C 10mg; Vit. E 1 IU.

MAPLE SUGAR ALMOND COOKIES

This recipe works for: Sugar Imbalances, Women's Health, Hair and Skin
For 24 cookies: Preheat oven to 325°F. Use a Canola Oil sprayed baking sheet.

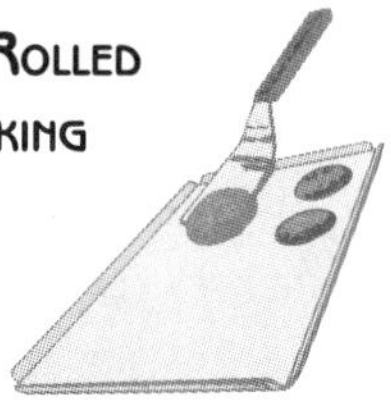

Process in a food processor to fine: 1 cup Toasted Almonds, 1 cup Rolled Oats, 1 cup Unbleached Flour, 3 TBS Maple Sugar Granules, $^1/_2$ tsp. Baking Powder, $^1/_4$ tsp. Baking Soda and $^1/_4$ tsp. Sea Salt.

—In a bowl blend: $^1/_2$ cup Almond Butter, $^1/_4$ cup Maple Syrup, $^1/_2$ tsp. Cinnamon, $^1/_2$ tsp. Allspice and 2 tsp. Vanilla. Blend both wet and dry ingredients together with a fork. Wrap in plastic wrap and chill.

—Roll out dough into a rectangle (trim sides and press extra dough back in to be re-rolled). Cut lengthwise, then horizontally to make 24 strips. Transfer to baking sheets. Press tops with fork tines. Bake about 20 minutes until light brown.

—Frost if desired with BUTTERSCOTCH CANDY FROSTING. The frosting holds very well for cookies, hardening to a candy-like substance. Bring $^1/_3$ cup Honey and 2 TBS Butter to a simmer. Cook 10 minutes over low heat until color begins to darken. Remove from heat and let bubbles die. Spoon over cookies and let harden. Cool, then refrigerate to store.

Nutrition; 117 calories; 3gm protein; 12gm carbo.; 2gm fiber; 6gm total fats; 0mg choles.; 44mg calcium; 1mg iron; 41mg magnesium; 115mg potass.; 44mg sodium; Vit. A 1 IU; Vit. C trace; Vit. E 2 IU.

DOUBLE GINGER MOLASSES COOKIES

This recipe works for: Sugar Imbalances, Heart Health, Hair, Skin and Nails
For 24 cookies: Preheat oven to 350°F. Use a Canola Oil sprayed baking sheet.

Combine in a pan until melted: $^1/_2$ cup Maple Sugar Granules, 4 TBS Butter, 4 TBS Canola Oil, $^1/_2$ cup Molasses, 2 TBS Lemon Juice and 2 TBS Honey Crystallized Ginger.

—Stir together: 2 cups Whole Wheat Pastry Flour, 1 teasp. Ground Ginger, 1 teasp. Baking Powder, $^1/_2$ teasp. Baking Soda, 1 teasp. Allspice, 1 teasp. Cinnamon, 1 teasp. Ground Cloves and $^1/_2$ teasp. Sea Salt.

—Combine mixtures together. Roll out into a dough; decorate with Raisins, chopped Nuts and Nutmeg dashes. Cover with plastic wrap and chill. Then cut with a cookie cutter, saving and reworking in scraps. Bake for 15 minutes. Cool on racks.

CRUNCHY GRANOLA COOKIES

This recipe works for: Waste Management, Heart Health, Sports Nutrition
For 36 cookies: Preheat oven to 350°F.

Mix all ingredients together: 6 TBS Peanut Butter, $1^1/_2$ cups nutty, crunchy Granola, $^1/_2$ cup Honey, $^1/_2$ cup Carob Chips and 1 teasp. Cinnamon. Drop onto oiled sheets, and bake for 10 minutes until edges brown.

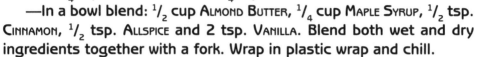

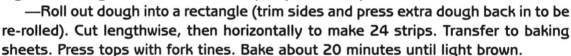

FROSTED LEMON TEA WAFERS

This recipe works for: Sugar Imbalances, Arthritis, Hair, Skin and Nails
For 24 cookies: Preheat oven to 350°F. Use a Canola Oil sprayed baking sheet.

Mix dry ingredients: 1 cup Unbleached Flour, 1/2 cup shredded Coconut, 1/3 cup crushed Almonds, 1/4 cup Rice Flour, 1 teasp. Baking Powder and 1/2 teasp. Baking Soda.
—Mix wet ingredients: 1 Egg, 1/2 cup Honey, 1/4 cup Oil, 1/4 cup Butter, 1/4 cup Lemon Yogurt, 1 tsp. Vanilla, 1/2 tsp. Cardamom, 1/4 tsp. Allspice, 2 TBS grated Lemon Zest.
—Combine both sets of ingredients to make a dough. Drop onto baking pans about 1-inch apart. They will spread. Bake for 10 minutes until edges are light brown. Cool. Do not stack. They will get soggy.
—Frost with LEMON CREAM CHEESE FROSTING: Whisk together 3-oz. Low Fat Cream Cheese, 2 TBS Honey and 1 teasp. grated Lemon Zest; frost just before serving.

Nutrition; 125 calories; 2gm protein; 14gm carbo.; 1gm fiber; 7gm total fats; 16mg choles.; 32mg calcium; 1mg iron; 12mg magnesium; 52mg potassium; 47mg sodium; Vit. A 30 IU; Vit. C 1mg; Vit. E 2 IU.

FRUIT JUICE BARS

This recipe works for: Sugar Imbalances, Weight Control, Overcoming Addictions
For 16 bars: Preheat oven to 350°F.

Blend in the blender to a puree: 1 cup chopped Dates, 1/2 cup Apple Juice, 1/2 cup Orange Juice, 3 TBS grated Orange Zest and 1 teasp. Vanilla; set aside.
—Grind 2 cups Rolled Oats in the blender to a coarse meal. Stir oats in a bowl with 2 cups Whole Wheat Pastry Flour and 1 TB Cinnamon. Stir in 1 1/2 cups Pear Juice.
—Press dough into a Canola Oil sprayed 8-inch square pan. Spread date puree on top. Bake for 35 to 45 minutes until crust is firm. Cool completely and cut in squares.

Nutrition; 144 calories; 4gm protein; 31gm carbo.; 4gm fiber; 1gm total fats; 0mg choles.; 24mg calcium; 1mg iron; 43mg magnesium; 221mg potass.; 3mg sodium; Vit. A 4 IU; Vit. C 6mg; Vit. E 1 IU.

MONSTER OATMEAL COOKIES

This recipe works for: Kid's Health, Sugar Imbalances, Allergies - Asthma
For 12 cookies: Preheat oven to 350°F.

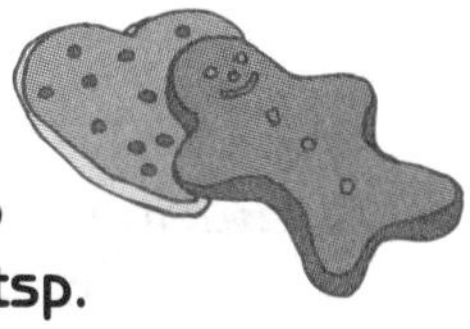

Mix together: 1/2 cup Canola Oil, 1/2 cup Whole Wheat Pastry Flour, 1 cup Toasted Wheat Germ, 1 cup Honey, 1 cup Rolled Oats, 1/2 cup Raisins, 1 cup shredded Coconut, 1 cup Blueberry Nut Granola, 1/2 tsp. Cinnamon, 1/4 teasp. Baking Powder and 2 TBS Orange Juice; let sit for 10 minutes to blend. Add more orange juice if needed to moisten. Divide into 12 balls. Place on greased sheets and flatten into big cookies, (about 3 or 4 on a sheet). Bake until golden, about 15 minutes.

Sugar-Free Treats

Nibbles and Surprises

Are you hooked on candy bars or sugar filled snacks for your late morning or afternoon energy lift? Try these portable, tasty goodies for energy and nutrition.

GLAZED ALMOND SQUARES

Surprisingly high in fiber and low in fat.

This recipe works for: Kid's Health, Sugar Imbalances, Allergies - Asthma

For 16 squares: Preheat oven to 350°F. Use an 8-inch square baking pan.

Make the cookie base: combine dry ingredients: $^3/_4$ cup Grapenuts Cereal, $^1/_2$ cup crunchy Almond Granola, 3 TBS Carob Powder, 1 TB Baking Powder and $^1/_2$ teasp. Baking Soda. Heat wet ingredients; simmer 1 minute: $^1/_3$ cup Canola Oil, $^1/_3$ cup Honey, 2 TBS Maple Syrup, $^1/_2$ teasp. Almond Extract, 1 TB Almond Butter.

—Mix both sets of ingredients together; add 3 TBS Vanilla Almond Milk for smoothness. Pour into a Canola Oil sprayed pan and bake for 35 minutes.

—Make the maple glaze while cookie base is still warm. Heat and stir in a pan until liquid and smooth: 4 teasp. Maple Syrup, 2 drops Almond Extract, 1 TB Carob Powder. Spread thinly over warm cake. Cut in squares.

Nutrition; 134 calories; 2gm protein; 21gm carbo.; 2gm fiber; 6gm total fats; 0mg choles.; 76mg calcium; 3mg iron; 19mg magnesium; 71mg potass.; 166mg sodium; Vit. A 106 IU; Vit. C trace; Vit. E 2 IU.

CHEWY GRANOLA DROPS

This recipe works for: Women's and Men's Health, Arthritis, Healthy Pregnancy

For 4 dozen drops: Preheat oven to 350°F. Use Canola Oil sprayed baking sheets.

Beat together: 2 Eggs, 1 cup Maple Sugar Granules, 2 TBS Canola Oil, $1^1/_2$ teasp. Vanilla and 1 teasp. Sea Salt. Mix in: 1 cup shredded Coconut, $^1/_4$ cup Raisins and 1 cup Coconut-Almond or other favorite Granola. Drop spoonfuls onto baking sheets; bake about 10 minutes until golden.

Nutrition; 51 calories; 1gm protein; 7gm carbo.; 2gm fiber; 6gm total fats; 0mg choles.; 76mg calcium; 3mg iron; 19mg magnesium; 71mg potass.; 166mg sodium; Vit. A 106 IU; Vit. C trace; Vit. E 2 IU.

CRISPY ALMOND BUTTER BALLS

This recipe works for: Men's- Kid's Health, Heart Health

For 4 dozen balls: Preheat oven to 350°F. Cool on racks.

Cream: $^1/_4$ cup Butter, $^1/_2$ cup Maple Syrup, $^2/_3$ cup Almond Butter. Mix in: $1^1/_3$ cups Whole Wheat Pastry Flour, 1 teasp. Baking Powder and $^1/_2$ teasp. Sea Salt. Roll into balls. Drop on Canola Oil sprayed baking sheets; bake 15 minutes until edges brown.

BUTTERSCOTCH COCONUT BALLS

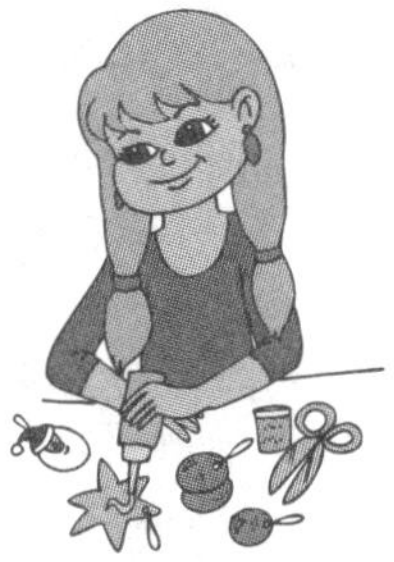

This recipe works for: Stress Reactions, Kid's Health
For 8 balls: Preheat oven to 250°F.

Brown 1 cup shredded Coconut until light gold. Pour in a mixing bowl. Blend with 1 cup Low Fat Cream Cheese, 1/2 cup Honey, 1 teasp. Vanilla and 2 TBS Butter. Roll into balls and press a Whole Almond into each. Chill.

Nutrition; 224 calories; 4gm protein; 22gm carbo.; 2gm fiber; 11gm total fats; 24mg choles.; 39mg calcium; 1mg iron; 12mg magnesium; 116mg potass.; 5mg sodium; Vit. A 95 IU; Vit. C 1mg; Vit. E 1 IU.

ALMOND BUTTER MEDJOOLS

This recipe works for: Overcoming Addictions, Allergies and Asthma, Hair and Skin
Stuffing for 8 big dates:

Cut open 8 big Medjool Dates and spread apart for stuffing. Mash and mix 1/2 teasp. Honey and 1/4 cup Almond Butter together. Stuff dates and roll in 1/4 cup toasted shredded Coconut. Serve chilled.

TOASTY BEE POLLEN SURPRISE

This recipe works for: Women's and Men's Health, Colds Recovery, Kid's Health
For 18 pieces:

Stir 1 cup Honey, 2 TBS Maple Syrup and 1 cup Peanut Butter in a pan until smooth.
—Remove from heat and mix in 2/3 cup toasted Coconut-Almond Granola (or your favorite granola), 1/2 cup chopped Toasted Walnuts, 1 cup Carob Powder, 1/2 cup shredded toasted Coconut, 1 cup toasted Sunflower Seeds, 4 TBS Bee Pollen Granules and 1/2 cup Raisins. Press into an 8-inch baking pan. Chill; cut in squares.

Nutrition; 294 calories; 8gm protein; 34gm carbo.; 3gm fiber; 16gm total fats; 0mg choles.; 30mg calcium; 2mg iron; 71mg magnesium; 261mg potass.; 16mg sodium; Vit. A 2 IU; Vit. C 1mg; Vit. E 6 IU.

HONEY CANDIED FRUITS

This recipe works for: Stress Reactions, Immune Health, Heart Health

Heat 2 cups Water, 1 1/2 cups Honey and 2 TBS Lemon Juice in a pan until blended.
—Dip in your choice of fruits, Pineapple, Pears, Figs, Apricots. Then dehydrate in a dehydrator, or on drying screens in the sun, until rubbery and chewy, but not too dry. Candied fruit can be stored airtight in the fridge for quite a while. Eat them just like they are, or use them in holiday fruit cakes, or to decorate cookies.

BAKED CANDY POPCORN

This recipe works for: Hair, Skin, Nails, Kid's Health, Sports Nutrition
For 12 servings: Preheat oven to 350°F.

Make a big batch of Popcorn. Turn into a large bowl. Stir in 1 $^1/_2$ cups Dry Roasted Peanuts. Melt 8-oz. Butter (1 stick) in a pan. Add $^1/_2$ cup Honey, $^1/_4$ cup Molasses and $^1/_2$ cup Maple Syrup. Simmer until bubbles form. Immediately pour over popcorn and peanuts, and toss to coat. Spread mixture on two Canola Oil sprayed baking sheets; bake until coating darkens, about 10 minutes. Cool completely before storing, so mix doesn't turn soggy.

APPLE BARS

This recipe works for: Overcoming Addictions, Allergies - Asthma, Illness Recovery
For 12 pieces: Preheat oven to 350°F.

Blend ingredients in a bowl: $^1/_2$ cup Applesauce, $^1/_2$ cup Apple Juice, 1 cup Raisins, 2 cups Whole Wheat Pastry Flour, 4 TBS Butter, 3 Eggs, 2 teasp. Baking Powder, 1 teasp. Baking Soda, 1 $^1/_2$ teasp. Cinnamon and 1 teasp. Nutmeg.

—Press into a Canola Oil sprayed square pan. Sprinkle with Apple Pie Spice or more Cinnamon and Nutmeg. Bake for 25 minutes.

Nutrition; 172 calories; 5gm protein; 28gm carbo.; 3gm fiber; 5gm total fats; 62mg choles.; 83mg calcium; 2mg iron; 35mg magnesium; 223mg potass.; 135mg sodium; Vit. A 60 IU; Vit. C 1mg; Vit. E 1 IU.

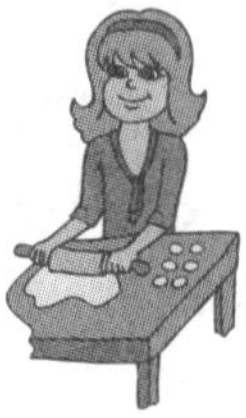

Sugar Free Cakes and Sweet Muffins

Have your cake and your health with these sugar free cakes muffins and sweet breads.

SWEET OAT BRAN MUFFINS

This recipe works for: Allergies, Sugar Imbalances, Waste Management
For 6 large (9 small) muffins: Bake at 400°F. for 20 minutes.

Mix in a bowl: 1 cup Oat Bran, 1 TB Lecithin Granules, 1 teasp. Baking Powder, 1 teasp. Cinnamon, $^1/_2$ teasp. Stevia Powder.

—Blender blend: $^1/_4$ cup Apple Juice. $^1/_2$ cup Raisins, 1 $^1/_2$ tsp. Vanilla, 1 Apple, 1 Egg.

—Stir both mixtures together gently. Spray muffin tins with Canola Oil Spray.

HONEY NUT CARROT CAKE

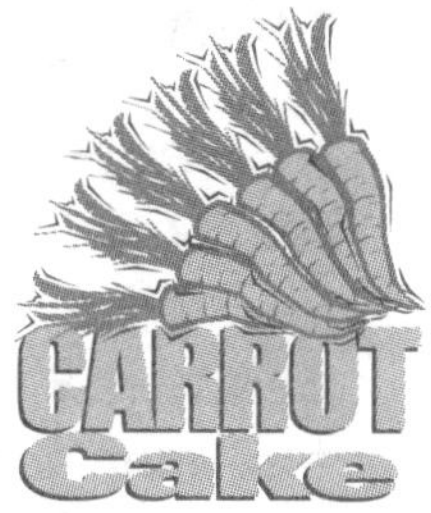

This recipe works for: Sugar Imbalances, Men's Nutrition
For 12 pieces: Preheat oven to 350°F.

Separate 6 Eggs. Beat yolks with: 1 cup grated Carrots, 1 cup chopped Walnuts, $^1/_2$ cup Honey, $^1/_2$ cup Unbleached Flour, $^1/_4$ cup Toasted Wheat Germ, $^1/_4$ cup crunchy Granola, 2 TBS Maple Syrup, 1 teasp. Cinnamon, $^1/_2$ teasp. Sea Salt, $^1/_4$ teasp. Nutmeg.

—Beat the 6 Egg Whites to stiff peaks and fold into cake. Pour into a Canola Oil sprayed square baking dish, and bake 45 minutes until very puffy and golden.

—Top with dollops of ALMOND HONEY ICING: beat 1 Egg White with 2 pinches Cream of Tartar to stiff peaks. Add $^1/_2$ cup Honey in a thin stream while beating. Add $^1/_4$ teasp. Almond Extract and beat until thick and fluffy.

SPICE INFUSED MUFFINS with MARMALADE WELLS

This recipe works for: Digestive Health, Men's Health, Weight Control
For 10 muffins: Preheat oven to 350°.

Stir dry ingredients together: $1^1/_2$ cups Whole Wheat Pastry Flour, 1 cup sliced Almonds, 1 teasp. Baking Powder, $^1/_2$ teasp. Baking Soda, 1 teasp. Cinnamon, $^1/_2$ teasp. Nutmeg and $^1/_2$ teasp. Cardamom Powder.

—Beat wet ingredients together: $^1/_2$ cup Honey, $^1/_4$ cup Plain Yogurt, $^1/_4$ cup Water, 4 TBS Canola Oil, 1 Egg, 1 teasp. grated Lemon Zest, and $^1/_2$ teasp. Allspice.

—Combine the two mixtures and stir until moistened. Fill 10 paper-lined muffin cups $^2/_3$ full. Gently press 1 rounded teaspoon of marmalade into the center of each muffin. Bake 20 minutes until golden and firm. Cool briefly in the pan, then remove to racks. Mix 2 TBS Date Sugar and $^1/_4$ teasp. Cinnamon and dust tops of muffins.

Nutrition; 282 calories; 6gm protein; 37gm carbo.; 3gm fiber; 9gm total fats; 21mg choles.; 82mg calcium; 2mg iron; 70mg magnesium; 223mg potass.; 99mg sodium; Vit. A 11 IU; Vit. C 1mg; Vit. E 3 IU.

BEST SUGAR FREE GINGERBREAD

This recipe works for: Heart Health, Kid's Health, Sports Nutrition
For 12 pieces: Preheat oven to 350°F. Use a Canola Oil sprayed square pan.

Sauté 3 TBS grated Ginger in 5 TBS Canola Oil til fragrant. Add $^1/_2$ cup Honey and $^1/_2$ cup Molasses and heat. Remove from heat; add $^1/_2$ cup Plain Yogurt and 1 Egg.

—Mix dry ingredients in a bowl: 2 cups Whole Wheat Pastry Flour, $1^1/_2$ teasp. Baking Soda, $^3/_4$ teasp. grated Orange Peel, $^1/_2$ teasp. Cinnamon, $^1/_2$ teasp. Ground Cloves, $^1/_2$ teasp. Allspice, $^1/_4$ teasp. Ginger Powder and $^1/_2$ teasp. Sea Salt. Stir into ginger-honey mixture just to moisten. Spread into baking pan. Bake for 30 minutes until top is springy and a toothpick inserted in the center comes out clean.

PIÑA COLADA MUFFINS

This recipe works for: Men's Health, Waste Management, Sugar Imbalances
For 8 muffins: Preheat oven to 375°F. Use paper-lined muffin cups.

Gently mix all ingredients in a bowl just to moisten: $1^{1}/_{2}$ cups Unbleached Flour, $^{1}/_{4}$ cup oven-toasted shredded Coconut, 2 teasp. Baking Powder, 1 Egg, $^{1}/_{2}$ cup Oat Bran, $^{1}/_{4}$ cup Canola Oil, $^{1}/_{2}$ cup Plain Yogurt, 1 can (8-oz.) Crushed Pineapple, $1^{1}/_{4}$ cups Pineapple-Coconut Juice. Spoon into muffin cups and bake for 20 minutes until a toothpick inserted in the center comes out clean. Sprinkle with oven-toasted, shredded Coconut and press into muffin top.

SWEET YAM MUFFINS

This recipe works for: Liver and Organ Health, Women's Health, Sports Nutrition
For 12 muffins: Preheat oven to 350°F. Use paper-lined muffin cups.

Bake until soft, then peel and mash 1 large Yam.

—Mix dry ingredients: 1 cup Unbleached Flour, $^{1}/_{3}$ cup Whole Wheat Pastry Flour, 2 tsp. Baking Powder, $^{1}/_{3}$ cup Fructose, $^{1}/_{2}$ cup Date Sugar, $^{1}/_{2}$ tsp. Cinnamon, $^{1}/_{4}$ tsp. Allspice, $^{1}/_{4}$ tsp. Nutmeg, $^{1}/_{4}$ tsp. ground Cloves, $^{1}/_{4}$ tsp. ground Ginger and $^{1}/_{2}$ tsp. Sea Salt.

—Combine wet ingredients: the mashed yam, 3 TBS Maple Syrup, $^{1}/_{4}$ cup Plain Yogurt, $^{1}/_{4}$ cup Water, 1 Egg, 4 TBS Butter and 2 TBS Canola Oil.

—Stir mixtures together; add $^{1}/_{4}$ cup chopped Walnuts and $^{1}/_{4}$ cup Raisins. Spoon into muffin cups. Mix 1 teasp. Fructose with $^{3}/_{4}$ teasp. Cinnamon and sprinkle a pinch on each muffin. Bake 25 minutes until muffin tops spring back when touched.

Nutrition; 226 calories; 4gm protein; 36gm carbo.; 2gm fiber; 8gm total fats; 28mg choles.; 95mg calcium; 1mg iron; 25mg magnesium; 231mg potass.; 163mg sodium; Vit. A 664 IU; Vit. C 7mg; Vit. E 1 IU.

GLAZED PEAR CAKE

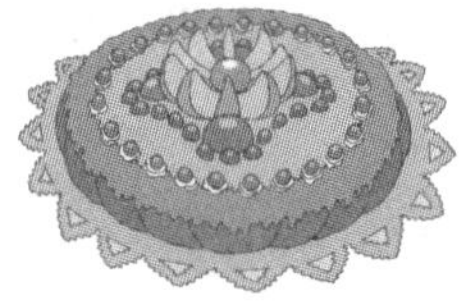

This recipe works for: Allergies and Asthma, Women's Health
For 10 pieces: Preheat oven to 350°F. Use

Separate 3 Eggs. Mix the yolks with: 1 cup Oat Flour, $^{1}/_{2}$ cup Barley Flour, 2 teasp. Baking Powder, $^{1}/_{2}$ teasp. Baking Soda. Melt together: 4 TBS Butter, $^{1}/_{2}$ cup Maple Syrup, 2 TBS Orange Juice Concentrate and 2 teasp. Vanilla.

—Blend mixtures together. Beat egg whites stiff with a pinch of Cream of Tartar. Fold into batter. Pour into a Canola Oil sprayed baking pan. Bake for 20 minutes.

—Make the PEAR GLAZE: Simmer 2 large thinly sliced Pears with 1 cup Frozen Apple Juice Concentrate until most juice is cooked off. Remaining amount should be thick and syrupy. Arrange pears on top of the cake decoratively. Spoon juice over.

Nutrition; 246 calories; 5gm protein; 42gm carbo.; 3gm fiber; 7gm total fats; 76mg choles.; 105mg calcium; 2mg iron; 32mg magnesium; 293mg potass.; 165mg sodium; Vit. A 75 IU; Vit. C 4mg; Vit. E 1 IU.

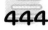

TENDER MOLASSES GINGERBREAD

Great for kids' snacks.

This recipe works for: Circulatory Health, Allergies, Kid's Health

For 9 pieces: Preheat oven to 350°F. Use a 9 x 9" square pan.

Stir together dry ingredients: $1\,^1/_4$ cups Whole Wheat Pastry Flour, $^3/_4$ teasp. Baking Soda, $^1/_2$ teasp. Cinnamon, $^1/_2$ teasp. ground Ginger, and $^1/_4$ teasp. Nutmeg. Mix the wet ingredients: 1 Egg, $^1/_4$ cup Canola Oil, $^3/_4$ cup Molasses, $^1/_2$ cup Hot Water, 2 TBS Honey, $^1/_4$ teasp. Allspice and $^1/_4$ teasp. Sea Salt. Combine the two mixtures, and beat smooth. Pour into baking pan and bake for 20 minutes until a toothpick comes out clean.

Nutrition; 198 calories; 3gm protein; 32gm carbo.; 2gm fiber; 6gm total fats; 23mg choles.; 248mg calcium; 6mg iron; 83mg magnesium; 759mg potass.; 187mg sodium; Vit. A 11 IU; Vit. C trace; Vit. E 2 IU.

SUGAR FREE GINGERBREAD HEAVEN

This recipe works for: Sugar Imbalances, Kid's Health, Digestive and Heart Health

Preheat oven to 350°F. Oil muffin tins or cake pans with Canola Oil spray.

Stir dry ingredients in a bowl: 2 cups Unbleached Flour, 2 tsp. Baking Powder, 1 tsp. Cinnamon, 1 TB minced Crystallized Ginger, $^1/_2$ tsp. Nutmeg and $^1/_2$ tsp. Sea Salt.

—Combine $^2/_3$ cup Rice Syrup, $^1/_3$ cup Barley Malt and 4 TBS Canola Oil and 3 TBS Orange Juice; stir into dry ingredients. Pour into baking pans and bake for 25 to 30 minutes (for muffins) or 35 to 40 minutes (for cake). When a toothpick inserted in the center comes out clean, cake is done.

—Make the ORANGE SESAME ICING: gently heat $^1/_2$ cup Rice Syrup, $^1/_3$ cup Barley Malt, 3 TBS Sesame Tahini, $^1/_2$ tsp. Vanilla. Add gradually about 6 to 8 TBS Orange Juice until icing reaches desired thickness. Add 2 teasp. Arrowroot Powder dissolved in 2 TBS Water. Stir gently; add $^1/_2$ cup chopped Walnuts and 1 teasp. grated Orange Peel.

SUGAR FREE ORANGE SCONES

Scones

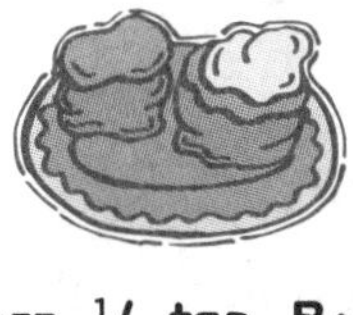

This recipe works for: Hair, Skin, Nails, Sugar Imbalances

Makes 8: Preheat oven to 350°F.

Make the scones: mix 2 cups Unbleached Flour, 2 tsp. Baking Powder, $^1/_2$ tsp. Baking Soda and $^1/_4$ tsp. Sea Salt. Stir in $^1/_4$ cup Canola Oil. Add $^1/_3$ cup Orange Honey, 2 TBS Maple Syrup, $^1/_2$ cup Frozen Orange Juice Concentrate thawed, $^1/_2$ cup Vanilla Soymilk and the grated Zest of 1 Orange. Mix lightly; allow to sit for 10 minutes. Pat dough into rectangles about $^1/_2$-inch thick. Place on a Canola Oil sprayed baking sheet.

—Make topping: Mix 2 TBS Frozen Orange Juice Concentrate thawed, $^1/_2$ tsp. Almond Extract and 2 TBS Orange Honey; brush onto scones. Sprinkle with sliced Almonds. Bake for 15 minutes.

Nutrition; 288 calories; 5gm protein; 50gm carbo.; 2gm fiber; 8gm total fats; 0mg choles.; 135mg calcium; 2mg iron; 21mg magnesium; 195mg potass.; 240mg sodium; Vit. A 5 IU; Vit. C 30mg; Vit. E 3 IU.

CRUMB TOP PUMPKIN BREAD

This recipe works for: Anti-Aging, Men's Health, Hair and Skin, Arthritis
Preheat oven to 350°F. Use a Canola Oil sprayed 8 x 12" baking pan.

Mix dry ingredients together until crumbly: 3 cups Whole Wheat Pastry Flour, 1/2 cup Fructose, 1/2 cup Date Sugar, 8-oz. (1 stick) Butter, 1/4 cup Canola Oil, 2 teasp. Ginger Powder, 1 teasp. Cinnamon, 1/2 teasp. Nutmeg, 1/4 teasp. Cardamom Powder. Set aside 2/3 cup of the mixture for topping.

—Mix wet ingredients: 1 can cooked Pumpkin, 1/2 cup Molasses, 2 Eggs, 2 TBS Plain Yogurt, 2 TBS Water, 1 1/2 teasp. Baking Soda. Mix the two ingredients together just to moisten, and turn into baking pan. Sprinkle crumble mix on top. Bake until top is firm, about 50 minutes. Cool slightly.

—Serve warm with CRUNCHY ALMOND TOPPING: Toast 1/2 cup sliced Almonds in the oven until brown, about 10 minutes. Bring 1/2 cup Maple Syrup to a boil. Stir in almonds. Bring to boil again. Pour onto oiled sheets. Let set for 10 minutes, and then break up into pieces. Sprinkle over pumpkin bread.

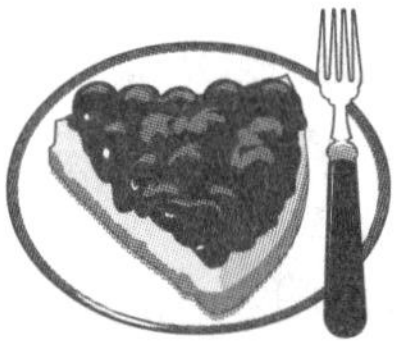

Sugar Free Cheesecakes and Pies

Sweet fruits and creamy soft cheeses are a perfect, soul-satisfying match. They've been a sweet pair since Greek and Roman times, centuries before sugar was even known. I've updated the original idea so you can enjoy them as sugar free desserts.

UPSIDE DOWN PEAR PIE

This recipe works for: Anti-Aging, Bone Health, Hair and Skin
Serves 12: Preheat oven to 375°F. Use a stove-to-oven 10-inch skillet.

Have ready 3 1/2-lbs. firm Pears, cored and thinly sliced; toss with 3 TBS Lemon Juice and set aside. Mix in a bowl with your fingers to a fine meal: 1/3 cup Butter, 4 TBS Maple Sugar Granules, 1 1/4 cups Whole Wheat Pastry Flour and 1 Egg. Pat into a 5-inch disc; wrap in plastic and chill while you make the rest.

—In an ovenproof skillet, melt 4 TBS Butter and blend with 3/4 cup Maple Sugar Granules and 2 TBS Fructose until mixture caramelizes, about 6 to 8 minutes. Watch closely. Remove from heat; spoon in pears, pressing together to fill pan compactly.

—Roll out dough between big sheets of plastic wrap to an 11-inch round. Remove top plastic sheet and invert dough over pears in the skillet. Remove plastic wrap and tuck 1-inch dough around edge between skillet and pears. Make 3 vents in dough. Bake 1 hour until pie is golden and juices are bubbly. Let stand for 24 hours so pears absorb all juices. To serve, loosen crust around edges with a thin knife, and invert on a large serving plate.

APPLE SPICE PIE

This recipe works for: Men's Health, Bone Health, Immune Enhancement
Serves 8: Preheat oven to 400°F.

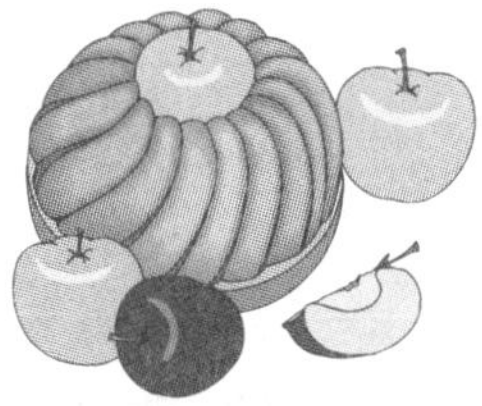

Make a crust: in a bowl mix $^3/_4$ cup Grapenuts Cereal and $^1/_2$ cup Rolled Oats. Simmer $^3/_4$ cup Raisins, $^1/_2$ cup Apple Juice and 2 TBS Maple Syrup until most of liquid is absorbed. Puree in a blender to smooth. Mix with grapenuts and press into a Canola Oil sprayed pie pan. Bake for 5 to 7 minutes until fragrant. Cool.

—Make the filling: Saute 6 cups sliced Granny Smith Apples in 2 TBS Butter for 3 minutes. Sprinkle with 1 teasp. Cinnamon, $^1/_2$ teasp. Nutmeg and $^1/_2$ teasp. Cardamom Powder. Mix in a bowl: $^1/_3$ cup Apple Juice, $^1/_3$ cup Water, 2 TBS Lemon Juice, $1^1/_2$ teasp. Arrowroot Powder and $^1/_2$ cup Maple Syrup. Pour over apples and simmer stirring until thickened, about 5 minutes. Turn into pie crust. Bake until pie is bubbly, about 30 minutes. Run under the broiler to crisp top. Sprinkle with 6 TBS Maple Sugar Granules and dot with 6 dollops of Frozen Vanilla Honey Yogurt to serve.

ALMOND SCENTED CHEESECAKE BITES

This recipe works for: Women's Health, Weight Control, Sugar Imbalances
For 24 individual cakes: Preheat oven to 300°F.

Make the batter: place 12-oz. Low Fat Cottage Cheese in a strainer over the sink and drain for 30 minutes. Put drained cottage cheese in a blender and blend until smooth with: 3 Eggs, $^1/_4$ cup Frozen Apple Juice Concentrate, $^1/_4$ cup Pineapple Juice Concentrate, 3 TBS chopped Almonds, 1 teasp. Almond Extract and 1 teasp. Vanilla.

—Fill paper-lined muffin tins $^2/_3$ full with batter. Bake 35 minutes until a toothpick inserted in the center comes out clean. Cool on rack, and then chill.

—Combine $^1/_3$ cup Low Fat Vanilla Yogurt and 3 TBS Maple Syrup. Drizzle on cakes.

MAPLE SYRUP PUMPKIN PIE

This recipe works for: Men's Health, Overcoming Addictions, Sugar Imbalances
Serves 12: Preheat oven to 325°F. Use a 9" springform pan.

Make the crust: crumb in the blender, Honey-sweetened Gingersnaps to make $^3/_4$ cup crumbs. Combine with 2 TBS melted Butter, 2 drops Stevia Extract or 1 pinch Stevia Powder, and $^1/_2$ teasp. Cinnamon; bake for 10 to 12 minutes. Remove and cool.

—Make the filling: with a mixer, blend 16-oz. Low Fat Cream Cheese, 2 Eggs, $^1/_2$ cup Maple Sugar Granules, $^1/_4$ cup Maple Syrup and 2 teasp. Chinese 5-Spice Powder. Remove one half cup for the topping. Blend in 1 can (16-oz.) cooked Pumpkin to the rest. Pour over crust. Spread with the half cup of topping layer.

—Bake for an hour until center just barely jiggles when moved. Run a thin knife around perimeter to separate cake from pan and chill for 3 hours. Remove pan rim.

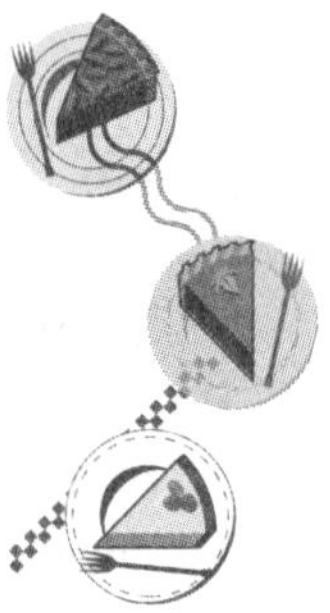

SUGAR FREE LEMON LIME PIE

This recipe works for: Bone Health, Overcoming Addictions, Arthritis
Serves 12: Preheat oven to 325°F. Use a 9" pie pan.

Make the crust: mix $^{3}/_{4}$ cup Honey-sweetened Graham Crackers crumbs with 2 TBS melted Butter and $^{1}/_{2}$ teasp. Allspice; bake for 10 to 12 minutes. Remove and cool.

—Make the filling: in a pan, sprinkle 1 packet Gelatin over 2 TBS Apple Juice Concentrate. Let sit 5 minutes to soften, then heat gently until gelatin dissolves. Remove from heat. Put in a blender and blend until smooth with: 1 cup Low Fat Cream Cheese, 1 cup Kefir Cheese and $^{1}/_{2}$ cup Lemon-Lime Yogurt. Add 4 TBS Maple Sugar Granules, 2 pinches Stevia Powder (or 6 drops Stevia Extract), 2 teasp. grated Lemon Zest and 2 teasp. grated Lime Zest, 4 TBS Lemon Juice and 4 TBS Lime Juice. Pour into crust. Chill until somewhat set. For the topping, mix $^{1}/_{2}$ cup Lemon-Lime Yogurt with 2 drops Stevia Extract or 1 pinch Stevia Powder and spread on top.

RASPBERRY BANANA CREAM PIE

This recipe works for: Kid's Health, Overcoming Allergies, Sugar Imbalances
Serves 8: Preheat oven to 400°F. Use a Canola Oil sprayed round baking dish.

Soften 1 packet of gelatin in $1^{1}/_{4}$ cups Raspberry Juice for 10 minutes. Then heat gently to dissolve for 10 minutes. Whisk in 1 cup Vanilla Rice Milk, $^{1}/_{2}$ cup unsweetened Cocoa, and 4 TBS Powdered Maple Sugar or Maple Sugar Granules. Dissolve 1 TB Arrowroot Powder in 2 TBS Lemon Juice and whisk in for 5 minutes to thicken. Add 1 TB Vanilla. Pour into prepared baking dish and cool. Chill in the fridge.

—In a pan, melt $^{1}/_{2}$ cup Sugar Free Raspberry Jam. Slice in 1 Banana thinly and stir gently to coat, Set aside. Toast $^{1}/_{2}$ cup chopped Almonds til golden in the oven. Cover top of chilled pie with jam-banana mix and sprinkle with almonds.

PEAR TART

This recipe works for: Female Balance, Overcoming Addictions, Immune Health
Serves 8: Preheat oven to 350°F. Make in a Canola Oil sprayed round baking pan.

Make a crust: mix together $1^{1}/_{4}$ cups Rolled Oats, $1^{1}/_{4}$ cups Unbleached Flour, $^{1}/_{4}$ cup Canola Oil, $^{1}/_{3}$ cup Maple Syrup, $^{1}/_{4}$ teasp. Baking Soda, $^{1}/_{4}$ teasp. Baking Powder, $^{1}/_{2}$ teasp. Nutmeg and 2 teasp. grated Lemon Zest. Mix well; chill for 15 minutes. Roll dough into a circle and fit into baking pan. Trim edges and bake 10 minutes.

—Make the filling: blender blend 1 large peeled pear with 2 TBS Orange Marmalade, 1 teasp. grated Ginger and 1 teasp. Vanilla. Spread over crust. Slice 3 ripe Pears thinly; arrange in an overlapping wheel to cover filling entirely. Bake for 20 minutes. Reduce heat to 325°F and leave in oven. Heat 3 TBS Orange Marmalade with 2 TBS Lemon Juice and brush on sliced pears. Bake 5 more minutes. Cool and then slice.

FRUIT TOP CHEESECAKE

This recipe works for: *Liver Health, Overcoming Addictions, Immune Health*
Serves 10: Preheat oven to 350°F. Use a 9" springform pan.

Make the crust: heat 1 cup crushed Honey-sweetened Gingersnaps, 3 TBS Butter and 6 TBS minced Honey Crystallized Ginger until bubbly and fragrant. Press into bottom and slightly up the sides of springform pan. Bake 10 minutes. Remove and cool.

—Blender blend until smooth and thin: 16-oz. Ricotta Cheese, 4 Egg Whites and 2 TBS Lemon Juice. Turn into a bowl and mix with 1 cup Low Fat Cream Cheese, 1 TB grated Lemon Zest, 1 teasp. Vanilla, 1 cup Maple Sugar Granules and 2 to 4 drops Stevia Extract (or $^1/_4$ teasp. Stevia Powder extract).

—Pour over crust. Bake for an hour until center just jiggles when moved. Run a thin knife around edge to separate cake from pan and chill for 3 hours. Remove pan rim. Peel and dice 1-lb mixed Fresh Fruits... good choices are Kiwi, Apricots, Peaches and Nectarines. Drain well. Toss with 3 TBS minced Honey Crystallized Ginger and spread on top of cake. (Note: a mix of dried diced fruits is also delicious.)

Nutrition; 371 calories; 11gm protein; 54gm carbo.; 1gm fiber; 11gm total fats; 36mg choles.; 190mg calcium; 2mg iron; 26mg magnesium; 335mg potass.; 194mg sodium; Vit. A 161 IU; Vit. C 6mg; Vit. E 2 IU.

APRICOT CHEESECAKE

This recipe works for: *Sugar Imbalances, Heart Health*
Serves 12: Preheat oven to 350°F. Use a 9" springform pan.

Make the crust: mix $^3/_4$ cup crushed Sugar Free Carob or Chocolate Cookies, and 2 TBS melted Butter; bake for 10 to 12 minutes. Remove and cool.

—Blend in a blender: 16-oz. Low Fat Ricotta Cheese and 8-oz. Low Fat Cream Cheese, 1 teaspoon Stevia Powder (or 30 drops Stevia Extract), 4 TBS Date Sugar, 1 cup Maple Sugar Granules, 4 Eggs, $^3/_4$ cup unsweetened Cocoa, $^1/_4$ cup Orange Juice, $^1/_2$ cup Honey Carob Chips and 2 teasp. grated Orange Zest. Pour into crust.

—Bake for an hour until center just jiggles when moved. Run a thin knife around edge to separate cake from pan; chill for 3 hours. Remove pan rim. Decorate with thin slices of Fresh Apricots (absorb excess moisture on paper towels first) to cover top of cheesecake. Serve in thin wedges.

Nutrition; 308 calories; 11gm protein; 38gm carbo.; 3gm fiber; 12gm total fats; 104mg choles.; 182mg calcium; 2mg iron; 46mg magnesium; 356mg potass.; 96mg sodium; Vit. A 138 IU; Vit. C 3mg; Vit. E 1 IU.

Fruit Sweetened Desserts

The natural way to end (or even begin) a meal.... fruit sweetened desserts and fruit-based sweets offer all the goodness of sweets without all the sugar.

SUGAR-FREE LEMON CARAMEL FLAN

This recipe works for: Liver and Organ Health, Weight Control, Skin and Hair
For 6: Preheat oven to 325°F. Use 6 oven-ready custard cups in a baking pan.

Make the caramel: Cut large strips Fresh Lemon Peel into slivers. Place 3 or 4 in the bottom of each custard cup. Dissolve 1/2 cup Honey and 2 TBS Lemon Juice in a pan and stir until bubbly. Add 2 TBS Water, stir to blend and divide over lemon slivers.

—Make the custard: In a pan, simmer until bubbles form: 2 cups Vanilla Rice Milk, 1 TB grated Lemon Zest, 4 Whole Cloves and 1 Whole Cinnamon Stick. Remove from heat and let steep for 15 minutes covered. Remove cinnamon and cloves.

—Whisk 3 Eggs, 4 TBS Maple Syrup and 1 teasp. Vanilla in a bowl. Whisk in custard; pour over caramel in cups. Place cups in baker; place on center oven rack and pour water around to come halfway up sides. Bake for an hour until a knife inserted in the center comes out clean. Remove, let cool, then cover cups with plastic and chill overnight. Loosen edges, invert on dessert plates and sprinkle with Nutmeg.

SUGAR-FREE CRUSTY HONEY ALMOND CREAM

This recipe works for: Digestive Problems, Women's Health, Allergies - Asthma
Enough for an 8 x 8" square pan:

Soften 1 packet Unflavored Gelatin in 1/4 cup Vanilla Yogurt and 1/2 cup Water. Separate 2 Eggs.

—Combine 1 cup Vanilla Yogurt and 1/2 cup Water in the top of a double boiler. Add Egg Yolks and a pinch Sea Salt. Cook custard gently until mixture coats a spoon. Remove from heat and add gelatin mixture. Stir to blend, then chill til custard begins to set. Whip Egg Whites to stiff peaks. Whip in 4 TBS Honey and 1/4 teasp. Almond Extract. Fold into gelatin mixture; turn into baking pan rinsed in cold water.

—Toast in the oven until golden, then sprinkle over top: 1 1/2 cups Wheat Germ and 1/2 cup sliced Almonds. Chill until firm; cut in squares to serve.

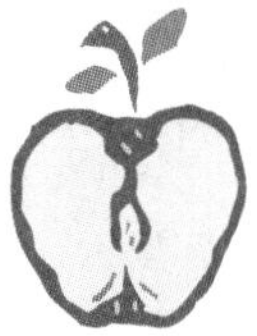

MAPLE SYRUP BAKED APPLES

This recipe works for: Liver Health, Weight Control, Immunity
Serves 8: Preheat oven to 350°F.

Core 8 Fuji Apples and place in a baking dish. Mix and fill core with: 2 TBS minced Honey Crystallized Ginger, 1 cup chopped Walnuts, 1/2 teasp. Cinnamon and 2 TBS grated Lemon Zest. Pour over 1 cup Maple Syrup. Bake for 35 minutes. Serve hot.

EASY FRUIT SLUSH

This recipe works for: Liver and Organ Health, Weight Control, Sugar Imbalances
Serves 4:

Blender blend: 1 cup bottled Honey Lemonade or bottled Green Tea (with honey and lemon), $^1/_2$ cup Orange Juice, 1 cup Crushed Pineapple with juice, 1 cup fresh Berries (any kind), 1 cup Fresh Strawberries, 2 Bananas. Freeze for 3 hours until firm but still slushy. Blender blend briefly and pour into parfait glasses. Top wih Fresh Mint Sprigs.

SUGAR FREE ORANGE SORBET

This recipe works for: Cancer Control, Weight Control, Sugar Imbalances
Serves 4:

Blender blend: 5 peeled Oranges, 1 TB grated Orange Peel, $1^1/_2$ cups Vanilla Rice Milk, 4 TBS frozen Orange Juice Concentrate. Freeze right in the blender for about 2 hours. Blend again while still slushy. Pour into parfait glasses and refreeze 1 hour.

PEARS in RASPBERRY SAUCE

This recipe works for: Anti-Aging, Weight Control, Sugar Imbalances
For 4 to 6 servings: Preheat oven to 350°F.

Slice 3 Pears; place in a baking dish. Blender blend: $^1/_4$ cup Honey-sweetened Raspberry Jelly, $^1/_2$ cup Orange Juice and $^1/_2$ cup Fresh Raspberries. Pour over pears. Cover with foil; bake for 30 minutes. Put in a serving dish and spoon sauce on top. Sprinkle on more Fresh Raspberries and chopped Toasted Almonds.

HONEY MANGO SORBET

This recipe works for: Hair, Skin and Nails, Weight Control, Sugar Imbalances
For 3 cups:

Blender blend the fruit of 2 large Mangoes. Turn into a pan and add $^1/_2$ cup Orange Honey, 2 TBS Lime Juice and 4 TBS Orange Juice. Freeze covered for 1 hour. Stir to reblend and freeze solid. Top with Coconut Shreds.

STRAWBERRIES BALSAMICO Great with biscotti.

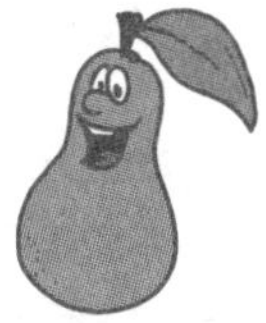

This recipe works for: Arthritis, Weight Loss, Healthy Pregnancy
Serves 8:

Cut 2 baskets Fresh Strawberries in half. Toss with 3 TBS Balsamic Vinegar and 1 teasp. Stevia Powder or 10 drops Stevia Liquid Extract.

PINEAPPLE-APRICOT MOUSSE

This recipe works for: Anti-Aging, Weight Control, Sugar Imbalances
Serves 8:

Bring 2 cups Pineapple Juice to a simmer with 1 TB Grated Ginger and 1 TB Honey, or 1 TB Ginger Syrup. Add 1 cup dried Apricots and simmer 5 minutes to soften. Puree in the blender til smooth. Transfer to a bowl and fold in 2 cups Vanilla Yogurt. Cool and layer in a serving bowl with 2 cups Lemon Yogurt. Sprinkle Nutmeg on top.

WATERMELON ICE with CAROB CHIP SEEDS

This recipe works for: Detoxification, Weight Control, Bladder-Kidney Problems
Makes about 6 servings. Serve within 30 minutes of blending for best texture.

Freeze 4 cups Watermelon Cubes solid. Freeze 1 small basket Raspberries (or use 1/2 package (12-oz.) frozen). Put in a blender and pulse until mixture resembles shaved ice. Add 1/3 cup Lemon-Lime Yogurt and process until smooth and creamy. Freeze for 30 minutes or longer. Mound into a serving bowl and stud with Carob Chips.

Nutrition; 112 calories; 2gm protein; 21gm carbo.; 2gm fiber; 4gm total fats; trace choles.; 39mg calcium; 1mg iron; 31mg magnesium; 232mg potass.; 11mg sodium; Vit. A 45 IU; Vit. C 18mg; Vit. E 1 IU.

RAISIN PECAN ICE CREAM

This recipe works for: Sugar Imbalances, Men's Health, Sports Nutrition
For 6 to 8 servings:

Chop 2 cups Fresh Mixed Fruit of your choice and 2 cups sliced Bananas. Freeze solid. —Blender blend with 1 cup Pineapple or Orange Juice and blend until stiff. Stir in 1 cup Raisins and 3/4 cup chopped Toasted Pecans. Serve immediately.

Nutrition; 201 calories; 2gm protein; 34gm carbo.; 4gm fiber; 8gm total fats; 0mg choles.; 23mg calcium; 1mg iron; 38mg magnesium; 441mg potass.; 3mg sodium; Vit. A 102 IU; Vit. C 14mg; Vit. E 3 IU.

HAWAIIAN PUNCH DESSERT

This recipe works for: Detoxification, Sugar Imbalances, Weight Loss
For 4 servings:

Toss together in a bowl: 1 peeled, cored Ripe Pineapple in 1" cubes, 1 peeled seeded Mango in 1" cubes, 1/4 cup Lime Juice, 1/4 cup Honey, 1/2 teasp. Lime Zest, and 3 TBS snipped Fresh Mint Leaves. Serve in dessert glasses topped with 4 Mint Sprigs.

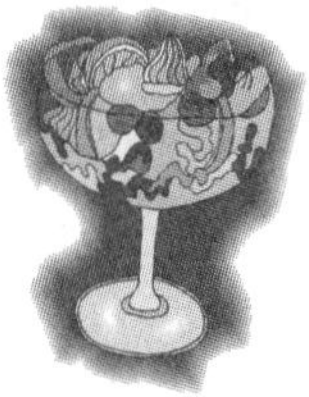

STRAWBERRY MOUSSE Great with raspberries or bing cherries, too.

This recipe works for: Hair and Skin, Digestive Health, Sugar Imbalances
For 4 to 5 servings:

Separate 3 Eggs. Set yolks and whites aside in separate mixing bowls.
—Cook 1-qt. Strawberries, 4 TBS Honey and 2 TBS Orange Juice in a saucepan for 10 to 15 minutes until syrupy. Save 10 strawberry halves for decoration.
—Mix a little hot syrup with 3 TBS Arrowroot Powder until dissolved. Mix into the reserved Egg Yolks. Return to the strawberries and beat for 2 minutes til combined.
—Beat Egg Whites to stiff peaks with a pinch Cream of Tartar. Fold into strawberry mix and chill for at least 2 hours.
Beat 1 cup Kefir Cheese or Low Fat Cream Cheese with 3 TBS Orange Juice until fluffy. Mix gently with chilled mousse and chill another 2 hours. Serve in individual mousse or custard cups and top each with a Strawberry Half.

Nutrition; 266 calories; 10gm protein; 31gm carbo.; 2gm fiber; 7gm total fats; 155mg choles.; 89mg calcium; 2mg iron; 21mg magnesium; 348mg potass.; 41mg sodium; Vit. A 170 IU; Vit. C 73mg; Vit. E 1 IU.

CINNAMON RICE PUDDING Kids love it!

This recipe works for: Kid's Health, Sugar Imbalances, Allergies and Asthma
For 6 to 8 servings: Preheat oven to 325°F.

Have ready 3 cups cooked Jasmine Rice. Mix rice with 2 cups Lemon Yogurt, 1/2 cup Honey, 1/2 cup Water, 2 TBS Maple Syrup, 5 Eggs, 2 TBS grated Orange Zest, 1 teasp. Vanilla, 1 teasp. Cinnamon, 3/4 cup Raisins and 2 chopped Fuji Apples.
—Turn the pudding into a deep Buttered baking dish, and bake for 1 hour until custard sets, and browns slightly at the edges. Stir occasionally while baking if it is looking too dry. Remove and let set for 10 minutes, while you make the topping.
—Make the FRUIT and JELLY TOPPING: Melt 1/2 cup Sugar Free Raspberry Jam in a saucepan. Slice in strawberries, or a peach or nectarine and spoon over pudding.

BERRY BERRY CUSTARD Perfect for summer berries of any kind.

This recipe works for: Women's Health, Sugar Imbalances, Bone Building
For 4 servings: Preheat oven broiler.

In a saucepan, whisk over medium heat: 1 Egg, 2 teasp. Arrowroot Powder, 1 TB Unbleached Flour, 6 TBS Maple Syrup, 1/2 teasp. Vanilla and 1 cup Vanilla Rice Milk. Stir constantly until mixture thickens. Remove from heat and transfer to a mixing bowl.

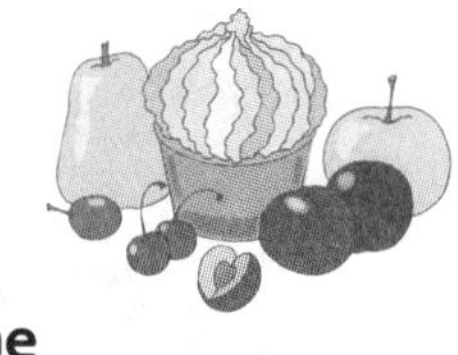

—Whisk in 3-oz. Low Fat Cream Cheese or Kefir Cheese. Chill in the fridge. Spoon into oven-proof custard cups. Run under broiler just to brown tops, 2 minutes. Sprinkle with Maple Sugar Granules to cover and broil again to melt.

Holiday Feasts & Parties

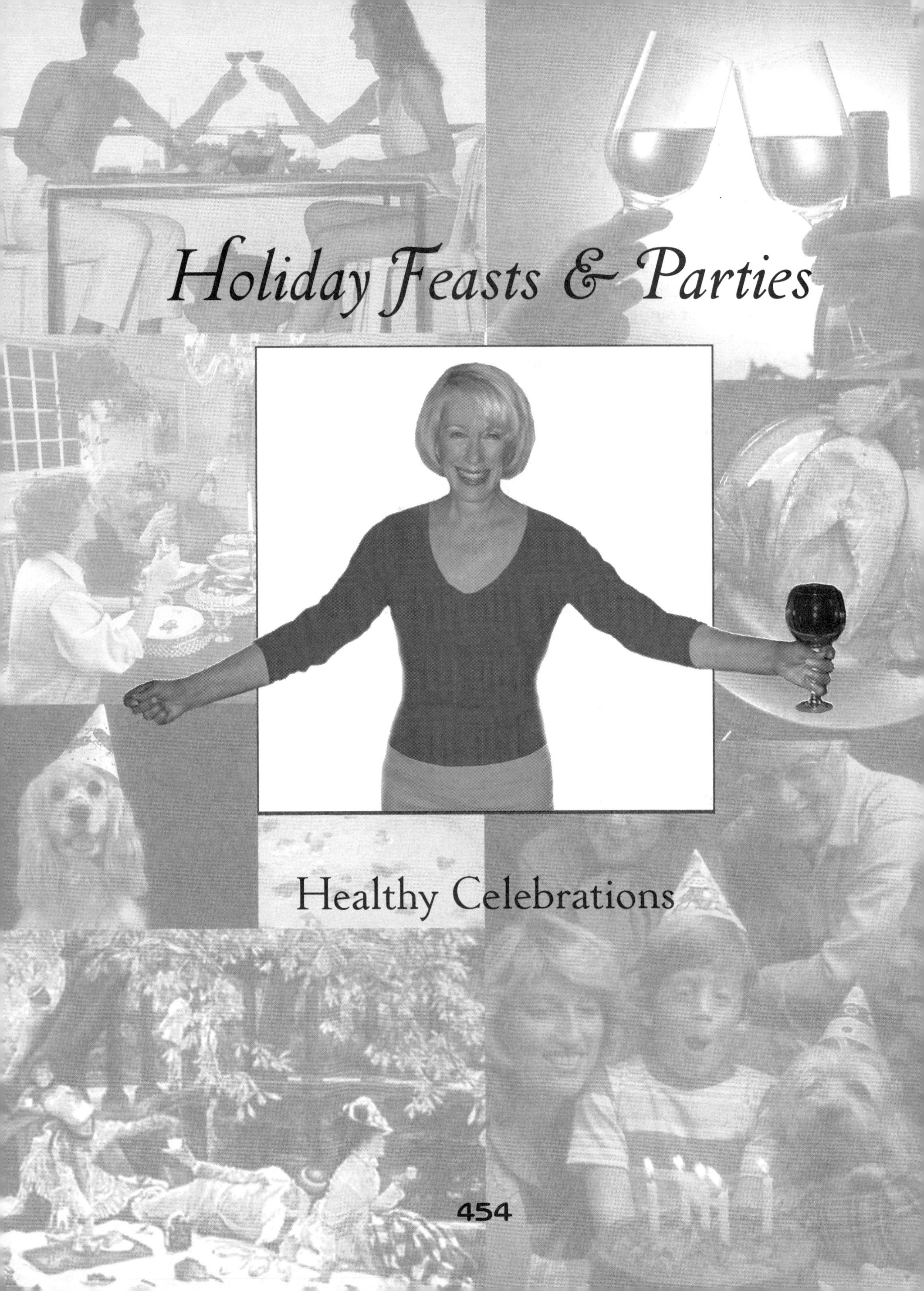

Healthy Celebrations

Healthy Holidays

Parties and Entertaining

America's holiday tradition began as a harvest celebration, full of the best foods to be had all year! The great American excuse for going off a healthy diet because of holidays and celebrations doesn't have to be yours. Returning to our roots, so to speak, is the best way I know to stay healthy in a season that's loaded today with fat, sugar, additives and preservatives.

Check out the great low-fat, low sugar recipes for parties and gatherings. Everyone can enjoy them; you can easily keep friends and family happy, roll out favorite holiday foods, and still stay reasonably close to your diet program. It just takes a small effort and a few changes to conventional cooking methods and ingredients.

A few recipes in this section use sugar as a sweetener. For occasional treats at holiday times, a small amount of sugar can be handled by most people. A little sugar clearly adds to the pleasure of special festive foods, and won't jeopardize your healing program for long. A small sweet treat every now and then is better for social and emotional balance than weeks of feeling deprived, and at risk for a possible "sugar orgy" later.

Healthy Tips for Holidays and Celebrations:

1: Take only small portions of anything.
2: Keep fats and calories as low as possible in whatever you fix.
3: Make only 3 or 4 recipes, including breads and desserts, for each meal. Today's "groaning board" means everybody will be overstuffed and groaning later.
4: Keep up your exercise and fitness program during the holidays.
5: Continue with your diet for all meals except the special ones.
6: After the holidays, return to your optimum diet right away.

Healthy Holidays Recipe Sections

These recipes will help keep you leaner, cleaner and healthier at a time of year when it's easy to forget a good diet.

Great Beginnings

Healthy Appetizers, Starters and Snacks

Holidays and celebrations mean parties. Giving a "healthy food" party may seem almost impossible. We're all so used to party foods loaded with fat, sugar and salt. It doesn't have to be that way. With a little thought and the recipes in this chapter, you can stay on your healthy healing diet, celebrate, have a good time, and please your guests. The foods offered here are especially appropriate for winter holiday parties.

NO ALCOHOL CRANBERRY MAPLE NOG Delicious hot

This recipe works for: Women's Health, Cancer Protection, Liver Health
For 8 servings:

Stir in a large soup pot: 2 cups Apple Cider, 2 cups Orange Juice, 2 Cinnamon Sticks, $^1/_2$ cup Maple Syrup, 1 quart (32-oz.) Green Tea (any flavor, Lemon or Peach are good), 1 can (8-oz.) Frozen Cranberry Juice, 1 Lemon cut in wheels and 12 Whole Cloves. Simmer 1 hour. Remove spices and lemon wheels. Serve with extra maple syrup and cinnamon swizzle sticks.

Nutrition; 164 calories; 1gm protein; 40gm carbo.; 2gm fiber; 1gm total fats; 0 choles.; 65mg calcium; 1mg iron; 16mg magnesium; 387mg potassium; 22mg sodium; Vit. A 14 IU; Vit. C 185mg; Vit. E trace.

BANANA DAIRY FREE NOG Great for kid's group celebrations

This recipe works for: Kid's Health, Healthy Pregnancy, Illness Recovery
For 4 servings:

Blender blend: 2 large ripe peeled Peaches, 3 Ripe Bananas, $1^1/_2$ cups Vanilla Almond Milk or Vanilla Rice Milk, 2 TBS Maple Syrup, $^1/_2$ teasp. Vanilla, 1 TB Honey and $^1/_2$ teasp. Cinnamon. Chill and top each glass with Nutmeg sprinkles.

Nutrition; 159 calories; 2gm protein; 39gm carbo.; 3gm fiber; 1gm total fats; 0 choles.; 54mg calcium; 1mg iron; 32mg magnesium; 475mg potassium; 4mg sodium; Vit. A 36 IU; Vit. C 12mg; Vit. E 1 IU.

NOT BUTTERED RUM

This recipe works for: Women's Health, Digestive Health, Stress and Relaxation
For 10 mugs:

Heat $^1/_2$ cup Maple Syrup with 1 $^1/_2$ teasp. Chinese 5-Spice Powder until fragrant. Remove from heat and set aside. Heat in a large pan, 10 cups Apple Cider; add spice mixture. Divide between individual mugs. Add 1 Cinnamon Stick and 2 to 3 TBS Dark Rum to each mug.

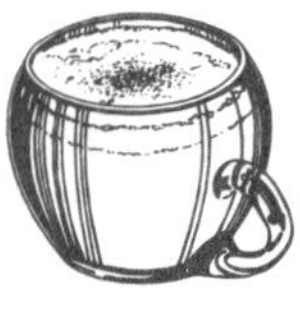

GREEK KISSES

This recipe works for: Men's Health, Hair, Skin and Nails, Bone Building
For 50 kisses: Preheat oven to 325°F.

Melt 1 stick Butter for the phyllo pastry. Remove phyllo from the freezer and let thaw in the package. Do not open until the filling is ready.

—Puree the filling in a food processor: 1 small bag Baby Spinach Leaves, 16-oz. Low Fat Ricotta Cheese, 8-oz. Feta Cheese, 1 small Red Onion, 2 TBS snipped Dill Weed, $^1/_4$ teasp. Nutmeg, 2 teasp. Cracked Pepper and Sea Salt to taste.

—Discard inner phyllo wrap and unfold phyllo sheets on sheets of wax paper. Cover with a damp dish towel. Remove one phyllo sheet from the original stack and lay on another sheet of wax paper; brush with melted butter, top with a second sheet of phyllo, brush it with butter and repeat til you have 4 sheets in a layer. With kitchen shears, cut layers all together into 3" squares. On each square, place 2 TBS filling. Bring up corners of squares and twist at the top to form a kiss. Brush with melted butter and place on an Olive Oil sprayed baking sheet. Repeat until you have about 50 kisses. Bake in the lower half of the oven until golden, about 10 minutes. Keep well refrigerated and reheat; or serve immediately.

BLACK BEAN CAVIAR

This recipe works for: Men's Health, Hair, Skin and Nails, Bladder-Kidney Health
Serves 12:

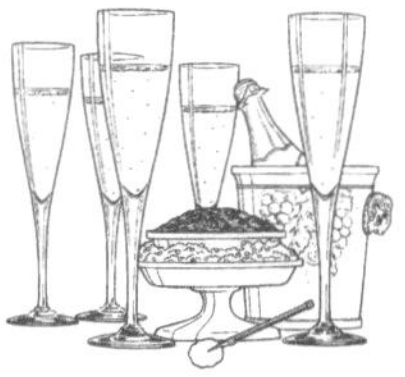

Blender blend all to smooth with some small chunks: 2 cups pitted Black Olives, $^1/_2$ cup Hoisin Sauce (Black Bean Paste), 1 teasp. Garlic Granules, 2 teasp. grated Lemon Zest and 1 teasp. Lemon Juice. Add 1 TB Dry Red Wine if more liquid is needed. Spread on water crackers topped with thin Cucumber slices, or add small Cucumber chunks and fill Endive Spears.

SMOKED SALMON APPETIZER ROLL-UPS

This recipe works for: Women's Health, Hair, Skin and Nails, Heart Health
For 12 servings: Use 2 large soft crackerbreads, available at deli counters.

Have ready 6-oz. thinly sliced Smoked Salmon. Cut into thin strips.

—Blend the filling: $^1/_3$ the smoked salmon slices, 1 carton, (8-oz.) Low Fat Cream Cheese, $^1/_4$ teasp. Cracked Pepper and 1 TB Lemon Juice. Spread half the cream cheese mix over the bottom two-thirds of each cracker bread. Divide salmon strips over the cream cheese. Divide 1 matchstick-cut Red Bell Pepper and 1 thinly sliced Cucumber over salmon. Cover everything with Baby Spinach or Arugula Leaves. Roll up from the bottom. Wrap in plastic and chill until firm, about 4 hours. Slice in rounds and serve.

VEGETABLE PATÉ with SWEET and SOUR GLOSS

This recipe works for: Men's Health, Hair, Skin and Nails, Bone Building
For about 8 to 10 people: Preheat oven to 375°F.

Mix the paté in the blender: 12-oz. Firm Silken Tofu, $1^1/_2$ cups chopped Mushrooms, 2 TBS Peanut Butter, 3 TBS Tamari, 8 chopped Green Onions. Turn into a bowl and add: 1 diced Red Bell Pepper, 1 can (7-oz.) diced Water Chestnuts, $^1/_4$ cup snipped Cilantro Leaves and $^1/_2$ teasp. Cracked Pepper. Oil a decorative mold. Line with waxed paper, and oil the paper. Pack in paté; bake 45 minutes. Remove and cool in the mold. Chill until ready to serve.

—Make the SWEET and SOUR GLOSS at serving time. Mix in a saucepan: $1^1/_2$ cups Pineapple-Orange Juice, $^1/_4$ cup Honey, $^1/_2$ cup Brown Rice Vinegar, $^1/_4$ cup Tamari and $^1/_4$ teasp. Garlic Powder. Bring to a boil and let simmer for 5 minutes while you unmold the paté on a Baby Spinach covered plate. Stir in 2 TBS Arrowroot dissolved in 2 TBS Sherry. Simmer until glossy. Spoon over paté. Looks like a big, shiny glazed jewel sitting on a bed of green ruffles. Surround with Apple Slices and Pumpernickle Toasts.

Nutrition; 148 calories; 9gm protein; 20gm carbo.; 2gm fiber; 4gm total fats; 0 choles.; 104mg calcium; 5mg iron; 62mg magnesium; 374mg potassium; 217mg sodium; Vit. A 132 IU; Vit. C 41mg; Vit. E 1 IU.

APPETIZER CREAM CHEESE HERB TORTA

This recipe works for: Men's Health, Hair, Skin and Nails, Bone Building
For 16 servings: Preheat oven to 325°. Bake in a Canola Oiled springform pan.

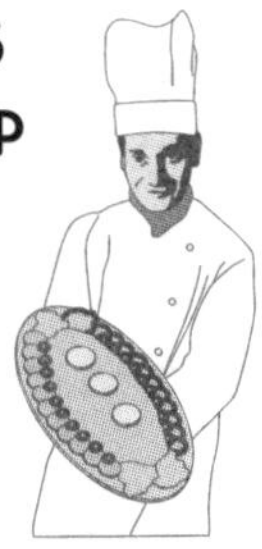

Make the crust: heat 1 cup crushed Gingersnaps, 3 TBS Butter and 6 TBS minced Honey Crystallized Ginger til fragrant. Press on bottom and slightly up the sides of springform pan; bake 10 minutes. Remove and cool.

—Blender blend 1 can Cream of Asparagus Soup, 16-oz. Ricotta Cheese, 1 carton (8-oz.) Low Fat Cream Cheese, 1 carton (8-oz.) Kefir Cheese, 1 cup grated Parmesan Cheese and 2 Eggs. Add $^1/_4$ tsp. Thyme and $^1/_4$ tsp. Tarragon and $^1/_2$ teasp. Basil. Turn into springform pan, Bake for $1^1/_2$ hours until puffy and light brown. Cool in pan. Chill in fridge. Spread with diced Walnuts, snipped Cilantro and chopped Hard Boiled Egg. Serve with Water Crackers.

WASABI NUTS

This recipe works for: Men's Health, Digestive Health, Liver and Organ Health
For 3 cups: Preheat oven to 400°F.

Pan roast 3 cups mixed Walnut Halves, Pecan Halves, shelled Hazelnuts, and Whole Almonds in 1 TB Canola Oil, 1 tsp. Wasabi Paste and 3 TBS bottled Teriyaki Sauce. Sprinkle with $^1/_2$ tsp. Cracked Pepper. Place on a Canola Oil sprayed baking sheet and bake until golden, five minutes. Cool and break into candy size chunks.

CHEESE TREES

Kids can help with these. They like to eat 'em, too.

This recipe works for: Men's Health, Sports Nutrition, Sugar Imbalances

For 24 trees: Preheat oven to 400°F. Use Canola Oil sprayed baking sheets.

Trim crusts from soft Whole Wheat Bread Slices slices, and roll flat with a rolling pin. Cut out bread with cookie cutters into 24 trees or other shapes. (Save scraps and crusts for stuffings and croutons.)

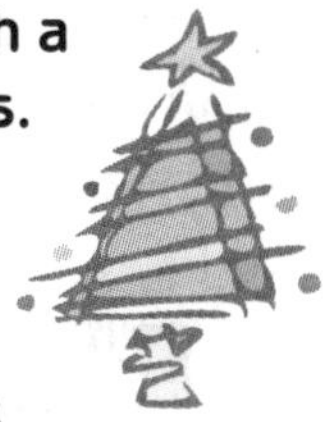

—Make the sauce: combine $^3/_4$ cup grated Parmesan Cheese, $^1/_4$ cup Low Fat Cream Cheese, $^1/_4$ cup Low Fat Mayonnaise, 2 TBS minced Green Onion and $^1/_4$ teasp White Pepper. Spread on bread; top tree with a small chunk of Dried Fruit or an Olive. Bake on prepared sheets until golden and bubbly.

VEGGIE PIZZAS on RICE CAKES

This recipe works for: Men's and Kid's Health, Heart Health, Sports Nutrition

Enough for 24 small rice cakes:

Toast Small Rice Cakes (any flavor) on a baking sheet in the oven until crisp.

—Sauté until aromatic: 2 TBS Olive Oil, 1 diced Red Onion, 1 minced Clove Garlic and 1 teasp. Italian Seasoning Herbs. Add $^1/_2$ slivered Red Bell Pepper, 1 cake Extra Firm Tofu, crumbled with your fingers and extra water squeezed out. Sizzle until golden. Divide mixture between rice cakes. Top with 1 thin Tomato slice, Low Fat Mozarrella Cheese chunks, and sprinkle with Parmesan Cheese. Run under broiler to melt the cheese.

CHEESE FILLED APRICOT HALVES

This recipe works for: Sugar Imbalances, Overcoming Addictions, Weight Control

For 32 halves:

Toast 32 Walnut Halves in the oven until fragrant. Remove and cool.

—Blender blend the filling: 3-oz. Low Fat Cream Cheese, 5-oz. Feta Cheese, $1^1/_2$ teasp. White Pepper, 1 teasp. Honey and $^1/_4$ teasp. Nutmeg. Fill 32 dried Apricot Halves. Press a walnut half on top of each. Place 3 to 4 TBS snipped Fresh Mint Leaves on a dish. Press apricots cheese side down into mint to coat. Cover and chill.

CHEESY NUT CRISPS

This recipe works for: Sugar Imbalances, Overcoming Addictions, Weight Control

For 15 to 20 crisps: Preheat oven to 350°F. Use a Canola Oil sprayed baking sheet.

Toss together: 1 cup shredded Low Fat Swiss Cheese, $^1/_2$ cup slivered Almonds, $^1/_2$ teasp. Cumin and 2 pinches Sweet Paprika. Drop in tablespoon mounds on the baking sheet. Bake for 12 to 15 minutes until golden brown. Serve warm around a small bowl of Salsa for dipping.

SPICY APPLE DIP

This recipe works for: Women's Health, Heart Health, Bone Building
For 6 servings:

Blender blend: $^1/_2$ cup Cottage Cheese, $^1/_4$ cup Low Fat Cream Cheese, 1 teasp. Brown Rice Vinegar, 1 large Fuji Apple, $1^1/_2$ teasp. Honey, 1 teasp. Wasabi Paste, $^1/_2$ teasp. Allspice and $^1/_4$ teasp. White Pepper. —Turn into a bowl and mix in 1 chopped Green Onion, $^1/_4$ cup snipped Parsley, and $^1/_4$ cup Raisins. Snip green onions on top, and serve with raw vegetable dippers like Cauliflower Florets, Jicama slices, Celery and Carrot Sticks.

Nutrition; 79 calories; 4gm protein; 12gm carbo.; 1gm fiber; 1gm total fats; 6mg choles.; 35mg calcium; 1mg iron; 8mg magnesium; 137mg potassium; 80mg sodium; Vit. A 40 IU; Vit. C 5mg; Vit. E 1 IU.

TINY CHICKEN ALMOND PITA SANDWICHES

This recipe works for: Men's Health, Respiratory Health, Hair and Skin
For 24 pita halves: Preheat oven to 400°F.

Have ready 12 Appetizer Size Pita Breads, cut in half. Warm slightly in the oven.
—Have ready 4 Organic Chicken Breast Halves, cooked and diced.
—Mix the sauce in a bowl: 1 cup Almond Butter, 3 TBS Soy Bacon Bits, 3 TBS Tamari, 2 teasp. Garlic-Lemon Seasoning, 1 TB White Wine Vinegar, 1 TB Sweet Hot Mustard, 1 cup Water and $^1/_4$ teasp. Hot Pepper Sauce; set aside to blend flavors.
—Stuff pitas with bits of thin sliced Red Onion, Alfalfa Sprouts, Tomato slivers, shredded Baby Spinach Leaves and diced Chicken. Stand upright in a shallow dish with sides touching. Spoon on sauce. Cover and chill to set stuffing. Bake for 25 minutes until browned and bubbly.

CHEESE and NUT TARTS

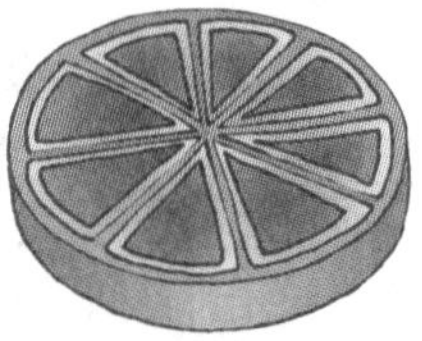

This recipe works for: Sugar Imbalances, Overcoming Addictions
Makes 48 tarts: Preheat oven to 300°F.

Have ready $^1/_2$ cup finely chopped oven-toasted Walnuts and 8-oz. Feta Cheese with rind removed. Cut cheese into 48 pieces.
—In a food processor, coarse chop 1 cup Red Seedless Grapes and 2 pinches Sea Salt. Put in a sieve to drain and set aside.
—In a bowl mix: 1 finely minced Scallion, 1 TB Raspberry Vinegar, 2 teasp. Walnut Oil or Grapeseed Oil, 4 pinches Garlic-Lemon Seasoning and 2 pinches minced Rosemary Leaves. Drain, add grapes and combine. Let stand again to release excess moisture.
—Place 48 mini pastry shells on a baking sheet. Divide walnuts and cheese among shells. Drain grape mixture again before dividing among shells. Bake just until cheese melts, 5 minutes ONLY. Serve hot and gooey.

Festive Healthy Menus

For All Kinds of Parties

Focusing on a healthy holiday doesn't have to take the fun out of celebrating. Like others, you have more energy to really enjoy this special time of year if you're on a healthy healing diet.

Thanksgiving Feast Menus

Thanksgiving is a uniquely American family holiday. True to the American nature, each family celebrates Thanksgiving a little differently.... a combination of our diverse heritage and special family traditions overlaid with the American experience.

Here are three different, healthy Thanksgiving feasts, each with lots to choose from, that express just that quality.... living in America in the 21st century.

A Word About Turkey:

Naturally-raised, free-run turkeys, like those from the Diestel and Shelton farms, are high grade sources of protein, free of hormone injections and antibiotics. Not only are these turkeys more ecologically responsible as they run and scratch for food, but they are allowed a longer life span, so their meat develops much more flavor. Turkey meat is leaner, lower in saturated fat and cholesterol, with more available vitamins and minerals, than chicken. One serving of cooked, skinless white meat is approximately 180 calories, with less total fat than any other meat. Turkey is a practical diet food, as well as a feasting food, all year round. To lower fat calories even more, roast your turkey with the skin on to keep the meat from drying out. Then, remove the skin before you eat it. Back meat, giblets and wings are mostly fat. Either discard these pieces, or use them in a strained stock for gravy.

A Traditional Pilgrim Thanksgiving

Part of the charm of an early American feast are the native American harvest foods that come into our gardens and Farmers Markets at this time of year.... corn, all kinds of squashes, pumpkins, yams and potatoes, apples, pears, berries, dried fruits, nuts, late harvest greens, cranberries and maple syrup. You don't even have to decide which of these tasty foods to choose; they all go well together. Like a wild potluck, everything is good.

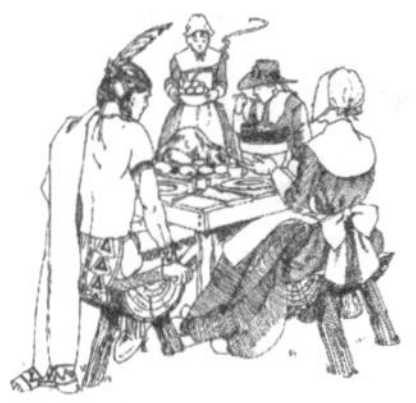

CRANBERRY WALNUT RELISH For 8 or more.

For 8 or more:

Simmer 12-oz. Fresh or Frozen Cranberries in $^1/_4$ cup Water, $^1/_4$ cup Honey and 1 cup Turbinado Sugar for 5 minutes only. Remove from heat and add $^1/_2$ cup Raisins and 2 TBS grated Ginger. Add 1 cup diced Green Apples, $^1/_2$ cup toasted diced Walnuts, 2 TBS Lemon Juice, 1 teasp. Cinnamon, $^1/_4$ teasp. Nutmeg and $^1/_4$ teasp. Cloves.

CRANBERRY-CIDER GLAZE Seals in turkey juices and flavor.

Heat in a saucepan: 1 cup Cranberry Nectar Frozen Concentrate, 6 TBS Butter, $^1/_2$ cup Apple Cider, $^1/_2$ cup Currant Jelly, $^1/_2$ teasp. Cinnamon and $^1/_2$ teasp. Allspice. Spread on turkey to cover before roasting and baste during roasting.

ROAST TURKEY with OYSTER STUFFING

This recipe works for: Mental Health, Overcoming Addictions

Preheat oven to 325°F. Enough for a 12-lb. Turkey.

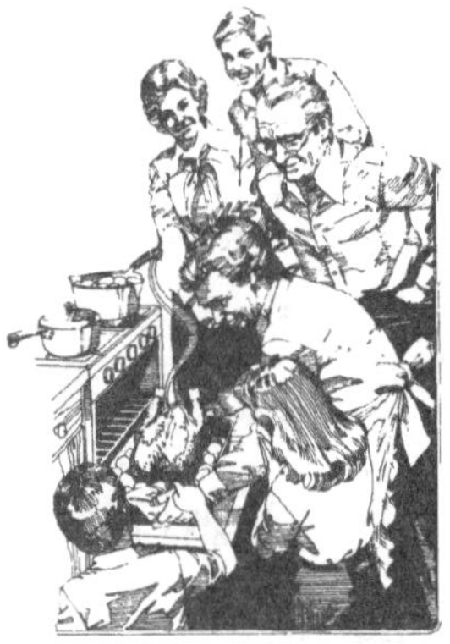

Roast turkey in a shallow open pan, 25 minutes per pound, until juices run clear. Scatter $^1/_2$ cup chopped Onions around turkey so they can roast along with it and be ready for the pan gravy.

—Make the OYSTER STUFFING: Put 8 cups diced Corn Bread in a large bowl. Sizzle in a large skillet about 5 minutes: 2 TBS Butter, 1 large diced Onion, 4 diced Shallots, 1 diced Red Bell Pepper, 3 diced Celery Ribs, $^1/_4$ cup Walnuts, 1 teasp. Lemon Pepper, $^1/_2$ teasp. Ground Sage, $^1/_4$ teasp. Ground Rosemary and 1 teasp. Tarragon Leaves. Add 1 pint Oysters, with their liqueur, 1 cup Turkey Broth (boil water with giblets, then strain out giblets), and $^1/_2$ cup Whiskey or Sherry. Toss to coat and heat. Toss with corn bread. Either stuff turkey or turn into a Canola Oil sprayed 3-qt. casserole dish. Lightly tent with foil and bake for 30 minutes until crusty at the edges. Makes 12 servings.

Nutrition; 675 calories; 75gm protein; 40gm carbo.; 3gm fiber; 32gm total fats; 25 4choles.; 173mg calcium; 8mg iron; 90mg magnesium; 858mg potassium; 510mg sodium; Vit. A 81 IU; Vit. C 16mg; Vit. E 2 IU.

MUSHROOM-ONION GRAVY for TURKEY

After roasting, pour off 2 TBS drippings into a skillet. Add 1 sliced Onion and 1 cup sliced Brown Cremini Mushrooms, add 2 TBS Whole Wheat Flour; stir over high heat for 3 minutes. Add 1 cup Water and 1 cup Sherry and stir until gravy comes to a boil and thickens smooth. Stir in 1 teasp. Cider Vinegar, $^1/_2$ teasp. Sea Salt and $^1/_4$ teasp. Pepper. Serve hot over turkey slices.

TURKEY PAN SAUCE: Put turkey on a carving/serving plate. Scrape drippings into a saucepan (or use the roasting pan on low heat). Sprinkle with 3 to 4 TBS Whole Wheat Flour; stir, scraping up browned bits into the sauce until everything is bubbly and well blended, 3 minutes. Add 1 cup Buttermilk, <u>or</u> $^1/_2$ cup Plain Yogurt and $^1/_2$ cup Water. Heat stirring, until bubbly and thickened. Add 1 cup Organic Chicken Broth and $^1/_4$ cup Sherry Wine. Bring to a boil and season with 1 teasp. Sea Salt and Pepper to taste.

SPOONBREAD DRESSING

This recipe works for: *Mental Health, Overcoming Addictions*
For 8 servings: Preheat oven to 350°F.

Heat 2 cups Organic Chicken Broth and 1 cup Kefir Cheese or Low Fat Cream Cheese in a large saucepan. Add 1$^1/_4$ cups Cornmeal. Stir until thick. Remove from heat. Stir in 6 beaten Eggs and set aside.

—Sauté for 10 minutes: 2 TBS Butter, 2 TBS Canola Oil, 2 diced Onions, and 1 diced Rib Celery. Stir in 2 TBS snipped Fresh Parsley, $^1/_2$ tsp. Oregano, $^1/_2$ teasp. Marjoram and 1 tsp. Sage Powder. Add to egg mixture, and stir in 2 tsp. Baking Powder. Beat vigorously about 5 minutes until smooth and light. Turn into a large Canola Oil-sprayed straight-sided baking dish and bake for 35 to 40 minutes til puffy and golden brown. Serve right away with spoonfuls of gravy. (See previous page.)

CORNMEAL BATTY CAKES A tradition since the first Thanksgiving.

This recipe works for: *Liver and Organ Health, Heart Health, Kid's Health*
For 24 batty cakes: Preheat griddle to hot; a drop of water skitters on the surface.

Combine $^3/_4$ cup Yellow Cornmeal, 1 Egg, $^1/_2$ tsp. Baking Powder, $^1/_2$ tsp. Sea Salt, $^1/_2$ tsp. Baking Soda and 1 cup Rice Milk until smooth. Coat hot griddle with a little Butter on a paper napkin. Ladle on 1 TB batter for each batty cake. Cook for 2 to 3 minutes on each side until brown. Keep batter stirred and finished cakes hot. Serve with honey to accompany roast turkey.

Nutrition per 4 cakes; 86 calories; 3gm protein; 15gm carbo.; 2gm fiber; 1gm total fats; 35mg choles.; 101mg calcium; 1mg iron; 21mg magnesium; 57mg potassium; 332mg sodium; Vit. A 23 IU; Vit. C 0mg; Vit. E trace

HARVEST BEANS and CORN

This recipe works for: *Men's Health, Sugar Imbalances, Illness Recovery*
For 6 servings:

Sizzle in a skillet for 3 minutes: 2 TBS Olive Oil, 2 minced Cloves Garlic, 2 minced Shallots, and 1 diced Red Onion. Add 2 cups Corn Kernels, and 1 cup <u>frozen</u> Lima Beans or Green Beans; simmer 3 minutes. Add 1 cup diced Tomatoes, $^1/_2$ cup diced Red Bell Pepper and 1 cup Blush Wine; simmer 15 minutes. Add 1 tsp. Sweet Paprika, $^1/_4$ tsp. Garlic Powder, $^1/_4$ tsp. White Pepper, $^1/_4$ tsp. Black Pepper, $^1/_4$ tsp. Dry Mustard, 2 TBS snipped Fresh Basil Leaves, 2 TBS Oregano Leaves, 2 TBS Thyme Leaves and 2 TBS fresh snipped Cilantro Leaves. Sprinkle on dashes Hot Pepper Sauce to taste.

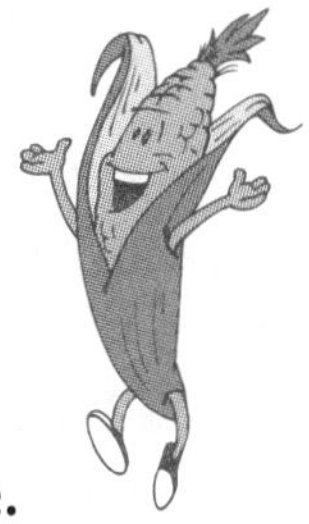

Nutrition; 149 calories; 4gm protein; 23gm carbo.; 4gm fiber; 2gm total fats; 0 choles.; 51mg calcium; 1mg iron; 39mg magnesium; 351mg potassium; 80mg sodium; Vit. A 147 IU; Vit. C 36mg; Vit. E 1 IU.

ROASTED BUTTERNUT SQUASH and CHESTNUT SOUP

This recipe works for: Allergies and Asthma, Respiratory Illness, Skin and Hair
Makes 6 servings: Preheat oven to 400°F.

Prick 2 large Butternut Squash with tip of a knife, place on baking sheets, and roast until a knife penetrates squash easily, about 1 hour. Let squash cool and cut in half lengthwise. Discard seeds and fibers; scoop out pulp into a bowl. Set aside.

—In a skillet, sizzle 3 TBS Butter, 3 TBS Canola Oil, 2 diced Yellow Onions and 2 pinches Rubbed Sage, stirring occasionally for 10 minutes. Add 6 cups Organic Low Fat Chicken Broth and squash pulp; bring to a boil. Reduce heat to low and simmer for 3 minutes. Remove from heat, let cool slightly, then purée in a blender and return soup pan. Stir in 1/2 cup canned Chestnut Purée, Sea Salt, Cracked Pepper and Nutmeg.

—Mix a CHESTNUT TOPPER: 1/2 cup Chestnut Purée, 2 TBS snipped Parsley, 2 TBS grated Parmesan Cheese, 1 pinch Rubbed Sage, 1 pinch Marjoram, and 1 pinch Cardamom Powder. Ladle soup into warmed bowls; top each with a big dollop of topper.

NEW ENGLAND STEAMED MOLASSES BREAD

This recipe works for: Allergies and Asthma, Illness Recovery, Skin and Hair
For 2 round molds (16 servings). Use a wok steamer rack.

Mix 1 cup Whole Wheat Flour, 1 cup Corn Meal, 1 cup Rye Flour, 3 tsp. Baking Powder, 1 tsp. Sea Salt and 1/2 teasp. Cardamom Powder. Stir in 2 cups Molasses and 1 cup Rice Milk.

—Spray molds with Canola Oil, line with waxed paper and spray waxed paper. Fill molds 2/3 full. Cover and steam on a wok steamer 3 1/2 hours. Remove covers and bake in moderate oven until top is dry.

Nutrition; 178 calories; 3gm protein; 42gm carbo.; 3gm fiber; 1gm total fats; 0 choles.; 429mg calcium; 9mg iron; 129mg magnesium; 1133mg potassium; 227mg sodium; Vit. A 4 IU; Vit. C 0mg; Vit. E trace.

GINGER YAMS

This recipe works for: Heart Health, Respiratory Illness, Men's Health
For 8 servings: Preheat oven to 450°F.

Peel and cube 4-lbs Yams. Thinly slice 4 Fuji Apples. In a large rectangular baking pan, melt 3 TBS Butter. Stir in yams, half the apple slices, 1 teasp. Sea Salt, 1/2 teasp. White Pepper and 1 TB grated Lemon Zest. Roast 30 minutes.

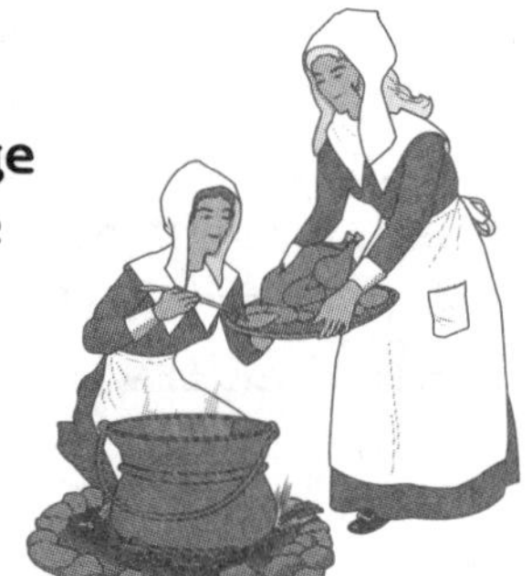

—In a bowl, combine 1 cup Crystallized Ginger cubes, rest of the apple wedges, 1/2 cup Sherry or Brandy, 1 TB Lemon Juice and 2 TBS Maple Syrup. Pour over yams and apples; roast 15 minutes until apples are tender.

OLD FASHIONED MOLASSES PIE

This recipe works for: Arthritis, Sugar Imbalances, Skin and Hair
For one 8" pie or 6 tarts: Preheat oven to 375°F. Have an unbaked pie shell ready.

Make the filling in the blender: 4 TBS WHOLE WHEAT PASTRY FLOUR, 4 TBS HONEY, 3 EGGS, 1/2 cup APPLE JUICE, 1/3 cup MOLASSES, 2 TBS BUTTER, 2 teasp. VANILLA, 1/2 teasp. SEA SALT. Pour into prepared shell, and bake until almost firm, but still slightly wobbly in the center when shaken. Remove and cool before serving.

Nutrition; 186 calories; 4gm protein; 29gm carbo.; 1gm fiber; 6gm total fats; 110mg choles.; 174mg calcium; 4mg iron; 50mg magnesium; 533mg potassium; 221mg sodium; Vit. A 84 IU; Vit. C 1mg; Vit. E 1 IU.

PINE NUT COOKIES

This recipe works for: Women's Health, Respiratory Illness, Skin and Hair
For 24 balls: Preheat oven to 350°F. Bake on a CANOLA OIL sprayed baking sheet.

Toast 1 cup PINE NUTS on a baking sheet in the oven for 5 minutes. Set aside.
—Mix cookie dough in a large bowl: 3 cups UNBLEACHED FLOUR, 1 1/2 teasp. BAKING POWDER, 1/4 teasp. BAKING SODA, 1 TB FENNEL SEED, 1 cup MAPLE SYRUP, 1/2 cup CANOLA OIL, 1 teasp. VANILLA, 1 teasp. ALMOND EXTRACT. Form and place balls on baking sheets. Flatten with a fork dipped in water, spacing cookies about 3" apart. Bake 25 minutes. Press an ALMOND HALF on top of each cookie and cool on racks.

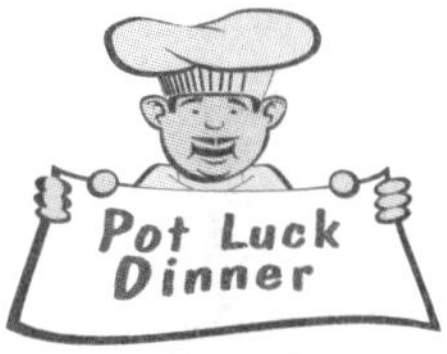

Thanksgiving Night Leftovers

In our family, the leftovers are just as enjoyable as the Thanksgiving meal itself.

BAKED TURKEY SANDWICHES

This recipe works for: Men's - Kid's Health, Allergies - Asthma, Stress Reactions
For 6 servings: Preheat oven to 350°F.

Scatter 4 cups HERB STUFFING CUBES over a large rectangular baking dish. Sizzle in a skillet 4 cups diced cooked Turkey, 1/2 cup diced ONION, 1/2 cup diced CELERY, 1/2 teasp. SEA SALT and 1/4 teasp. PEPPER. Distribute mixture over top of stuffing cubes. In a bowl, mix 1 1/2 cups PLAIN ALMOND MILK, 1 can CREAM OF MUSHROOM SOUP, 1 cup shredded MOZARRELLA CHEESE, 2 EGGS and 1 TB YELLOW MUSTARD. Pour over turkey and bake 40 minutes until a knife inserted in the center comes out clean.

HARVEST SUPPER PIE Perfect for leftovers.

This recipe works for: Allergies and Asthma, Respiratory Illness, Skin and Hair
For 8 slices: Preheat oven to 450°F.

Have ready $1^1/_2$ cups packed leftover cooked squash and carrots.

—Make the POPPY SEED CRUST: Mix together to form a dough, $^3/_4$ cup Whole Wheat Pastry Flour, $^1/_2$ cup Cornmeal, 2 TBS Butter, 2 TBS Poppy Seeds, $^1/_2$ teasp. Sea Salt and 3 TBS Ice Water. Press into a pie plate. Set aside.

—Blender blend the filling: the cooked squash-carrot mixture, 3 Eggs, $^3/_4$ cup Maple Syrup, $^3/_4$ cup Plain Yogurt, $^1/_2$ teasp. Ginger, 1 teasp. Cinnamon, $^1/_2$ teasp. Allspice and $^1/_4$ teasp. Sea Salt.

—Pour into poppy seed shell and bake in the lower third of the oven 10 minutes. Reduce heat to 325°F, and bake 45 minutes until center is almost set, but still wobbly. Remove and cool before cutting.

Nutrition; 238 calories; 6gm protein; 40gm carbo.; 3gm fiber; 6gm total fats; 89mg choles.; 119mg calcium; 2mg iron; 51mg magnesium; 309mg potassium; 255mg sodium; Vit. A 318 IU; Vit. C 2mg; Vit. E 1 IU.

MAPLE SYRUP BAKED APPLES

This recipe works for: Liver Health, Weight Control, Immune Power
Serves 8: Preheat oven to 350°F.

Core 8 Fuji Apples and place in a baking dish. Mix and fill core with: 2 TBS minced Honey Crystallized Ginger, 1 cup chopped Walnuts, $^1/_2$ teasp. Cinnamon and 2 TBS grated Lemon Zest. Pour over 1 cup Maple Syrup. Bake for 35 minutes. Serve hot.

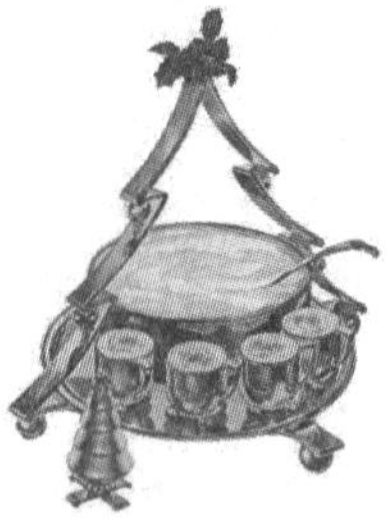

A Lavish Victorian Holiday Feast

The whole idea was opulence in the nineteenth century, as America began to reap the rewards of a century of hard labor and nation building. Prosperity meant lavish celebration feasts. Choose among the recipes in this menu for a sumptuous feeling without the calories, fat or sugar.

FRAGRANT TURKEY GLAZE

Heat in a saucepan: 6 TBS Butter, 3 TBS Madeira or Sherry, 1 TB Lemon Juice, $^1/_2$ teasp. Cinnamon and $^1/_2$ teasp. Allspice. Brush on turkey to cover before roasting.

CIDER EGGNOG

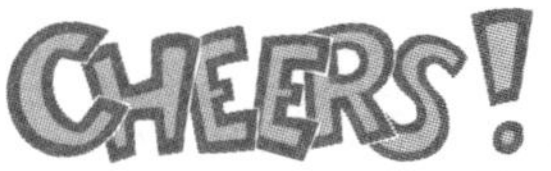

This recipe works for: Stress and Exhaustion, Men's Health, Illness Recovery
Serves 10:

Stir in a bowl: 2 Eggs, 3 TBS Maple Syrup, 3 TBS Brandy, 1 TB Lemon Juice, $^1/_4$ tsp. Cinnamon and $^1/_4$ tsp. Nutmeg. Whisk in another bowl: 1 carton (8-oz.) Kefir Cheese or Low Fat Cream Cheese with 1 TB Lemon Juice, $^1/_4$ tsp. Allspice and $^1/_4$ tsp. Cardamom Powder.

—Heat 1 qt. Apple Cider; remove from heat. Whisk in egg mixture. Put serving bowl. Plop in 10 dollops cream cheese mix. Ladle into cups; sprinkle with Nutmeg.

CRANBERRY RELISH

This recipe works for: Women's Health, Heart Health, Digestive Health
Serves 8:

Simmer 12-oz. Fresh or Frozen Cranberries in $^1/_4$ cup Water and $1^1/_4$ cups Turbinado Sugar for 5 minutes <u>only</u>. Remove from heat and add $^1/_2$ cup Raisins and 1 to 2 TB minced Crystallized Ginger. Add 1 cup diced Fuji Apples, $^1/_2$ cup diced Celery, $^1/_4$ cup Red Wine Vinegar, 1 tsp. Cinnamon, $^1/_2$ tsp. Nutmeg and $^1/_4$ tsp. Allspice. Chill and serve.

BRANDY POTATO STICKS Serve these very hot.

This recipe works for: Men's Health, Respiratory Health, Hair and Skin
For 4 people:

Cut $1^1/_2$-lbs. Yellow Dutch Potatoes in matchsticks. Sizzle in a skillet for 10 minutes in 2 TBS Butter. Add $^1/_2$ cup Brandy and $^1/_2$ cup Organic Chicken Broth. Cover and simmer until tender, about 15 minutes. Add $^3/_4$ cup Plain Low Fat Yogurt and $^1/_4$ cup Water. Cook over high heat for 5 minutes. Season with Sea Salt, Pepper and Nutmeg.

SQUASH and CIDER SOUP for WINTER WARMTH

This recipe works for: Heart Health, Waste Management, Fatigue Syndromes
Serves 6:

Drizzle Whole Wheat Bread Cubes with Olive Oil. Sprinkle with Sesame Seeds and season with Garlic-Lemon Seasoning. Toast and set aside.

—Sizzle in a soup pot 10 minutes: 1 TB Olive Oil, 1 diced Onion, 2 minced Cloves Garlic, 2 tsp. Chinese 5-Spice Powder, 1 teasp. Sea Salt and 1 diced Granny Smith Apple.

—Add 4 cups Organic Chicken Broth and 2 cups Apple Cider. Simmer 25 minutes til tender. Remove from heat, cool slightly and puree half the soup in a blender til smooth. Add back to the pot. Stir in 2 cups shredded cooked Turkey. Heat briefly and ladle into wide soup bowls. Top with swirls of Kefir Cheese and the toasted croutons.

CARROT GINGER SOUP

This recipe works for: Women's Health, Heart Health, Liver and Organ Health
For 4 servings:

Combine ingredients in a soup pot: sizzle 2 TBS Olive Oil, 1 TB minced Crystallized Ginger and 1 cup diced Onions for 5 minutes. Add 1 cup diced Carrots and 1 cup diced Yellow Dutch Potatoes; sizzle for 8 minutes. Add 4 cups Water, bring to a boil and simmer for 20 minutes. Remove from heat and add $^1/_2$ cup sliced Almonds, 2 TBS Orange Juice and 1 TB Honey. Puree in a blender; pour in a soup tureen and stir in 1 TB minced Crystallized Ginger, and $^1/_2$ cup Sherry.

CRANBERRY MOLDED SALAD

This recipe works for: Heart Health, Waste Management, Fatigue Syndromes
Serves 6:

Drain and reserve juice from 1 can (11-oz.) Mandarin Oranges and 1 can (18-oz.) Sliced Peaches. Add enough Sherry and Water to make $1^1/_4$ cups liquid. Heat in a pan just to boiling. Remove from heat and stir in 1 pkg. (3-oz.) Orange Gelatin.

CHESTNUT STUFFED TURKEY

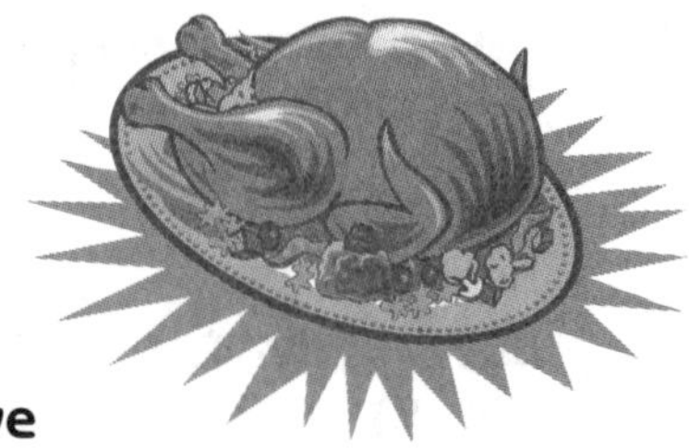

This recipe works for: Men's Health, Stress Reactions
Stuffing serves 8. Preheat oven to 325°F.

Crack and remove meats from 2-lbs. Chestnuts. Drop meats into boiling water; boil 5 minutes. Drain and remove skins. (Wear rubber gloves; skins come off easier while they're very hot.) Chop meats. Bring 2 cups Organic Chicken Broth to a boil and add chestnuts. Simmer 8 minutes. Drain and set aside. Reserve broth.

—Sizzle in a skillet: 2 TBS Olive Oil, 6 diced Celery Ribs and 2 diced Yellow Onions for 5 minutes. Add $1^1/_2$ cups reserved broth and simmer until liquid is reduced by half. Add 4 TBS Butter, 6 TBS Olive Oil, 2 teasp. Marjoram, and 1 teasp. each: Thyme, Sage, Sea Salt and Pepper. When butter melts, stir in remaining broth and 10 cups diced Whole Wheat Bread Cubes to coat.

—Prepare turkey: Remove giblets and neck. Rinse turkey inside and out. Rub with cut Lemon, Sea Salt and Pepper. Stuff fresh herb sprigs, like Sage, Rosemary, Thyme or Oregano under breast skin. Stuff turkey and close openings with skewers or twine.

—Roast turkey, basting every hour with the glaze on page 466. Roasting time is about 25 minutes per pound. When meat thermometer in center registers 180°F, turkey is done; or when a cut in a meaty part shows white instead of pink, or when a drumstick moves easily. Remove stuffing in the kitchen and place on a serving platter. Present whole turkey at the table and then carve. Note: Use any size turkey with this stuffing recipe. Bake any extra stuffing and serve on the side.

ROSEMARY ONION FLOWERS

This recipe works for: Brain Health, Respiratory Health, Hair, Skin, Nails
6 servings: Preheat oven to 400°F. Bake in an Olive Oil sprayed rectangular pan.

Peel and trim off top and root ends of 4 large Red Onions to flatten. Set each onion on its root end. Starting at the top, cut through the middle to 1/2" from the bottom; turn onion and cut through the middle to 1/2" from the bottom. You'll have 4 quarters. Repeat again and you'll have 12 attached wedges of the onion.
—Set onions upright in a baking pan. Drizzle with 4 TBS Olive Oil. Season with Sea Salt and Cracked Pepper; bake covered with foil for 1 hour until tender. Uncover, sprinkle with 4 TBS Spiced Brown Rice Vinegar, 2 teasp. snipped Fresh Rosemary Leaves and Pine Nuts or chopped Walnuts. Bake uncovered for 15 minutes to brown tips and sprinkle with snipped Fresh Parsley to serve.

BABY PUMPKINS with CORN PUDDING FILLING

This recipe works for: Men's Health, Overcoming Addictions
Serves 8: Preheat oven to 325°F.

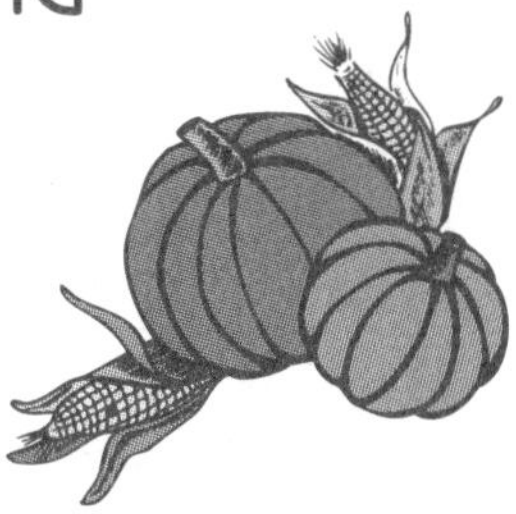

Place 8 Baby Pumpkins on a wok steamer rack. Cover and steam for 20 minutes. Remove from wok and let cool; then slice off top quarter, scoop out seeds and enough flesh to make a nice filling shell. Rub each pumpkin and top with Canola Oil.
—Make the filling: in a skillet, sizzle 1 diced Onion in 2 TBS Butter for 5 minutes. Add 1 pkg. (10-oz.) frozen Corn Kernels, 2 TBS bottled Chipotle Chili Sauce, 1/2 tsp. Tarragon and 1/2 tsp. Sage. Sizzle 5 minutes. Remove from heat; whisk in 1/2 cup Plain Almond Milk or Rice Milk, 1/2 cup Low Fat Cream Cheese, Sea Salt to taste and 3 Eggs.
—Place pumpkins and tops on baking sheets. Fill pumpkin shells with pudding and bake for 25 to 30 minutes until center is almost firm. Cover with tops to serve.

Nutrition; 190 calories; 8gm protein; 25gm carbo.; 4gm fiber; 6gm total fats; 96mg choles.; 94mg calcium; 2mg iron; 38mg magnesium; 734mg potassium; 35mg sodium; Vit. A 2760 IU; Vit. C 15mg; Vit. E 3 IU.

LOW FAT CANDIED SWEET POTATOES

This recipe works for: Men's and Women's Health, Weight Control, Hair and Skin
8 servings: Preheat oven to 400°F. Spray a baker-serving dish with Canola Oil spray.

Pierce, then bake 8 Sweet Potatoes for 1 1/4 hours until soft. Scrape out potato flesh into a bowl. Mash while hot with 2 TBS Butter, 3 TBS Maple Syrup, 1/4 teasp. Cinnamon, 1/4 teasp. White Pepper, 1/4 teasp. Nutmeg and 2 teasp. grated Orange Zest. Beat with electric mixer until smooth. Make the topping: mix 3 TBS Maple Sugar Granules, 1/4 teasp. Allspice and 1/4 teasp. Cinnamon. Sprinkle over potatoes. Bake at 350°F for 30 minutes. Serve steaming hot.

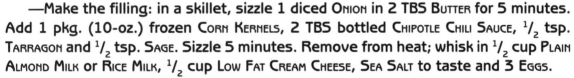

VICTORIAN GINGER PUDDING

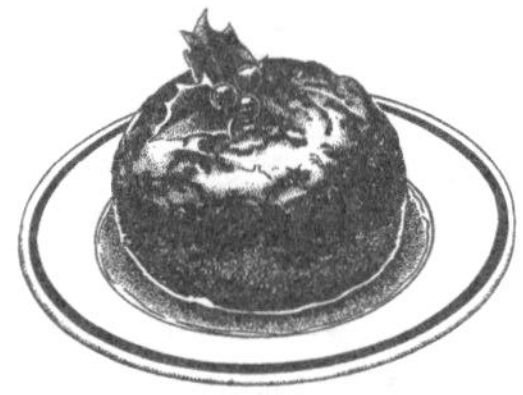

This recipe works for: *Men's Health, Fatigue, Colds and Flu*
12 -14 dessert slices: Preheat oven to 350°F.

Have ready in the oven, a shallow pan of simmering water.

—In a food processor: blend enough pitted prunes to make $^3/_4$ cup Prune Butter; add 5 Eggs, $^3/_4$ cup Turbinado Sugar, $^1/_4$ cup Maple Syrup, 1 stick Butter, the juice of 1 Orange and the grated Zest of the Orange. Turn into a bowl and stir in 2 cups Whole Wheat Pastry Flour, 1 cup Unbleached Flour, 2 TBS Ground Ginger, 1 cup Crystallized Ginger and $1^1/_2$ teasp. Baking Soda.

—Spray a $2^1/_2$ qt. baking dish with Canola Oil. Spoon in batter. Cover with foil; put in the oven pan of simmering water. Bake $1^1/_2$ hours. Turn onto a serving plate.

—Make the LEMON SAUCE: in a pan, stir 2 thin-sliced unpeeled Lemons, 2 teasp. grated Orange Zest, $^1/_4$ cup Turbinado Sugar, $^1/_4$ cup Maple Syrup, 6 TBS Orange Juice and 4 TBS Sherry. Boil on high heat until liquid is almost gone - 8 minutes. Watch closely. Add 4 more TBS Orange Juice and 2 TBS Brandy. Bring to a rolling boil. Remove from heat. Cover and chill until ready to serve on the Ginger Pudding.

VICTORIAN FRUIT CAKE A rich no-sugar cake, Serve in thin sliver pieces.

This recipe works for: *Sugar Imbalances, Women's Health, Waste Management*
For 12 servings: Preheat oven to 350°. Use a Canola Oil sprayed 9 x 12" baker.

Have ready a blend of: $^1/_2$ cup chopped Walnuts, $^1/_2$ cup Sesame Seeds, $^1/_4$ cup Shredded Coconut and $^1/_4$ cup Toasted Wheat Germ, toasted in the oven and set aside.

—Combine cake ingredients: $^1/_2$ cup Honey, $^1/_2$ cup Canola Oil, 2 Eggs, $^1/_2$ cup Rice Flour, $1^1/_4$ cups Whole Wheat Pastry Flour, 8 Pitted Prunes blender blended to a butter, 2 teasp. grated Orange Zest. Spread into baker; bake for 15 minutes. Cool slightly.

—Mix the topping: $^3/_4$ cup Maple Syrup, $^1/_2$ cup Raisins, $^1/_2$ cup diced Dry Pineapple, $^1/_4$ cup chopped Dry Apricots, 1 teasp. Vanilla, $1^1/_2$ teasp. Nutmeg, $^1/_2$ teasp. Cinnamon, $^1/_4$ teasp. Allspice. Stir in toasted ingredients. Spread on cake and return to the oven for 20 more minutes until light brown. Cool, cut and serve.

Nutrition; 390 calories; 7gm protein; 55gm carbo.; 4gm fiber; 17gm total fats; 35mg choles.; 98mg calcium; 3mg iron; 81mg magnesium; 344mg potassium; 17mg sodium; Vit. A 48 IU; Vit. C 5mg; Vit. E 5 IU.

HOT GINGER PEAR WINE

This recipe works for: *Heart Health, Digestive Health, Colds and Flu*
Serves 8:

Heat on very low heat for 5 minutes: 6 cups canned Unsweetened Pear Nectar, 2 cups White Wine, 4 TBS Honey, 2 TBS minced Crystallized Ginger and 2 TBS Lemon Juice. Pour into mugs. Top with Lemon Wheels and Cinnamon Sticks.

A Modern Low Fat Thanksgiving

The hallmarks of holiday feasts today are carefully chosen fresh ingredients, exquisite low fat desserts, fragrant drinks and sauces. It all speaks to a less is more idea; less quantity, more quality, less fat and sugar, more seasonings and taste.

HOT WASSAIL Non-alcoholic punch for everybody.

This recipe works for: Kid's Health, Digestive Health, Colds and Flu
Serves 12:

Simmer on low heat: 6 cups Apple Cider, 2 cups Pineapple Juice, $^1/_2$ cup Orange Juice, 5 TBS Maple Syrup, 3 TBS Lemon Juice, 1 teasp. grated Lemon Zest, 3 Cinnamon Sticks, and $^1/_4$ teasp. Nutmeg. Pour into mugs. Stick Whole Cloves into the skin of 16 Orange Wedges and float on top of each mug.

Nutrition; 124 calories; 1gm protein; 30gm carbo.; 1gm fiber; trace total fats; 0 choles.; 36mg calcium; 1mg iron; 15mg magnesium; 281mg potassium; 6mg sodium; Vit. A 9 IU; Vit. C 24mg; Vit. E trace

WILD RICE and MUSHROOM SOUP

This recipe works for: Cancer Protection, Stess Reduction, Weight Control
Makes 8 servings:

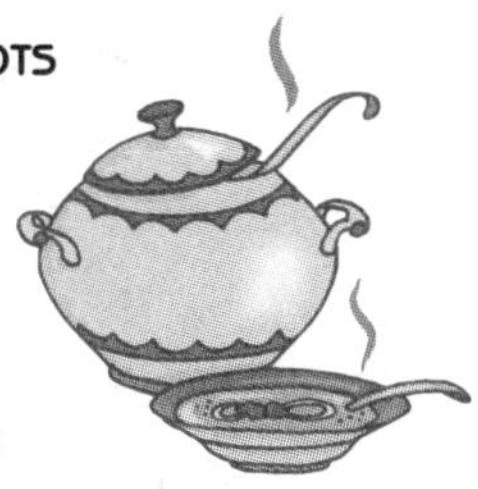

In a large soup pot, sizzle 1 TB Olive Oil and 3 cups diced Shallots for 5 minutes. Add 1 teasp. Dulse Flakes, 1 teasp. Sesame Salt, 1 cup pre-soaked, drained Wild Rice and 8 cups Low Fat Organic Chicken Broth. Bring to a boil, then reduce to simmer.

—In a skillet, sizzle 1 TB Olive Oil, 1 diced Carrot and 3 cups mixed, sliced Fresh Mushrooms (Portobellas, Porcinis, Brown Cremini and White Button). Sauté for 5 minutes.

—Remove from heat and blender blend the carrot and mushrooms with enough liquid from the soup pot to make a purée. Add the purée to the soup pot.

—Reheat the skillet. Sizzle 1 TB Olive Oil. Add 2 cups sliced White Button Mushrooms and 2 cups slivered Fresh Shiitake Mushrooms, 2 TBS Brown Rice Vinegar, 2 TBS Sherry, 3 TBS Lemon Juice and 2 teasp. Herbs de Provence (or $^1/_2$ tsp. <u>each</u>: dried Oregano, Marjoram, Thyme, Tarragon and Basil). Simmer until the mushrooms have released their juice. Remove mushrooms with a slotted spoon and add them to the simmering soup pot. Add 2 TBS Sherry to the skillet, stir and cook to reduce the liquid and thicken it slightly, about 5 minutes.

—Remove from heat and scrape into the soup pot. Simmer soup for 20-30 minutes, until the wild rice is very tender. Garnish with snipped Parsley.

Nutrition; 172 calories; 9gm protein; 27gm carbo.; 3gm fiber; 2gm total fats; 0 choles.; 48mg calcium; 2mg iron; 40mg magnesium; 677mg potassium; 175mg sodium; Vit. A 266 IU; Vit. C 13mg; Vit. E 1 IU.

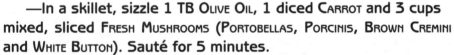

ROASTED GARLIC SOUP

This recipe works for: Heart Health, Digestive Health, Colds and Flu
Makes 4 to 6 servings: Preheat oven to 450°F. Oil a baking sheet with Olive Oil.

Brush 15 large peeled Garlic Cloves with Olive Oil and arrange on baking sheet. Bake for 10 to 15 minutes, until soft and browned around edges. Don't allow to get too brown or they will be bitter in the soup. When cloves are done, process in blender with 1 cup of Organic Chicken Broth to make a smooth puree. Set aside.

—In a soup pot, bring 1 cup Organic Chicken Broth and $^1/_2$ cup Golden Rice to a boil. Cover; cook for 12 minutes. Add 3 cups more Organic Chicken Broth, 1 cup Water and $^1/_2$ cup White Wine. Lower heat; add 1 tsp. Dry Thyme, 1 tsp. Dry Tarragon, the reserved garlic purée, Sea Salt and Cracked Black Pepper to taste. Add $^1/_2$ cup Frozen Peas. Cover, remove from heat and let stand 10 minutes for peas to thaw before serving.

SCRUMPTIOUS CORN CASSEROLE

This recipe works for: Liver and Organ Health, Men's and Kid's Health
Makes 6 to 8 servings: Preheat oven to 350°F.

Sizzle 1 diced Onion and 1 diced Red Bell Pepper in 1 TB Butter and 1 TB Canola Oil for 5 minutes. Stir in 1 package (16-oz.) Frozen Corn Kernels, 1 carton (8-oz.) Low Fat Cream Cheese, $^1/_2$ cup grated Low Fat Cheddar Cheese, 1 diced Tomato, 1 TB Dry Cilantro, Sea Salt and Pepper to taste, and 2 TBS Arrowroot Powder dissolved in 2 TBS Sherry. Bake for 30 to 40 minutes. Sprinkle with Sweet Paprika and serve hot.

Nutrition; 239 calories; 10gm protein; 24gm carbo.; 3gm fiber; 8gm total fats; 31mg choles.; 166mg calcium; 2mg iron; 32mg magnesium; 316mg potassium; 69mg sodium; Vit. A 209 IU; Vit. C 31mg; Vit. E 1 IU.

GARLIC MASHED POTATOES

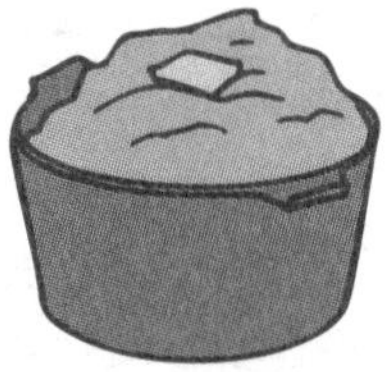

This recipe works for: Heart Health, Colds and Flu, Anti-Aging
Makes 8 servings:

Peel and quarter 3-lbs. Yellow Dutch Potatoes. Bring to boil in 2-qts. Salted Water. Simmer for 20-25 minutes until soft. Move pan off heat. Sizzle 2 TBS minced Garlic in 2 TBS Butter. Add $^1/_2$ cup Water, $^1/_2$ cup Plain Yogurt or Kefir Cheese, $^1/_2$ teasp. Sea Salt and $^1/_2$ teasp. Lemon-Pepper. Simmer until thickened and liquid is reduced by $^1/_3$.

—Drain potatoes and add Garlic mixture. Beat with electric mixer to peaks.

RASPBERRY ORANGE GLAZE for the TURKEY

Heat in a pan: 2 cups Raspberries, 1 cup Orange Juice, 6 TBS Honey, 2 teasp. grated Orange Zest, $^1/_2$ teasp. Ground Sage, $^1/_2$ teasp. Chinese 5-Spice Powder, $^1/_2$ teasp. Thyme. Brush on turkey before roasting. Baste every 20 minutes during roasting.

ROAST TURKEY with VEGETABLE STUFFING

This recipe works for: Women's Health, Overcoming Addictions, Bone Building
12 servings: For about a 16-lb. Turkey. Preheat oven to 450°F.

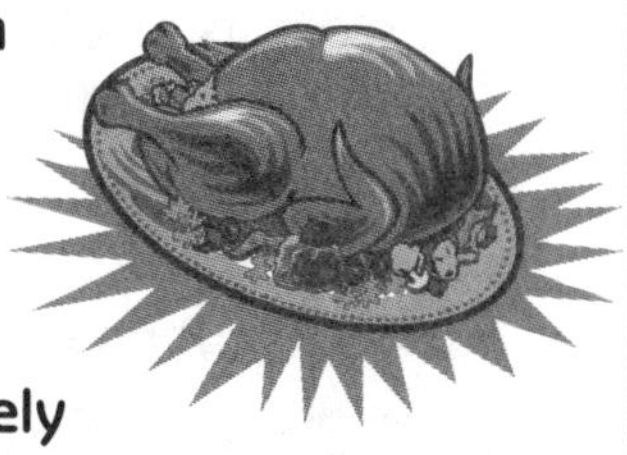

Tenderize the turkey: Remove giblets and place turkey in a large tub. Cover with water; pour in 1-lb. Kosher Salt or Coarse Salt. Chill 8 to 12 hours. Remove, rinse turkey well and pat dry.

—Make vegetable stuffing: mix 8 TBS Butter, 1 diced Onion, 1 diced Rib Celery, 1 diced Carrot, 4 Baby Turnips, 4 sprigs each Thyme, Sage, and Rosemary. Pack body cavity and neck cavity loosely with veggies. Tie legs together with twine; secure neck flap to back with a skewer.

—Rub outside of turkey with Raspberry Glaze (page 472). Set turkey on its side on a rack in a roasting pan. Roast 15 minutes. Turn on other side and roast 15 minutes. Reduce heat to 325°F, turn breast side up; cover with a foil tent. Add 3 TBS Sherry and water to the roasting pan. Baste with glaze every 20 minutes until juices run clear, 3 hours total time. Baste and let rest 20 minutes before carving.

UN-STUFFING

Bake this stuffing as a separate dish along with the turkey.
This recipe works for: Men's Health, Overcoming Addictions, Sexuality
Enough for 4 people: Preheat oven to 325°F.

Place 8 cups Whole Wheat Bread Cubes or diced Corn Bread in a large bowl.

—Sauté in a large skillet for about 5 minutes til fragrant: 1 large chopped Onion 1 chopped Red Bell Pepper, 2 Ribs Celery, 1 teasp. Sea Salt, 1 teasp. Lemon Pepper, 1/2 teasp. ground Sage, 1/4 teasp. ground Rosemary, 1/4 teasp. Nutmeg. Add either 1 pint Oysters, or 1 can (7-oz.) Sliced Water chestnuts and 1 cup Sliced Mushrooms.

—Add 1/2 cup Turkey Broth (simply boil bones in water for broth), and 1/2 cup Sherry. Toss to coat and heat. Mix with bread cubes and toss. Turn into an oiled 3-qt. casserole. Cover and bake for 30 minutes until crusty at the edges.

THANKSGIVING PUMPKIN BREAD

This recipe works for: Men's Health, Overcoming Addictions, Sexuality
Serves 12: Preheat oven to 375°F. Spray a square pan with Canola Oil.

Beat together 6 TBS Butter, 2 TBS Canola Oil, 1 cup Maple Sugar Granules, 2 Eggs and 1/2 cup Honey. Stir together, 1 cup Unbleached Flour, 1 cup Whole Wheat Pastry Flour, 2 1/2 teasp, Baking Powder, 1/2 teasp. Sea Salt, 1/2 teasp. Baking Soda. Blend dry mix with wet mix. Add 1 teasp. Cinnamon, 2 TBS minced Crystallized Ginger and 1/2 teasp. Ground Cloves. Add 4 TBS Almond Milk or Rice Milk, 1 cup canned Pumpkin and 1/2 cup chopped Walnuts. Pour batter into prepared pan and bake for 35 to 40 minutes until cake pulls away from sides of pan. Cool and slice.

SHERRY SCENTED WILD RICE and NUTS

This recipe works for: Heart and Artery Health, Anti-Aging, Stress Relaxation
For 8 servings:

In a pan, heat 1 cup Raisins and 1/2 cup Sherry to boiling. Reduce heat, simmer for 5 minutes, remove from heat and set aside. Toast 1 cup Slivered Almonds in the oven until golden. Remove and set aside.

—Boil turkey bones in 6 cups water 20 minutes for broth. Put 1 cup Wild Rice in a pot with 2 cups turkey broth and 1 TB Butter. Cook over low heat for 1 hour.

—Bring 3 cups turkey broth to a boil in another pot; add 1 cup Golden or Short Grain Brown Rice and 1 TB Butter. Reduce heat and cook until liquid is absorbed, about 45 minutes. Combine all ingredients in a serving dish. Season with Sea Salt and Lemon-Pepper. Snip on 1/2 cup Fresh Parsley over top.

Nutrition; 347 calories; 10gm protein; 47gm carbo.; 4gm fiber; 12gm total fats; 7mg choles.; 71mg calcium; 2mg iron; 109mg magnesium; 490mg potassium; 86mg sodium; Vit. A 46 IU; Vit. C 6mg; Vit. E 6 IU.

SWEET POTATO SOUFFLÉ

This recipe works for: Men's Health, Weight Control, Stress Relaxation
For 6 servings: Preheat oven to 450°F. Spray a casserole with Canola Oil.

Separate 4 Eggs. Put the whites in a large mixing bowl and set aside.

—Peel 1 large Sweet Potato; cube and set aside.

—Blender blend smooth: 4 Egg Yolks, 1/2 cup Maple Syrup, 1 cup Plain Yogurt, 2 TBS Lemon Juice, 2 cups Organic Chicken or Turkey Broth, 1 tsp. grated Lemon Zest, 1/2 tsp. Sea Salt, 1/2 tsp. Sweet Tooth Baking Mix (pg.487), and the cubed sweet potato.

—Beat the egg whites to stiff peaks with 2 teasp. Honey. Fold into squash mix. Turn into casserole, and bake for 10 minutes. Lower heat to 325°F. and bake for 45 minutes until sweet potatoes are tender and a toothpick comes out clean.

Nutrition; 227 calories; 9gm protein; 38gm. carbo.; 2gm. fiber; 4gm total fats; 144mg choles.; 128mg calcium; 1mg iron; 22mg magnesium; 375mg potassium; 267mg sod.; Vit. A 1037 IU, Vit. C 13mg; Vit. E 1 IU.

THANKSGIVING PUMPKIN PARFAIT

This recipe works for: Men's Health, Weight Control, Sugar Imbalances
For 6 servings:

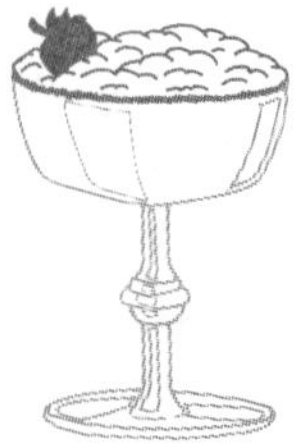

Blender blend in batches: 8 sliced Bananas, 1/3 cup Maple Syrup, 1 TB Chinese 5 Spice Powder and 2 cups canned Pumpkin. Freeze in ice cube trays. Ten minutes before you're ready to serve, remove frozen cubes from trays, reblend until creamy; spoon into parfait glasses and top with minced Crystallized Ginger.

FANCY MOLDED DESSERT with SWEET WINE

This recipe works for: Heart and Artery Health, Weight Control, Stress Relaxation
Make ahead and chill airtight 4 hours for best results: For 6 servings:

Have ready $1^1/_2$ cups sliced Strawberries and 1 cup sliced Seedless Red Grapes.

—In a 2 quart pan, mix 2 envelopes Unflavored Gelatin, 3 TBS Fructose and $^1/_2$ cup Dessert Wine like Muscat, French Colombard or Johannisberg Reisling. Stir over medium heat until fructose and gelatin dissolve. Add 2 more cups wine and 1 TB Lemon Juice. Pour $^2/_3$ cup of the mixture into a loaf pan. Arrange half the strawberry slices on top in a single layer. Chill until firm to the touch, about 45 minutes. Pour on another $^2/_3$ cup gelatin-wine mix, and arrange half the grapes on top in a layer. Chill 45 minutes. Repeat layers and gelatin wine mix.... chilling 45 minutes <u>between each layer</u>.

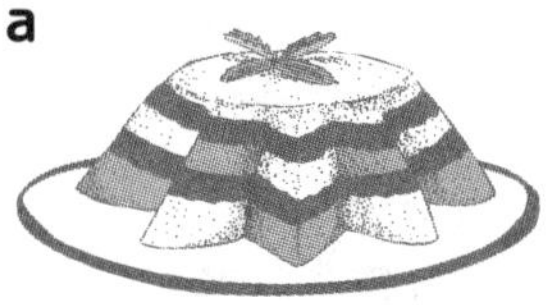

—To unmold, dip pan in very hot water until gelatin just begins to soften at edges, 4 or 5 seconds. Lift from water, dry pan with a cloth and invert a flat plate over the pan. Holding plate and pan together, invert and remove pan (if mold does not slip out, slide a thin knife between sides and dessert to release it). Cut and serve on dessert plates with Mint Sprigs or Chocolate Mint Shavings.

SUGAR FREE, FRESH FESTIVE FRUITCAKE

This recipe works for: Heart Health, Weight Control, Allergies and Asthma
Makes 3 large or 6 small fruitcakes for 48 servings: Preheat oven to 300°F. Lightly oil and flour 3, 2-quart or 6, 1-quart loaf pans. To keep fruitcakes from cracking on top, place a pan of water on oven rack below fruitcake pans.

In a large bowl, combine $^1/_2$ cup chopped dried Unsweetened Pineapple, 1 cup Raisins, 1 cup chopped dried Calmyrna Figs, 1 cup chopped dried Nectarines or Peaches, 1 cup pitted chopped Dates, 1 cup chopped dried Apricots, $^1/_4$ cup grated Orange Zest, 2 cups Brandy or Orange Juice, 1 cup Sherry or Pineapple Juice and 1 cup Apple Juice. Cover bowl with a clean dish towel and let fruit macerate for 4 days. Stir twice a day.

—In a large bowl, blend 3 cups Whole Wheat Pastry Flour and 3 cups Unbleached Flour, $1^1/_2$ TBS Baking Powder, 1 tsp. Allspice and 1 tsp. Nutmeg. In another bowl combine $^1/_2$ cup Canola Oil, 4 Egg Whites, lightly beaten, 2 Whole Eggs, lightly beaten and 2 cups Maple Syrup. Stir soaked fruit into flour mixture and coat well. Add egg mixture, then stir in $^1/_4$ cup chopped Almonds and $^1/_4$ cup chopped Walnuts.

—Divide batter evenly into pans. Bake fruitcakes 2 hours. When a toothpick comes out clean, remove fruitcakes from oven and cool. If a fruitcake is still gooey in center, bake as long as 30 minutes more. Baking time depends on how much liquid the dried fruit has absorbed.

Nutrition; 171 calories; 3gm protein; 33gm carbo.; 2gm fiber; 3gm total fats; 8mg choles.; 64mg calcium; 1mg iron; 27mg magnesium; 226mg potassium; 44mg sodium; Vit. A 22 IU; Vit. C 7mg; Vit. E 1 IU.

CHINESE PEARS and GINGER DESSERT

This recipe works for: Liver and Organ Health, Digestive Health, Fatigue
Serves 4:

Make VANILLA SUGAR: Mix 2 TBS Turbinado Sugar with the seeds scraped out of 1 split Vanilla Bean. Let sit overnight. Cut the Vanilla Pod into 1" pieces.

In a skillet, bring Vanilla Pod pieces, 6 TBS Turbinado Sugar, 2 TBS Maple Syrup and 1 cup Water to a boil. Simmer 5 minutes. Remove pod. Add 2-lbs. firm sliced Pears, the vanilla sugar and 1 TB Lemon Juice. Simmer 5 minutes. Stir in 3 TBS Butter and 3 TBS minced Crystallized Ginger. Turn off heat. Let sit for 5 minutes. Serve warm.

FRESH HOMEMADE CRANBERRY CANDY

This recipe works for: Women's Health, Skin and Hair, Colds and Flu
For 24 pieces:

In a pan, combine 2 cups Cranberries, $1^1/_2$ teasp. grated Orange Zest, 2 TBS minced Crystallized Ginger and $^3/_4$ cup Orange Juice. Heat until berries begin to pop. Remove from heat to cool slightly, and purée in the blender until smooth. Add back to the saucepan with $^3/_4$ cup Maple Sugar Granules and 3 TBS Unflavored Gelatin. Cook over stirring constantly for 15 minutes, until you can see the bottom of the pan when a spoon is drawn across it. Stir in $^1/_2$ cup chopped Walnuts, and spread mixture in a Canola Oil sprayed loaf pan. Let stand uncovered overnight. Cut in squares.

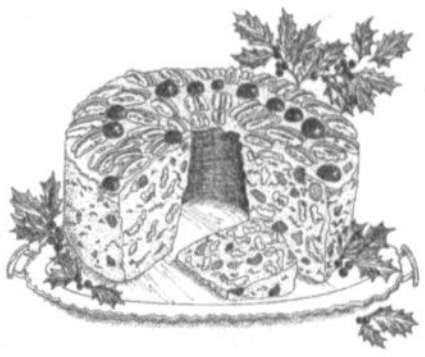

A Memorable Holiday Brunch

Brunch has become a perfect relaxing meal for holidays, celebrations and vacations. Everything goes at brunch... sweets, breakfast foods, salads, quiches, and decadent (but healthy) drinks.

EASY FRUIT PARFAIT

This recipe works for: Liver and Organ Health, Weight Control, Sugar Imbalances
Serves 4:

Blender blend: 1 cup bottled Honey Lemonade or Green Tea (with honey and lemon), $^1/_2$ cup Orange Juice, 1 cup Crushed Pineapple with juice, 1 cup fresh Berries (any kind), 1 cup Fresh Strawberries, 2 Bananas. Freeze for 3 hours until firm but still slushy. Blender blend briefly and pour into parfait glasses. Top with Fresh Mint Sprigs.

FRENCH ONION SOUP

This recipe works for: Liver - Organ Health, Hair and Skin, Respiratory Infections
Serves 6

In a large soup pot, heat 1 TB Olive Oil and 1 cup Dry Sherry until bubbling. Add 8 minced Cloves Garlic and 4 large Yellow Onions, thinly sliced in circles; sizzle slowly, stirring frequently for 20 minutes, until they become pasty. Add 1 TB Whole Wheat Pastry Flour, and stir 2 minutes. Add 4 cups Mineral Rich Enzyme Broth (page 33); bring to a boil, reduce heat and simmer 20 minutes. Season with Sea Salt, Cracked Pepper and 1 TB Tamari Sauce. Ladle soup into bowls and float a slice of toasted French Bread on top of each.

Nutrition; 161 calories; 4gm protein; 23gm carbo.; 3gm fiber; 3gm total fats; 0 choles.; 49mg calcium; 1mg iron; 24mg magnesium; 244mg potassium; 198mg sodium; Vit. A trace; Vit. C 8mg; Vit. E 1 IU.

BRUNCH FRENCH TOAST

This recipe works for: Men's and Kid's Health, Hair and Skin, Sugar Imbalances
Serves 6 to 8:

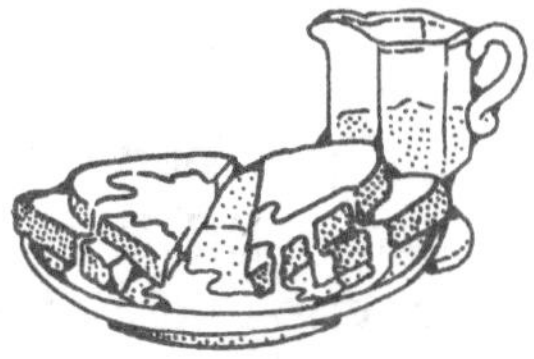

Thinly slice 1 Fuji Apple. Sprinkle with Lemon Juice and set aside.

—Make the sauce in a shallow dish: whisk 4 Eggs, 1 cup Vanilla Rice Milk, 1 TB Maple Sugar Granules, 1/4 teasp. Cinnamon, 1/4 teasp. Nutmeg and 1/4 teasp. Vanilla.

—In a large skillet sizzle about 1 TB Butter. Coat both sides of 2 slices Whole Wheat Sourdough Bread with sauce. Lay in the skillet, and cook 3 minutes on each side to brown. Repeat until all slices are browned. Keep warm on a plate in the oven.

—In a bowl mix 1/3 cup Maple Syrup with 1/2 cup Vanilla Yogurt. In a saucepan heat 1/3 cup Maple Syrup with 1/2 cup Almond Butter until melted.

—To serve place 1 or 2 slices of French Toast on each plate. Divide apple slices over toast. Sprinkle on toasted Granola or toasted Shredded Coconut and spoon on dollops of maple-yogurt mix and almond butter sauce.

BRUNCH SCRAMBLED EGGS with SMOKED SALMON

This recipe works for: Women's Health, Stress, Brain Boosting, Recovery
Makes 6 brunch servings: Use a non-stick skillet.

Whisk in a bowl: 12 Eggs, 1/2 tsp. Salt, 1/2 tsp. Lemon-Pepper.

Heat 3 TBS Canola Oil over medium-high heat. Add eggs. Using wooden spoon, stir until eggs are almost set, about 5 minutes. Gently fold in 6-oz. Thinly Sliced Smoked Salmon, cut into 1/2-inch wide strips. Stir just until eggs are set, about 1 minute. Transfer eggs to platter. Dot hot eggs with 8-oz. well-chilled Low Fat Cream Cheese, cut in small cubes. Sprinkle with Snipped Fresh Chives.

PARTY ARTICHOKE QUICHE

This recipe works for: Arthritis, Liver and Organ Health, Female Balance
Preheat oven to 325°F.

Make a simple crust: mix 1 $^1/_4$ cups Unbleached Flour with 2 TBS Canola Oil, 2 TBS Butter, and 1 Egg until crumbly. Press into a quiche pan and bake at 350°F for 5 to 8 minutes. Remove and cool.

—Grate your choice of Low Fat Cheeses onto the crust to one-inch thickness. Slice 1 large (11-oz.) jar of water packed Artichokes and arrange on top of the cheeses.

—Sauté in 2 TBS Butter, 1 teasp. Dijon Mustard, 6 sliced Mushrooms and 2 sliced Scallions. Layer on top of artichokes.

—Make the sauce in the blender: 3 Eggs, $^1/_2$ cup Low Fat Cream Cheese, $^1/_4$ cup Water, 2 TBS Sherry and $^1/_2$ teasp. Chinese 5-Spice Powder. Pour over quiche. Lightly sprinkle with nutmeg and bake until firm. Serve warm.

MARVELOUS MUFFINS Everybody loves these party muffins.

This recipe works for: Men's and Kid's Health, Sports Nutrition
For 18 melt-in-your-mouth muffins: Preheat oven to 375°F.

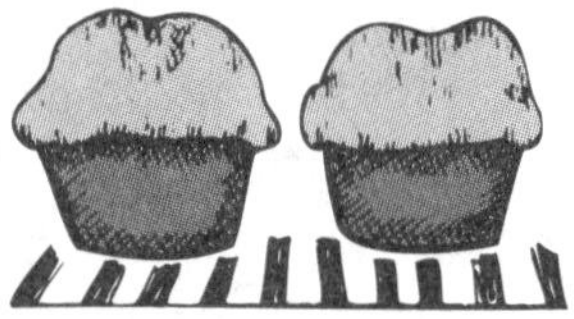

In a food processor, grate into a large bowl: 2 large Carrots and 1 large Fuji Apple. Mix in $^3/_4$ cup shredded Coconut, $^1/_2$ cup chopped Pecans, $^1/_2$ cup chopped Dates, 3 Eggs, $^3/_4$ cup Canola Oil and $^1/_2$ teasp. Vanilla.

—Add dry ingredients, mixing gently after each addition: 1 cup Whole Wheat Pastry Flour, 1 cup Unbleached Flour, 1 cup Turbinado Sugar, $^1/_4$ cup Maple Sugar Granules, 1 teasp. Baking Powder, 1 teasp. Baking Soda, 1 teasp. Cinnamon and 1 teasp. Nutmeg. Spoon into Canola Oil sprayed muffin cups or paper lined muffin cups, and bake for 18-20 minutes until a toothpick comes out clean. Cool.

Nutrition; 248 calories; 3gm protein; 29gm carbo.; 2gm fiber; 13gm total fats; 35mg choles.; 47mg calcium; 2mg iron; 27mg magnesium; 188mg potassium; 109mg sodium; Vit. A 242 IU; Vit. C 2mg; Vit. E 4 IU.

LEMON POPPYSEED DESSERT BREAD

This recipe works for: Men's and Kid's Health, Sports Nutrition
For 2 loaves: Preheat oven to 350°F. Use 2 Canola Oil sprayed loaf pans.

Stir together dry ingredients: 4 cups Unbleached Flour, $^1/_2$ cup Oat Flour, 1 TB Baking Powder, 1 teasp. Sea Salt and $^1/_2$ cup Poppy Seeds. Mix wet ingredients: 5 Eggs, 1 cup Canola Oil, $^1/_2$ cup Turbinado Sugar, $^1/_4$ cup Maple Sugar Granules, $^1/_2$ cup Honey, 1 cup Plain Rice Milk, 3 TBS grated Lemon Zest. Mix both ingredients together. Turn into loaf pans and bake for 40 minutes until a toothpick comes out clean.

FANCY COUSCOUS RING WITH GOLDEN PEPPER SAUCE

This recipe works for: Cancer Protection, Weight Control, Illness Recovery
Serves 6 to 8: Use an Olive Oil sprayed ring mold.

Make the GOLDEN PEPPER - ONION SAUCE first. Mix in a bowl: $^1/_2$ cup diced Onion and $^1/_2$ cup Yellow Bell Pepper. Combine in a pan and bring to a boil: $^1/_4$ cup Water, $^1/_4$ cup Balsamic Vinegar, $^1/_4$ cup Olive Oil, 1 teasp. Honey and 2 dashes Hot Pepper Sauce. Let cook for 3 minutes and pour over peppers and onions. Cover and chill.

—Meanwhile, bring $2^1/_2$ to 3 cups Salted Water to a boil. Add 1 package (12-oz.) Couscous and 4 TBS Olive Oil. Cover, remove from heat and let sit 10 minutes. Fluff with a fork. Set aside.

—Drain peppers and onions. Add 1 cup finely diced Tomatoes to sauce; season with Lemon-Pepper to taste and mix into couscous. Add 1 cup Fresh Tomato Salsa (page 198). Turn into ring mold, smooth top and chill well.

—Before serving, bring 6 cups Water to boil with 1 teasp. Herbal Seasoning Salt. Add 1 cup diced Broccoli and blanch 2 minutes until color changes. Remove with a slotted spoon. Add 1 cup diced Cauliflower and blanch 7 minutes, remove with slotted spoon. Add 1 cup diced Red Onion; cook for 5 minutes to crunchy tender.

—Unmold couscous ring onto a plate; fill with broccoli, cauliflower and onion.

Nutrition; 281 calories; 5gm protein; 32gm carbo.; 3gm fiber; 12gm total fats; 0 choles.; 73mg calcium; 1mg iron; 21mg magnesium; 266mg potassium; 144mg sodium; Vit. A 100 IU; Vit. C 43mg; Vit. E 3 IU.

NO-SUGAR FRUIT CAKE with HONEY GLAZED FRUITS

This recipe works for: Sugar Imbalances, Allergies and Asthma
For 24 small slices: Preheat oven to 325°F. Use a Canola Oil sprayed loaf pan.

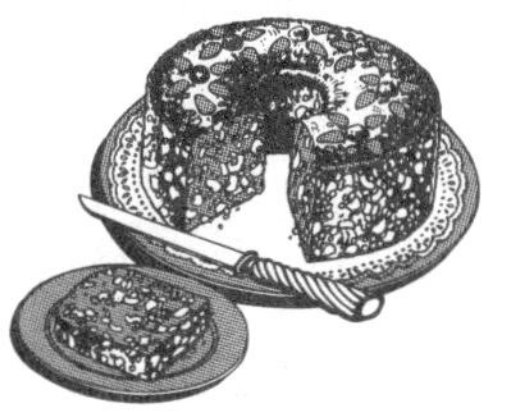

Simmer in a large pot for about 15 minutes: $^1/_2$ cup Water, $^1/_2$ cup any Fruit Juice, $^1/_2$ cup Maple Sugar Granules, $^1/_2$ cup Honey, $^1/_2$ cup Butter, 1 TB Maple Syrup. Remove from heat and add 1 cup Whole Wheat Pastry Flour, 1 cup Unbleached Flour, $^3/_4$ cup chopped Dates, $^1/_2$ cup chopped Walnuts, 1 teasp. Baking Soda, 1 cup Raisins, 1 teasp. Sweet Tooth Baking Spice (pg. 487) and 2 TBS Port Wine. Turn into loaf pan and bake until firm.

—Remove, cool, invert onto a serving plate covered with greenery.

—Make the HONEY GLAZED FRUITS: Bring 1 cup Honey and $^1/_2$ cup Water or Sweet Sherry to a boil until syrupy. Mix in 4 cups diced Dried Mixed Fruits, $^1/_2$ cup shredded Coconut, $^1/_2$ cup Walnuts Halves, and $^1/_2$ cup sliced Almonds. Cook in syrup until tender.

—Remove the fruits and nuts with a slotted spoon and top the cake. Or cut the cake in half lengthwise. Fill it, and then top it with the fruits. Chill before slicing.

Nutrition; 305 calories; 4gm protein; 57gm carbo.; 3gm fiber; 9gm total fats; 10mg choles.; 36mg calcium; 1mg iron; 38mg magnesium; 365mg potassium; 59mg sodium; Vit. A 52 IU; Vit. C 3mg; Vit. E 2 IU.

SUNDAY SQUASH

This recipe works for: Skin and Hair, Men's Health, Illness Recovery
For 6 - 8 servings: Preheat oven to 350°F.

Slice 2-lbs. Yellow Crookneck Squash in rounds. Sauté in 1 TB Butter with 1 small Sweet Yellow Onion until fragrant, about 5 minutes.

—Blend squash and onions in the blender with 4 TBS Butter, 1 Egg, 4 TBS Kefir Cheese or Low Fat Cream Cheese, $^1/_2$ teasp. Sea Salt. Pour in a mixing bowl and add 1 cup grated Low Fat Cheddar Cheese and $^1/_2$ cup crumbled Cornbread. Turn into a shallow casserole and top with grated Parmesan Cheese and crumbled Cornbread. Bake for 20 minutes until steaming. Serve hot.

TRIPLE GINGER CHEESECAKE

This recipe works for: Overcoming Addictions, Heart Health
Serves 8: Preheat oven to 350°F. Make in a Canola Oil sprayed springform pan.

Make the crust: heat 1 cup crushed Gingersnaps, 3 TBS Butter and 6 TBS minced Honey Crystallized Ginger until bubbly and fragrant. Press into bottom and slightly up the sides of springform pan; bake 10 minutes. Remove and cool.

—Make the filling: blend 2 cartons (8-oz.) Low Fat Cream Cheese, 4 TBS Maple Sugar Granules, 4 TBS Orange Marmalade, 2 Eggs, 2 TBS Orange Juice and 1 TB grated Ginger. Turn into pan and bake for 25 minutes.

—Mix the topping: 1 cup Low Fat Cream Cheese, $^1/_2$ cup Kefir Cheese or Low Fat Sour Cream, 4 TBS Maple Sugar and 3 TBS minced Crystallized Ginger. Spread over hot cheesecake; return cake to oven and turn off heat. Let sugars melt; remove, cool and chill.

SWEET INDULGENCE

Healthy Holiday Desserts

Every one of these recipes is very low in fat sugar and calories. Enjoy holiday desserts while you guard your health.

HOLIDAY CRANBERRY MOUSSE

This recipe works for: Weight Control, Liver Health, Women's Health
For 4 to 6 servings:

Blender blend smooth: $^1/_2$ cup Low Fat Cream Cheese, 2 TBS Rosé Wine, 2 TBS Honey, 1 8-oz. jar Sugar Free Cranberry Preserves, $^1/_4$ teasp. Cinnamon, $^1/_4$ teasp. Nutmeg. Beat 4 Egg Whites to stiff peaks, and fold into the cheese/wine mix. Spoon into parfait glasses or mousse cups and chill overnight.

AMBROSIA CHEESECAKE

This recipe works for: Sugar Imbalances, Liver Health, Women's Health
For 16 small rich servings: Preheat oven to 350°F. Use a springform pan.

Combine 2 cups Sugarless Graham Crackers and 4 TBS melted Butter and pat onto the bottom and part of the sides of a Canola Oil sprayed pan. Chill until ready to fill.

—Blender blend the filling: 4-oz. Low Fat Cream Cheese, 1 carton (8-oz.) Kefir Cheese, 3 Eggs, 1/2 cup Honey, 2 teasp. Orange Juice, 1 teasp. Lemon Juice and 1 teasp. grated Lemon Zest. Pour into shell, and bake for 20 minutes only. Remove from the oven and cool for 10 minutes while you make the topping.

—Blender blend the topping: 1 cup Plain Yogurt, 2 TBS Honey, 1 teasp. Vanilla, 1 TB Lemon Juice and 1 teasp. grated Lemon Zest. Pour over cheesecake and bake for 10 to 15 more minutes. Remove, cool and chill until ready to serve. Decorate with drained Mandarin Orange slices if desired.

CARROT RAISIN SPICE CAKE

This recipe works for: Sugar Imbalances, Anti-Aging, Digestive Health
Serves 12: Preheat oven to 350°F. Use a Canola Oil sprayed 9" springform pan.

Mix together: 1 1/2 cups Unbleached Flour, 1/2 cup Whole Wheat Pastry Flour, 1 teasp. Baking Powder, 1 teasp. Baking Soda, 1/2 teasp. Sea Salt, 2 teasp. Cinnamon, 1/2 teasp. Nutmeg, 1/2 teasp. Ginger Powder, 1/2 teasp. Ground Cloves. In another bowl, soak 3/4 cup Raisins in 1/2 cup Orange Juice until they plump. Then add 7 TBS Canola Oil, 1 cup Maple Syrup, 1/2 cup Vanilla Rice Milk (or Vanilla Almond Milk), 2 TBS grated Orange Zest and 2 cups shredded Carrots.

—Gently mix both sets of ingredients. Batter will be stiff. Spread into springform pan and bake for 35 to 40 minutes, until sides shrink from pan and a toothpick comes out clean. Cool in pan then remove sides. Lightly brush top of warm cake several times with a mixture of 6 TBS Maple Syrup, 2 TBS Orange Juice, 2 TBS Sherry, 1 TB grated Orange Zest, 1/2 tsp. Vanilla and 1/2 tsp. Cinnamon. Cool before cutting.

EASY HOLIDAY DATE SQUARES

This recipe works for: Kid's and Men's Health, Allergy and Asthma
For 16 squares: Preheat oven to 350°F. Use a 9" Canola Oil baking pan.

Mix in a bowl: 3 Eggs, 1 cup crushed Granola, 1 cup Maple Sugar Granules, 1 cup chopped Dates, 1/4 cup Wheat Germ, 1 cup chopped Walnuts, 1 tsp. Baking Powder, 1 tsp. Vanilla and 1/4 tsp. Sea Salt. Press into pan; bake for 45 minutes. Cut in squares while warm. Press a candied fruit piece onto the top of each.

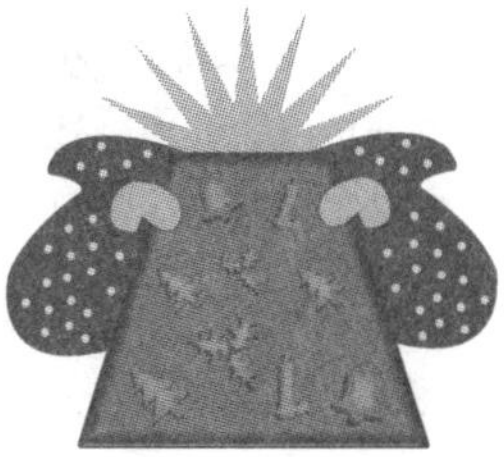

GINGER CHRISTMAS CAKE

This recipe works for: Sugar Imbalances, Heart Health, Overcoming Addictions
Serves 12: Preheat oven to 325°F. Use a Canola Oil sprayed springform pan.

Mix fruits and nuts: 1 cup diced Dates, 1 cup minced Crystallized Ginger, 1 cup diced Walnuts, $^1/_2$ cup Hazelnuts and $^1/_2$ cup Raisins. Sift on $^1/_2$ cup Whole Wheat Pastry Flour, 1 cup Unbleached Flour, $^1/_2$ tsp. Nutmeg and 1 tsp. Baking Powder. Set aside.

—With an electric mixer, beat 1 stick Butter with $^1/_2$ cup Maple Sugar Granules, 1 TB grated Orange Zest, 3 TBS Orange Juice and 1 tsp. Vanilla. Fold in fruit and flour mix.

—Turn into prepared pan, smooth top and decorate with Crystallized Ginger Cubes, Walnut Halves and Date Halves. Bake for $1^1/_4$ hours. Turn off oven and let bake for 15 more minutes. Remove and let stand for 15 minutes. Poke 6 to 8 holes all the way through the cake with a skewer and drizzle in Sherry. Wrap cake in cheesecloth, then in foil; store in an airtight container for several days before serving for best results.

APPLE PIE with RAISIN COOKIE CRUST

This recipe works for: Stress and Exhaustion, Liver Health, Waste Management
Serves 10: Preheat oven to 350°F. Make in a Canola Oil sprayed pie pan.

Make the cookie crust: heat $1^1/_2$ cups crushed Oatmeal Raisin Cookies, 3 TBS Butter, 1 Egg and $^1/_4$ cup Applesauce 5 minutes. Press into bottom and up the sides of the pan; bake 10 minutes. Remove and cool.

—Make the filling: in a pan heat 6 to 8 peeled, sliced Fuji Apples, $^1/_2$ cup Maple Sugar Granules, $^1/_2$ cup Apple Juice, 2 teasp. Cinnamon and 2 teasp. Vanilla. Mix 1 TB Arrowroot Powder with $^1/_4$ cup Apple Juice and stir about 4 minutes. Turn into baked crust; set pie on baking sheet to catch drips and bake for 10 more minutes.

CRANBERRY PUDDING CAKE

This recipe works for: Bladder-Kidney Health, Bone Building, Women's Health
For one 9" square pan: Makes 9 servings. Preheat oven to 325°F.

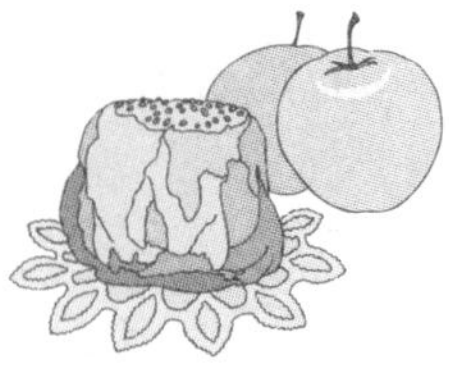

Sprinkle the bottom of a Canola Oil sprayed baking pan with $^1/_2$ cup Turbinado Sugar, 2 cups Cranberries and $^1/_2$ cup chopped Walnuts. Put in the oven to melt for 10 minutes. Remove and cool for filling.

—Beat together: 2 Eggs, $^1/_2$ cup Whole Wheat Pastry Flour, $^1/_2$ cup Honey and 3 TBS Canola Oil. Pour over berries and shake to settle. Bake until top is golden and springs back when touched, about 45 minutes to 1 hour. Serve hot or cold.

Nutrition; 219 calories; 4gm protein; 31gm carbo.; 2gm fiber; 9gm total fats; 47mg choles.; 22mg calcium; 1mg iron; 28mg magnesium; 131mg potassium; 19mg sodium; Vit. A 24 IU; Vit. C 4mg; Vit. E 2 IU.

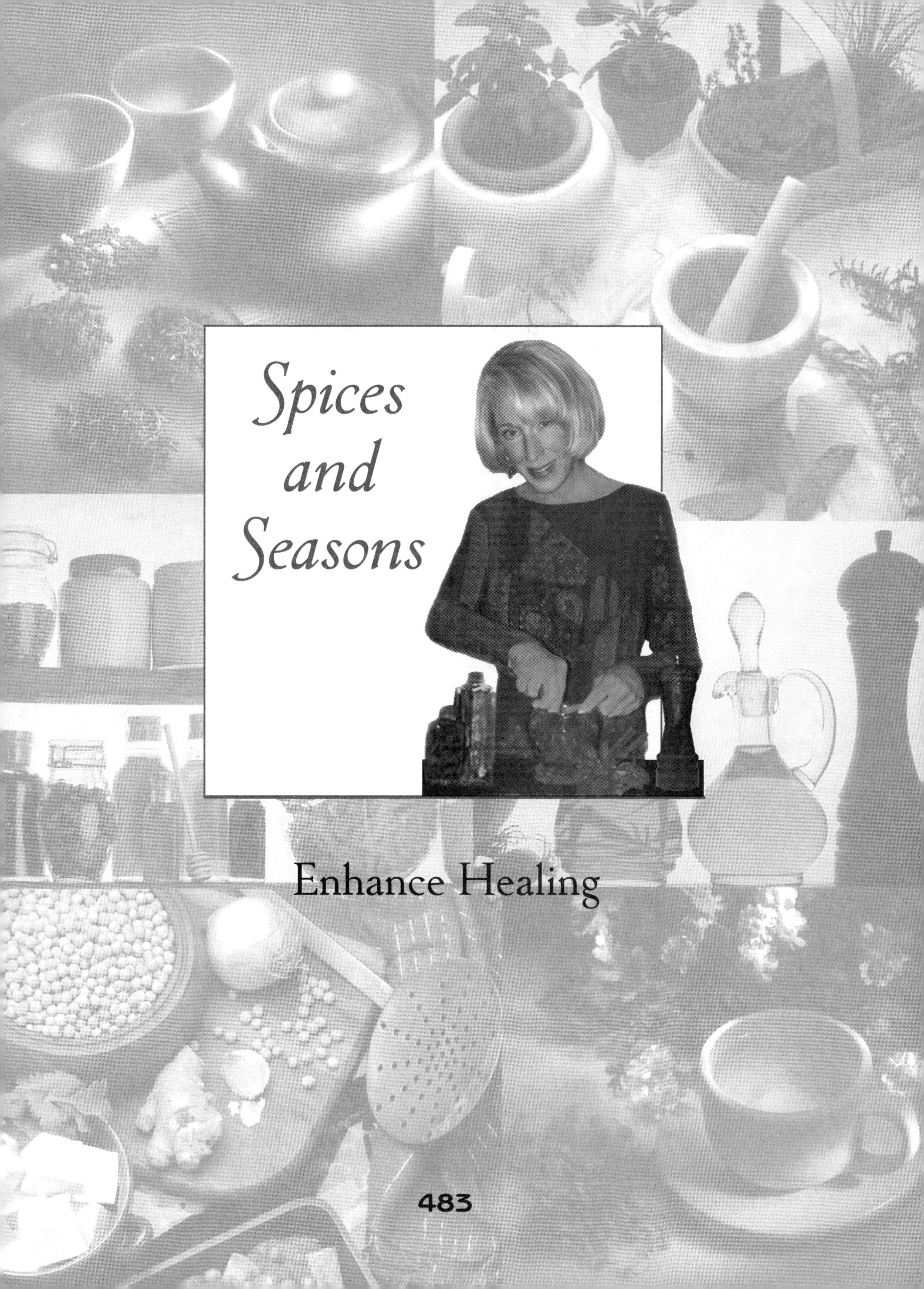

Spices and Seasons

Enhance Healing

Make Your Food Sing!

Healing Spices and Seasonings

Make your own kind of music with food.

Seasoning defines the character of a recipe. When we remember a delicious dish, we remember the flavor instead of the contents. Spices and herbs contain fragrant volatile oils, whose scents not only trigger memories, but also stimulate, calm, or revive us. I call spices "aromatherapy that you can eat."

Spices contradict the general opinion that what tastes good can't be good for you. Most spices contain powerful antioxidants and other phytochemicals that aid digestion, lower cholesterol and high blood sugar, reduce inflammation, stimulate glands and organs, even fight cancer.... healing benefits that come directly from highly complex compounds in the spice oils.

America's grocery shelves are awash in convenience foods loaded with chemicals to prolong shelf life, boost taste buds and enhance food appearance. None of the chemicals have a role in nutrition; many play a detrimental role in health. Making your own seasonings and condiments assures you of the highest quality ingredients tailored to your healthy diet, with no hidden additives.

For example, pre-prepared foods are usually full of salt. America's tastebuds have become over-tolerant of salt... more and more has to be added to stimulate our taste, so many of us consume too much table salt for good body balance. Restricted circulation, water retention, even chronic migraines are involved with salt balance in the body. Heart problems, high blood pressure and hypertension are regularly a result of excessive salt. Salt substitutes from herbs and spices can help normalize body fluid salinity, and restore intestinal tone, healthy glands and organs.

Seasonings and Condiments Recipe Sections

Herbal Salts and Seasonings

Get good salts from foods like tamari, shoyu, miso, umeboshi plums, sauerkraut and other fermented foods, and herbs rich in potassium and iodine like sea greens; these are all foods with enzyme properties that make the salts usable.

Herbal salts and seasonings can play a healthy part in an ongoing balanced diet. Use them as they are here, or experiment and create your own, starting with these recipes as a basis. They will definitely make a difference to your cooking.

Amounts given here are small enough for a container you can handle easily in the kitchen, but large enough so you don't have to make them up very often.

Natural Seasoning Tips for Enhancing Your Cooking:

1: Toast nuts, seeds and grains to bring out their full flavor. Dry roast grains in the cooking pot before adding water or stock. Toast nuts and seeds in a 400° oven on baking sheets until golden brown.

2: Use grated fresh lemon or lime zest to bring out food flavor. Rub the peel against a hand grater, or peel with a vegetable peeler and sliver. Squeeze a little fresh lemon juice (or balsamic vinegar) over a dish just at serving to heighten flavor.

3: Use fresh herbs when you can. Chop and stir them in at the last minute for the most intense taste. Use a mortar and pestle when pounding herbs and spices for the most flavor.

4: Begin a sauté with the strongest seasonings of a recipe. Add them to a dry heated pan, or with the oil, and sauté for a few minutes until their fragrance is released. Then continue with your recipe. This one little change will make a big difference in the robustness of a recipe's flavor.

FRESH LEMON-PEPPER

There is a noticeable taste difference between this and other lemon pepper you may have used. The secret is in the lemon oil. Just a few drops from a small bottle of essential pharmaceutical grade lemon oil..... inexpensive, well worth the investment.

Whirl ingredients in the blender briefly for consistency and flavor: 1-oz. Sea Salt, $2^1/_2$-oz. Coarse Grind Black Pepper, 2 TBS Sesame Seeds, 2 TBS Soy Nuts, 2 teasp. Lemon Peel Powder, 2 teasp. dry Parsley Flakes, $^1/_4$ teasp. Stevia Powder, $^1/_2$ teasp. Garlic Powder, $^1/_2$ teasp. Onion Powder and drops of Lemon Oil to taste. Store tightly covered.

SEA VEGGIE SUPREME

Both a flavor enhancer and a nutritional part of your recipe. Crumble into a bowl, then just whirl briefly in the blender into a coarse grind. Dry sea veggies expand with the liquid in your recipe. Use freely as a salt substitute on salads, soups, rice, anything.

Blend $^3/_4$ cup snipped dried Dulse, $^1/_4$ cup chopped dry Wakame, $^1/_4$ cup chopped dry Kombu, $^1/_4$ cup chopped Nori or Sea Palm, $^1/_2$ cup White Sesame Seeds.

SESAME SALT DELIGHT

A delicious way to wean yourself away from salt, and never miss the salty taste. Very high in nutrients. Store covered in the fridge.

Stir 1 cup Brown Sesame Seeds, 1 cup Black Sesame Seeds and $^1/_2$ cup chopped Walnuts in a heavy dry skillet on low heat until seeds pop. Add 1-oz. snipped Dry Dulse, 1 TB Sea Salt, 1 teasp. snipped dry Sea Palm, and 1 teasp. granulated Kelp. Stir, heating until aromatic. Turn into a blender or seed mill and grind.

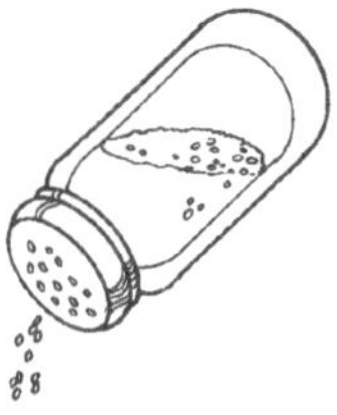

ZEST SEASONING SALT

A bold, smoky seasoning salt, good in soups, potatoes, grills of all kinds. Buy many of the ingredients in bulk from your health food store.

Whirl ingredients in the blender to granular consistency: $^1/_4$ cup Sea Salt, 2 teasp. Dry Basil, 1 TB Soy Bacon Bits, 1 TB Smoky Flavor Nutritional Yeast, 1 TB Onion Granules, 1 TB Dry Chopped Chives, 1 TB Dry Parsley Flakes, 1 TB Diced Dry Tomato, 1 teasp. Dry Grated Lemon Peel, 1 teasp. Garlic Granules, $^1/_2$ teasp. Oregano, $^1/_2$ teasp. Savory, $^1/_2$ teasp. Horseradish Powder, $^1/_2$ teasp. Black Pepper, $^1/_2$ teasp. Paprika.

ASIAN COOKING SPICE

A good base seasoning for stir-fries, in baking, or sprinkle on steamed veggies.

Whirl in a blender: 2 TBS minced Ginger, 1$^1/_2$ TB Star Anise, 1 tsp. Fennel Seed, $^1/_2$ tsp. Ground Cardamom, $^1/_2$ tsp. Cinnamon, $^1/_2$ tsp. Oriental Mustard Powder, $^1/_4$ tsp. Cloves, $^1/_4$ tsp. Paprika, $^1/_4$ tsp. Black Pepper, $^1/_4$ tsp. Orange Peel Powder, $^1/_8$ tsp. Stevia Powder.

SPICY ITALIAN HERBS

Store airtight for long lasting flavor.

Stir together in a bowl: 3 TBS Dry Basil, 1$^1/_2$ TBS Oregano, 1 TB dry crushed Rosemary, 1 TB Dry Parsley, 1 teasp. Garlic Powder, $^1/_2$ teasp. Fennel Seed, $^1/_2$ teasp. Rubbed Sage, $^1/_2$ teasp. Marjoram

GARLIC LEMON SESAME SEASON

A very popular universal, healthy seasoning. Excellent in a sauté in place of chopped garlic for aroma, adds a complex flavor to Italian and European cooking.

Whirl in a blender until aromatic: 6-oz. TOASTED WHITE SESAME SEEDS, 2-oz. BROWN SESAME SEEDS, $^1/_4$ cup dry PARSLEY FLAKES, 2-oz. DRIED CHOPPED ONION, 2 TBS dry BASIL, 2 tsp. minced GINGER, 2 tsp. GARLIC GRANULES, 2 tsp. DRY GRATED LEMON PEEL, 1 tsp. PAPRIKA, $^1/_2$ tsp. TARRAGON, $^1/_2$ tsp. CELERY SEED, drops LEMON OIL to taste, $^1/_8$ tsp. STEVIA POWDER.

SALTERNATIVE HERB SALT

Herbs only, no salt at all, this blend relies instead on dried sea vegetables for its "saltiness." It is delicious, particularly tasty for healing recipes.

Whirl in the blender to sprinkling consistency: 2 TBS KELP GRANULES, 2 TBS DRY WAKAME FLAKES, 2 TBS DRY DULSE FLAKES, 2 TBS ONION GRANULES, 2 TBS BASIL, 1 TB GARLIC GRANULES, 1 teasp. DRY DILL WEED, $^1/_2$ teasp. DRY CHOPPED CHIVES, $^1/_2$ teasp. THYME, $^1/_2$ teasp. CELERY SEED, $^1/_2$ teasp. MARJORAM, $^1/_2$ teasp. PAPAYA LEAF.

GREAT 28 MIX Try it; you'll love this popular seasoning blend.

A delicious seasoning; mix with kefir cheese or cream cheese as a dip, sauté it in butter as the base of a soup or sauce, flavor broth to cook grains; mix with mayonnaise for a sandwich spread, with yogurt, or oil and vinegar as a salad dressing.

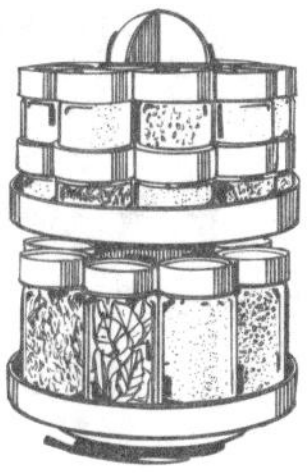

Whirl in a blender: 3 TBS chopped TOASTED WALNUTS, 3 TBS DRY ONION GRANULES, 3 TBS TOASTED SESAME SEEDS, 2 TBS DRY CHOPPED TOMATOES, 2 TBS DRY CHOPPED MUSHROOMS, 2 TBS SOY BACON BITS, 2 TBS NUTRITIONAL YEAST FLAKES, $1^1/_2$ TBS DULSE GRANULES, 1 TB KELP GRANULES, 1 TB MISO SOUP POWDER, 1 TB DRY BASIL, 1 TB DRY PARSLEY FLAKES, 1 TB DRY CHOPPED CHIVES, 1 TB CHILI POWDER, 1 teasp. dry GRATED LEMON PEEL, 1 teasp. CELERY SEED, 1 teasp. BLACK PEPPER, $^1/_2$ teasp. GARLIC GRANULES, $^1/_2$ teasp. DRY GRATED ORANGE PEEL, $^1/_2$ teasp. OREGANO, $^1/_2$ teasp. PAPRIKA, $^1/_2$ teasp. DRY DILLWEED, $^1/_2$ teasp. SAGE, $^1/_2$ teasp. ROSE HIPS, $^1/_2$ teasp. TARRAGON, $^1/_2$ teasp. CURRY POWDER, $^1/_2$ teasp. SAVORY, $^1/_4$ teasp. STEVIA POWDER.

SWEET TOOTH BAKING MIX Just right for spicing sweet baked things.

A great "convenience mix" to save time and proportion measuring.

Measure into a jar. Cover and shake: 4 TBS CINNAMON, 2 TBS NUTMEG, $1^1/_2$ teasp. GINGER POWDER, 2 teasp. GROUND CLOVES, 1 teasp. ORANGE PEEL POWDER, 1 teasp. LEMON PEEL POWDER, 1 teasp. ALLSPICE and 1 teasp. MACE

HEALING SALAD HERBS Store airtight.

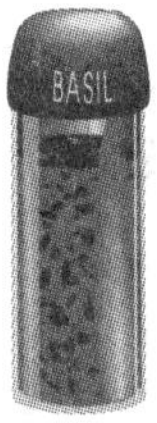

Mix 3 TBS Dry Basil, 2 TBS Toasted Sesame Seeds, 1 TB Dry Thyme, 1 1/2 TB Dry Parsley, 1 tsp. Garlic Granules, 1 TB Dry Dill, 2 tsp. Dry Mint, 1 tsp. Marjoram, 1/2 tsp. Tarragon, 1/2 tsp. Chervil, 1/2 tsp. Celery Seed, 1/2 tsp. snipped Dulse.

GREEK SESAME SEASONING

Recall those fabulous memories of the Greek islands and pungent Greek cooking. Try it on fresh Mediterranean foods... roma tomatoes, dark greens, sautéed zucchini.

Measure into a jar. Cover and shake to blend: 3 TBS Sea Salt, 2 TBS Toasted White Sesame Seeds, 2 TBS Brown Sesame Seeds, 2 TBS Black Sesame Seeds, 2 TBS Toasted Walnuts, 1 TB Oregano, 1/2 TB Basil, 1 TB Onion Powder, 1/2 teasp. Garlic Powder, 1/2 teasp. Paprika, 1 TB Dry Grated Lemon Peel, 1/4 teasp. Stevia Powder, drops of Lemon Oil to taste.

HOT CHILI SPICE

The proportions are just right for spicy Mexican dishes.

Whirl in the blender til fragrant: 3 TBS Cornmeal, 3 TBS Chili Pepper Flakes, 3 TBS Chili Powder, 2 TBS Onion Powder, 1 TB Dried Chopped Bell Pepper, 2 teasp. Sea Salt, 1 teasp. Cumin Powder, 1/2 teasp. Dry Minced Garlic, 1/2 teasp. Cayenne, 1/2 teasp. Oregano.

SPICY SALT for VEGGIES Especially good for macrobiotic dishes.

In a skillet, stir for 3 minutes: 1 TB Sea Salt, and 1 teasp. each- White Sesame Seeds, Black Sesame Seeds, Chopped Almonds, and 1/2 teasp. each- Cumin Seeds, Coriander Seed, Coarse Black Pepper and Mustard Seed. Whirl in the blender if desired to a powder.

HEALING CURRY POWDER

Did you know that curry is thought to have begun its life as a medicinal? A remedy for swelling and inflammation, a natural antibiotic, a healer for a congested liver, a digestive tonic, curry has these and many more healing properties. Curry is also effective for increased calorie burning after a meal, a good aid to a weight loss diet.

In a dry skillet, cook for 5 minutes: 2 TBS Coriander Seed, 2 TBS Cumin Seed, 1 TB Caraway Seed, 2 teasp. Mustard Seed, 2 teasp. Fennel Seed, 2 teasp. Anise Seed, 1/2 teasp. Fenugreek Seed, 1/4 teasp. Cardamom Seed, 1/4 teasp. Whole Cloves, 2 pinches Chili Powder, 1 pinch Stevia Powder, 1 pinch Black Pepper, 1 pinch Cinnamon. Remove from heat. Stir in 2 TBS Turmeric Powder. Blender blend to a powder.

Custom Diet Flour and Grain Blends

A mix of flour grains lends lightness, taste interest, and more health benefits.

LIGHT, NUTTY FLOUR MIX

Mix 3 cups UNBLEACHED FLOUR, $1^1/_2$ cups WHOLE WHEAT PASTRY FLOUR, $^1/_2$ cup OAT FLOUR, $^1/_2$ cup BARLEY FLOUR.

HIGH NUTRIENT GRAINS

Versatile, healthy, non-fattening, high fiber. Buy the ingredients at your health food store.

Mix in a large bowl: 2 cups BROWN RICE, $1^1/_2$ cups WINTER WHEAT BERRIES, $1^1/_4$ cups WHOLE RYE BERRIES, 1 cup BUCKWHEAT BERRIES, 1 cup OAT GROATS (uncut oats), 1 cup PEARL BARLEY, 1 cup MILLET, 1 cup TRITICALE, 1 cup WHITE SESAME SEEDS.

—To cook: dry roast 1 cup of the grains in a pot over medium heat until fragrant, about 5 minutes. Add 2 cups boiling water. Let bubble for a minute. Cover and reduce heat. Steam for about 25 minutes until water is absorbed.

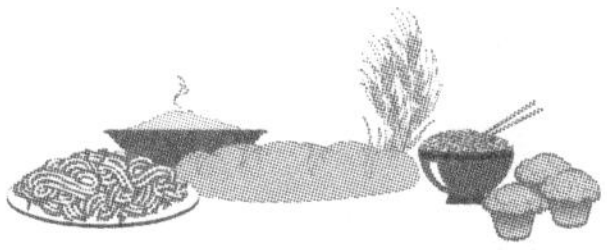

Naturally Cultured Condiments

Commercial condiments are one of the worst offenders for adding chemicals, preservatives and colorings. It's easy to make your own fresh natural condiments.

HOMEMADE MAYONNAISE

It only takes a minute to make, and the taste difference from commercial brands is amazing. Add variations like an AVOCADO or a SCALLION, or 2 TBS PARMESAN CHEESE.

Blender blend: 1 EGG, 1 teasp. DIJON MUSTARD, 1 TB LEMON JUICE, 1 TB TARRAGON VINEGAR, 1 TB HONEY, $^1/_2$ teasp. SEA SALT. Whirl briefly, and with the motor running, add 1 cup CANOLA OIL in a thin steady stream until mayonnaise thickens to consistency.

QUICK HONEY KETCHUP

Easy to make, with a fresh no-salt taste.

Whirl in the blender until smooth and thick: 1 cup pureed PLUM TOMATOES, 1 chopped GREEN ONION, $^1/_4$ cup CANOLA OIL, 2 TBS HONEY, 1 TB minced ONION, 1 TB LEMON JUICE and pinches of BASIL, OREGANO, TARRAGON and THYME to taste.

AMAZINGLY DELICIOUS KETCHUP Store in glass jars. Freeze extra.

Make this in a large pot and cook slowly, all day if necessary, until ketchup consistency is reached. It is a sweet, spicy, complex condiment that needs a long cooking time for flavors to meld. Make it when the tomato harvest is in, and freeze in pint jars for later use. The recipe makes 5 pints.

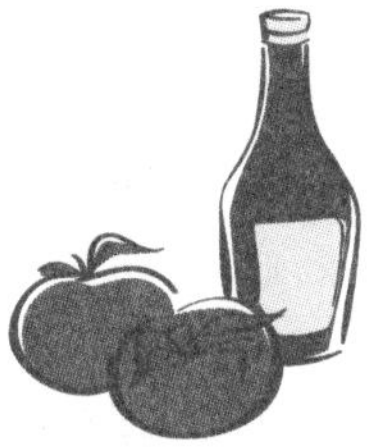

Sizzle in 4 TBS Olive Oil until very brown: 1-lb. Onions, $^1/_2$ cup Maple Sugar Granules, 2 teasp. Dry Mustard, $^1/_2$ teasp. Hot Pepper Sauce. Add and bring to a simmer: 1 diced Tart Apple, 2 diced Red Bell Peppers, 2 diced Ribs Celery, 7-lbs. peeled chopped Plum Tomatoes, $^1/_4$ cup Molasses, 1 teasp. Cinnamon, $^1/_2$ cup Raspberry Vinegar, $^1/_2$ cup Rosé Wine and 4 teasp. Sea Salt. Add seasonings: $^1/_2$ teasp. Ground Cloves, $^1/_4$ teasp. Allspice, $^1/_4$ teasp. Nutmeg. Simmer slowly, partially covered until thick.

SWEET and SOUR MUSTARD Makes 4 cups; stores beautifully.

Mix and let stand for 1 hour: $1^1/_3$ cups Champagne Vinegar, $1^1/_3$ cups Dry Mustard (4-oz.). Add 6 Eggs, 1 cup Honey, $^1/_4$ cup Maple Sugar Granules and $^3/_4$ cup Turbinado Sugar; whisk until smooth. Pour into a saucepan; heat and stir until thickened and bubbling, about 10 minutes. Remove from heat and pour into jars. Cool and chill.

QUICK and EASY SALSA Make your tacos fast.

Chunky chop in a food processor: 4 Tomatoes, 4 to 6 Green Onions, 1 Clove Garlic, 1 can (4-oz.) Diced Green Chilies, $^1/_2$ teasp. Chili Powder, 4 Sprigs Cilantro Leaves.

CHILI-LIME SALSA

Peel and dice 2 Plum Tomatoes and 1 Cucumber. Mix in a bowl with 2 TBS minced Fresh Jalapeño Chilies, $^1/_4$ cup Red Onion, the diced meat of 1 Lime, $^1/_2$ teasp. Balsamic Vinegar and 2 TBS Lime Juice.

SUMMER HARVEST RELISH Makes 8 cups; stores well.

Roast, blacken and peel 1 large Red Bell Pepper under a broiler, or use 1 jarred Red Bell Pepper. Peel, seed and chop pepper. Whisk in a bowl, $^1/_4$ cup Brown Rice Vinegar, 3 TBS Maple Syrup, $2^1/_2$ teasp. Hot Pepper Sauce, $1^1/_2$ teasp. Turmeric, $^1/_2$ teasp. Ground Cumin and 1 teasp. Sea Salt. Whisk in 4 TBS Teriyaki Sauce and 2 packages (16-oz.) Frozen Corn, thawed and drained. Stir in Red Pepper and $^1/_2$ cup minced Red Onion.

SAUERKRAUT A premier cultured healing food.

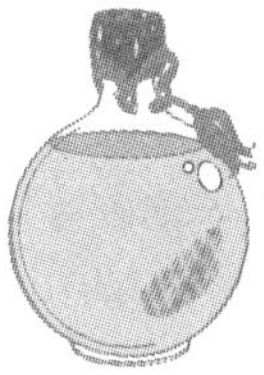

Rinse and drain 2 cups bottled sauerkraut in a colander to remove excess salt. Sizzle in a skillet: 1 TB Olive Oil, 1/2 Red Onion and 2 minced Cloves Garlic for 5 minutes. Add sauerkraut, 1 1/4 cups Johannisberg Riesling Wine, 1/4 cup Balsamic Vinegar, 6 Dry Juniper Berries, and Cracked Pepper to taste. Simmer 30 minutes; serve chilled.

HOT PINEAPPLE DAIKON RELISH Makes about 1 1/2 cups.

Mix in a bowl: 1/2 cup diced FRESH Pineapple, 2 TBS diced Lime, 1 TB minced Ginger, 1 TB Dry Mustard mixed in 1 TB Water, 2 teasp. Horseradish and 1/2 teasp. Sesame Salt. Add 4-oz. peeled, shredded Fresh Daikon Radish. Cover and chill.

LEMON PEEL RELISH For 2 cups: Excellent with chicken and fish.

Peel yellow skin from 6 Lemons. Mince the peel, trim pith from lemons and remove seeds. Cut 2 of the lemons in chunks. (Save other 4 lemons for another use.)

—Sauté 1/2 cup minced Onion in 1 TB Canola Oil until limp but not brown, about 7 minutes. Add the lemon and the lemon peel, 1/2 cup White Wine, 4 TBS Fructose and 1 teasp. White Pepper. Stir until most of the liquid is evaporated and mixture is syrupy, about 15 minutes. Let cool. Cover and chill.

CRANBERRY GINGER RELISH For about 3 cups

Cut 2 large Tangerines or Mandarin Oranges in chunks. Whirl briefly in the blender with 1/4 cup minced Crystallized Ginger, 12-oz. Cranberries and 1/3 cup Fructose. Chill.

SUGAR-FREE APPLE GINGER CHUTNEY For about 6 cups.

Peel 4 Oranges and 1 Lemon, leaving white pith intact. Mince peel in a food processor. Remove pith and seeds from oranges and lemon and dice. Put minced peel and diced fruit in a large pot. Add 4 cored and diced Granny Smith Apples, 1 diced large Red Onion, 4 minced Cloves Garlic, 1/4 cup minced Crystallized Ginger, 1 cup Raisins, 1 1/2 cups Apple Cider Vinegar, 1 can (6-oz.) Frozen Orange Juice Concentrate, 1 can (6-oz.) Frozen Apple Juice Concentrate and 2 TBS Curry Powder. Bring to a boil, then reduce heat and simmer for 90 minutes until thickened stirring occasionally. Pour into 3 pint jars. Cover tightly.

GOLDEN HARVEST PICKLES

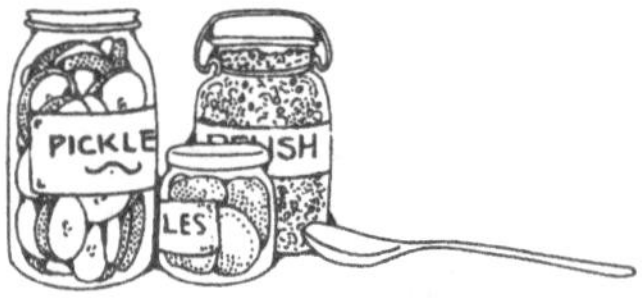

In a pot, simmer for 5 minutes: 4 cups Water with $^{1}/_{2}$ cup Apple Cider Vinegar, 3 TBS Sea Salt, 1 TB minced Garlic, 2 teasp. Turmeric, 2 teasp. Cumin Seeds, 2 teasp. Fennel Seeds and 1 minced, seeded Chipotle Chili.

—Cut 8 cups veggies like Cauliflower, Carrots, Green Beans, Pearl Onions, Radishes, Baby Turnips or Cucumbers into shapes. Layer attractively in 1 qt. glass jars. Divide contents of brine pot between jars. Cover and chill for 3 days before serving.

LEMON CUCUMBER PICKLES

Slice 7 or 8 Lemon Cucumbers in rounds and place in a colander. Sprinkle with Sea Salt and let drain 1 hour.

—In a saucepan, combine 1 cup Tarragon Vinegar, 1 cup Water, 4 TBS Fructose, 1 teasp. Stevia Powder, 1 teasp. Sea Salt, 1 teasp. Mustard Seed, $^{1}/_{2}$ tsp. Celery Seed, $^{1}/_{2}$ teasp. Turmeric and 1 pinch Cinnamon. Bring to a simmer; taste. Add more sweetener or vinegar if needed. Remove from heat. Rinse and add cucumbers. Sprinkle with pinches of Dill Weed. Let stand until cool; then cover and chill 2 days befor serving.

Healthy Sauces and Dressings

Sauces and dressings can make or break a recipe. Usually they're loaded with fat and calories, so they can make or break your diet, too. Here are some healthy ones:

MUSTARD-HERB SAUCE

Sizzle 6 TBS Olive Oil, 1 minced Clove Garlic, 1 minced Shallot and 1 minced Scallion for 3 minutes. Remove from heat and add 3 TBS White Wine Vinegar, 2 TBS Dijon Mustard, 2 teasp. minced Fresh Tarragon Leaves ($^{3}/_{4}$ teasp. dry) and Lemon-Pepper to taste. Spoon onto steamed veggies, chicken or fish.

TROPICAL GRILLING SAUCE for SALMON Enough for 8 people.

Toss together: 1 cup diced FRESH Pineapple, 1 diced, peeled Papaya, 4 diced Nectarines, 2 diced peeled Tomatoes, 6 snipped Scallions, 1 minced seeded Jalapeño Pepper, 2 TBS Lemon Juice, $^{2}/_{3}$ cup Olive Oil, $^{1}/_{3}$ cup White Wine and 1 TB Honey. Brush on salmon during grilling. Serve on the side.

LOW FAT ROASTED RED PEPPER SAUCE For 2 cups.

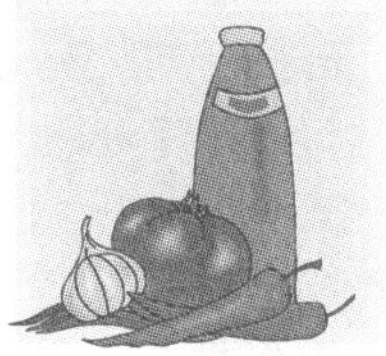

Sliver 4 jarred Roasted Red Bell Peppers. Pour 1 TB oil from the jar into a skillet. Heat and sizzle $^1/_2$ cup diced Onion, 2 minced Cloves Garlic and $^1/_2$ cup White Wine for 20 minutes until onion is tender. Turn mixture into a blender; add $^1/_2$ cup Organic Low Fat Chicken Broth. Puree, return mixture to skillet; simmer, stirring for 15 minutes. Add red peppers and 1 tsp. Herbs de Provence. Season with Cracked Pepper.

GINGER PECAN SAUCE Great for veggie kebabs.

Pulse 1 cup Pecans in a food processor until they're chunky. Set aside.

—In a saucepan, sizzle 1 TB Toasted Sesame Oil, 3 minced Scallions, 2 minced Cloves Garlic and 1 minced TB Crystallized Ginger for 1 minute. Stir in pecans, 4 TBS Tamari, 4 TBS Shredded Coconut, $^1/_4$ cup Rice Milk and 2 to 4 shakes Hot Pepper Sauce. Simmer for 30 minutes until thickened. Add 2 TBS Sherry and spoon on veggies.

FUJI APPLESAUCE with RAISINS For about 6 cups.

Core and chop 6 Fuji Apples. Put in a heavy pan on the lowest possible heat. Add 1 cup Water and 1 cup Apple Juice. Partially cover and simmer slowly until apples begin to soften. Add 1 cup Honey (or $^1/_2$ cup Honey and $^1/_2$ cup Maple Syrup), and 2 teasp. Sweet Tooth Baking Mix (page 487). Cook until soft and fragrant. Remove from heat; puree in the blender. Add 2 TBS Lemon Juice and $^1/_2$ teasp. Sea Salt to intensify flavor. Stir in $1^1/_2$ cups Raisins.

ETHIOPIAN DRESSING Great for respiratory problems.

Whisk together: $^1/_2$ cup Lemon Juice, 3 minced Cloves Garlic, a 1-inch piece Ginger, shredded, 1 tsp. Paprika, $^1/_2$ tsp. Hot Pepper Sauce, 1 tsp. Cumin Seed, 1 tsp. Anise Seed, $^1/_2$ cup snipped Fresh Parsley, $^1/_3$ cup snipped Fresh Cilantro, 2 TBS snipped Fresh Mint, $^3/_4$ cup Olive Oil, 1 TB Sesame Seeds, $^1/_2$ tsp. Sea Salt, $^1/_2$ tsp. Cracked Pepper.

BASIL-MISO DRESSING Immune enhancing.

Blender blend: $^1/_4$ cup diced Red Onion, $1^1/_2$ cups packed <u>fresh</u> Basil Leaves, 4 TBS Plain Yogurt, 4 TBS Olive Oil, 4 TBS Brown Rice Vinegar, 1 TB Orange Honey (or $^1/_4$ teasp. Stevia Powder), 2 teasp. Chickpea Miso, 1 teasp. Dijon Mustard, 1 teasp. Italian Blend Herbs. Add Water or White Wine to make a good consistency if too thick.

ORANGE-SESAME DRESSING
Skin beautifying. For $^3/_4$ cup.

Whisk together: 2 TBS Light Miso, 3 TBS Toasted Sesame Seeds, 1 TB Hot Water, 1 TB Sherry or Sake, $^1/_4$ cup Orange Juice, $1^1/_4$ TB Canola Oil, 2 TBS Brown Rice Vinegar, 2 teasp. Fructose (or $^1/_4$ teasp. Stevia Powder), 2 teasp. Tamari and 1 teasp. minced Crystallized Ginger.

CHIPOTLE CHILI SAUCE
Great for salmon, veggies, or potato salad.

Soak 1 or 2 dry Chipotle Chilies in water for 10 minutes; drain, puree in the blender. Whisk together: 2 TBS Raspberry Vinegar, 4 TBS Lime Juice, 1 teasp. Dijon Mustard, the pureed chilies, 1 minced Clove Garlic, 1 teasp. Sea Salt, $^1/_2$ cup Olive Oil.

YOGURT DIPPING SAUCE
Good for raw veggies, pitas, olives, more.

Make the YOGURT CHEESE: Set a strainer lined with cheesecloth over a large bowl. Let cheesecloth drape over sides of bowl. Dump in 4 cups Plain Yogurt, fold cheesecloth completely over yogurt. Chill overnight. Yogurt whey will drain out and yogurt cheese will remain in strainer.

—Place cheese into a bowl and stir in 2 TBS Olive Oil, $^1/_2$ teasp. Turmeric, $^1/_2$ teasp. Sea Salt, $^1/_4$ teasp. Ground Cumin, $^1/_8$ teasp. Marjoram, $^1/_8$ teasp. Cayenne Pepper.

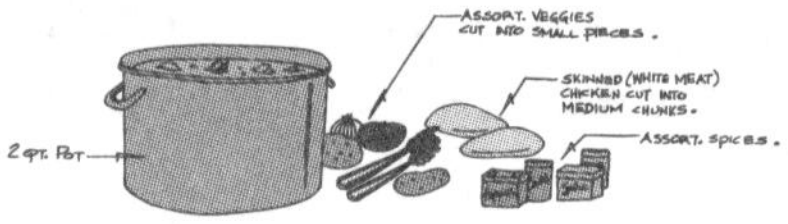

Broths, Broth Powders and Marinades

The broth is the essence of a soup or sauce. Fresh homemade broths have the best flavor and healing qualities. Canned boths are often over-salted, or full of chemical enhancers. Broths freeze nicely - even in ice cube trays, so you can make up a large batch, and use a little or a lot at a time. When making a purifying soup for a healing diet, shred the greens and veggies beforehand, and heat the broth just long enough for the vegetables to become tender crisp.

RICH BROWN BROTH
A hearty soup and broth. Makes about 8 cups.

Sizzle 4 sliced Red Onions in 2 TBS Butter and 2 TBS Olive Oil in a large soup pot until very brown and aromatic. Add 1 cup Red Wine, 6 cups Water and 3 TBS Miso Paste; bring to a boil. Simmer to concentrate flavors, and add snipped Fresh Parsley and snipped Chives. Strain if using as a stock.

SAVORY ONION-VEGGIE BROTH Makes about 6 cups.

Sauté in a large soup pot 5 minutes until aromatic: 2 TBS Olive Oil, 4 cups chopped Yellow Onions, 1 TB Sea Salt, 1 teasp. Dry Basil, $^1/_2$ teasp. Oregano, $^1/_2$ teasp. Dry Thyme, $^1/_2$ teasp. Rosemary, $^1/_2$ teasp. Dry Sage and $^1/_2$ teasp. Pepper.

—Add 1 cup mixed chopped Celery, Carrots and Greens, and $^1/_4$ cup snipped Fresh Parsley; toss 5 minutes. Add 1-qt. Water; cover and simmer 30 minutes. Strain if using as a stock.

V-8 VEGETABLE BROTH Makes about 8 cups

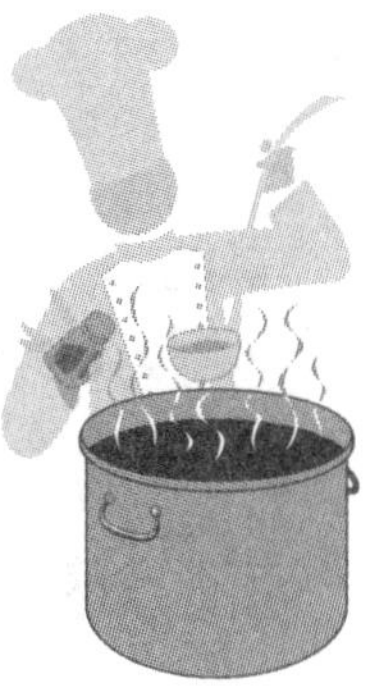

Sauté in a large soup pot 5 minutes until aromatic: 2 TBS Olive Oil, $^1/_4$ cup chopped Garlic, $^1/_2$ cup chopped Yellow Onions. Add 1 teasp. Sea Salt, $^1/_2$ cup chopped Carrots, $^1/_2$ cup chopped Celery, $^1/_2$ cup chopped Turnips, $^1/_2$ cup chopped Spinach, $^1/_2$ cup chopped Green Onions and $^3/_4$ cup chopped Tomatoes. Sizzle 10 minutes.

—Add 4 cups Water, $^3/_4$ cup Tomato Juice, 2 TBS snipped Parsley, 2 TBS snipped Fresh Basil (1 tsp. dry), 1 TB Nutritional Red Star Yeast, $^1/_2$ tsp. Savory, $^1/_2$ tsp. Oregano and $1^1/_2$ cups Miso Soup. Partially cover and let simmer until aromatic, about 30 minutes. Use this broth as a soup or strain and use as a base for a soup or sauce

ROASTED VEGGIE BROTH Intense flavor. Preheat oven to 425°F.

In a large roasting pan, toss with 3 TBS Olive Oil and 3 TBS Balsamic Vinegar: 2 Whole Heads Garlic, cloves peeled and chopped, 1-lb. sliced Red Onions, 1-lb. sliced Yellow Onions, 1-lb. chopped Carrots, 1-lb. chopped Acorn Squash, 1-lb. chopped Potatoes, 1 chopped Daikon White Radish, 4 chopped Baby Turnips and 1 cup Crystallized Ginger Chunks. Roast, stirring occasionally for 30 minutes.

—Turn into a large soup pot; add 4-qts. Water, bring to a boil, reduce heat and simmer gently for 1 hour. Press broth liquid out through a strainer. Discard solids.

GINGER BROTH Boosts circulation and energy right away. About 9 cups.

Sauté in a large soup pot 5 minutes until aromatic: 2 TBS Olive Oil, $^1/_4$ cup chopped Garlic and 2 cups chopped Yellow Onions. Add 1-lb. chopped Carrots, 4 TBS shredded Ginger Root and 4 TBS chopped Crystallized Ginger.

—Add 2-qts Water and 1-qt. Roasted Veggie Broth (above). Add Sea Salt and Pepper to taste, and snipped Fresh Herbs, like Parsley, Basil, Sage and Thyme. Strain broth through a sieve or cheesecloth and discard solids.

RICH BROWN BROTH A hearty soup and broth. Makes about 8 cups.

Sizzle 4 sliced Red Onions in 2 TBS Butter and 2 TBS Olive Oil in a large soup pot until very brown and aromatic. Add 1 cup Red Wine, 6 cups Water and 3 TBS Miso Paste; bring to a boil. Simmer to concentrate flavors, and add snipped Fresh Parsley and snipped Chives. Strain if using as a stock.

SPICY VEGETABLE BROTH MIX A dry soup mix to make and store.

Whirl briefly in the blender so there are still recognizable chunks: $^1/_4$ cup Dry Onion Flakes, 4 TBS chopped Dried Tomatoes, 3 TBS Soy Nuts, 3 TBS chopped Dried Carrots, 2 TBS chopped Dried Mushrooms, 2 TBS Nutritional Red Star Yeast Flakes, 1 TB Tamari Powder or Miso Powder, 1 TB Soy Bacon Bits, $^1/_2$ teasp. Celery Seed, $^1/_2$ teasp. Chili Powder, $^1/_2$ teasp. Italian Blend Herbs, $^1/_2$ teasp. Garlic-Lemon Seasoning (page 487).

—For a quick delicious broth, sauté 2 teasp. Mix in 2 teasp. Butter til fragrant. Add $1^1/_2$ cups Water and $^1/_2$ cup White Wine; simmer for 10 minutes.

HERBAL BROTH POWDER Boost digestibility of any dish.

Mix in a large batch: 1 cup Dry Basil, $^1/_3$ cup Dry Thyme, $^1/_4$ cup Garlic Granules, $^1/_4$ cup Dry Parsley Flakes, $^1/_3$ cup Dry Dulse Flakes, 2 TBS Dry Marjoram, 3 TBS Dry Oregano and $^3/_4$ cup Toasted Sesame Seeds. Store tightly covered and use as desired.

HIGH SIERRA RANCH MIX Make fresh dressing whenever you want it.

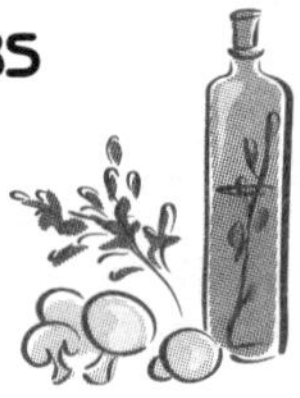

Make the mix: $^3/_4$ cup Dry Onion Flakes, $^1/_4$ cup dry Parsley Flakes, 2 TBS Chia Seeds, 2 TBS Poppy Seeds, 2 TBS Garlic Powder, 2 TBS Sea Salt, 2 TBS Lemon-Pepper, 2 TBS Onion Powder, $^1/_8$ teasp. Cayenne.

—To make a ranch dressing, mix in a bowl: $1^1/_4$ cup dry HIGH SIERRA MIX, 2 TBS Lemon Juice, 1 cup Low Fat or Lemon Mayonnaise, $^1/_2$ cup Plain Yogurt and $^1/_2$ cup Water.

—To make up a ranch vinaigrette dressing, whisk in a bowl: $^1/_4$ cup dry HIGH SIERRA MIX, $^1/_2$ cup Olive Oil, $^1/_4$ cup Lemon Juice. Chill for pasta salads or greens.

SESAME MARINADE For about $^1/_2$ cup.

Shake in a jar to blend: 2 TBS Tamari, 2 TBS Toasted Sesame Seeds, 2 TBS Brown Sesame Oil, 1 TB Brown Rice Vinegar, $^1/_2$ teasp. Black Pepper, $^1/_4$ teasp. Hot Pepper Sauce $^1/_2$ teasp. Sesame Salt.

SWEET CAESAR MARINADE For $1^1/_2$ cups:

Whirl briefly in the blender: $^1/_4$ cup Lemon Juice, $^1/_4$ cup Balsamic Vinegar, 3 TBS Romano Cheese, 2 TBS Water, 1 TB Tomato Paste, 2 TBS White Wine, 1 teasp. Fructose or Honey, $^1/_2$ teasp. Lemon-Garlic Seasoning, $^1/_4$ teasp. Black Pepper. Add $^3/_4$ cup Olive Oil slowly in a steady stream while blending until thickened. Chill to blend flavors.

TERIYAKI MARINADE Especially good for grilled seafood and poultry.

Whisk together: 1 TB shredded Ginger, 2 minced Cloves Garlic, 3 snipped Green Onions, 4 TBS Tamari, 4 TBS Sherry, 1 TB Toasted Sesame Oil, 1 TB Olive Oil, 2 TBS Honey, $^1/_4$ teasp. Cinnamon, $^1/_4$ teasp. Black Pepper.

HERB GARDEN MARINADE For chicken, tofu or seafood.

Whisk together: $^1/_4$ cup Lemon Juice, $^1/_4$ cup Tarragon Vinegar, 2 minced Cloves Garlic, 3 minced Shallots, 2 TBS Olive Oil, 2 seeded, minced Jalapeño Peppers, $^1/_2$ cup mixed minced Fresh Herbs (Basil, Dill, Rosemary, Tarragon, Oregano), $^1/_2$ teasp. Sea Salt, $^1/_4$ teasp. Black Pepper.

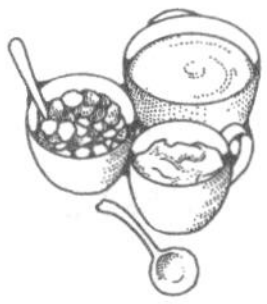

Healthy Pestos and Butter Spreads

Intense flavors... a little goes a long way. Pestos and butters freeze well in ice cube trays. Just pop out as much as needed.

SWEET WINE BUTTER Especially good for thick fish like Salmon or Ahi.

Heat briefly in a pan: $^1/_2$ cup Gewertztraminer or Sauterne Wine, 1 teasp. White Wine Vinegar, 1 minced Shallot, 2 TBS Butter, 2 TBS minced Fresh Herbs like Basil, Savory and Marjoram and $^1/_4$ teasp. Lemon-Pepper. Stir in until glossy $^1/_8$ teasp. Arrowroot Powder mixed in 1 teasp. Water.

ROSEMARY BUTTER Good for Swordfish, Salmon or Ahi and poultry.

Cream 2 sticks soft Butter with 1 TB snipped Fresh Rosemary, 1 minced Shallot, 1 minced Clove Garlic, and 2 TBS snipped Fresh Parsley. Store in a crock; use as needed.

BASIL PESTO For $1^1/_2$ cups.

Whirl in the blender: 2 cups packed Fresh Basil Leaves (or Cilantro Leaves for a new taste), 1 cup grated Parmesan Cheese, $^1/_2$ to $^2/_3$ cups Olive Oil, 1 teasp. Garlic Granules.

BASIL LEMON BUTTER Particularly good on steamed vegetables.

Cream 2 sticks soft Butter with $^1/_3$ cup minced Fresh Basil, 1 teasp. Lemon-Garlic Seasoning, and 1 TB Lemon Juice. Store in a crock and use as needed.

FRESH HERB PESTO

Whirl in the blender: $^1/_2$ cup Fresh Basil, $^1/_2$ cup Cilantro, 3 TBS Fresh Oregano, 3 TBS Fresh Thyme, 1 TB Fresh Rosemary, 1 TB Fresh Mint, 4 TBS chopped Walnuts, 2 TBS Chickpea Miso, Lemon-Pepper to taste. With motor running, drizzle in 4 TBS Olive Oil.

HOT PEPPER PESTO

Whirl in the blender: $^1/_2$ cup packed Fresh Basil Leaves, $^1/_2$ cup packed Cilantro Leaves, $^1/_4$ cup chopped, seeded Red Serrano Chilies, 2 TBS Lime Juice, 2 TBS Water, $^1/_4$ cup Olive Oil, $1^1/_2$ TBS minced Garlic, 1 teasp. Sea Salt and 1 teasp. Ground Cumin.

BASIL-TOMATO BUTTER

Whirl in a blender: $^1/_4$ cup drained Dried Tomatoes packed in oil, 2 sticks soft Butter and 1 TB Fresh Basil, 1 teasp. Lemon-Garlic Seasoning, and 1 teasp. Cracked Pepper.

LEMON BUTTER

Cream 1 stick soft Butter with $^1/_4$ cup minced Green Onions, 2 TBS Lemon Juice, 1 teasp. Thyme, 1 teasp. grated Lemon Zest and $^1/_2$ teasp. Lemon-Garlic Seasoning.

CHILI-GARLIC BUTTER Great on grilled Corn or Potatoes.

Cream 2 sticks soft Butter with $^1/_3$ cup minced Fresh Cilantro, 1 minced, seeded Jalapeño Chili, 1 teasp. Garlic Salt.

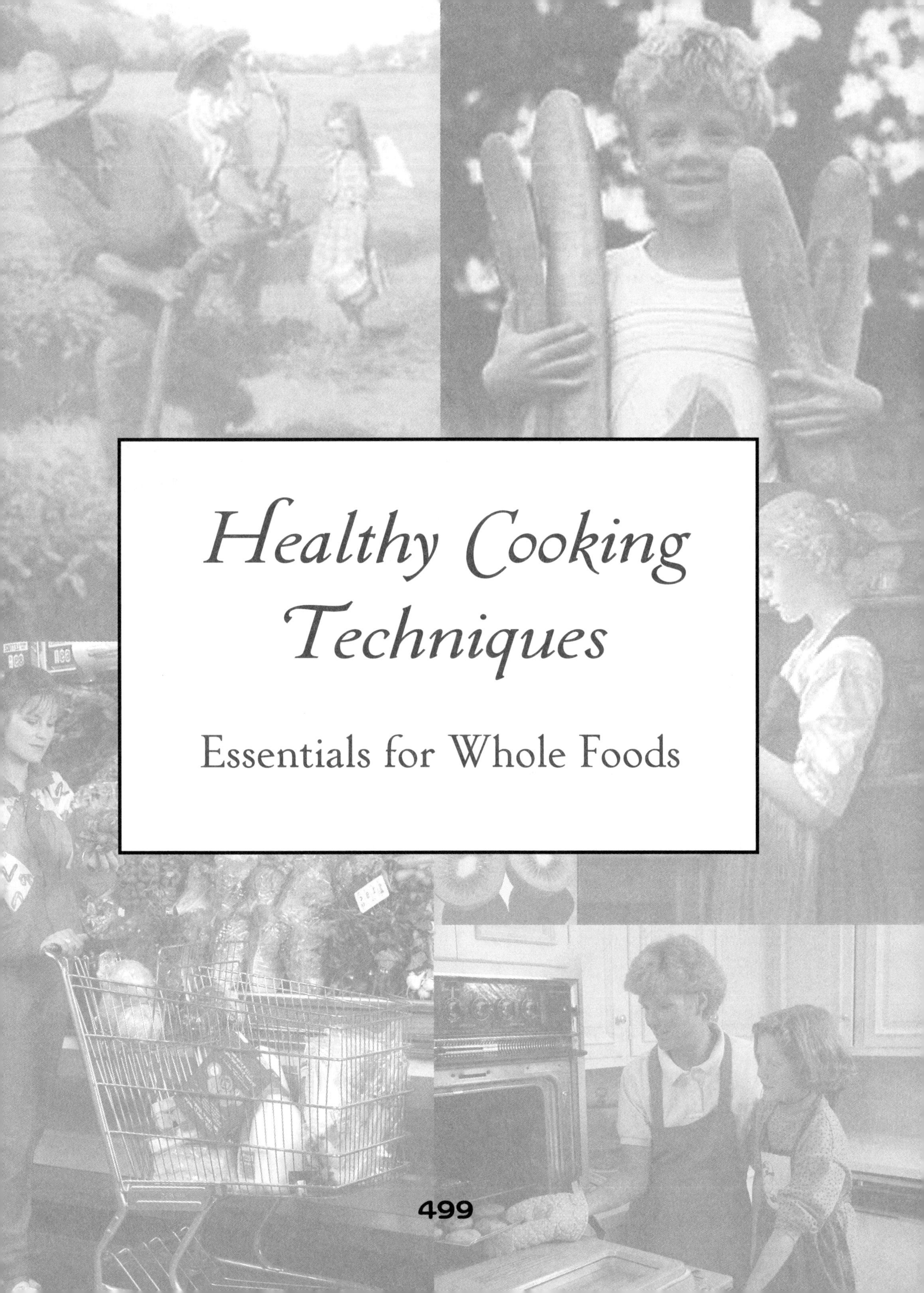

Healthy Cooking Techniques

Essentials for Whole Foods

Cooking Techniques and Essentials with Whole Foods

**Sometimes it isn't just what you eat.....
the way you cook it can mean success for a healing diet.
This section includes the best methods for getting the optimum nutrition
and healing benefits from your food.**

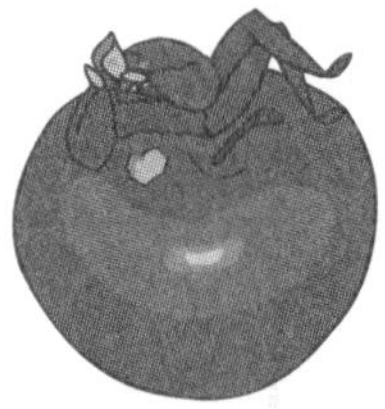

Healthy Techniques with Vegetables:

–When steaming vegetables, always have water boiling first. Add 1 teasp. Miso paste, or a few liquid smoke drops to the water for an outdoor grill taste if desired, then add the veggies.

–Parboil vegetables in seasoned water or a light broth for crunchiness, color and flavor. Simmer liquid first, add veggies and just simmer until color changes. (Save cooking liquid for use in the recipe.) Drain immediately, run under cold water to set color, then chill for a salad, or toss in a hot pan with a little butter, broth or tamari to heat through. Squeeze a little lemon juice over for tang.

–Concentrate flavors of zucchini, tomatoes and eggplant by sprinkling with sesame or herb salt. Let sit in a colander over the sink for 10 to 15 minutes, then press out moisture. It makes a real difference in the sweetness of the vegetables.

–Dry salad greens thoroughly after washing by rolling them in paper towels, or by using a salad spinner. The greens will be crisper, and need less dressing for taste.

–Invest in a food processor. It makes your salad ingredients look and taste elegant. Today these appliances are smaller, easy to clean, and encourage you to have a salad every day.

–When stir-fry/steaming, heat the wok first; then add oil, and heat to very hot. Then add veggies and stir-fry fast to seal in nutrients. Turn heat to low, add sauce, cover, and steam til sauce bubbles.

–Are you juicing carrots and apples in your healing diet? Use the carrot and apple pulp from juicing in place of grated apples or carrots in baked recipes, like muffins or quick breads. You can even use the pulps in place of all or part of the sugar or honey in other baked dishes.

–Some foods release more of their nutrients when lightly cooked: Lightly steaming carrots releases bio-available carotenes (cancer preventing substances) better. Simmering tomatoes enhances lycopene activity, a cancer protective. Heating spinach leaves until just wilted improves its carotene assimilation.

Healthy Techniques with Poultry:

–Have poultry at room temperature before cooking. Pat meat dry.

–Oven roast poultry bones and carcasses to enhance flavor richness. Then freeze in plastic bags to use for making homemade broth.

–When baking stuffings or cornbread separately for a roast turkey or chicken dinner, use a cast iron skillet for increased flavor and texture.

Healthy Techniques for Eggs:

–The secret for lightness in soufflés, dumplings, crepes, and omelets is simply gentleness. Work with a light hand when you work with eggs - no vigorous stirring or beating.

–When beating eggs to "stiff but not dry," always add a pinch of cream of tartar to maintain lightness and puff.

–Poach eggs in a light miso or chicken broth, or bouillon instead of water for better flavor and to maintain shape.

Healthy Techniques with Pasta:

–Mushy, or tough pasta can ruin a meal. Attention is the key once pasta cooking has started. I like to make the pasta sauce first if possible. Just keep it warm til pasta is ready.

–Use a very large pot; probably the largest one you have. Use a lot of water, so pasta can swim and separate when cooking. The more water, the less gummy the pasta. Add 1 TB Olive Oil or Canola Oil so water won't boil over and pasta strands will separate after cooking. Bring water to a rolling boil. Add 1 tsp. Sea Salt to lift pasta flavor. Your sauce is ready by this point.

–Add pasta in batches to the water slowly, so water doesn't stop boiling. Stir after each batch to keep pasta separated. Keep the water at a fast boil, covering it briefly to insure continuous boiling.

–Fresh pasta cooks very fast, in 2 to 6 minutes. Watch it closely, and start testing for doneness in 2 or 3 minutes. Dry pasta cooks in about 8 to 20 minutes, depending on its size and shape. Start testing for doneness at about 6 to 7 minutes. Remove a strand or piece with a fork and bite into it. If it isn't still hard, and it isn't mushy, it's al dente (to the tooth) and it's done.

–Drain immediately, adding a little cold water to the pot first to stop the cooking. Draining into a colander is the easiest way. Do not rinse unless pasta is to be used for a cold salad.

–Add sauce right away and serve. If sauce can't be added right away, toss with a little oil. (To re-heat pasta before saucing, put it in a bowl of hot water, and stir to let pieces gently separate.)

The Healthy Way to Use Oils: *(Never deep-fat fry when you are on a healing program.)*
–Use only vegetable, nut or seed oils, mechanically, expeller, or cold pressed.

–Use oils for quick sautées, salad dressings, and as a replacement for butter in baking and sauces.

–Don't re-use cooking oils that have been heated.

–Store all cooking oils in the refrigerator after they have been opened.

Healthy Crusts, Toppings, and Coatings:
Crusts, toppings, sprinkles and coatings are an important part of a recipe. The foundation should be as healthy as the filling. A quiche, pie, or casserole is a layered dish, to be built from the bottom up. (See index for individual crust and topping recipes).

Low-fat, thin crusts for pizzas, quiches, and vegetable tarts:
–Use crushed, whole grain cracker crumbs, either plain, or sprinkled with a little low oil dressing or tamari. Bake until crispy - about 10 minutes at 375° - then fill.

–Split chapatis or pita bread halves horizontally, or use whole wheat or corn tortillas. Toast briefly for crispiness; lay on the bottom of your baking dish and top with filling.

–Thin-slice tofu blocks horizontally. Bake with a little oil at 350° for firmness before filling.

–Spread crispy Chinese noodles on the bottom of the baking dish. Toast in the oven; then fill.

–Sprinkle toasted nuts and seeds to cover bottom of the baking dish. Add seasoning salt and fill.

–Spread cooked brown rice to cover the bottom and sides of a lecithin-sprayed baking dish. Toast at 375° to crisp and dry slightly, then fill.

–For the ultimate easy crust, use any cooked whole grain or vegetable leftovers, and whirl in the blender to a paste. Press into a lecithin-sprayed baking dish, crisp in a 400° oven for 10 minutes, and voila! you have an original, easy crust for a new quiche, casserole, or savory pie.

Low-fat crusts for dessert pies, tarts and custards: (See page 489 for a light flour mix if you wish to make a conventional crust. Whole grains produce a lighter, slightly nutty pastry.)

–Toast wheat germ in the oven. Mix with a little date sugar or honey to sweeten, and spread on bottom and sides of baking dish. Toast again briefly and fill.

—Use toasted nuts and seeds, ground and sweetened with a little date sugar or honey. Spread on the bottom and sides of baking dish. Toast again briefly for crunch, and fill.

• Use juice-sweetened, sugarless cookie crumbs. Press onto bottom and sides of baking dish. Toast briefly and fill.

• Sprinkle date sugar (ground up dates), or maple syrup granules, or maple sugar on bottom of a custard or dessert dish. Broil briefly to caramelize; then fill and bake as usual. Yum.

Casserole foundations - a unique cooking art:

Avoid the calories and density of a crust with a casserole foundation. Quiches and casseroles become new dishes, but still give a favorite fillings something good to rest on. Cover the bottom of the baking dish with any of the following:

- Hard boiled eggs;
- Left over cooked brown rice or other whole grain;
- Spaghetti squash, cooked and briefly toasted;
- Zucchini or tomato rounds.

For both bottoms and toppings:

- Chinese-noodles, toasted;
- Whole grain granola, toasted;
- Whole grain chips, crushed slightly and toasted.

Healthy low-fat, low salt coatings for seafood, poultry and veggies:

Mix any of the following with yogurt, or egg and water; coat food and chill briefly before baking.

- Toasted wheat germ;
- Crushed whole grain chips;
- Falafal or tofu burger mix.

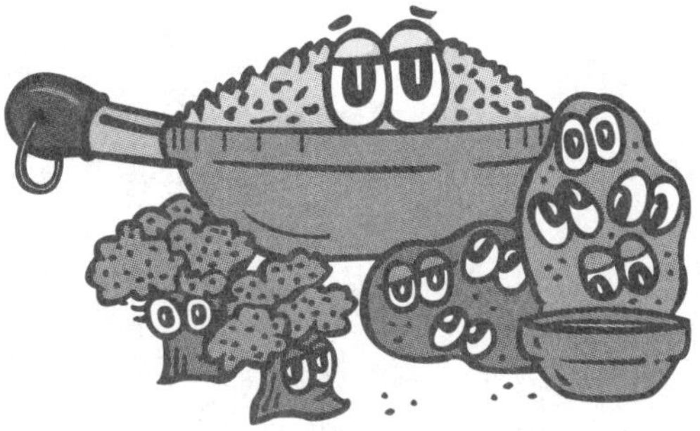

Index

Using this index..........

This extensive index maximizes your healing choices. Each recipe is listed in a number of categories that can fit in with your healing goals, as well as your meal planning needs. Two examples: 1) you want to give a party, and you're on a weight loss program that limits your fat intake and boosts your metabolism. Check out the Appetizers, Seafood, Fish and Low Fat recipe sections; 2) you're on a macrobiotic diet to curb disease progression. Check out the Macrobiotics, Rice and Grains and Vegetable recipe sections.

A

C

D

F

G

H

I

J

K

L

M

Q

U

V

X
Y
Z

Bibliography

Bon Appetit- 1999-2001

Bricklin, Mark & Sharon Claessens. *The Natural Healing Cookbook.* Rodale Press, 1981.

Calbom, Cherie & Maureen Keane. *Juicing For Life.* Trillium Health Products, 1992.

Carper, Jean. *The Food Pharmacy.* Bantam Books, 1988.

Carper, Jean. *Food: Your Miracle Medicine.* HarperCollins, 1993.

Cheraskin, E. M.D., D.M.D. et al. *Diet & Disease.* August 1987.

Cichoke, Dr. Anthony J. *The Complete Book of Enzyme Therapy.* Avery Pub., 1999.

Delicious! 1999-2001

Editors of Prevention Magazine. *The Healing Foods Cookbook.* Rodale Press, 1991.

First For Women Magazine- 1999-2001

Kirschmann, Gayla J. and John D. Kirschmann. *Nutrition Almanac.* McGraw-Hill, 1996.

Haas, Elson M., M.D. *The Detox Diet.* Celestial Arts, 1996.

Page, Linda, N.D., Ph.D. *Healthy Healing 11th Edition: A Guide To Self-Healing For Everyone.* Traditional Wisdom, Inc. 2000, 2001.

Sunset Magazine- 2000-2001

Total Health Magazine- 2000-2001

Turner, Lisa. *Meals That Heal.* Healing Arts Press, 1996.

Vegetarian Times Magazine - 1988-2001.

Whole Foods Magazine - 1989-2001.

Wittenberg, Magaret M. *Experiencing Quality: A Shopper's Guide to Whole Foods.* Whole Foods, 1981.

Product Resources

Where you can get what we recommend.....

The following list is for your convenience and assistance in obtaining further information about the products I recommend in the Cook Book Set. The list is unsolicited by the companies named. Each company has a solid history of testing and corroborative data that is invaluable to me and my staff, as well as empirical confirmation by the stores that carry these products who have shared their experiences with us. We hear from thousands of readers about the products they have used. I consider their information in every one of my books on natural health. I realize there are many other fine companies and products who are not listed here, but you can rely on the companies who are, for their high quality products and good results.

- Alacer Corp., 19631 Pauling, Foothill Ranch, CA 92610, 800-854-0249
- All One, 719 East Haley St., Santa Barbara, CA 93103, 800-235-5727
- Aloe Life International, 4822 Santa Monica Ave. #231, San Diego, CA 92107, 800-414-2563
- Alta Health Products, Inc., 1979 E. Locust Street, Pasadena, CA 91107, 626-796-1047
- America's Finest, Inc., 140 Ethel Road West, Suites S & T, Piscataway, NJ 08854, 800-350-3305
- Anabol Naturals, 1550 Mansfield Street, Santa Cruz, CA 95062, 800-426-2265
- Arise & Shine, P.O. Box 1439, Mt. Shasta, CA 96067, 800-688-2444
- Ark Naturals Products for Pets, 6166 Taylor Road #105, Naples, FL 34109, 941-592-9388
- Barleans Organic Oils, 4936 Lake Terrell Rd., Fern Dale, WA 98248, 800-445-3529
- BD Herbs, 14000 Tomki Road, Redwood Valley, CA 95470, 800-760-3739
- Beehive Botanicals, Route 8, Box 8257, Hayward, WI 54843, 800-233-4483
- BHI (Heel Inc.) 11600 Cochiti Road SE, Albuquerque, NM 33376, 800-621-7644
- Biotec Foods / BioVet, 5152 Bolsa Ave. Suite 101, Huntington Beach, CA 92649, 800-788-1084
- Bodyonics (Pinnacle), 140 Lauman Lane, Hicksville, NY 11801, 800-899-2749
- Boericke & Tafel Inc.,(B & T) 2381 Circadian Way, Santa Rosa, CA 95407, 800-876-9505
- Bragg/Live Food Products, Inc., Box 7, Santa Barbara, CA 93102, 805-968-1028
- CC Pollen Co., 3627 East Indian School Rd., Suite 209, Phoenix, AZ 85018-5126, 800-875-0096
- Champion Nutrition, 2615 Stanwell Dr., Concord, CA 94520, 800-225-4831
- Coenzyme-A Technologies Inc., 12512 Beverly Park Road B1, Lynnwood, WA 98037, 425-438-8586
- Country Life, 28300 B Industrial Blvd., Hayward, CA 94545, 800-645-5768
- Creations Garden, 25269 The Old Road, Suite B, Newhall, CA 91381, 661-254-3222
- Crystal Star Herbal Nutrition, 21602 North 21st Ave., Phoenix, AZ 85027, 800-736-6015
- Dancing Paws, 8659 Hayden Place, Culver City, CA 90232, 888-644-7297
- Dr. Diamond/Herpanacine Associates, P.O. Box 544, Ambler, PA 19002, 888-467-4200
- Dr. Goodpet, P.O. Box 4547, Inglewood, CA 90309, 800-222-9932
- EAS, 555 Corporate Circle, Golden, CO 80401, 800-923-4300
- East Park Research, Inc., 2709 Horseshoe Drive, Las Vegas, NV 89120, 800-345-8367 (orders)
- Eidon Products, 9988 Hibert St. #104, San Diego, CA 92131, 800-700-1169
- Enzymatic Therapy, Dept. L, P.O. Box 22310, Green Bay, WI 54305, 800-783-2286
- Enzymedica, 1970 Kings Hwy., Punta Gorda, FL 33980, 888-918-1118
- Earth's Bounty/Matrix Health Products, 9316 Wheatlands Road, Santee, CA 92071, 800-736-5609
- Esteem Products Ltd., 15015 Main St., Suite 204, Bellevue, WA 98007, 800-255-7631
- Ethical Nutrients/Unipro, 971 Calle Negocio, San Clemente, CA 92673, 949-366-0818
- Flint River Ranch, 1243 Columbia Avenue B-6, Riverside, CA 92507-2123, 888-722-4589
- Flora, Inc., 805 East Badger Road, P.O. Box 73, Lynden, WA 98264, 800-446-2110, 604-451-8232

- Futurebiotics, 145 Ricefield Lane, Hauppauge, NY 11788, 800-367-5433
- Gaia Herbs, Inc., 12 Lancaster County Road, Harvard, MA 01451, 800-831-7780
- Golden Pride, 1501 Northpoint Pkwy., Suite 100, West Palm Beach, FL 33407, 561-640-5700
- Green Foods Corp., 320 North Graves Ave., Oxnard, CA 93030 800-777-4430
- Green Kamut Corp., 1542 Seabright Ave., Long Beach, CA 90813, 800-452-6884
- Grifron/Maitake Products, Inc., P.O. Box 1354, Paramus, NJ 07653, 800-747-7418
- Halo-Purely For Pets, Inc. 3438 East Lake Road #14, Palm Harbor, FL 34685, 800-426-4256
- Herbal Answers, Inc., P.O. Box 1110, Saratoga Springs, New York 12866, 888-256-3367
- Health from the Sun/Arkopharma, 19 Crosby Drive, Bedford, MA 01730, 800-447-2229
- Healthy House, P.O. Box 436, Carmel Valley, CA 93924, 888-447-2939
- Heart Foods Company, Inc., 2235 East 38th Street, Minneapolis, MN 55407, 612-724-5266
- Herbal Magic, Inc., P.O. Box 70, Forest Knowlls, CA 94933, 415-488-9488
- Herbal Products & Development, P.O. Box 1084, Aptos, CA 95001, 831-688-8706
- HerbaSway Laboratories,342 Quinnipiac St., Wallingford, CT 06492, 800-672-7322
- Herbs Etc., 1340 Rufina Circle, Santa Fe, NM 87505, 505-471-6488
- Herbs For Life, P.O. Box 40082, Sarasota, FL 34278, 941-362-9255
- Highland Laboratories, P.O. Box 199 110 South Garfield, Mt. Angel, OR 97362, 888-717-4917
- Imperial Elixir, P.O. Box 970, Simi Valley, CA 93062, 800-423-5176
- Jarrow Formulas, 1824 South Robertson Blvd., Los Angeles, CA 90035, 310-204-6936
- Jones Products Int'l, Inc./ Sport Star, 4069 Wedgeway Court, Earth City, MO 63045, 800-736-6015
- Lane Labs, 25 Commerce Drive, Allendale, NJ 07401, 800-526-3005
- MagneLyfe/Encore Technology, Inc., 80 Fifth Ave., Suite 1104, New York, NY 10011, 877-624-6353
- Maine Coast Sea Vegetables, RR1 Box 78, Franklin, Maine 04634, 207-565-2907
- Maitake Products, Inc., P.O. Box 1354, Paramus, NJ 07653, 800-747-7418
- Medicine Wheel, P.O. Box 20037, Sedona, AZ 86341-0037, 800-233-0810
- M.D. Labs, 1719 W. University, Suite 187, Tempe, AZ 85281, 800-255-2690
- Mendocino Sea Vegetable Co., P.O. Box 1265, Mendocino, CA 95460, 707-937-2050
- Metabolic Response, 2633 W. Coast Hwy, Suite B, Newport Beach, CA 92663, 800-948-6296
- Mezotrace Corporation, 415 Wellington St., Winnemucca, NV 89445, 800-843-9989
- Monas Chlorella, 8815 South Decatur Blvd., Las Vegas, NV 89139, 800-275-0343
- Moon Maid Botanicals, 13870 SW 90 Ave., MM104, Miami, FL 33176, 877-253-7853
- Motherlove Herbal Co., P.O. Box 101, Laporte, CO 80535, 970-493-2892
- MRI (Medical Research Institute), 2160 Pacific Ave., Suite 61, San Francisco CA 94115, 888-448-4246
- Natren Inc., 3105 Willow Ln., Westlake Village, CA 91361, 800-992-3323
- Natural Animal Health Products, Inc., 7000 U.S. 1 North, St. Augustine, FL 32095, 800-274-7387
- Natural Balance (Pep Products), 3130 N. Commerce Ct., Castle Rock, CO 80104-8002, 303-688-6633
- Natural Energy Plus, 4630 N. Paseo De Los Cerritos, Tucson, AZ 85745, 888-633-9233
- Natural Labs Corporation (Deva Flowers), P.O. Box 20037, Sedona, AZ 86341-0037, 800-233-0810
- Nature's Apothecary, 6350 Gunpark Drive #500, Boulder, CO 80301, 800-999-7422
- Nature's Path, P.O. Box 7862, Venice, FL 34287, 800-326-5772
- Nature's Plus, 548 Broadhollow Road, Melville, NY 11747-3708, 631-293-0030
- Nature's Secret/Irwin Naturals, 10549 West Jefferson Blvd., Culver City, CA 90232, 310-253-5305
- Nature's Way, 10 Mountain Springs Parkway, Springville, UT 84663, 800-962-8873
- Nelson Bach, Wilmington Technology Park, 100 Research Dr., Wilmington, MA 01887, 800-319-9151
- New Chapter, P.O. Box 1947, Brattleboro, VT 05302, 800-543-7279
- No-Miss Nail Care 6401 E. Rogers Circle Suite 14, Boca Raton, FL 33487, 800-283-1963
- Noni of Beverly Hills, Inc., 16158 Wyancotte Street, Vans Nuys, CA 91406, 310-271-7988
- Nova Homeopathics, 5600 McLeod NE, Suite F, Albuquerque, NM 87109, 800-225-8094

- NOW, 395 S. Glen Ellyn Rd., Bloomingdale, IL 60108, 800-999-8069
- Nutramedix Inc., 212 N. Hwy One, Tequesta, FL 33469, 800-730-3130
- NutriCology /Allergy Research Group, 30806 Santana St., Hayward, CA 94544, 800-545-9960
- Omega Nutrition/Body Ecology, 6515 Aldrich Road, Bellingham, WA 98226, 404-350-8420
- Orthomolecular Specialties, P.O. Box 32232, San Jose, CA 95152-2232, 408-227-9334
- Oshadhi, 1340 G Industrial Ave., Petaluma, CA 94952, 888-674-2344
- Pines International, Inc., 992 East 1400 Road, Lawrence, KS 66044, 800-697-4637
- Planetary Formulas, P.O. Box 533 Soquel, CA 95073, 800-606-6226
- Premier Labs, 27475 Ynez Rd., Suite 305, Temecula, CA 92591, 800-887-5227
- Prime Pharmaceutical, 1535 Yonge St. Suite 200, Toronto, Ontario, Canada M4T 1Z2,800-741-6856
- PureForm, 3240 West Desert Inn Rd., Las Vegas, NV 89103, 888-363-9817
- Quantum, Inc., P.O. Box 2791, Eugene, OR 97402, 800-448-1448
- Rainbow Light, P.O. Box 600, Santa Cruz, CA 95061, 800-635-1233
- Rainforest Remedies, Box 325, Twin Lakes, WI 53181, 800-824-6396
- Real Life Research, Inc., 14631 Best Ave., Norwalk, CA 90650, 800-423-8837
- Rejuvenative Foods, P.O. Box 8464, Santa Cruz, CA 95061, 800-805-7957
- Solaray, Inc., 1104 Country Hills Dr., Suite 300, Ogden, UT 84403, 800-669-8877
- Sonne's Organic Foods, Inc., P.O.Box 2160, Cottonwood, CA 96022, 800-544-8147
- Source Naturals Inc., 23 Janis Way, Scotts Valley, CA 95066, 800-777-5677
- Spectrum Essentials, 133 Copeland St., Petaluma, CA 94952, 707-778-8900
- Springlife Inc., 4630 N. Paseo De Los Cerritos, Tucson, AZ 85745, 888-633-9233
- Sun Wellness, 4025 Spencer St. #104, Torrance, CA 90503, 800-829-2828
- Transformation Enzyme Corporation, 2900 Wilcrest, Suite 220, Houston, TX 77042, 800-777-1474
- Transitions For Health, 621 SW Alder, Suite 900, Portland, OR 97205, 800-888-6814
- Trimedica International, Inc, 1895 South Los Feliz Drive. Tempe AZ 85281-6023, 480-998-1041
- UAS Laboratories, 5610 Rowland Road, Suite 110, Minnetonka, MN 55343, 952-935-1707
- Vibrant Health, 432 Lime Rock Rd., Lakeville, CT 06039, 800-242-1835
- Vitamin Research Products, 3579 Highway 50 East, Carson City, NV 89701, 800-877-2447
- Waddell Creek Organic Bee Pollen, 654 Swanton Road, Davenport, CA 95017
- Wakunaga / Kyolic, 23501 Madero, Mission Viejo, CA 92691, 800-421-2998 / 800-825-7888
- Wisdom of the Ancients, 640 South Perry Lane, Tempe, AZ 85281, 800-899-9908
- Wyndmere Naturals, Inc., 153 Ashley Road, Hopkins, MN 55343, 800-207-8538
- Y.S. Royal Jelly and Organic Bee Farm, RT. 1, Box 91-A, Sheridan IL 60551, 800-654-4593
- Zand Herbal Formulas, P.O. Box 5312, Santa Monica, CA 90409, 360-384-5656
- Zia Natural Skincare, 1337 Evans Ave., San Francisco, CA 94124, 800-334-7546

Bonus Healing Diets from Dr. Linda Page

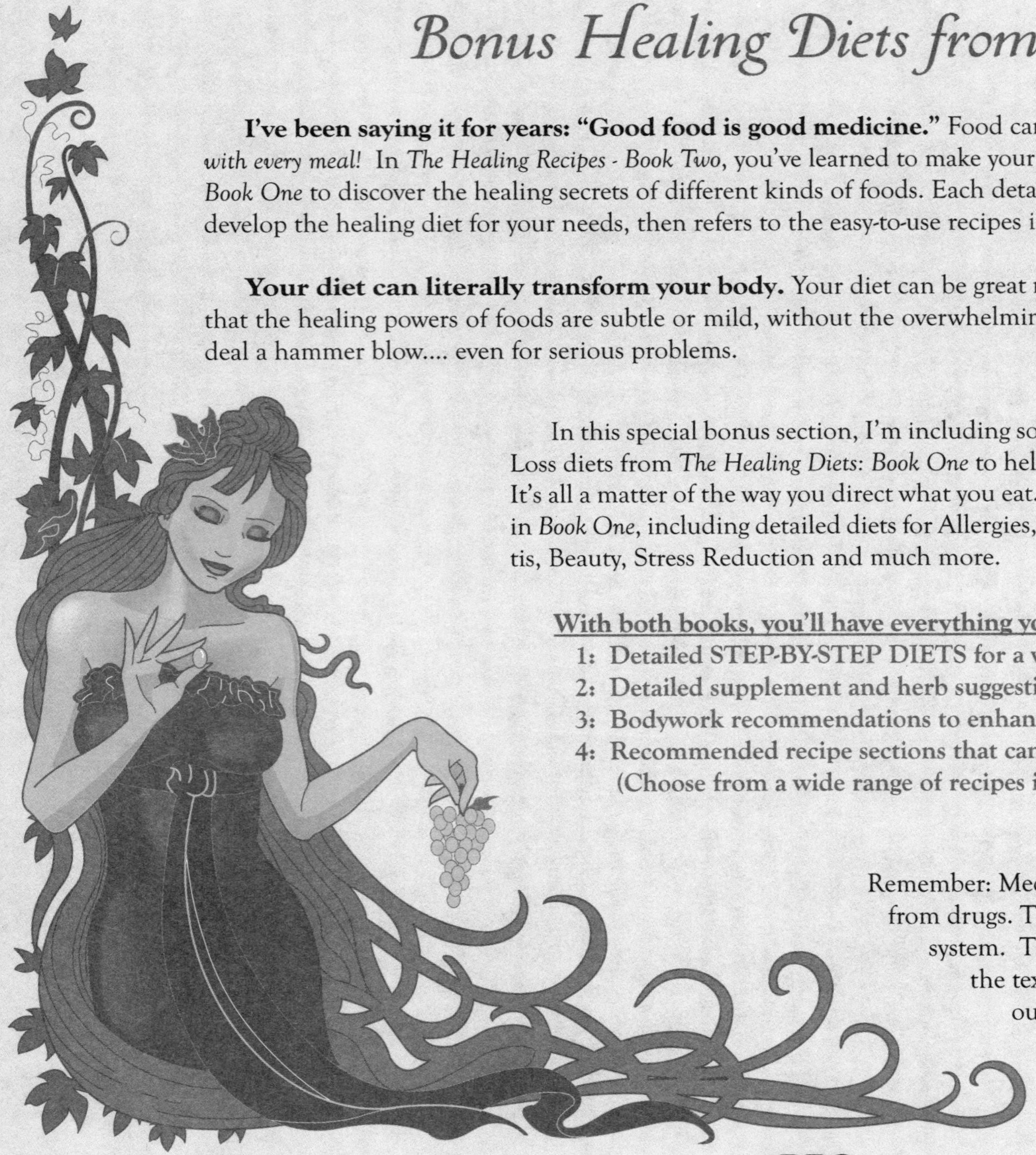

I've been saying it for years: "Good food is good medicine." Food can even be your best medicine. You can literally, *heal with every meal!* In *The Healing Recipes - Book Two*, you've learned to make your own food medicines. Now, use *The Healing Diets - Book One* to discover the healing secrets of different kinds of foods. Each detailed program in *The Healing Diets* shows how to develop the healing diet for your needs, then refers to the easy-to-use recipes in *The Healing Recipes.*

Your diet can literally transform your body. Your diet can be great medicine.... even for serious diseases. We tend to think that the healing powers of foods are subtle or mild, without the overwhelming potency of drugs. Yet healing doesn't always need to deal a hammer blow.... even for serious problems.

In this special bonus section, I'm including some of the most requested Detoxification and Weight Loss diets from *The Healing Diets: Book One* to help you navigate the healing path easily and effectively. It's all a matter of the way you direct what you eat. There are over 90 more healing diets to choose from in *Book One*, including detailed diets for Allergies, Cancer Control, Chronic Fatigue Syndrome, Arthritis, Beauty, Stress Reduction and much more.

With both books, you'll have everything you need to do it yourself, day by day, and succeed.

1: Detailed STEP-BY-STEP DIETS for a wide range of illnesses and health problems.
2: Detailed supplement and herb suggestions to enhance your healing progress.
3: Bodywork recommendations to enhance your healing program.
4: Recommended recipe sections that can help your diet the most.
(Choose from a wide range of recipes in each section to keep your diet interesting.)

Remember: Medicines from foods and herbs work the opposite from drugs. They nourish the body and enhance the immune system. The food you eat changes your weight, your mood, the texture of your skin, the shape of your body, your out look on life.... and therefore your future.

A healing diet is the first step to the health and balance of your universe.

Do You Need to Detoxify?

What is detoxification? Our bodies naturally do it every day. Detoxification is a normal body process of eliminating or neutralizing toxins through the colon, liver, kidneys, lungs, lymph and skin. In fact, internal detoxification is one of our body's most basic automatic functions. Just as our hearts beat nonstop and our lungs breathe continuously, so our metabolic processes constantly dispose of accumulated toxic matter. It's a perfect natural set-up.... the catch is that today, body systems and organs that were once capable of cleaning out unwanted substances are now completely overloaded with toxic material from our environment.

We long for yesterday's pollution-free environment, whole foods and pure water. Today, we control our environment even less. But, since humans are born with a "self-cleaning system," this ideal probably never existed. Our bodies try to protect us from dangerous material by surrounding it with mucous or fat so it won't cause imbalance or trigger an immune reaction. **The body stores foreign substances in fatty deposits – a significant reason to keep your body fat low.** Some people carry around 15 extra pounds of mucous that harbors this waste! Keep pollutants to a minimum and periodically get rid of them through detoxification.

Detoxification through special cleansing diets may be the missing link to disease prevention, especially for immune-compromised diseases like cancer, arthritis, diabetes and fatigue syndromes like candida albicans. Our chemicalized, genetically altered foods radically alter our internal ecosystems, (that's not even counting too much animal protein, too much fat, too much caffeine and alcohol). Even if your diet is good, a body cleanse can restore your vitality against environmental toxins that pave the way for disease.

A detox program aims to remove the cause of disease before it makes us ill. It's a time-honored way to keep immune response high, elimination regular, circulation sound, and stress under control so your body can handle the toxicity it encounters. In the past, detoxification was used either clinically for recovering from addictions, or as a once-a-year "spring cleaning" for general well-being. Today, a regular detox program two or three times a year makes a big difference not only for health, but for the quality of our lives.

Should you detoxify? Today Americans are exposed to chemicals of all kinds on an unprecedented scale. Industrial chemicals and their pollutant run-offs in our water, pesticides, additives in our foods, heavy metals, anesthetics, residues from drugs, and environmental hormones are trapped within the human body in greater concentrations than at any other point in history.

Many chemicals are so widespread that we are unaware of them. But they have worked their way into our bodies faster than they can be eliminated, and are causing allergies and addictions in record numbers. **More than 2 million synthetic substances are known, 25,000 are added each year, and over 30,000 are produced on a commercial scale.** Only a tiny fraction are ever tested for toxicity. A lot of them come to us from developing countries that have few safeguards in place.

The molecular structure of some chemicals interacts with human DNA, so long term exposure may result in genetic alteration that affects cell functions. World Health Organization research implicates environmental chemicals in 60 to 80% of all cancers. Hormone-disrupting pesticides are linked to hormone problems, psychological disorders, birth defects, still births and now breast cancer.

As toxic matter saturates our tissues, antioxidants and minerals in vital body fluids are reduced, so immune defenses are thrown out of balance. Circumstances like this are the prime factor in today's immune compromised diseases like candidiasis, lupus, fibromyalgia, chronic fatigue syndrome, even arthritis (which now impairs over 50 million Americans).

Chemical oxidation is the other process that allows disease. The oxygen that "rusts" and ages us also triggers free radical activity, a destructive cascade of incomplete molecules that damages DNA and other cell components. If you didn't have a reason to reduce your animal fat intake before, here is a critical one: **oxygen combines with animal fat in body storage cells and speeds up the free radical process.**

Almost everyone can benefit from a cleanse. It's one of the best ways to remain healthy in dangerous surroundings. Not one of us is immune to environmental toxins, and most of us can't escape to a remote, unpolluted habitat. Technology is now seriously able to harm the health of our entire planet, even to the point of making it uninhabitable for life. We must develop our culture further and take larger steps of cooperation. Mankind and the Earth must work together – to save it all for us all.

What can we do?

We can start by keeping our own body systems in good working order so that toxins are eliminated quickly. We can take a closer look at our own air, water and food, and keep an ever watchful eye on the politics that control our environment. Legislation on health and the environment follows two pathways in America today.... the influence of business and profits, and the demands of the people for a healthy habitat and responsible stewardship of the Earth. (See "Fluoridation – An Unnecessary Poison in our Drinking Water," pg. 61.)

Is your body becoming toxic? Body signs can tell you that you need to detoxify.

We all have different "toxic tolerance" levels. Listen to your body when it starts giving you those "cellular phone calls." If you can keep the amount of toxins in your system below your toxic level, your body can usually adapt and rid itself of them.

Do you have:

—Frequent, unexplained headaches, back or joint pain, or arthritis?
—Chronic respiratory problems, sinus problems or asthma?
—Abnormal body odor, bad breath or coated tongue?
—Food allergies, poor digestion or chronic constipation with intestinal bloating or gas?
—Brittle nails and hair, psoriasis, adult acne, or unexplained weight gain over 10 pounds?
—Unusually poor memory, chronic insomnia, depression, irritability, chronic fatigue?
—Environmental sensitivities, especially to odors?

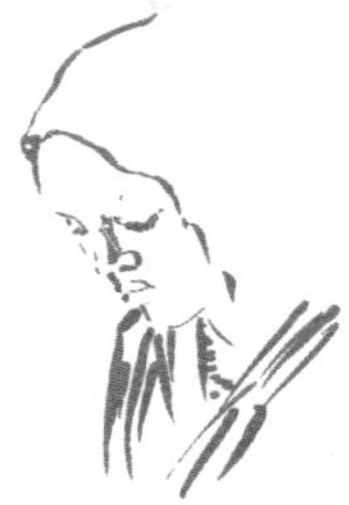

Laboratory tests like stool, urine, blood or liver tests, and hair analysis can also shed light on the need for a detox.

What benefits can you expect from a good detox?

A detox frees your body of clogging waste deposits, so you aren't running with a dirty engine or driving with the brakes on. Cleansing lets your body rebalance, so energy levels rise physically, psychologically and sexually, and creativity begins to expand. You start feeling like a different person – because you are. Your outlook and attitude change, because your actual cell make-up changes.

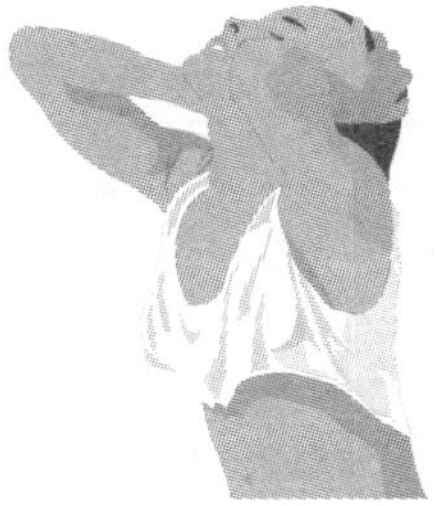

1: You'll clean your digestive tract of accumulated waste and fermenting bacteria.
2: You'll clear your body of excess mucous and congestion.
3: You'll purify your liver, kidney and blood, impossible under ordinary eating patterns.
4: You'll enhance mental clarity, impossible under chemical overload.
5: You'll be less dependent on sugar, caffeine, nicotine, alcohol or drugs.
6: You'll turn around bad eating habits... your stomach can reduce to normal size for weight control.
7: You'll release hormones that couple with essential fatty acids to stimulate your immune system.

You've decided your body needs a cleanse.

How long can you give out of your busy lifestyle to focus on a cleansing program so that all the processes can be completed? 24 hours, 2 or 3 days, or up to ten days? The time factor is important – you'll want to allocate your time ahead of time, to prepare both your mind and your body for the experience ahead.

A good detox program is in 3 steps – cleansing, rebuilding and maintaining.

Years of experience with detoxification have convinced me that if you have a serious health problem, a brief 3 to 7 day juice cleanse is the best way to release toxins from your body. Shorter cleanses can't get to the root of a chronic problem. Longer cleanses upset body equilibrium more than most people are ready to deal with except in a clinical environment. A 3 to 7 day cleanse can "clean your pipes" of systemic sludge – excess mucous, old fecal matter, trapped cellular and non-food wastes, or inorganic mineral deposits that are part of arthritis.

A few days without solid food can be an enlightening experience about your lifestyle. It's not absolutely necessary to take in only liquids, but a juice diet increases awareness and energy availability for elimination. Fresh juices literally pick up dead matter from the body and carry it away. Your body becomes easier to "hear," telling you via cravings what foods and diet it needs – for example, a desire for protein foods, or B vitamin foods like rices or minerals from greens. This is natural biofeedback.

A detox works by self-digestion. During a cleanse, the body decomposes and burns only the substances and tissues that are damaged, diseased or unneeded, such as abscesses, tumors, excess fat deposits, and congestive wastes. Even a relatively short fast accelerates elimination, often causing dramatic changes as masses of accumulated waste are expelled.

You will know your body is detoxing if you experience a short period of headaches, fatigue, body odor, bad breath, diarrhea or mouth sores that commonly accompany accelerated elimination. However, digestion usually improves right away as do many gland and nerve functions. Cleansing also helps release hormone secretions that stimulate immune response and encourages a disease-preventing environment.

Is a water fast the fastest way to cleanse? I don't recommend it. Here's why:

Juice cleansing is a better evolution in detoxification methods. Detoxification experts agree that fresh vegetable and fruit juice cleansing is superior to water fasting. Fresh juices, broths and herb teas help deeply cleanse the body, rejuvenate the tissues and guide you to a faster recovery from health problems better than water fasting.

A traditional water fast is harsh and demanding on your body, even in times past before huge amounts of food and environmental toxins were part of the picture. Today, a water fast can be dangerous. Deeply buried pollutants and chemicals may be released into elimination channels too rapidly during a water fast. Your body is essentially "re-poisoned" as the chemicals move through the bloodstream all at once. Sometimes, the physical and emotional stress of a water fast even overrides the healing benefits.

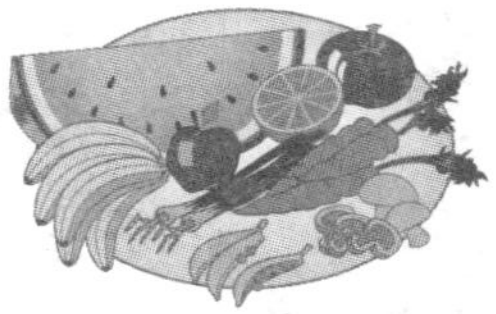

Vegetable and fruit juices are alkalizing, so they neutralize uric acid and other inorganic acids better than water, and increase the healing effects. Juices support better metabolic activity, too. (Metabolic activity slows down during a water fast as the body attempts to conserve dwindling energy resources.) Juices are better for digestion – easily assimilated into the bloodstream. They don't disturb the detoxification process.

Step one: elimination. Clean out mucous and toxins from the intestinal tract and major organs. Everything functions more effectively when toxins, obstructions and wastes are removed.

Step two: rebuild healthy tissue and restore energy. With obstacles removed, activate your body's regulating powers to rebuild at optimum levels. Eat only fresh, simply prepared, vegetarian foods during the rebuilding step. Include supplements and herbal aids for your specific needs.

Step three: keep your body clean and toxin-free. Modify your lifestyle habits for a strong resistant body. Rely on fresh fruits and vegetables for fiber, cooked vegetables, grains and seeds for strength and alkalinity, lightly cooked sea foods, soy foods, eggs and low fat cheeses for protein, and a little dinner wine for circulatory health. Include supplements, herbs, exercise and relaxation techniques.

What Type of Cleanse Do You Need?

Cleanses come in all shapes and sizes. You can easily tailor a cleanse to your individual needs. Unless you require a specific detox for a serious illness, or recovery from a long course of drugs or chemical therapy, I recommend a short cleanse twice a year, especially in the spring, summer or early autumn when sunshine and natural vitamin D can help the process along.

The short detox program on the next two pages is a general cleanse that you can return to again and again, whenever your body needs a "wash and brush." Check out the rest of this detox chapter to access cleanses for specific body systems and problems.

3-Day Body Stress Cleanse

Do you need an overall body stress cleanse?

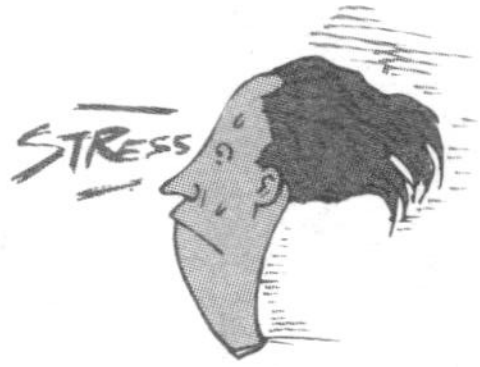

You change the oil in your car to make it run smoother and last longer. You plunge into spring cleaning to rid your home of health hazards. You buy air and water filters to clean out environmental toxins. You sink into a hot bath to cleanse your skin. If you stop there, you've left out an important part of the cleansing job. Cleansing on the inside improves everything on the outside. A stress cleanse revitalizes your whole body. It clears the junk out of body pathways so that wholesome nutrients can get in to rebuild energy and strength. I believe that much of the "food" in America's supermarkets doesn't really have much that your body can translate into nutrition. Some "foods" like designer fake fats or hormone-treated animal foods may even contribute to illness.

Is your body showing signs that it needs a stress cleanse?

—Is your immune response low? Are you catching every bug that comes down the pike?
—Are you unusually tired? Do you feel mentally dull? Do you feel like you need a pick-me-up?
—Have you had unusual body odor or bad breath lately? Have you gained weight even though your diet hasn't changed?

Stress Cleanse Detox Diet

Start with a 3 day juice-liquid diet like this one and follow with 4 days of fresh foods. Eat plenty of fresh veggies and fruits, and fiber foods like whole grains and beans. Avoid trans fats (page 74), but get plenty of essential fatty acids from sea greens, and herbs like ginger, ginseng or evening primrose oil. Drink plenty of water.

—On rising: take a glass of 2 fresh squeezed lemons, and 1 TB maple syrup in 8-oz. of water.

—Breakfast: have a nutrient-dense Kick-Off Cleansing Cocktail: juice 1 handful fresh wheat grass or parsley – extremely rich in chlorophyll and antioxidants, 4 carrots, 1 apple, 2 celery stalks with leaves, $^1/_2$ beet with top.

—Mid-morning: have a glass of fresh carrot or fresh apple juice. Add 1 TB. of a green superfood like Crystal Star ENERGY GREEN™ drink mix; Green Kamut GREEN KAMUT; Vibrant Health GREEN VIBRANCE.

—Lunch: have a Salad-In-A-Glass: juice 4 parsley sprigs, 3 tomatoes, $^1/_2$ bell pepper, $^1/_2$ cucumber, 1 scallion, 1 lemon wedge.

—Mid-afternoon: have a cup of Crystal Star CLEANSING & PURIFYING™ tea, green tea or mint tea.

—Dinner: have a warm Potassium drink for mineral electrolytes (page 568). Or Super Antioxidant Soup: 1 cup broccoli florets, 1 sliced leek, 2 cups peas, $^1/_2$ cup sliced scallions, 4 cups chard leaves, $^1/_2$ cup diced fennel bulb, $^1/_2$ cup fresh parsley, 6 garlic minced cloves, 2 tsp. astragalus extract (or $^1/_4$ cup broken astragalus bark), 6 cups vegetable stock, pinch cayenne, 1 cup diced green cabbage, $^1/_4$ cup dry, snipped sea greens. Bring ingredients to a boil. Simmer 10 min. Let sit 20 minutes. Strain and use broth only.

In the Recipe Book: See Detoxifocation and Cleansing Foods, and Healing Drinks for more info.

Herb and Supplement Choices

Choose 2 or 3 stress cleansing enhancers.

• **Cleansing boosters:** Crystal Star DETOX™ caps with goldenseal stimulates the body to eliminate wastes rapidly; or Crystal Star CLEANSING & PURIFYING™ tea.

• **Cleansing support formulas:** New Chapter LIFE SHIELD; or Futurebiotics OXY-SHIELD. When solid food is re-introduced, use Nature's Secret ULTIMATE CLEANSE.

• **Enzyme support:** Prevail DETOX ENZYME FORMULA; Transformation EXCELLZYME.

• **Antioxidants help remove toxins:** Biotec CELL GUARD; Rainbow Light MULTI CAROTENE COMPLEX.

• **Probiotics restore a friendly intestinal environment:** Jarrow Formulas JARRO-DOPHILUS+FOS; Wakunaga KYO-DOPHILUS; Prevail INNER ECOLOGY.

• **Electrolytes dramatically boost energy levels:** Nature's Path TRACE-LYTE LIQUID MINERALS.

• **Green superfoods:** Crystal Star ENERGY GREEN™ drink; Vibrant Health GREEN VIBRANCE.

• **Detoxing flower remedies:** Natural Labs STRESS/TENSION; Nelson Bach RESCUE REMEDY.

Bodywork and Lifestyle Techniques

Bodywork techniques accelerate your cleanse:

• **Enemas:** Flushing your colon on the first and the last day of your stress detox quickly releases toxins.

• **Especially helpful:** Guided imagery, biofeedback and aromatherapy techniques.

• **Stretch:** Body stretch daily during your cleanse. Repeat 5 times: Stand tall; raise your hands above your head. Stretch your arms and fingers to reach for the sky; move your hands and fingers as if you are climbing up into the sky. Rise on your toes as you reach; inhale deeply through your nostrils. Exhale slowly; gradually return to your starting position, arms loose at your sides. Follow your stretch with a brisk walk.

• **Deep Breathing:** Deep, relaxed breathing removes stress, composes the mind, improves mood and increases energy. 1. Take a full breath. Exhale, slowly. Slowly. 2. Take another deep, full breath. Release slowly. 3. And again. 4. Maintain a quiet rhythm, exhaling more slowly than you inhale.

• **Massage:** A massage therapy treatment further removes toxins and stimulates cleansing circulation.

Benefits that you may notice as your body responds to a body stress cleanse:

- **Your digestion noticeably improves as your digestive tract is cleansed of accumulated waste.**
- **You'll feel lighter (most people lose about 5 pounds on this cleanse) and more energized.**
- **You'll feel less dependent on substances like sugar, caffeine, nicotine, alcohol and drugs as your bloodstream purifies.**
- **You'll feel healthier. Most people have noticeably better resistance to common colds and flu.**
- **You'll feel more mentally alert, less space-y, more emotionally balanced. Creativity begins to expand.**
- **You'll feel energized as your body rebalances. Energy levels rise physically, psychologically and sexually.**

Can't find a recommended product? Call the 800 number listed in Product Resources for the store nearest you and for more info.

Controlling Your Weight

The latest statistics are shocking. **One out of every two Americans is overweight.** This doesn't count kids who are rapidly becoming an overweight generation. Right now, two-thirds of Americans are trying to lose weight. Amazingly, of those, only 20% are actually reducing their calories or exercising. Next to smoking, obesity is the second leading preventable cause of death in the United States, contributing to an excess of 300,000 deaths each year. The natural recommendations presented on this page can be used successfully for a wide variety of men and women struggling with their weight. Notes: Yo-yo dieting increases the risk of gallstones. For the best results, start slowly on your weight loss program and stick with it. The four keys to an effective weight control diet: low fat, high fiber, regular exercise, lots of water.

The Six Most Common Weight Loss Blockers

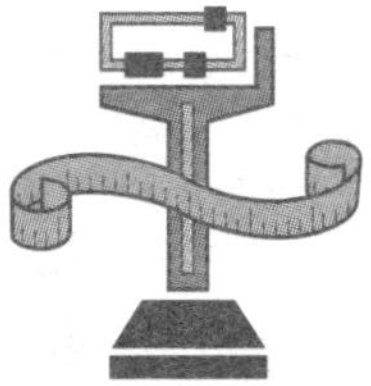

There are almost as many different weight loss problems as there are people who have them. I've identified six of the most common and developed comprehensive programs to address them. Each of the six plans has years of success behind it. Once you make the decision to be a thin person, identify your most prominent weight control problem, especially if there seems to be more than one. When results in the primary area begin to pay off, secondary problems are often overcome in the process. Take additional supplements after the first program is well underway if lingering problem spots exist.

1: Lazy Metabolism and Thyroid Imbalance. If you've experienced weight gain after 40 or after menopause, thyroid malfunction and lowered metabolism may be to blame. Huge new studies reveal that as many as 1 in 10 women over 65 have the early stages of hypothyroidism!

The signs: 1) General weakness and fatigue, especially in the morning; 2) Digestive disturbances like heartburn, unusual bad breath or body odor; 3) Unexplained depression and anxiety; 4) Breast fibroids; 5) Hair loss, especially in women.

Recommendations: To boost metabolism and support your thyroid, add seaweeds like kelp, dulse and nori, rich in natural iodine, to your daily diet. Sea greens are also available in capsules or extracts, like New Chapter OCEAN HERBS and Crystal Star's IODINE POTASSIUM™ caps. Add thermogenic spices like cinnamon, cayenne, mustard and ginger to speed up your fat burning process. Try dipping raw veggies in mustard throughout the day. One teasp. of mustard can increase metabolism 25% for up to 3 hours!

Note: if you have the slightest tendency to wheat or gluten allergies (you'll bloat when you eat them), avoid breads and pastries.

2: Sugar Craving and Blood Sugar Imbalances. Dieters who cut their fat intake to almost zero often try to make up for the missing fats by adding more sugar for better taste. But, sugary foods are usually empty calories... the downfall of dieters. And they raise insulin levels too much – your body's signal to make fat, no good for weight loss.

The signs: 1) Moodiness, being easily frustrated with a tendency towards crying spells; 2) Great fatigue (especially after sugar binges); 3) Having a wired feeling that is only relieved by eating sweets.

Recommendations: Increase your intake of healthy essential fatty acids (EFA's) from sources like seafood, sea greens, spinach or flax seed oil to reduce the cravings. Take EVENING PRIMROSE OIL, an easy-to-use EFA source, 3000mg daily. Eat more fiber. You'll have less cravings for sugar. High fiber foods improve the control of glucose metabolism and help promote weight loss and regularity. Target excess sugar in the blood with herbs for weight loss. Crystal Star GINSENG-LICORICE ELIXIR™ or Herbal Magic HYPOGLY-HERBAL. Take a dry sauna every day possible for 15 minutes. Raising your body temperature with dry heat really helps balance sugar levels and accelerate weight loss.

3: Overeating Fat and Calories. Overeating and eating too much fat are big reasons why it's so hard for Americans, particularly men, to lose weight. Men are often encouraged to dip into second, even third helpings as a sign of manliness or approval for the cook. Men also tend to overeat when they're under stress, tired, or on-the-run.... circumstances under which many American men eat today. Our lifestyles don't help. 45% of every food dollar is spent on eating out, and restaurant portions are bigger than ever as consumers demand more food for their money.

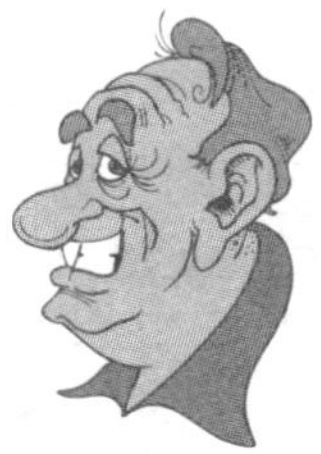

The signs: 1) Binging on junk foods, especially fatty, sugary foods, about every ten days; 2) Eating all your calories at one meal and then trying to eat nothing for the rest of the day when you're dieting (most people can't do it); 3) Having second and third helpings at a meal but still feeling hungry.

Recommendations: Control your portions so you don't overeat. Reduce fats to no more than 20% of your food intake. (Don't replace fats with fat substitutes like Olestra.) An herbal appetite suppressant with St. John's wort can curb cravings for fatty foods. Hypericin, one of St. John's wort's constituents, makes the user feel full, much the same way the drug fenfluramine does, but without the hazards of heart valve damage. Try Crystal Star APPE-TITE™ caps with St. John's Wort, Nature's Secret THINSOLUTION or Natural Balance SEROTHIN.

4: Liver Malfunction and Cellulite Formation. Your liver is responsible for fat metabolism. Liver malfunction is also directly related to sugar metabolism. Add to that the fact that most of us have a liver that's overloaded with toxic build-up today and you have three reasons why liver health is related to weight problems. A poorly functioning liver is almost always involved in cellulite formation, too. Women are hardest hit by cellulite because their skin fibers are thinner than a man's. Fatty wastes become lodged beneath the skin's surface more easily in a woman when the liver or lymphatic system is sluggish.

The signs: 1) Extreme, unrelenting fatigue; unusual depression and sadness; 2) Unexplained, pudgy weight gain; 3) Heartburn and constipation that worsen after fatty meals; 4) Food and chemical sensitivities; 5) Bulging, dimply, skin on hips, buttocks, thighs and knees (women); torso and stomach (men).

Recommendations: A two-week course of herbal bitters can regenerate the liver by increasing bile production. Try Crystal Star BITTERS & LEMON™ extract, or Gaia Herbs SWEETISH BITTERS ELIXIR. Detox your liver with Monas CHLORELLA. Add B complex, like Nature's Secret ULTIMATE B to assist liver detoxification and fat metabolism. Cellulite Tip: Seaweed body wraps are especially good because they also squeeze cellulitic waste back into the working areas of the body so it can be eliminated. Check out your nearest day spa for a good program.

5: Poor Circulation and Low Energy. A lifestyle with little exercise slows down circulation, metabolism and elimination, factors which impede successful weight loss. For some dieters, initial weight loss is rapid, but then a plateau is reached and further weight loss becomes difficult. Restricted food intake slows down metabolism, and affects circulation.

The signs: 1) Hands, feet, face and ears become cold regularly; 2) Poor memory; 3) Ringing in the ears.

Recommendations: For circulation stimulation: Futurebiotics CIRCUPLEX or Rosemary Gladstar's BUTCHER'S BROOM caps, or add CoQ-10, 100mg daily. Mineral electrolytes, like Nature's Path TRACE-LYTE turn body energy circuits back on. Dry brush your skin before showers to speed up circulation.

6: Poor Elimination. An astounding 30 million Americans have chronic constipation.... and it can be a major factor in weight control. If your colon is sluggish, your body hangs on to toxins and wastes that would normally be removed through elimination channels. This build-up of waste materials in your blood and bowel slows down all systems and your weight loss program.

The signs: 1) frequent bad breath, body odor and coated tongue; 2) infrequent bowel movements.

Recommendations: Try an easy fiber drink. Take 2 TBS of aloe vera juice concentrate in juice each morning. Add 2 capsules of an herbal formula like Crystal Star FIBER & HERBS CLEANSE™, or Herbal Magic COL-LIV HERBAL. Use massage therapy on your lower back (near the kidneys) to relieve colon congestion. If you get backaches when you're constipated, your transverse colon is probably blocked up by impacted wastes. Sometimes a little light massage work can help to break up the congestion and release the accumulated materials.

Note: Changing diet composition is the key. The importance of cutting back on saturated fat cannot be overstated. Saturated fats are hard for the liver to metabolize. Focus on healthy fats from seafood, sea greens, nuts and seeds which curb cravings by initiating a satiety response.

Watchwords:

—**Fat isn't all bad.** It's your body's chief energy source. Most overweight people have too high blood sugar and too low fat levels. This causes constant hunger; the delicate balance between fat storage and fat utilization is upset; and your ability to use fat for energy decreases. Eating fast, fried, or junk foods aggravates this imbalance. You wind up with empty calories and more cravings. Fat becomes non-moving energy; fat cells become fat storage depots. But don't replace fats with fat substitutes like Olestra. Fake fats fool your tastebuds, not your stomach. In one study, people who replaced 20% of their fat with fake fats were still hungry at the end of the day and they ate twice as much food as normal! Fake fats are nutrition thieves. Eating a one ounce portion of olestra potato chips on a daily basis reduces blood carotene levels by 50%!

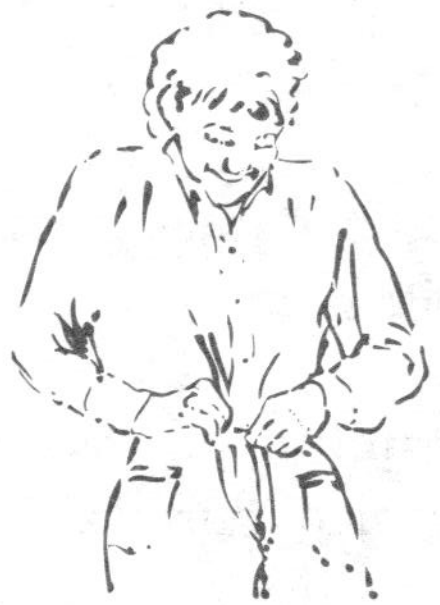

—**Water can get you over diet plateaus.** Dehydration slows resting metabolic rate (RMR) and can cause waste products like ketones to build up in tissues. Drink juices or green tea in the morning to wash out waste products.

—**A little caffeine after a meal raises thermogenesis** (calorie burning) and boosts metabolic rate. Use fat burning spices like ginger, cinnamon, garlic, mustard and cayenne.

—**High fiber fruits and veggies are a key to successful body toning.** Have an apple every day!

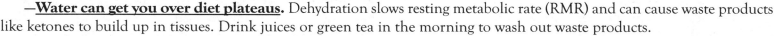

Herb and Supplement Choices

• **Stimulate BAT thermogenesis:** Evening Primrose oil 3000mg daily; Carnitine 3000mg daily; Crystal Star THERMO-CITRIN® GINSENG™ caps; Source Naturals DIET PHEN; Natural Balance ULTRA DIET PEP; Nature's Secret ULTIMATE WEIGHT LOSS; Diamond Herpanacine DIAMOND TRIM.

—**Deficiencies can lead to food binges:** B-complex with extra B-6 200mg (boosts serotonin and metabolizes carbohydates); lack of minerals leads to sugar craving: Crystal Star MINERAL SPECTRUM™ or ZINC SOURCE™ caps.

• **Control food cravings:** Crystal Star APPE-TITE™ caps with St. John's Wort; Nature's Secret THIN SOLUTION; 5-HTP as directed; chromium picolinate (400mcg); L-glutamine 2000mg, spirulina and bee pollen for sugar cravings; Natural Balance SEROTHIN caps with 5-HTP.

• **Natural fat blockers:** Health from the Sun CLA (conjugated linoleic acid) up to 2000mg daily; fat digesting enzymes, like Prevail FAT ENZYME; garcinia cambogia in formulas like Now's CITRI-MAX or Natrol CITRI-MAX PLUS; Pyruvate aids in transforming blood sugar into energy, 5 grams daily; Twin Lab PYRUVATE FUEL; Chitosan reduces absorption of fats; Natural Balance FAT MAGNET. *Note: Gastrointestinal problems may result from excessive use of pyruvate or chitosan.*

• **Good fats help burn bad fats:** Barleans OMEGA-3 FLAX OIL or Omega Nutrition ESSENTIAL BALANCE help overcome binging; Co-enzyme A Technology BODY IMAGE; Richardson Labs CHROMA-SLIM - a lipotropic-carnitine formula.

• **Boost metabolism:** Enzymatic Therapy THYROID/TYROSINE caps; for compulsive eating, tyrosine 1000mg with zinc 30mg daily. Enzymatic Therapy 7-KETO NATURAL LEAN.

Bodywork and Lifestyle Techniques

• **Daily exercise is the key to permanent, painless weight control.** Exercise releases fat from the cells. (Exercising early in the day can raise metabolism as much as 25%! Exercising before breakfast is best because the body dips into its fat stores for quick energy.)

—Even if eating habits are just slightly changed, you can still lose weight with a brisk hour's walk, or 15 minutes of aerobic exercise.

—One pound of fat represents 3500 calories. A 3 mile walk burns up 250 calories. In about 2 weeks, you'll lose a pound of real extra fat. That's 3 pounds a month and 30 pounds a year without changing your diet. It's easy to see how cutting down even moderately on fatty, sugary foods in combination with exercise can still provide the look and body tone you want.

• **Exercise promotes an afterburn effect,** raising metabolic rate from 1.00 to 1.05-1.15 per minute up to 24 hours afterwards. Calories are used up at an even faster rate after exercise.

• **Weight training exercise increases lean muscle mass,** replacing fat-marbled muscle tissue with lean muscle. Muscle tissue burns calories; the greater the amount of muscle tissue you have, the more calories you can burn. This is very important as aging decreases muscle mass. Exercise before a meal raises blood sugar levels and thus decreases appetite, often for several hours afterward.

• **Deep breathing exercises increase metabolic rate.** See pg. 472 of this book.

Can't find a recommended product? Call the 800 number listed in Product Resources for the store nearest you and for more info.